Advances in Periodontics

Edited by

Thomas G. Wilson, Jr, DDS
Private Practice of Periodontics and Dental Implants, Dallas, Texas
Clinical Associate Professor, University of Texas at San Antonio Dental School
Affiliate Assistant Professor, University of Washington, Seattle, Washington

Kenneth S. Kornman, DDS, PhD
Clinical Professor and Former Chairman, Department of Periodontics
University of Texas Health Science Center at San Antonio, San Antonio, Texas

Michael G. Newman, DDS
Adjunct Professor of Periodontics
University of California at Los Angeles, School of Dentistry, Los Angeles, California

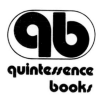

quintessence
books

Quintessence Publishing Co, Inc
Chicago, London, Berlin, São Paulo, Tokyo, and Hong Kong

Library of Congress Cataloging-in-Publication Data

Advances in periodontics / edited by Thomas G. Wilson, Jr., Kenneth S.
  Kornman, Michael G. Newman.
       p. cm.
     Includes bibliographical references and index.
     ISBN 0-86715-250-8
     1. Periodontics. I. Wilson, Thomas G. II. Kornman, Kenneth S.
III. Newman, Michael G.
     [DNLM: 1. Periodontal Diseases — therapy. 2. Periodontics. WU 240 A244]
RK361.A34 1992
617.6'32 — dc20
DNLM / DLC
for Library of Congress   91-32558
                                                                CIP

quintessence books

© 1992 by Quintessence Publishing Co, Inc, 551 North Kimberly Drive, Carol
Stream, Illinois.

Composition: Graphic World, St. Louis, MO
Lithography, printing, and binding: Toppan Printing Co Pte, Ltd, Jurong Town,
Singapore
Printed in Singapore

DEDICATIONS

I would like to dedicate this book first to my family for providing the strength and time to complete my work. So thank you Penny, Trey, John, and especially, my mother. And next, to the teachers who guided my way and allowed me the freedom to make my own decisions and mistakes. Thank you Jim Clark, Cliff Ochsenbein, Leonard Tibbetts, and most of all, Saul Schluger.

Thomas G. Wilson, Jr

This book and all my other professional activities are possible because of the love and support of my family: Bonnie, Seth, Lisa, and my parents, Rachel and Morris. Thank you for all you have given over the years to make these activities a reality.

This book is also dedicated to Sigurd Ramfjord, Harald Löe, Saul Schluger, and all of my former graduate students. Drs Ramfjord and Löe provided philosophical concepts and scientific principles that continually influence my work, but more importantly, they have dictated the direction of periodontal practice for the last 25 years. This book attempts to reflect the transitions in thought that are challenging today's practitioners. These exciting new developments in periodontics are possible because of the solid base established by these two innovators.

Much of my professional thought today is also the result of the wonderful opportunity to have been challenged intellectually by so many bright and energetic graduate students. We hope that this book and future revisions will reflect our graduate students who represent the continuously changing leading edge of our profession.

It seems most appropriate that former students of Drs Schluger and Ramfjord have collaborated on a book that attempts to conceptualize how the strong ideas and debates of the 1960s and 1970s have combined with emerging knowledge to guide the practitioner of the 1990s.

Kenneth S. Kornman

To our families and colleagues for their support, encouragement, patience, and love.

Michael G. Newman

Contents

Contributors

Oded Bahat, BDS, MSD
Private Practice of Periodontics, Beverly Hills, California

Erwin P. Barrington, DDS, PhD
Professor of Periodontics, University of Illinois at Chicago; Private Practice of Periodontics, Chicago, Illinois

Raul G. Caffesse, DDS, MS, Dr Odont
Professor and Chairman, Director of Advanced Education, Department of Periodontics, University of Texas Health Science Center at Houston, Houston, Texas

Thomas J. Fleszar, DDS, MS
Private Practice of Periodontics, Sterling Heights, Michigan

Joseph A. Giovannitti, Jr, DMD, FADSA
Private Practice of Dental Anesthesiology, Dallas, Texas; Adjunct Associate Professor, Department of Pharmacology, Division of Pain and Anxiety Control, Baylor College of Dentistry, Dallas, Texas; Consultant, Olin E. Teague Veterans' Center, Temple, Texas

Mark Handelsman, DDS
Private Practice of Periodontics, Beverly Hills, California; Clinical Assistant Professor, University of Southern California Dental School, Los Angeles, California

Vincent J. Iacono, DMD
Professor and Director, Postgraduate Periodontics, School of Dental Medicine, State University of New York at Stony Brook, Stony Brook, New York

Marjorie Jeffcoat, DMD
James R. Rosen Professor of Dental Research and Chairman, Department of Periodontics, University of Alabama at Birmingham, School of Dentistry, Birmingham, Alabama

Wayne B. Kaldahl, DDS
Professor, Department of Periodontics, University of Nebraska Medical Center — Dentistry; Private Practice of Periodontics, Lincoln, Nebraska

Kenneth L. Kalkwarf, DDS, MS
Professor of Periodontology and Dean, University of Texas Health Science Center at San Antonio Dental School, San Antonio, Texas

Kenneth S. Kornman, DDS, PhD
Clinical Professor and Former Chairman, Department of Periodontics, University of Texas Health Science Center at San Antonio, San Antonio, Texas

Niklaus P. Lang, DDS, MS, PhD
Professor and Chairman, Department of Comprehensive Dental Care, University of Berne, School of Dental Medicine, Berne, Switzerland

Burton Langer, DDS, MSD
Private Practice of Periodontics and Oral Diagnosis, New York, New York

Laureen Langer, DDS
Private Practice Limited to Periodontics and Oral Diagnosis; Assistant Clinical Professor, Columbia University School of Dental and Oral Surgery; Attending — Columbia Presbyterian Medical Center, New York, New York

Howard N. Livers, DDS
Private Practice of Prosthodontics, New York, New York

Dan M. Loughlin, DDS, MS
Private Practice of Periodontics, Arlington, Texas

Ingvar Magnusson, DDS, Dr Odont
Professor, Periodontal Disease Research Center, Department of Oral Biology, College of Dentistry, University of Florida, Gainesville, Florida

Michael K. McGuire, DDS
Private Practice of Periodontics, Houston, Texas; Clinical Associate Professor, University of Texas at San Antonio Dental School; Clinical Associate Professor, University of Texas at Houston Dental Branch, Houston, Texas

James T. Mellonig, DDS, MS
Associate Professor of Periodontics, Director, Graduate Periodontics, University of Texas at San Antonio, San Antonio, Texas

Michael G. Newman, DDS
Private Practice of Periodontics; Adjunct Professor of Periodontics, School of Dentistry, University of California at Los Angeles, Los Angeles, California

Joan Otomo-Corgel, DDS, MPH
Adjunct Assistant Professor University of California — Los Angeles School of Dentistry, Department of Periodontics; Staff Periodontist — Veterans Administration Medical Center, West Los Angeles (Graduate Periodontics), Rancho Los Amigos Hospital; Private Practice Limited to Periodontics, Los Angeles and Montebello, California

Terry D. Rees, DDS
Professor and Chairman, Department of Periodontics, Director of the Stomatology Center, Baylor College of Dentistry, Dallas, Texas

Bengt G. Rosling, DDS, Dr Odont
Associate Professor, Department of Periodontology, University of Göteborg, Sweden; Research Associate, PDCRC, Department of Oral Biology, New York State University, Buffalo, New York

John S. Sottosanti, DDS
Associate Professor, University of Southern California; Private Practice, San Diego, California

Bjorn Steffensen, DDS, MS
Assistant Professor, Department of Periodontics, University of Texas Health Science Center at San Antonio, San Antonio, Texas

Henry H. Takei, DDS, MS
Clinical Professor of Periodontics, School of Dentistry, University of California, Los Angeles; Private Practice of Periodontics, Los Angeles, California

Ray C. Williams, DMD
Associate Professor and Chairman, Department of Periodontology, Harvard School of Dental Medicine, Boston, Massachusetts

Richard D. Wilson, DDS, FACD
Private Practice of General Dentistry; Clinical Professor, Department of Periodontics, Virginia Commonwealth University School of Dentistry, Richmond, Virginia

Thomas G. Wilson, Jr, DDS
Private Practice of Periodontics and Dental Implants, Dallas, Texas; Clinical Associate Professor, University of Texas at San Antonio Dental School; Affiliate Assistant Professor, University of Washington, Seattle, Washington

Preface

This book is designed to facilitate the flow of information from the researcher to the practitioner. As such, it does not attempt to serve as an encyclopedia of periodontology or periodontics, but rather focuses on the application of leading-edge concepts, technologies, and techniques that are likely to represent the core of the specialty practice of periodontics for the next several years. We use the term "leading-edge" specifically to denote the exciting interface between research and practice and the application of new knowledge to patient care. Two concepts are implicit in the use of this term. The first is that a true leading edge in not stationary, but is continually moving forward. This book therefore represents our view of the edge in the early 1990s and will most certainly eventually change. The second implication of the term is that it represents a transition in practice. Transitions by definition are uncomfortable. This book attempts to present realistic and practical views of our current state of the art in the hope of assisting the practitioner in managing these transitions. To this end we chose academicians and clinicians highly respected in their subspecialties to write about their areas of expertise. Most chapters have a review of current concepts, followed by a clinician's synthesis of the material and how he or she transfers the knowledge gathered in the first section to therapy for patients.

The format features "Quick Reviews" at the end of each chapter to provide the reader with an overview of the material. They are designed as guides to areas of interest. Most of the clinical sections are designed to serve as an atlas for those who wish information about the specific clinical skills discussed.

This book is written to the level of a knowledgeable practitioner in periodontics, be he or she a periodontist, general practitioner, or dental hygienist. The combination of well-referenced reviews with practical clinical applications makes it especially appropriate for the dental student in the clinical phase of training and the graduate student in periodontics.

The editors sincerely thank the contributors to this book for their untiring efforts to produce a work of quality. Also, thanks go to the many who have helped along the way, including Dr Dan Buser, Dr George Merijohn, and Dr Paul Tannebaum. Our special gratitude goes to two people without whom this project would never have reached completion, Georgia Wright and Karen Pevehouse.

Getting Started: A Guide to the Use of *Advances in Periodontics*

First, some preliminaries...

This book speaks to advances in traditional approaches to therapy as well as new methods for treating inflammatory periodontal lesions. It is divided into four major sections:

Part I — Examination, disease activity, and treatment planning
Part II — Therapy for chronic inflammatory periodontal diseases
Part III — Adjunctive therapy
Part IV — Advances in implant dentistry

Our premise in the examination and therapy sections is that the vast majority of inflammatory periodontal lesions can be divided into two broad categories. The first category contains chronic problems such as gingivitis (seen in both children and adults) and chronic adult periodontitis. These diseases make up the large majority of periodontal lesions and are predictably responsive to current conventional therapy. The second category contains more aggressive lesions that manifest as periodontitis and includes diseases presently termed prepubertal, localized juvenile, generalized juvenile, rapidly progressive, and refractory periodontitis. These diseases are seen in all age groups. Until recently, this latter group of diseases has at best been difficult to manage and is less predictable in their response to conventional therapy. Their diagnosis and treatment are covered in chapter 6.

Therapy for the aggressive group is aimed at managing host factors that may contribute to the periodontal conditions and at reducing the type or relative percentage of specific bacteria that seem to play a role in the etiology for these problems. Once this goal has been achieved and the bacterial disease has been controlled, the patient is then placed into the chronic group and treated according to the remaining manifestations of disease activity. *Therapy for these problems is divided by disease severity, not procedure,* with sections on chronic gingivitis, mild periodontitis, moderate periodontitis, and severe periodontitis (covered in Part II). Patients in the aggressive category should not be considered for esthetic procedures or implants until the disease has been controlled. Therapy for types of gingivitis other than the chronic form is covered in chapter 5.

A suggestion on how to use this book

For ideas concerning patients with periodontal diseases, first read Part I, then read Part II. The flow diagram provides an overview of the organization of the book (see page 13).

Parts III and IV can be used independently.

Finally, some thoughts to chew on...

In the previous 20 years, efforts to better define the determinants of successful periodontal care led to great progress in our understanding of therapy. Today, it is generally accepted that for the chronic diseases, control of the subgingival bacterial load and establishment and maintenance of a clean supragingival environment achieves predictable control of periodontal diseases. Prior to our understanding of the dominance of this unifying principle, there was much focus on the details of different surgical procedures, and graduate students devoted extensive time to learning the uses and limitations of each procedure. Although this book provides some examples of how outstanding clinicians apply the principle, the unifying principle itself is the most critical feature of successful periodontal therapy. For example, although the senior authors come from very different therapeutic backgrounds, we have found that given a specific patient, our practical therapy would be very similar. Such practical similarities are often obscured by the use of terminology intended to distinguish one surgical procedure from another. As with the management of all diseases, once the key therapeutic principles have been discovered, previous therapeutic distinctions become less relevant.

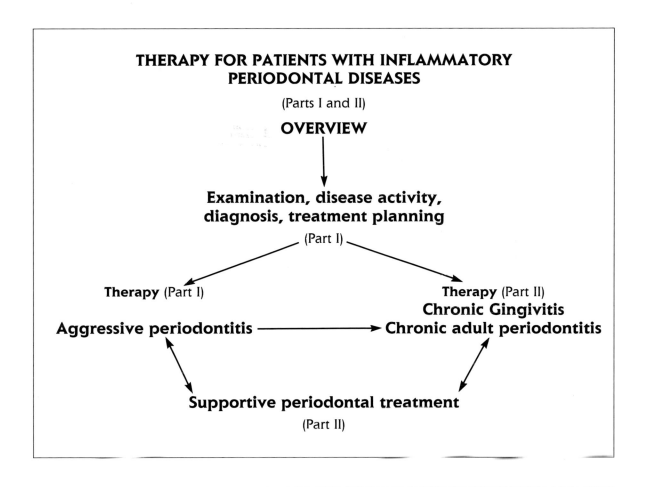

**THERAPY FOR PATIENTS WITH INFLAMMATORY
PERIODONTAL DISEASES**

(Parts I and II)

OVERVIEW

**Examination, disease activity,
diagnosis, treatment planning**

(Part I)

Therapy (Part I)

Therapy (Part II)
Chronic Gingivitis

Aggressive periodontitis ⟶ **Chronic adult periodontitis**

Supportive periodontal treatment

(Part II)

ADJUNCTIVE CARE FOR PERIODONTAL PATIENTS

(Part III)

**Enhancing esthetics
Medically compromised patients**

IMPLANT DENTISTRY

(Part IV)

**Presurgical treatment planning
Radiographic techniques
Choice of system
Clinical management and maintenance**

PART I
Examination, Disease Activity, Diagnosis, and Treatment Planning

Examination of Patients With Periodontal Diseases

CURRENT CONCEPTS by Ingvar Magnusson

CLINICAL APPLICATION by Thomas G. Wilson, Jr

C U R R E N T   C O N C E P T S

Descriptive indices of oral health and oral hygiene are used to evaluate the need for periodontal therapy and the effect of different therapeutic regimens. The individual response to periodontal therapy is evaluated by recording and documenting differences in indices and measurements. Such documentation helps improve the accuracy of the diagnosis and reduces the risk for over- or undertherapy. It is probable that the practitioner of the future will devote more time to diagnosis and documentation than to actual therapy. Before any data are collected, however, it is important to understand what the data indicate and the validity of that information.

EXAMINATION OF SOFT TISSUES

The index system most commonly used to evaluate gingival status is the system (or modifications thereof) devised by Löe and Silness,[1] in which the gingival units are scored as follows: 0 = healthy gingiva; 1 = slight inflammation; 2 = moderate inflammation with bleeding at pressure; and 3 = severe inflammation with spontaneous bleeding. Later, Löe[2] modified the system by changing the score of 2 from bleeding at pressure to bleeding upon probing. The index was modified further by Gordon et al,[3] who used a noninvasive scoring system

ranging from 0 to 4. The Löe-Silness score of 1 was divided into two categories: mild inflammation of any portion of the gingival unit, and mild inflammation of the whole gingival unit. This modified index was recommended by Lobene[4] for use in clinical trials. Lobene et al[5] showed that this modified gingival index had a high correlation with the Löe-Silness index; these authors then listed the advantages of this system as follows:

1. It is noninvasive, thereby eliminating concerns about the disruption of soft tissue or plaque in the gingival region, as well as obviating the need for infection control practices that

would be required if sulcular probing were done.

2. It is logistically simpler. Decision-making is simplified if bleeding considerations do not have to be superimposed on visual determinations.

3. There is less variability in its implementation if bleeding on pressure or probing is excluded. This feature, in combination with item 2, can result in greater accuracy in interexaminer calibration.

4. It affords greater sensitivity in detecting therapeutic efficacy. The expansion of the scale at its low end makes this index more sensitive to improvements in gingival health following treatment.

A particular index should probably not be recommended for general use; it may be that different indices suit different examiners; the most important issue is that the examiner be consistent. Although visual inflammation gives us information regarding marginal inflammation, bleeding on probing gives us information about the status of the bottom of the pocket, that is, the epithelium / connective tissue interface.

Often, gingival inflammation is described by bleeding only. Lang et al[6] studied bleeding on probing as a predictor for the progression of periodontal disease and found that bleeding was a limited but useful indicator in clinical diagnosis for patients in the periodontal maintenance phase. Different methods to record bleeding have been described, the most simple being just the presence or absence of bleeding on probing at a particular site. The percentage of bleeding sites can then be calculated. Saxer and Mühlemann[7] described a Papillary Bleeding Index (PBI) in which the sulcus is swept with a blunt periodontal probe and the amount of papillary bleeding is recorded 20 to 30 seconds after each quadrant has been probed. The amount of bleeding is scored from 1 (minimal) to 4 (profuse), and the PBI is calculated by adding up all the bleeding scores and dividing by the number of papillae examined.

Histologically, it has been shown that parallel with the increase of the PBI there is an increase of the inflammatory infiltrate. Loesche[8] introduced the Papillary Bleeding Score in which bleeding was evaluated from 0 to 5 after a Stimudent interdental cleaner (Johnson & Johnson) was inserted interproximally. This scoring system, which was related to the Löe-Silness Gingival Index (Table 1-1), was simplified by Caton and Polson[9] in the Eastman Interdental Bleeding Index, in which the presence or absence of bleeding was recorded after a Stimudent interdental cleaner had been inserted and removed four times. Caton et al[10] reported that the Eastman Interdental Bleeding Index was a more reliable clinical indicator for detecting interdental inflammatory lesions than was the Papillary Bleeding Index.

In a calibration study, Magnusson et al[11] assessed the intra- and interexaminer variability of 11 previously calibrated examiners with regard to a noninvasive gingival index (Gordon et al[3]) and the Papillary Bleeding Score (Loesche).[8] The results are illustrated in Fig 1-1. The intraexaminer correlation coefficient between two examination visits was 0.94 for the Papillary Bleeding Score and 0.68 for the gingival index. The interexaminer correlation coefficient was 0.96 for the Papillary Bleeding Score and 0.64 for the gingival index. It can thus be concluded that the Papillary Bleeding Score is highly reproducible and suitable for use in the evaluation of periodontal therapy.

Earlier, a classification system for the appearance of gingival inflammation was described by Schour and Massler.[12] In 1956, Russell[13] described a periodontal index (which has been widely used in descriptive studies) of the occurrence and severity of peri-

TABLE 1-1 *Papillary Bleeding Score (PBS) compared to Löe-Silness Gingival Index (GI)*

PBS	GI	COMPARISON
0	0	Healthy gingiva; no bleeding upon insertion of Stimudent interproximally
1	1	Edematous, reddened gingiva; no bleeding upon insertion of Stimudent interproximally
2	2	Bleeding without flow upon insertion of Stimudent interproximally
3	2	Bleeding with flow along gingival margin upon insertion of Stimudent interproximally
4	2	Copious bleeding upon insertion of Stimudent interproximally
5	3	Severe inflammation, marked redness, and edema; tendency to spontaneous bleeding

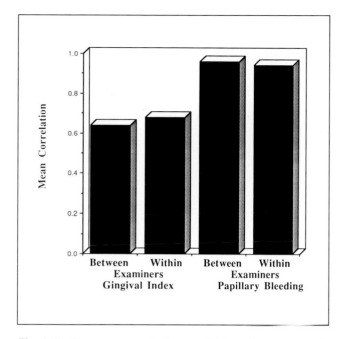

Fig 1-1 *Pearson correlation coefficient between and within examiners for the Papillary Bleeding Index and the gingival index.*

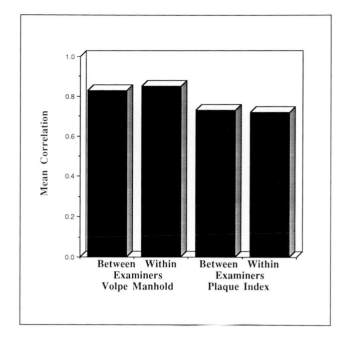

Fig 1-2 *Pearson correlation coefficient between and within examiners for the Volpe-Manhold index and the Quigley-Hein index.*

odontal disease. His periodontal index consists of both qualitative and quantitative criteria. Qualitatively, the presence of gingival inflammation is recorded. Quantitatively, the tooth is scored as 1 if the inflammation is present only in localized areas and 2 if inflammation is present around the whole circumference of the tooth. A score of 6 is given if the tooth has deepened pockets and a score of 8 if it has lost its function.

All of the index systems described above are reversible and can be returned to 0 after successful periodontal therapy. In order to get an indication of the amount of lost attachment, it was recommended by Ramfjord[14] that the lost attachment be measured in millimeters from the cementoenamel junction to the bottom of the pocket and be used in a Periodontal Disease Index. This type of index is irreversible because lost attachment is rarely completely regained after periodontal therapy.

EVALUATION OF ORAL HYGIENE

Ramfjord[14] suggested the use of an index to evaluate oral hygiene status, and Greene and Vermillion[15] devised an Oral Hygiene Index to relate oral hygiene status to the presence of disease. This index consists of both a debris index, scored 0 to 3 (a score of 1 would indicate that one third of the surface was covered, etc), and a calculus index, also scored 0 to 3. It was shown that 90% of the periodontal disease could be related to the amount of plaque and calculus present and to the subject's age.[16] The increase of the Oral Hygiene Index with age was explained mainly by an increase of calculus.

Quigley and Hein[17] modified the Oral Hygiene Index to develop an index for the evaluation of different oral hygiene measures. This modified index used a scoring range from 0 to 5 by in-

serting two low values between scores 0 and 1 in the Oral Hygiene Index system. The extended score permits a more sensitive assessment of therapeutic efficacy.

Silness and Löe[18] developed a Plaque Index system that has been widely used in epidemiological studies. This system evaluates the thickness of the plaque at the gingival margin as follows: 0 = no plaque; 1 = nonvisible plaque that can be scraped from the tooth surface with a probe; 2 = visible plaque; and 3 = abundant plaque. To evaluate calculus formed during shorter clinical trials, Ennever et al[19] developed a Calculus Surface Index to be used on the lingual surface of the four mandibular incisors. The tooth surface was divided into four fields by two intersecting diagonal lines and the presence (1) or absence (0) of calculus was then registered in each field. Volpe and Manhold,[20] in studying development of calculus over longer periods of time, measured the amount of calculus along two intersecting diagonal lines on the lingual surfaces of mandibular incisors and canines and added together the resulting 12 numbers.

Magnusson et al[11] studied the reproducibility of the Volpe-Manhold index and the Quigley-Hein index. The intra- and interexaminer correlation was calculated for 11 calibrated examiners (Fig 1-2). The intraexaminer correlation coefficient was 0.85 for the Volpe-Manhold index and 0.72 for the Quigley-Hein index. The interexaminer correlation coefficient was 0.88 for the Volpe-Manhold index and 0.73 for the Quigley-Hein index, indicating that these indices are acceptably reproducible.

EVALUATION OF TOOTH MOBILITY

Registration of tooth mobility is an important part of a periodontal examination, because it represents a function of the persisting height of the alveolar bone and the width of the periodontal ligament. Presence of inflammation will affect the coronal part of the periodontal ligament. The inflammatory status has to be considered in the evaluation of mobility. However, because tooth mobility may be attributable to causes other than periodontal disease (such as periapical lesions and trauma), it is essential to determine its cause. Increased mobility often occurs in a reduced but healthy periodontium and usually does not require therapy as long as mobility is not continuing to increase. To determine if changes in mobility have occurred as a result of either therapy or disease, it is important to document and record both initial and posttherapy data. Tooth mobility may be recorded as follows[21]:

Degree 1: movability of the crown of the tooth 0.2 to 1 mm in a horizontal direction.

Degree 2: movability of the crown of the tooth more than 1 mm in a horizontal direction.

Degree 3: movability of the crown of the tooth in a vertical direction as well.

Fleszar et al[22] devised a similar system for recording tooth mobility, as follows[23]:

Degree 1: slightly increased mobility.

Degree 2: definite to considerable increase in mobility, but no impairment of function.

Degree 3: extreme mobility; a "loose" tooth that would be uncomfortable in function.

Measuring tooth mobility manually as described above is the easiest and most practical method for use in a clinical setting. For research purposes, however, there are more sophisticated and exacting methods that use various mechanical devices. The macroperiodontometer (devised by Mühlemann[24]), which provides rapid and reproducible assessment of horizontal tooth mobility, is the instrument most commonly used by clinical researchers. The macroperiodontometer permits only the measurement of single-rooted teeth, although an improved modification of the instrument, described by O'Leary and Rudd,[25] may be used to take measurements on all tooth types. Persson and Svensson[26] constructed a device for measuring

tooth mobility using loads below 100 p in a buccolingual direction on anterior maxillary teeth. Strain gauges and a differential transformer are used as sensors of force and displacement. The displacement is recorded at the same location on the tooth surface and in the same direction as the loading force. A two-channel potentiometric recorder is used to document signals.

The Periotest (Siemens Ltd) is a compact, handheld clinical instrument that measures tooth mobility by delivering a repeated mechanical impulse. A small metal slug is used to deliver the pulse, the deceleration of which is automatically recorded by the microprocessor that controls the device. The duration of the deceleration signal (tooth-to-slug contact time) is used to compute the Periotest value. In a recent study[27] it was concluded that the Periotest appears to provide a reasonable measurement of tooth mobility but that readings from very loose teeth should be interpreted with care.

COMPUTERIZED DATA COLLECTION

Currently, computers are routinely used in many dental offices only for accounting and billing. There is, however, enormous potential for the use of computers for clinical data collection. Using existing software, indices that describe gingival condition, plaque, and calculus can be entered and stored in a computer either manually via the keyboard or by examiner-operated multiple foot switches (a system developed for the Florida Probe by Gibbs et al[28]). The printout illustrated in Fig 1-3a shows full-mouth data, including recession, pocket depth, bleed-

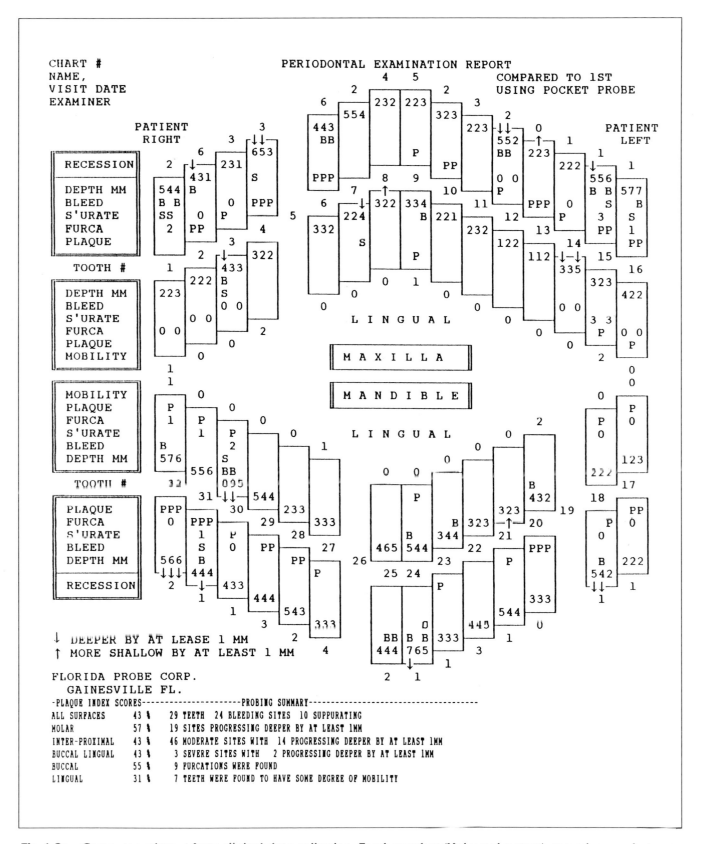

Fig 1-3a *Computer printout from clinical data collection. Tooth number (Universal system), recession, pocket depth, bleeding, suppuration, furcation involvement, and plaque are indicated.*

```
CHART #
NAME,
EXAMINER
VISIT DATE

TESTS PERFORMED <RECESSION> <PROBING,BLEEDING,SUPPURATION> <FURCATION> <PLAQUE> <MOBILITY> USING POCKET PROBE
```

	SITE DB	B	MB	ML	L	DL	
TOOTH 1	5.1 BS	4.1 S F=2	4.1 B	3.0 F=0	2.1	2.1 F=0	M=1 R= 2.0
TOOTH 2	4.1 B	P 2.9 F=0 P	1.1	2.2 F=0	1.9	2.2 F=0	M=0 R= 6.0
TOOTH 3	2.1	P 3.0 F=0	1.0	2.9 F=0	2.9	3.8 BS F=0	M=0 R= 3.0
TOOTH 4	5.4 S	P 4.3	P 3.1	P 2.1	2.1	2.9	M=2 R= 3.0
TOOTH 5 XX	0.0 F=0	0.0	0.0 F=0	0.0	0.0	0.0	M=0 R= 0.0
TOOTH 6	4.1	P 4.1 B	P 3.1 B	P 2.1	3.0	3.0	M=0 R= 6.0
TOOTH 7	4.3	4.3	3.3	4.1 S	1.8	1.9	M=0 R= 2.0
TOOTH 8	2.2	3.1	1.9	1.9	1.9	2.9	M=0 R= 4.0

	SITE MB	B	DB	DL	L	ML	
TOOTH 9	2.0	2.0	P 2.9	3.3 B	2.4	P 2.4	M=1 R= 5.0
TOOTH 10	3.1	2.1	P 3.2	P 1.2	2.2	1.9	M=0 R= 2.0
TOOTH 11	2.1	2.1	2.8	2.0	2.3	2.1	M=0 R= 3.0
TOOTH 12	4.3 B F=0	P 4.3 B	2.1 F=0	2.0	1.7	1.1	M=0 R= 2.0
TOOTH 13	2.0	P 2.0	P 2.8	P 2.1	1.2	0.9	M=0 R= 0.0
TOOTH 14	1.9	P 1.9 F=0	1.9	5.0 F=0	3.1	3.1 F=0	M=0 R= 1.0
TOOTH 15	5.1 B	5.1 F=3	P 5.9 BS	3.1 F=3	2.1	P 2.3 F=3	M=2 R= 1.0
TOOTH 16	5.1	6.9 S F=1	P 7.0 B	P 2.1 F=0	2.1	P 3.5 F=0	M=0 R= 1.0
TOOTH 17	2.0	1.7 F=0	P 1.9	P 2.7	1.9 F=0	P 1.2	M=0 R= 1.0
TOOTH 18	4.3	3.8 B F=0	1.9	P 2.1	2.1 F=0	P 2.1	M=0 R= 1.0
TOOTH 19 XX	0.0	0.0 F=0	0.0	0.0	0.0 F=0	0.0	M=0 R= 0.0
TOOTH 20	3.1	P 2.7	P 3.0	P 2.1	2.9	3.4 B	M=2 R= 0.0
TOOTH 21	5.1	3.7	P 4.0	2.3	2.0	3.1	M=0 R= 1.0
TOOTH 22	3.3	3.9	4.9	2.7	1.9	3.1	M=0 R= 3.0
TOOTH 23	3.2	P 3.2	3.2	3.8 B	3.9	2.8	M=0 R= 1.0
TOOTH 24	6.9 B	5.9	4.7 BS	3.9	4.0	P 4.8 B	M=0 R= 1.0

	SITE DB	B	MB	ML	L	DL	
TOOTH 25	3.3	3.8 B	4.0 B	4.5	5.4	4.0	M=0 R= 2.0
TOOTH 26 XX	0.0	0.0	0.0	0.0	0.0	0.0	M=0 R= 0.0
TOOTH 27	3.1	P 3.1	3.1	2.8	3.1	2.9	M=1 R= 4.0
TOOTH 28	5.0	3.7	P 3.0	P 3.1	2.9	2.0	M=0 R= 2.0
TOOTH 29	3.3	3.6	P 3.6	P 3.3	3.7	4.3	M=0 R= 3.0
TOOTH 30	3.9	3.2 F=0	P 3.2	4.8	9.1 B F=2	P 8.1 BS	M=0 R= 1.0
TOOTH 31	4.2	P 4.1 BS F=1	P 3.7	P 5.9	5.1 F=1	P 4.6	M=0 R= 1.0
TOOTH 32	4.9	P 6.0 F=0	P 6.0	P 6.0	6.3 F=1	P 4.6 B	M=1 R= 2.0

```
-PLAQUE INDEX SCORES---------------------PROBING SUMMARY-----------------
ALL SURFACES    43 %   29 TEETH  24 BLEEDING SITES  10 SUPPURATING
MOLAR           57 %   19 SITES PROGRESSING DEEPER BY AT LEAST 1MM
INTER-PROXIMAL  43 %   46 MODERATE SITES WITH  14 PROGRESSING DEEPER BY AT LEAST 1MM
BUCCAL LINGUAL  43 %    3 SEVERE SITES WITH    2 PROGRESSING DEEPER BY AT LEAST 1MM
BUCCAL          55 %    9 FURCATIONS WERE FOUND
LINGUAL         31 %    7 TEETH WERE FOUND TO HAVE SOME DEGREE OF MOBILITY
```

Fig 1-3b *Same data as in Fig 1-3a, shown in table format.*

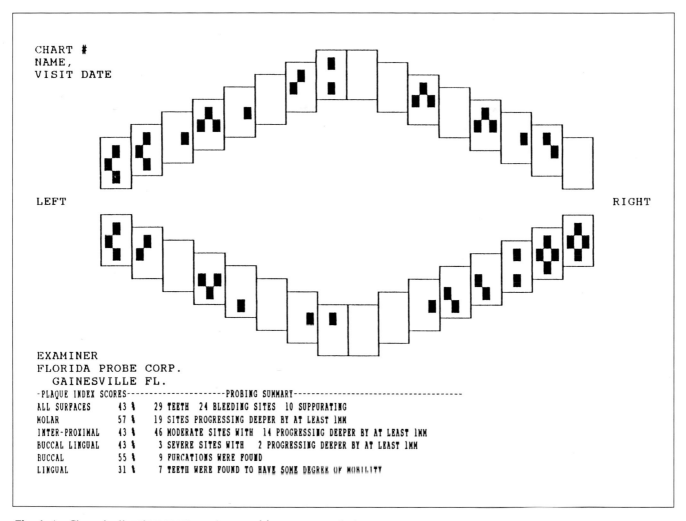

CHART #
NAME,
VISIT DATE

LEFT   RIGHT

EXAMINER
FLORIDA PROBE CORP.
    GAINESVILLE FL.
-PLAQUE INDEX SCORES---------------------PROBING SUMMARY--------------------------------
ALL SURFACES   43 %   29 TEETH 24 BLEEDING SITES 10 SUPPURATING
MOLAR   57 %   19 SITES PROGRESSING DEEPER BY AT LEAST 1MM
INTER-PROXIMAL   43 %   46 MODERATE SITES WITH 14 PROGRESSING DEEPER BY AT LEAST 1MM
BUCCAL LINGUAL   43 %   3 SEVERE SITES WITH   2 PROGRESSING DEEPER BY AT LEAST 1MM
BUCCAL   55 %   9 FURCATIONS WERE FOUND
LINGUAL   31 %   7 TEETH WERE FOUND TO HAVE SOME DEGREE OF MOBILITY

Fig 1-4 *Chart indicating tooth surfaces with presence of plaque.*

ing, furcation involvement, suppuration, plaque, and mobility, which have been entered by the use of multiple foot switches. Figure 1-3b shows the same data in table format.

Tooth mobility data also can be entered and stored in a computer, again, either via the keyboard or by an examiner-operated foot switch.[28] If measurements are taken by means of a mechanical instrument, this can be connected to a computer by a linear transducer. Separate charts can then be generated to illustrate, for instance, the patient's plaque situation from visit to visit (Fig 1-4), or to illustrate any differences between current measurements and those taken at the first or the previous visit.

PERIODONTAL PROBING TECHNOLOGY

Even though pocket probing depth measurements yield important information regarding periodontal status and response to therapy, currently, in clinical research, the "gold standard" for "active" disease at a site is a measurable *loss of attachment*. A number of studies have attempted to correlate attachment level with other clinical parameters. For example, Badersten et al[29] tried to relate probing level changes in treated subjects to other clinical characteristics in an attempt to determine if any other clinical parameter could be used to predict disease activity (ie, loss of attachment). Sites with a deep initial probing depth demonstrated a higher incidence of gain and a lower incidence of attachment loss than did shallower sites. All other investigated characteristics, including plaque, bleeding, suppuration, tooth surface, and tooth position, showed either weak association or no association with probing attachment change following therapy.

Currently, then, it appears that the only reliable clinical method for assessing progression or remission of periodontal disease is to monitor longitudinal changes in probing attachment level measurements recorded from a fixed reference point. The aim of probing attachment level measurements is to determine the most coronal connective tissue fibers of the periodontal ligament. Several studies evaluating the location of the probe tip in both healthy and diseased conditions[30-34] have shown that in a healthy periodontium, the probe tip usually stops short of the connective tissue attachment, whereas when gingival inflammation is present, the probe tip penetrates past the apical termination of the junctional epithelium and into the connective tissue.

Studies have also shown that the penetration of the probe is positively correlated with probing forces,[35-37] indicating that to obtain reproducible measurements it is important to probe with a standardized force. Badersten et al[38] studied the reproducibility of probing attachment level measurements using a manual probe and found that approximately 90% of the recordings could be repeated within ±1 mm difference. This was found for intra- and interexaminer comparisons of two calibrated examiners. The level of reproducibility varied notably between patients and was improved following nonsurgical periodontal therapy.

Automatic Constant-Force Probes

Following a workshop on the Quantitative Evaluation of Periodontal Diseases by Physical Mea-surement Techniques, the National Institute for Dental Research (NIDR) issued a request for proposals to develop and clinically evaluate an improved periodontal pocket depth attachment level measurement system.[39] The new periodontal probe system was to meet the following criteria:

1. A precision of ±0.1 mm
2. A range of 10 mm
3. Constant probing force
4. Noninvasive; lightweight for comfortable use over an extended period of time; easy to use
5. Able to access any location around all teeth
6. A guidance system to ensure that measurements are taken from the same part of the sulcus each time (desirable but not mandatory)
7. Complete sterilization of all portions entering or nearing the mouth (cold sterilization not acceptable)
8. No biohazard from material or electric shock
9. Digital output

The above criteria were more or less met by Gibbs et al,[40] who developed the Florida Probe system (Florida Probe Corporation), which combined the advantages of constant probing force with precise electronic measurement and computer storage of the data. The Florida Probe (Fig 1-5) eliminates the potential errors associated with visual reading. The system, which consists of a probe handpiece, a digital readout, a foot switch, a computer interface, and a computer, was studied by Magnusson et al[41] and correlated to standard probe measurements. They concluded that the reproducibility of pocket depth measurements obtained with the electronic probe was significantly superior to the reproducibility of

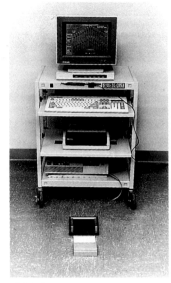

Fig 1-5 *The Florida Probe system. The probe handpiece is connected to the computer and a foot switch.*

those obtained with a standard probe. There was no difference in time consumption between the two methods; however, data from the electronic probe are entered into the computer automatically, thereby eliminating the need for an assistant to record the measurements.

An electronic probe using an optical encoder transduction element was evaluated by Goodson and Kondon.[42] These authors reported somewhat higher reproducibility with the electronic probe compared to conventional probing and a correlation coefficient of 0.82 between the two different methods. This probe has now been named Interprobe (Bausch & Lomb).

To detect progression of periodontal disease over a shorter time period, Haffajee et al[43] recommended the tolerance method, in which the difference between replicate attachment level measurements was used to calculate a standard deviation for all the measurement pairs made in an individual. The subject threshold for attachment loss in an individual site is considered to be three standard deviations of the mean differences between all the paired measurements. For 22 subjects studied, standard deviation values varied from 0.52 to 1.30 mm, giving a mean subject threshold for attachment loss of 2.46 mm (range: 1.56 to 3.90 mm). This means that in some patients a considerable loss of attachment is needed to determine progression of disease.

Magnusson et al[44] also investigated the reproducibility of attachment level measurements taken with the Florida Probe. With the use of the constant-force electronic probe and fixed reference points on custom-made acrylic resin stents, a high level of agreement was achieved for attachment level measurements made by different examiners (mean standard deviation = 0.28 mm) or by a single examiner during different visits (mean standard deviation = 0.33 mm). The highest agreement between attachment level measurements was achieved when the measurements were performed at the same visit, even though the measurements were performed by two different examiners (a periodontist and a dental hygienist). It is significant that by using the tolerance method,[43] Magnusson et al[44] established that the probe used in this study was significantly more sensitive in detecting a threshold for attachment loss than was the standard periodontal probe. For the 10 subjects, the standard deviations varied from 0.25 to 0.33 mm, with an average of 0.28 mm. With the standard manual probe, Haffajee et al[43] reported an average of 0.82 mm, with a range of 0.52 to 1.30 mm. Using three standard deviations as a threshold for attachment

loss, the average threshold in the Magnusson study would be 0.84 mm, compared to 2.46 mm for Haffajee and coworkers. Thus, it appears that progressive periodontal disease could be detected more quickly by the constant-force electronic probe used in the Magnusson study. Several reports[37,45-47] indicate that measurements of deeper pockets are more variable. In the study by Haffajee et al,[43] subjects were classified as having advanced periodontal disease; the Magnusson study dealt with subjects having minimal to early disease. However, when the same constant-force probe was used in subjects with severe periodontal disease, the standard deviations were found to be of the same magnitude or lower in that group of subjects.[44]

Jeffcoat et al[48] have described a new electronic periodontal probe that can automatically detect the cementoenamel junction. The Jeffcoat probe provided highly reproducible measurements when tested in beagle dogs (mean standard deviation for repeated measurements was 0.18 mm). In a recent study by Jeffcoat et al,[49] 10 human subjects with attachment loss ranging between 0.5 and 7.5 mm were measured 10 times over 2 weeks. The overall mean standard deviation of the repeated measurements was 0.17 mm. Using the same threshold of three standard deviations of attachment loss to indicate significant change, the average threshold with the Jeffcoat probe would be 0.51 mm.

Two other electronic probes (the Birek Probe[50] and the Florida Disk Probe[51]) have been designed to measure changes in attachment level using the occlusal surface or the incisal edge as a reference point. The Birek Probe works on constant air pressure and mea-

sures attachment level from the occlusal surface. In a study of duplicate measurements in nine subjects, it was found that 82% of the measurements were within a 1-mm difference. The standard deviation for all teeth was 0.46. The Florida Disk Probe was recently used independently by Low et al[51] and Osborn et al[52] to assess reproducibility of repeated measurements of the same sites in two groups of subjects. Both studies produced highly reproducible measurements with low standard deviation between replicate measurements (mean standard deviations = 0.26 and 0.18 mm, respectively). This probe does not require a prefabricated acrylic resin stent.

The Low study[51] compared two models of the Florida Probe (Fig 1-6): the stent model and the new disk model. The two probes are similar in design (both have a probe tip diameter of 0.4 mm and are preset at a constant 25-g force) but differ in the way they rest on a fixed reference point. The probe tip of the stent model runs through a metal sleeve which has a 1-mm collar that rests on the ledge of a fabricated vacuform stent (Fig 1-7). The disk model has a metal disk 11 mm in diameter that rests on the occlusal surface or incisal edge of the tooth (Fig 1-8). Both probes are connected to a digital readout. When the probe tip is in correct alignment with the tooth and the collar or disk is placed on the respective fixed reference point, a foot-activated rheostat is depressed to enter the measurement (to 0.1 mm) automatically into a computer.

The Low study to compare the stent and disk probe models consisted of two phases. In the first phase, 10 human skulls were probed, first with the stent probe, then with the disk probe. Two ex-

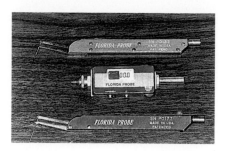

Fig 1-6 *The Florida Probe. Stent model probe (top), digital readout (middle), and disk model probe (bottom).*

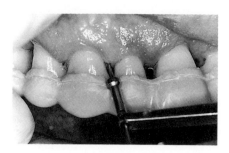

Fig 1-7 *Stent model probe in position with the collar of the probe on the ledge of the fabricated acrylic resin stent.*

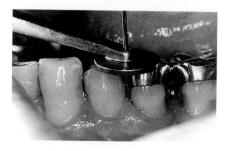

Fig 1-8 *Disk model probe in position with the disk resting on the incisal edge.*

aminers measured six sites around each tooth in each skull during one session and repeated the measurements at a second session 7 to 10 days later. All measurements were made with the probe tip parallel to the long axis of the tooth at the midbuccal and midlingual areas and as close as possible to the midinterproximal area from the buccal and lingual aspects.

In the second phase, the same protocol was used to probe four human subjects with early to moderate periodontitis. As before, two examiners measured six sites around each tooth, first with the stent probe, then with the disk probe. After 7 to 10 days, subjects returned and measurements were repeated by the same examiners. Sites showing differences over 1.0 mm were reexamined. This involved an average of 5 / 192 stent probe sites and 10 / 192 disk probe sites. Table 1-2 shows comparisons of the standard deviations of the differences between duplicate measurements.

The new electronic probes appear to be superior to manual probes. In the studies described above, the range of overall standard deviations for repeated measurements of individual sites in different subjects was 0.17 to 0.32 mm. Regarding the ability to de-

TABLE 1-2 *Standard deviations (SD) and range by subject calculated for two examiners on duplicate attachment level measurements in four human subjects*

PROBE TYPE	SD	SD RANGE BY SUBJECT
Disk	0.26	0.24–0.28
Stent	0.25	0.21–0.28

tect significant attachment level changes, this should still be an improvement over the 0.82 mm obtained by Haffajee et al[43] using the manual probe.

Even though probing attachment level is currently the "gold standard" for active disease at a site, changes in attachment level are not always easy to interpret because of the limitation of probing in assessing the histological attachment level. In monitoring attachment level changes on a monthly basis using the more sensitive electronic probes, we have noted attachment level fluctuations that exceed measurement error. Figure 1-9 shows duplicate measurements taken monthly at a single site that was scaled every 3 months but which received no other treatment. The site lost attachment from baseline to 3 months, showed a 1.5-mm gain between months 4 and 6 and at 7 months lost 1.5 mm. Though a change of 1.5 mm may seem insignificant when compared to

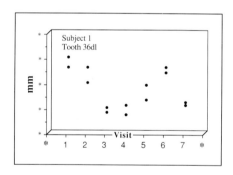

Fig 1-9 *Example of longitudinal variation in probing measurements over a period of 7 months. The graph illustrates duplicate monthly measurements at the distolingual aspect of a mandibular left first molar.*

changes of 2 to 3 mm required to detect change using the standard probe, the tolerance method suggests this is a significant change for this patient as probed by the Florida Probe. The standard deviation of the differences between measurement pairs was 0.24 mm for this patient. Using three standard deviations as the threshold for a significant change as suggested by Haffajee et al,[43] a 1.5-mm change is significantly more than the 0.72-mm change calculated for the threshold. We are not sure what these fluctuations mean, but for the present we must regard a loss of probing attachment level as indicative of active progressing disease and a gain as improvement or remission. Short-time changes, both loss and gain, may only reflect fluctuation in collagen content accompanied by changes in inflammatory status[30,31,34] and may not indicate real attachment changes. Watts[53] suggested that it is also possible that despite the best efforts of the clinician, these changes might also represent errors in probe placement or angulation. If attachment loss is confirmed at a later time, however, it probably represents a true loss, indicative of active and progressive periodontal disease.

During the next few years, we hope to improve our ability to assess disease activity. The electronic constant-force probes help to reduce the variability associated with probing and also facilitate the gathering and analysis of large volumes of longitudinal probing data, making large-scale field trials more feasible. Recently a probe for recording pocket temperature was described by Kung et al.[54] The basis for this instrument is that elevated temperature is normally a characteristic of inflammation. The results from a study of the probe suggested that site temperature is a diagnostic sign of inflammatory activity associated with periodontal disease. Thus, tooth-by-tooth analysis showed that diseased teeth have higher temperatures than anatomically equivalent healthy teeth ($P < .01$).

Probes and the Examination of Patients Considered for Implants

Over the last few decades, increased emphasis on both esthetics and function in regard to the edentulous or partly edentulous patient has created rapid development of dental implants. Of the wide variety of dental implants available, the Brånemark System is by far the best scientifically documented system. Developed in the late 1960s,[55] this system uses osseointegrated titanium fixtures. Several reports have documented high long-term success rates in edentulous jaws, especially for mandibular implants.[56-58] Albrektsson et al[58] followed 334 mandibular implants for 5 to 8 years and reported a success rate of 99.1%. In the maxilla, 106 implants, followed for a period of 5 to 7 years, had a success rate of 84.9%. Ericsson et al[59] reported cases where combinations of osseointegrated implants and natural teeth have been used to support fixed bridges with good clinical results. Adell et al[57] suggested the following indications for treatment with osseointegrated implants: *(1)* insufficient retention of a denture, generally due to extreme resorption of the alveolar process; *(2)* mental inability to accept a denture in cases of technically adequate or inadequate retention; and *(3)* functional disturbances (eg, severe nausea and vomiting reflexes) caused by a denture. Dental implants are contraindicated in patients at intraoperative or postoperative risk and in patients with conditions that compromise bone healing.[60] Such conditions include osteoporosis, connective tissue disorders, chronic steroids, immunosuppressives, and therapeutic irradiation of the implant site.

Osseointegrated implants can be used in almost any jaw, but of course the morphology of the bone will determine the implant design and size and the surgical approach. In cases where the residual ridge is too narrow, grafts can be considered before placement of implants, and in fact, Albrektsson et al[58] reported high success rates in such jaws as well as in irradiated jaws.

The examination of patients being considered for implants includes both clinical evaluation of soft tissues and a radiographic evaluation. When natural teeth are present, the soft tissue and oral hygiene are evaluated as are loss of attachment, pocket depth, and tooth mobility. This examination serves as a baseline for future followup and evaluation of therapy.

However, probing around implants is difficult for the following reasons: *(1)* the prosthetic construction may need to be removed for access, and *(2)* standard metal instruments are unsuitable. Instead, plastic or titanium probe tips should be used to avoid damage of the implant / tissue interface. If automatic probing is considered, the Florida Probe is available with a titanium tip that will not hurt the implant; also, the Interprobe system comes with disposable plastic tips.

CLINICAL APPLICATION

Periodontal diseases are found in all patient groups, regardless of age or socioeconomic status; therefore, a periodontal examination should be performed for every patient with teeth.[61] It is equally important for dental professionals to record the findings of these examinations. The question that must be asked is not *whether* to examine for inflammatory periodontal diseases, but to what *extent* the clinician chooses to examine each patient.

The extent of the examination should be determined by the amount of responsibility the individual clinician wishes to assume in the diagnosis, active treatment, and supportive periodontal treatment (maintenance) for that patient. In short, the more responsibility one intends to assume, the more extensive the initial and followup examinations must become. As mentioned, at present it is suggested that a complete examination be performed on every patient with teeth. For those clinicians who only want to screen and then refer patients, there are two simple screening tests that may be used: the Perio Access Screening Examination and the CPITN[62] (also called the Periodontal Screening and Recording [PSR]) (see pages 32 and 34).

COMPREHENSIVE PERIODONTAL EXAMINATION

It is of utmost importance to remember that the concepts detailed in this chapter are changing rapidly; continued updating of knowledge on the subject is strongly suggested.

To judge the efficacy of active and supportive periodontal treatment (maintenance), the clinician must have adequate and accurate baseline data; without this baseline against which to measure, it is impossible to define success. With accurate baseline data, however (gathered during proper examination and diagnosis), selecting the appropriate active and supportive periodontal treatment (SPT) becomes less problematic. Careful examinations for patients with periodontal diseases are critical, and adequate time must be found during all phases of therapy for this procedure. This phase of care will help to determine severity and disease activity (see chapter 4) and can prevent overtreatment or, as is often the case, undertreatment of these inflammatory lesions.

Health Histories

The initial periodontal examination starts with a questionnaire that the patient fills out. It should contain vital statistics (age, weight, etc), address, employment and marital status, a review of medical and dental histories, and the patient's chief complaint. Questions concerning present and past compliance to oral hygiene and SPT are included. The document should be signed and dated by the patient and the dentist and updated periodically. (An example of a long-form health history has been published elsewhere.[63]) The health history should be reviewed with the patient by the dentist. This is an appropriate time to determine both the patient's goals for therapy and motivation to seek care. In many cases these

goals will be unfocused and patients will need the assistance of the dental professional in formalizing their desired end points in therapy. Setting goals serves several purposes, including ameliorating concerns about the proposed care, helping the patient develop realistic expectations, and identifying and then overcoming barriers to the patient's undergoing therapy.

Compliance Data

Since most periodontal diseases are chronic, patient compliance is a major factor in successful therapy. Patients who do not clean their teeth well or who do not comply to suggested SPT usually have recurrent problems (see chapter 12). It is important to ask patients about past compliance, even though their responses are often unreliable.[64] More accurate data can usually be obtained from previous dentists if needed.

Radiographic Examination and Radiographic History

A set of appropriate radiographs is essential for making a proper diagnosis (see chapter 3). Each patient is unique, but most adults with teeth require a full-mouth series of periapical films accompanied by posterior vertical bitewing radiographs. These should be exposed using a parallel (right-angle) technique. The combination of panographic and bitewing radiographs rarely provides adequate coverage; this combination is not accurate enough to make a correct diagnosis.

Radiographs should be kept to a minimum but, for patients with active periodontal diseases, a full set of radiographs should be taken every 2 years. Vertical bite-wing films can provide optimal views of the coronal portions of the teeth and can be used as a screening tool between full-mouth sets of radiographs. A set of seven vertical bite-wings is preferred over four horizontal films in adults because this vertical position allows a view of the coronal portions of the alveolar bone in both the maxilla and the mandible.

Mounts are available that allow placement of several series of bite-wings in the same holder, thus permitting the clinician to follow bone patterns over time. The opportunity to make a correct diagnosis is improved with perspective. Perspective is improved by collecting the patient's old radiographs. Comparison of films can often give an indication of the rapidity of bone loss. As will be seen in chapter 5, patients with slow progressive deterioration will fit

into different diagnostic categories and receive therapy different from those patients in whom rapid loss has been documented.

CLINICAL CHARTING

Record Missing Teeth
(Fig 1-10)

Pocket Probing Depths

The manual periodontal probe remains an important diagnostic tool that the clinician can use to obtain information about the health of the soft tissues, bone loss, tissue tone, subgingival calculus deposits, furcations, and variations in root anatomy; however, it does have limitations. Pocket probing depths found with these devices can vary greatly depending on probe angulation, pressure applied, health of the tissue, diameter of the probe, and operator

variables. In inflamed tissue, the probe passes through the junctional epithelium (epithelial attachment) and into the connective tissue.[65] This means that one is not measuring the true histologic depth of the pocket. Consequently, the term *pocket probing depth* has begun to replace the more traditional term "pocket depth." Pocket probing depth has been described as the distance between the gingival margin and the apical depth of periodontal probe tip penetration.[66] Manual probing remains an art, and great diligence is needed to standardize one's technique and thereby ensure reproducible readings (Figs 1-11a and b).[35]

Proper force is important because the harder one pushes, the farther the probe tip penetrates into the periodontal tissues. Forces from 25[44] to 50[67] g have been suggested as appropriate. With manual probing and a thin (0.5 mm) probe, many patients find 50 g of force uncomfortable, but forces in the range of 25 g seem to be light, and some deeper areas in tight tissue may be misread. In practice it seems that the ideal manual force lies between these two extremes. To standardize one's probing force, the periodontal probe can be pushed against a metric scale, then this amount of force can be reproduced in the mouth. For increased accuracy or for calibration, electronic probes that deliver either a 25-g force or 50-g force are available (Vine Valley Research). The standard manual probe has the advantage of being readily available and significantly less expensive than the other probes described (see pages 21 to 25). In addition, devices (Dental Designs of Dallas) are available that attach to a manual probe and provide pressure-sensitive capabilities for increased consistency without excessive expense.

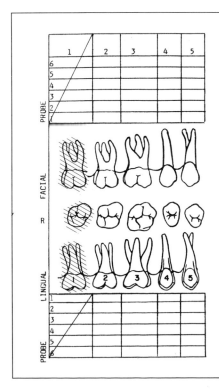

Clinical charting — record missing teeth
(Fig 1-10)

- Missing teeth are marked by slash.
- Unerupted teeth are circled.

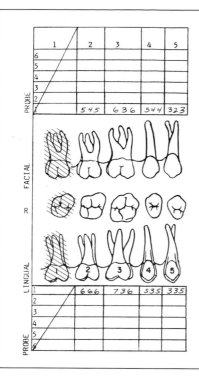

Probe selection and use (manual) (Figs 1-11a and b)

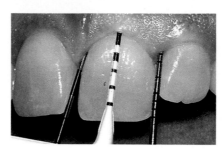

To obtain the most accurate manual readings, use a thin probe positioned as parallel to the long axis of the tooth as possible and drag it through the sulcus (pocket). Pictured here are thin probes (0.4 to 0.5 mm) with Williams markings (1, 2, 3, 5, 7, 8, 9, and 10 mm) on the left, CPITN markings (PSR) (0.5, 3.5, 5.5, 8.5, and 11.5 mm) in the center, and CP12 markings (3, 6, 9, and 12 mm) on the right.

Probe use (computerized) (Fig 1-12)

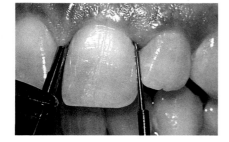

Computerized probes provide very accurate readings, a standardized force and probe tip diameter, and the convenience of computerized data storage. The current "gold standard" for these devices is the Florida Probe (Florida Probe Corporation). Its drawbacks for clinical practice are its expense, the extra time it takes to use the device, and the discomfort experienced by some patients. The device is best used by paralleling the probe to the long axis of the tooth (this is often difficult in posterior areas or on the lingual surface of anterior teeth with long clinical crowns), as shown on the left of the photograph. The sleeve is then depressed until it reaches the margin of the gingiva (at right in the photograph), then a foot switch is depressed to record the data.

Computerized probes (Fig 1-12) have been developed that give more accurate readings than the methods just detailed. Some measure from the soft tissue margin[68] and some detect the distance from the base of the probe tip to the cementoenamel junction.[48]

Clinicians must remember that probing depths, be they computerized or manual, can be misleading in the presence of excessively tight or flaccid tissue, when there are large deposits of calculus, or when visibility or placement of the probe is hindered. Even though these problems make it difficult to standardize probing depth readings, the information obtained makes it well worth the effort.

Prior to the initial examination is an excellent time to collect probing charts from the patient's previous dentists. Although probe readings can vary from office to office, the perspective these readings provide (especially when combined with previous radiographs) is of great value when establishing a correct diagnosis.

Gingival Recession or Hyperplasia

This parameter is measured from a set point on the tooth, usually the cementoenamel junction, the margin of a restoration, or the occlusal edge. It is an important measure because it provides perspective for pocket probing depth. In most cases midbuccal and midlingual (palatal) recessions are recorded (Figs 1-13a and b).

Bleeding Upon Probing; Suppuration; Bacterial Plaque (Figs 1-14a and b)

Bleeding upon probing can be found in two ways: *(1)* as an independent process by dragging the tip of a thin periodontal probe through the gingival sulcus, using a pressure of 25 g,[44] or *(2)* by recording any bleeding seen up to

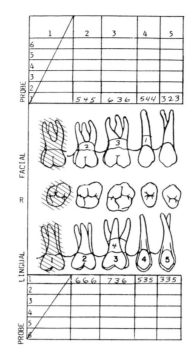

Clinical charting — gingival recession
(Figs 1-13a and b)

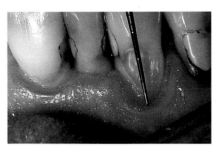

In this example, the pocket probing depth is 3 mm. If the amount of recession were not recorded, the fact that approximately 7 mm of attachment had been lost (equal to a 10-mm pocket probing depth) would have been overlooked when the chart was read.

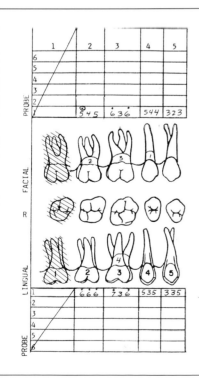

Clinical charting — bleeding upon probing, suppuration, and bacterial plaque (Figs 1-14a and b)

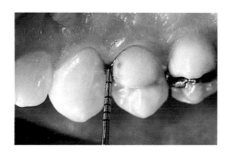

In clinical practice, these parameters are recorded as either present or absent:

- Bleeding upon probing, as noted in the clinical photo, can be recorded as a dot above the pocket probing depth or on a modified O'Leary chart.[69]
- Suppuration is found by pressing on the gingival tissues or is seen at the time pocket probing depths are recorded. It is recorded as a circle with a dot in the center.
- Supragingival bacterial plaque can be recorded on a modified O'Leary chart.

30 seconds after the pocket probing depth reading of a particular site has been taken.[69] The importance of this index may be found in its absence rather than its presence because absence of bleeding almost always indicates gingival health (see chapter 4).

At the same time that the clinician scores bleeding upon probing, any visible supragingival dental plaque also can be recorded. If time is limited, remember that bleeding on probing gives more information concerning tissue health than does the accumulation of plaque.

Suppuration can be found when using the periodontal probe or by exerting coronal pressure on the gingival tissues. This last approach is usually performed with a football-shaped burnisher.

Tooth Mobility

Tooth mobility is clinically measured in two simple ways: when pressure is placed on individual teeth while the jaws are apart (bidigital mobility) (Figs 1-15a and b), and that seen when the teeth are in function (fremitus)[70] (Figs 1-16a and b).

Furcations

Furcations can be clinically assessed in two ways. The first is to use a Nabers Probe. The second is to horizontally probe the depth in millimeters (Figs 1-17a to c).

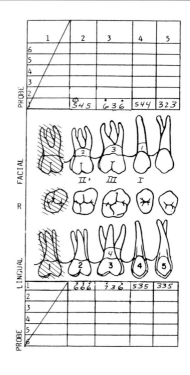

Clinical charting — tooth mobility (bidigital)
(Figs 1-15a and b)

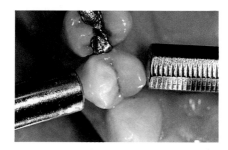

At present there is no simple, inexpensive, reproducible system for documenting bidigital mobility. This measurement is performed by pressing on the facial and lingual surfaces of the teeth with the nonworking ends of two instrument handles. The clinician can then use a modification of the "Miller scale" as recommended by Fleszar et al[22]:

Class 0: Physiologic mobility; firm tooth
Class I: Slightly increased mobility
Class II: Definite to considerable increase in mobility, but no impairment of function
Class III: Extreme mobility; a "loose" tooth that would be uncomfortable in function

(A " + can be used for intermediate values, eg, 1 +). This approach obviously leads to a great deal of individual variation. However, some degree of reproducibility is possible within one's own office.

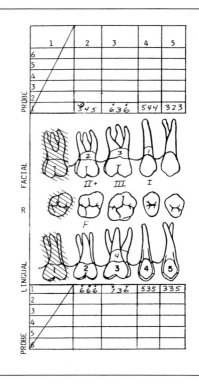

Clinical charting — tooth mobility (fremitus)
(Figs 1-16a and b)

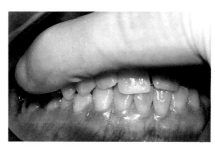

Fremitus (functional mobility) is the movement of teeth during function or parafunction. Fremitus can often be detected earlier than bidigital tooth mobility and has been associated in the presence of inflammation with increased bone and attachment loss (pocket formation) when compared to teeth without fremitus.[70] The clinical photo shows testing for fremitus. The index finger is placed on the labial surface of the maxillary teeth and the patient is asked to grind in lateral and protrusive movements. Any movement seen or felt is considered fremitus.

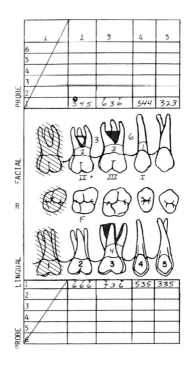

Clinical charting — furcations (Figs 1-17a to c)

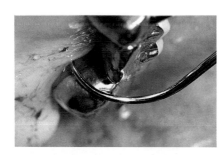

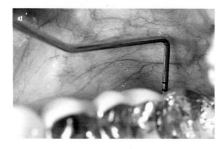

• Nabers Probes are best used in palatal furcas of maxillary molars and interproximal furcas of maxillary premolars.

The furcas found with the Nabers Probe can be classified in the following manner:

Class I : A depression that does not catch the probe

Class II : A furca deep enough to catch the probe but not contiguous with other furcas on the same tooth

Class III: Bone loss through and through

• Standard probes can be used horizontally in buccal and lingual furcas. When combined with vertical probing depths, this approach is an accurate way to quantify bone loss, but this form of analysis is usually only feasible in buccal furcations on the maxilla and in buccal and lingual furcations on the mandible.

Attached and Keratinized Gingiva

The keratinized tissue of the gingiva extends from the mucogingival junction to the most coronal aspect of the midfacial or midlingual surface of the free gingival margin. The amount of attached gingiva is found by subtracting the midfacial or midlingual pocket probing depth from the width of keratinized gingiva (Figs 1-18a and b). For additional information, see chapters 14 and 15.

MICROBIOLOGICAL EXAMINATION

Dentistry is moving away from the idea that the cause of all inflammatory lesions is the microbiological conglomerate commonly called *dental plaque.* Current thought holds that at least some of the forms of these diseases are associated with specific bacterial species or combinations of a few of these species. This belief has ushered in the need to detect specific microorganisms, which in turn has led to the development of tests for these microbes and their products (Figs 1-19a to d). More on these tests can be found in chapter 2.

At present there are several types of microbiological tests; they include: *(1)* culture of the viable bacteria and assessment of antimicrobial susceptibility; *(2)* DNA or antibody probes that detect specific bacterial DNA or cell wall components; and *(3)* detection of bacterial products such as specific enzymes. These tests are currently suggested for patients who are suspected of having aggressive types of periodontitis.

The following methods can be used as screening tests as a precursor to a full examination. In almost every instance a full examination is preferred over these approaches.

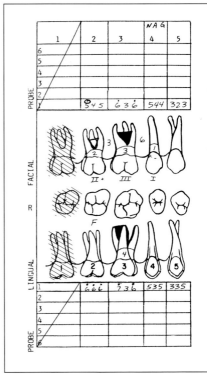

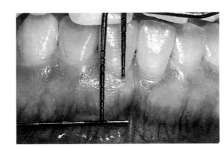

Clinical charting — attached and keratinized gingiva
(Figs 1-18a and b)

The horizontal probe has located the mucogingival junction (the most apical area where nonmovable tissue is found), while other probes measure the pocket probing depth (2 mm) and the width of the keratinized gingiva (7 mm). In this example the amount of attached gingiva would be 5 mm. *NAG* = no attached gingiva.

Microbiologic examination (Figs 1-19a to d)

- The area to be sampled should have deepened pocket probing depths and active signs of disease.

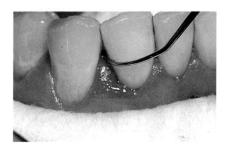

- The area should be isolated and dried with a cotton roll. Supragingival plaque is then removed with a sterile instrument.

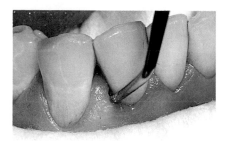

- The pocket is then sampled with a sterile curet.

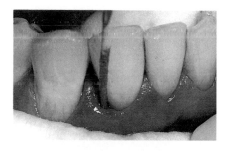

- When minimal subgingival bacteria are found, three paper points (10 seconds each) should be used.

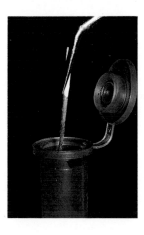

- The sample is then carried to the appropriate container and medium for shipment to the laboratory.

Screening Tests for Periodontal Diseases

Perio Access Quick Screen (Fig 1-20) The Perio Access Quick Screen is a sticker placed on the patient's treatment record form. It facilitates examination and establishes a preliminary diagnosis. It can be used for initial examination screening, summarizing comprehensive examination findings, and providing a chart record of the diagnosis, for existing patients in need of a screening / diagnosis.

The sticker indicates each criterion for the clinician to evaluate and provides a scoring / point system weighted in terms of the degree of periodontal treatment difficulty and the degree to which the amount of attachment loss will affect long-term prognosis. The clinician adds the point totals and then checks off the score which is adjacent to a particular diagnostic category. The form is preprinted with the term "preliminary diagnosis," which, from a medical legal standpoint, allows the dental hygienist to record the data.

Periodontal Screening and Recording (PSR) A second screening tool that is a variation of the Community Periodontal Index of Treatment Needs (CPITN Alternative II), which has been endorsed by the World Health Organization.[71] Recently this index has been modified by the American Academy of Periodontology. The Academy's modification is termed Periodontal Screening and Recording (PSR).

The PSR is designed to be used for patients age 18 years or older and assays every surface of every tooth. This examination involves the use of a thin periodontal probe with a colored strip (running from 3.5 to 5.5 mm) with a 0.5-mm ball at the tip. During this

PERIO ACCESS® Quick Screen							DIRECTIONS. Examine patient for each of the six categories listed and check off one box per category. Total the points (Pts.) for the checked boxes and locate the preliminary diagnosis.		
DATE: / /		✓ Pts.		✓ Pts.		✓ Pts.	TOTAL Pts.	PRELIMINARY CASE TYPE	PRELIMINARY DIAGNOSIS
1. SUBGINGIVAL FURCATIONS	CL I	☐ 5	Slt-CL II	☐ 20	Deep CL II-CL III	☐ 150	3-8	I	Gingivitis
2. POCKETS	4-5mm	☐ 20	5-6mm	☐ 50	> 6mm	☐ 150	10-20	II	Early Periodontitis
3. RECESSION	≤ 1mm	☐ 0	1-2mm	☐ 20	≥ 3mm	☐ 40	25-45	II	Early-Mod. Periodontitis
4. MOBILITY	None	☐ 0	Slight	☐ 10	Mod-Adv	☐ 40	45-75	II	Mod. Periodontitis
5. ATTACHED GINGIVA	Yes	☐ 0	No	☐ 35			75-190	III	Mod.-Adv. Periodontitis
6. BLEEDS ON PROBING	Isol/Slt	☐ 3	Yes	☐ 5			≥-190	IV	Adv. Periodontitis
©George K. Merijohn, D.D.S. 1986								V	Refractory Progressive Perio.

NOTE: This point system has been developed for generalized perio conditions. Higher total points from fewer teeth probably reflect an advanced localized condition requiring specialized care.

Fig 1-20 *Screening tests for periodontal diseases.*

examination, the entire sulcus (pocket) of each tooth or implant is probed and a reading is taken at six points on each tooth or implant. Readings are taken at the mesiofacial, midfacial, distofacial, and corresponding lingual/palatal areas. The probe is inserted into the crevice until resistance is met, then a reading is taken. The highest reading for each sextant is then recorded in a box specific for that sextant (Fig 1-21).

An *X* is used to indicate any sextant with no teeth and no dental implants, and the severity of the disease is indicated by a set of numbers ranging from 0 to 4 (Table 1-3). An * placed in the box indicates a clinical abnormality found in that sextant. These abnormalities include but are not limited to bone loss in a furcation, tooth mobility, and mucogingival problems or gingival recession that extends from the cementoenamel junction apically for 3.5 mm (into the colored area of the probe). If an abnormality exists (*) in codes 0 to 2, notation and/or treatment of that condition is warranted. If such an abnormality exists in codes 3 or 4, a comprehensive examination and treatment are necessary.

If a 3 is found, the entire sextant is probed and recorded. If a 4 is recorded, the entire mouth is examined using the approaches described in this chapter.

REEVALUATION
(Fig 1-22)

Health histories should be verbally updated at each visit and changes recorded. In addition, patients can review and re-sign their health history on a yearly basis. For patients with active periodontal disease, a full series of periapical and bite-wing radiographs should be taken every 2 years and seven vertical bite-wings exposed in intervening times. Patients with diseases other than chronic periodontal diseases may need radiographs more frequently. Probing pocket depths are optimally taken

```
           Maxilla

        Tooth numbers

Right  1–5    6–11   12–16  Left
      ─────┼──────┼─────
      32–28 27–22  21–17

          Mandible
```

Fig 1-21 *Sextant used for screening PSR.*

TABLE 1-3 *Scale used with periodontal screening and recording (PSR)*

PSR CODE	POCKET PROBING DEPTH	CALCULUS/DEFECTIVE MARGINS	BLEEDING UPON PROBING
0	Colored area visible	No	No
1	Colored area visible	No	Yes
2	Colored area visible	Yes	May be present
3	Colored area partially visible	May be present	May be present
4	Colored area not visible	May be present	May be present

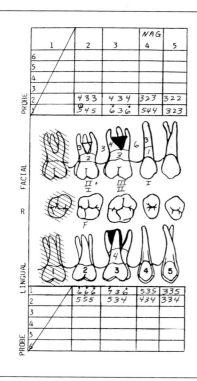

Reevaluation
(Fig 1-22)

The data collected are compared to information found at the initial visit and final diagnosis.

before treatment begins, at appropriate reevaluation visits during active therapy, within a few months after active therapy (to serve as a new baseline), and at each supportive periodontal treatment (SPT) visit. Bleeding upon probing, gingival recession, and fremitus are usually recorded at these same intervals. For more detail, see the clinical chapter on supportive periodontal treatment (chapter 12).

QUICK REVIEW

I. Examination of soft tissues
- The Löe and Silness index system, used to evaluate gingival status, has undergone several modifications, which, at least for some examiners, have improved its sensitivity and accuracy.
- Various indices have been devised to describe gingival inflammation by the amount of bleeding only. These include the Papilla Bleeding Index, the Papillary Bleeding Score, and the Eastman Interdental Bleeding Index. The Papillary Bleeding Score was found to be highly reproducible.
- Russell's Periodontal Index assesses the occurrence and severity of periodontal disease. Ramfjord's Periodontal Disease Index assesses attachment loss.
- Suppuration from the periodontal pocket is certainly a clear sign of the presence of inflammation. Whether it occurs both in established but stable disease or is a sign of disease activity will be discussed in chapter 4.

II. Evaluation of oral hygiene
- As for the gingival indices, it is probably not critical which one is used as long as it is consistent and is able to inform both examiner and patient about oral hygiene status.

III. Evaluation of tooth mobility
- Tooth mobility, which is not always attributable to periodontal disease, represents a function of the persisting height of the alveolar bone and the width of the periodontal ligament. It is important to record both initial and posttherapy mobility data to determine if changes have occurred as a result of either therapy or disease.

Quick Review continues on page 36.

QUICK REVIEW
(continued)

- Mobility may be measured manually or by various mechanical devices, the most common of which is the macro-periodontometer.

IV. Automatic constant force probes

- A measurable attachment loss represents the "gold standard" for determining "active" disease. To obtain reproducible measurements, standardized probing force is necessary.
- The Florida Probe was found to yield reproducible results.
- The Interprobe and Jeffcoat's probe can automatically detect the cementoenamel junction.
- The Birek Probe and the Florida Disk Probe measure attachment level changes using the occlusal surface or the incisal edge as a reference point.
- Electronic probes appear to be superior to manual probes; they help reduce probing variability and facilitate the acquisition of large volumes of data.
- A probe using temperature as a diagnostic sign for periodontal disease has been developed and is currently being studied.

V. Clinical application

- A periodontal examination should be performed for every patient with teeth.
- The more responsibility the therapist wishes to accept for the patient's therapy the more comprehensive the examination should be.

- Initial examination should include:
  — a written health history signed by the patient then reviewed and signed by the dentist
  — data on past compliance to suggested oral hygiene and supportive periodontal treatment (maintenance)
  — current radiographic examination and collection of previous radiographs
  — clinical charting
    (1) pocket probing depths
    (2) gingival recession
    (3) bleeding upon probing; bacterial plaque formation; and suppuration
    (4) tooth mobility: bidigital and fremitus
  — microbiologic monitoring is often indicated in patients with problems other than chronic diseases (chronic gingivitis and / or chronic adult periodontitis)
  — furcations
  — amount of attached and keratinized gingiva
- Reevaluations should occur:
  — during active therapy
  — approximately 3 months following cessation of active therapy
  — at each supportive periodontal treatment (maintenance) visit

REFERENCES

1. Löe H, Silness J: Periodontal disease in pregnancy. I. Prevalence and severity. *Acta Odontol Scand* 1963; 21:532-551.
2. Löe H: The Gingival Index, the Plaque Index and the Retention Index systems. *J Periodontol* 1967;38:610-616.
3. Gordon JM, Lamster IB, Seiger MC: Efficacy of Listerine antiseptic in inhibiting the development of plaque and gingivitis. *J Clin Periodontol* 1985; 12:697-704.
4. Lobene RR: Discussion: Current status of indices for measuring gingivitis. *J Clin Periodontol* 1986;13:381-382.
5. Lobene RR, Mankodi SM, Ciancio SG, Lamm RA, Charles CH, Ross NM: Correlations among gingival indices: A methodological study. *J Periodontol* 1989;60:159-162.
6. Lang NP, Joss A, Orsanic T, Gusberti FA, Siegrist BE: Bleeding on probing. A predictor for the progression of periodontal disease? *J Clin Periodontol* 1986;13:590-596.
7. Saxer UP, Mühlemann HR: Motivation and Aufklärung. *Schweiz Mschr Zahnheilk* 1975;85:905-919.
8. Loesche WJ: Clinical and microbiological aspects of chemotherapeutic agents used according to the specific plaque hypothesis. *J Dent Res* 1979;58:2404-2412.
9. Caton JG, Polson AM: The interdental bleeding index: A simplified procedure for monitoring gingival health. *Compend Contin Educ Dent* 1985;6:88-92.
10. Caton J, Polson A, Bouwsma O, Blieden T, Frantz R, Espeland M: Associations between bleeding and visual signs of interdental gingival inflammation. *J Periodontol* 1988;59:722-727.
11. Magnusson I, Marks RG, Taylor M, Clark WB, Clouser B, Maruniak J: Intra- and interexaminer correlation of some oral indices. *J Dent Res* 1990; 69(Abstr. no. 1970):355.
12. Schour I, Massler M: Gingival disease in postwar Italy (1945). I. Prevalence of gingivitis in various age groups. *J Am Dent Assoc* 1947;35:475-482.
13. Russell AL: System of classification and scoring for prevalence surveys of periodontal disease. *J Dent Res* 1956; 35:350-359.
14. Ramfjord SP: Indices for prevalence and incidence of periodontal disease. *J Periodontol* 1959;30:51-59.
15. Greene JC, Vermillion JR: The Oral Hygiene Index. A method for classifying oral hygiene status. *J Am Dent Assoc* 1960; 61:172-179.
16. Russell AL: International nutrition surveys: A summary of preliminary dental findings. *J Dent Res* 1963;42:233-244.
17. Quigley GA, Hein JW: Comparative cleansing efficiency of manual and power brushing. *J Am Dent Assoc* 1962;65:26-29.
18. Silness J, Löe H: Periodontal disease in pregnancy. II. Correlation between oral hygiene and periodontal condition. *Acta Odontol Scand* 1964; 22:121-135.
19. Ennever J, Sturzenberger OP, Radike AW: The calculus surface index method for scoring clinical calculus studies. *J Periodontol* 1961;32:54-57.
20. Volpe AR, Manhold JH Jr: Method of evaluating the effectiveness of potential calculus inhibiting agents. *NY State Dent J* 1962;28:289-290.
21. Lindhe J: *Textbook of Clinical Periodontology.* Copenhagen: Munksgaard, 1983.
22. Fleszar TJ, Knowles JW, Morrison EC, Burgett FG, Nissle RR, Ramfjord SP: Tooth mobility and periodontal therapy. *J Clin Periodontol* 1980;7:495-505.
23. Lindhe J: *Textbook of Clinical Periodontology.* 2nd ed. Copenhagen: Munksgaard, 1989.
24. Mühlemann HR: Periodontometry, a method for measuring tooth mobility. *Oral Surg Oral Med Oral Pathol* 1951;4:1220-1233.
25. O'Leary TJ, Rudd KD: An instrument for measuring horizontal tooth mobility. *Periodontics* 1963;1:249-254.
26. Persson R, Svensson A: Assessment of tooth mobility using small loads. I. Technical devices and calculations of tooth mobility in periodontal health and disease. *J Clin Periodontol* 1980;7:259-275.
27. Robertson G: The multiple impulse method of tooth mobility assessment — An evaluation of the Periotest. Third North Sea Conference on Periodontology. British, Dutch and Scandinavian Society on Periodontics, May 16-19, 1990:62.
28. Gibbs CH, Lee JG, Hirschfeld JW, Low SB, Magnusson I, Clark WB: Periodontal data collection using multiple foot switches. *J Dent Res* 1988;67:(Abstr. no. 1028)241.
29. Badersten A, Nilveus R, Egelberg J: Effect of nonsurgical periodontal therapy (VIII). Probing attachment changes related to clinical characteristics. *J Clin Periodontol* 1987; 14:425-432.
30. Armitage GC, Svanberg GK, Löe H: Microscopic evaluation of clinical measurements of connective tissue attachment levels. *J Clin Periodontol* 1977;4:173-190.
31. Magnusson I, Listgarten MA: Histological evaluation of probing depth following periodontal treatment. *J Clin Periodontol* 1980;7:26-31.
32. Polson AM, Caton JG, Yeaple RN, Zander HA: Histological determination of probe tip penetration into gingival sulcus of humans using an electronic pressure-sensitive probe. *J Clin Periodontol* 1980;7:479-488.
33. Jansen J, Pilot R, Corba N: Histologic evaluation of probe penetration during clinical assessment of periodontal attachment levels. An investigation of experimentally induced periodontal lesions in beagle dogs. *J Clin Periodontol* 1981;8:98-106.
34. Fowler C, Garrett S, Crigger M, Egelberg J: Histological probe position in treated and untreated human periodontal tissues. *J Clin Periodontol* 1982;9:373-385.
35. Hassell TM, Germann MA, Saxer UP: Periodontal probing: Interinvestigator discrepancies and correlations between probing force and recorded depth. *Helv Odontol Acta* 1973; 17:38-42.
36. Van der Velden U, de Vries JH: Introduction of a new periodontal probe: The pressure probe. *J Clin Periodontol* 1978;5:188-197.
37. Van der Velden U: Probing force and the relationship of the probe tip to the periodontal tissues. *J Clin Periodontol* 1979;6:106-114.
38. Badersten A, Nilvéus R, Egelberg J: Reproducibility of probing attachment level measurements. *J Clin Periodontol* 1984;11:475-485.
39. Parakkal PF: Proceedings of the workshop on quantitative evaluation of periodontal diseases by physical measurement techniques. *J Dent Res* 1979;58:547-553.
40. Gibbs CH, Hirschfeld JW, Lee JG, Low SB, Magnusson I, Thousand RR, Yerkin P, Clark WB: Description and clinical evaluation of a new computerized periodontal probe — The Florida Probe. *J Clin Periodontol* 1988; 15:137-144.
41. Magnusson I, Fuller WW, Heins PJ, Rau CF, Gibbs CH, Marks RG, Clark WB: Correlation between electronic and visual readings of pocket depth with a newly developed constant force probe. *J Clin Periodontol* 1988; 15:180-184.
42. Goodson JM, Kondon N: Periodontal pocket depth measurements by fiber optic technology. *J Clin Dent* 1988; 1:35-38.
43. Haffajee AD, Socransky SS, Goodson JM: Comparison of different data analysis for detecting changes in attachment level. *J Clin Periodontol* 1983;10:298-310.
44. Magnusson I, Clark WB, Marks RG, Biggs CH, Manouchehr-Pour M, Low SB: Attachment level measurements with a constant force electronic probe. *J Clin Periodontol* 1988;15:185-188.
45. Glavind L, Löe H: Errors in the clinical assessment of periodontal destruction. *J Periodont Res* 1967;9:180-184.

46. Löe H, Anerud A, Boysen H, Smith M: The natural history of periodontal disease in man. The rate of periodontal destruction before 40 years of age. *J Periodontol* 1978;49:607-620.

47. Goodson JM, Tanner ACR, Haffajee AD, Sornberger GC, Socransky SS: Patterns of progression and regression of advanced destructive periodontal disease. *J Clin Periodontol* 1982;9:472-481.

48. Jeffcoat MK, Jeffcoat RL, Jens SC, Captain K: A new periodontal probe with automated cemento-enamel junction detection. *J Clin Periodontol* 1986; 13:276-280.

49. Jeffcoat MK, Jeffcoat RL, Captain K, Reddy M, Williams RC: Attachment level probing with automated CEJ detection: Clinical trials. *J Dent Res* 1989;68:236.

50. Birek P, McCulloch CA, Hardy V: Gingival attachment level measurements with an automated periodontal probe. *J Clin Periodontol* 1987; 14:472-477.

51. Low SB, Taylor M, Marks RG, Gibbs C, Magnusson I, Clark WB: Measuring attachment level with an electronic disk probe. *J Dent Res* 1989;68:(Abstr. no. 1421) 359.

52. Osborn J, Stoltenberg J, Huso B, Aeppli D, Pihlstrom B: Comparison of measurement variability using a standard and constant force periodontal probe. *J Periodontol* 1990;61:497-503.

53. Watts TL: Probing site configuration in patients with untreated periodontitis. A study of horizontal positional error. *J Clin Periodontol* 1989;16:529-533.

54. Kung RT, Ochs B, Goodson JM: Temperature as a periodontal diagnostic. *J Clin Periodontol* 1990;17:557-563.

55. Brånemark P-I, Breine U, Adell R, Hansson BO, Lindstrom J, Olsson Å: Intraosseous anchorage of dental prostheses. I. Experimental studies. *Scand J Plast Reconstr Surg* 1969;3:81-100.

56. Brånemark P-I, Hansson BO, Adell R, Breine U, Lindstrom J, Hallen O, Ohman A: Osseointegrated implants in the treatment of the edentulous jaw. Experience from a 10-year period. *Scand J Plast Reconstr Surg* 1977;11:Suppl 16, pp 1-105. Also as a monograph from Almquist & Wiksell International, Stockholm.

57. Adell R, Lekholm U, Rockler B, Brånemark P-I: A 15-year study of osseointegrated implants in the treatment of the edentulous jaw. *Int J Oral Surg* 1981;10:387-416.

58. Albrektsson T, Dahl E, Ehnbom L, et al: Osseointegrated oral implants. A Swedish multicenter study of 8139 consecutively inserted Nobelpharma implants. *J Periodontol* 1988;59:287-296.

59. Ericsson I, Lekholm U, Brånemark P-I, Lindhe J, Glantz P-O: A clinical evaluation of fixed-bridge restorations supported by the combination of teeth and osseointegrated titanium implants. *J Clin Periodontol* 1986; 13:307-312.

60. Shulman LB: Surgical considerations in implant dentistry. *J Dent Educ* 1988;52:712-720.

61. American Dental Association Risk Management Series: *Diagnosing and Managing the Periodontal Patient.* Chicago: American Dental Association, 1986.

62. Cutress TW, Ainamo J, Sardo-Infirri J: The community periodontal index of treatment needs (CPITN) procedure for population groups and individuals. *Int Dent J* 1987;37:222-233.

63. Wilson TG: *Dental Maintenance for Patients with Periodontal Diseases.* Chicago: Quintessence Publ Co, Inc, 1989:18-21.

64. Wilson TG: Compliance. A review of the literature with possible applications to periodontics. *J Periodontol* 1987;58:706-714.

65. Listgarten MA, Mao R, Robinson PJ: Periodontal probing and the relationship of the probe tip to periodontal tissues. *J Periodontol* 1976;47:511-513.

66. Caton JG: Periodontal diagnosis and diagnostic aids. In: *Proceedings of the World Workshop in Clinical Periodontics.* Chicago: American Academy of Periodontology. 1989;I-1 to I-22.

67. Proye M, Caton J, Polson A: Initial healing of periodontal pockets after a single episode of root planing monitored by controlled probing forces. *J Periodontol* 1982;53:296-301.

68. Hugoson A: Gingival inflammation and female sex hormones. A clinical investigation of pregnant women and experimental studies in dogs. *J Periodont Res* 1970;5(Suppl):1-18.

69. O'Leary TJ, Drake RB, Naylor JE: The plaque control record. *J Periodontol* 1972;43:38.

70. Pihlstrom BL, Anderson KA, Aeppli D, Schaffer EM: Association between signs of trauma from occlusion and periodontitis. *J Periodontol* 1986; 57:1-6.

71. Ainamo J et al: Development of the World Health Organization Community Periodontal Index of Treatment Needs CPITN. *Int Dent J* 1982; 32:281-291.

The Role of Microbiology in Periodontal Therapy

CURRENT CONCEPTS by Kenneth S. Kornman / Michael G. Newman

CLINICAL APPLICATION by Thomas G. Wilson, Jr

CURRENT CONCEPTS	CLINICAL APPLICATION
Microbial testing	Recommendations for microbial analysis
Antibiotic susceptibility	Steps for successful microbial sampling
Practical uses of microbial information today	**QUICK REVIEW**
Microbial evaluations in private practice	**REFERENCES**
Local delivery of antimicrobials	

C U R R E N T   C O N C E P T S

In 1975, technological and conceptual advances allowed for the identification of an unusual collection of bacteria found in the subgingival plaque of patients with localized juvenile periodontitis.[1] During the 10 years that followed this revolutionary observation in LJP, numerous investigators from several laboratories* demonstrated that distinct subgingival microbiotas could be associated with different periodontal conditions (Table 2-1). The promise and hope of these exciting observations was that periodontitis could one day be diagnosed and treated like an infectious disease. Although it is strongly believed that the field will move in that direction, it has become clear in re-

*Much of this work was conducted in laboratories directed by Drs KS Kornman, MA Listgarten, WJ Loesche, WEC Moore, L Moore, MG Newman, SS Socransky, J Slots, ACR Tanner, and JJ Zambon.

TABLE 2-1 *Periodontal conditions associated with a distinct subgingival microbiota**

Gingival health
Gingivitis
Pregnancy gingivitis
Adult necrotizing ulcerative gingivitis
Prepubertal periodontitis
Localized juvenile periodontitis
Chronic adult periodontitis
HIV periodontitis
Diabetes-associated periodontitis

*Conditions are included only if comparable data are available from at least two laboratories.

cent years that the story is much more complicated than originally envisioned. The complexities of this approach should not deter practitioners and researchers from striving towards that promising goal, but these issues should strongly encourage a realistic view of the current situation. This chapter presents a short, practical

approach to microbial evaluations as a part of periodontal therapy. It is acknowledged that until very recently, efforts to study and treat periodontitis as if it were a simple bacterial infection have produced information that has oftentimes confused and frustrated practitioners. The guidelines contained in this chapter represent the best judgment of the authors at the time of publication, based on published data and clinical and laboratory experience. Many of the assumptions and much of the data relative to the role of specific bacteria in periodontal diseases have been recently reviewed[2] and will not be restated.

In order to effectively use microbial information in the treatment of periodontitis, it is important to understand some of the difficulties that have been routinely encountered in past attempts to treat periodontitis as a microbiologically simple infection.

The *first complicating factor* that has been realized in recent years is that periodontitis resembles complex chronic systemic diseases, such as cardiovascular disease and some of the viral diseases, rather than an acute single microorganism infectious disease such as streptococcal pharyngitis. In chronic systemic disease, although there are a few dominant etiologic factors that apply across the population, the appearance of diseases in a specific individual is influenced by multiple factors that must be viewed in the context of a specific patient. Accumulation of supragingival plaque appears to be one of the dominant factors that is related to periodontitis across the majority of the population. The relationship of certain specific bacteria to periodontitis appears at this time to be important to therapy in some groups of patients and less important, or even unimportant, in other patients. Our past attempts at finding one or two microorganisms that were dominant determinants of disease in all patients have been very frustrating.

The *second complicating factor* in attempting to treat periodontitis as a simple infection has been a lack of specific therapy that may be used selectively against specific bacteria in cases of periodontitis. Although practitioners often treat periodontitis with systemic antibiotics, there really are no antibiotics that are highly specific for selected segments of the subgingival microbiota. The use of antibiotics in many patients, therefore, is comparable to chemical scaling and root planing. Antibiotic susceptibility testing of subgingival plaque samples from patients with periodontitis invariably reveals that most, to all, of the microorganisms are susceptible to

penicillins and/or tetracyclines. There are of course exceptions to this finding, most prominently in patients who have been exposed repeatedly to tetracycline or multiple antibiotics. Metronidazole is the only antibiotic currently used in periodontal therapy that approaches specificity, because it selectively kills anaerobic bacteria. Although this would theoretically leave the facultative bacteria, it has been known for many years that metronidazole will also inhibit facultative bacteria very successfully if they are living in an anaerobic environment. The lack of truly selective therapies limits our ability to specifically target treatment based on specific microbial findings.

The *third complicating factor* is that periodontitis does not behave like a classic infection. Periodontitis, contrary to simple infections such as streptococcal pharyngitis, is associated with several microorganisms that have pathogenic potential. Because of host and environmental conditions, these microorganisms may inhabit the periodontal area for long periods of time prior to detectable disease initiation. In some patients certain bacteria such as *Actinobacillus actinomycetemcomitans* may behave more like classic pathogens, but in most individuals pathogenic microorganisms such as *Prevotella intermedia (Bacteroides intermedius*)* appear to require other factors in order to initiate disease. Much work is currently in progress on the microbial conditions and genetic differences between patients, as well as the genetic differences between strains of bacteria, that may

*The oral *Bacteroides* species are in the process of being reclassified because they are genetically different from some of the intestinal *Bacteroides*. *Bacteroides gingivalis* is now named *Porphyromonas gingivalis* and *Bacteroides intermedius* is now *Prevotella intermedia*. Other oral *Bacteroides* species will also be renamed.

contribute to the apparent pathogenicity that is observed in our patients.

In spite of the above complications, it is reasonable, based on current knowledge, to establish practical uses for microbiology in the therapy of patients with periodontitis. At this time current knowledge suggests that microbial information may be reasonably used in the following situations:

1. **As a risk factor.** Although the presence of *Porphyromonas gingivalis (Bacteroides gingivalis)* does not reliably predict disease initiation or progression, its presence does substantially increase the likelihood of future problems.[3] This of course should be viewed in the context of each specific site in each patient. In an adult patient who smokes and has clinical signs of plaque and calculus, the presence of *P. gingivalis* represents one additional risk factor for disease. Proper use of risk assessment in adult periodontitis patients can be a strong tool for modifying patient behavior and for focusing therapy on those individuals at greater risk.

2. **To monitor treatment.** Although the situation for an individual patient is complicated for the reasons described above, in general the elimination of *A. actinomycetemcomitans, P. gingivalis,* and *P. intermedia* are an indication that clinical improvement has or will occur following therapy.

3. **To target therapy.** The overchriding concept of infectious disease management is that knowledge of the specific microbial agent involved will guide selection of treatment and result in a better therapeutic outcome. The ultimate goal for using microbial information in periodontal therapy is to more effectively select

therapy to achieve a more predictable outcome. The complexities noted above for the disease, in particular the lack of specific therapies, have complicated our understanding and use of microbiology to target treatment. This should nevertheless continue to be our ultimate goal if we are to truly justify the acquisition of microbiological information.

MICROBIAL TESTING

In order to use information effectively in periodontal therapy, it is of course essential that the information be accurate and reliable. At present, limited options are available for microbial testing of subgingival plaque. The traditional method is to culture the viable bacteria in the sample. Culture of anaerobic bacteria is now a routine procedure in most medical microbiology laboratories. The most common periodontal pathogens, with the exceptions of *Bacteroides forsythus* and spirochetes, may be grown using conventional anaerobic techniques. Although most medical microbiology laboratories routinely grow these microorganisms, many of the commercially available identification techniques will result in a misidentification of many of the oral anaerobes. It is therefore advisable for the laboratory to have experience with oral anaerobes and their characterization. The optimal choice for culturing is a local laboratory experienced with oral microbial samples. If this is not available, a few national testing services routinely process periodontal samples. Transport of live samples always results in a substantial loss of anaerobes. Although this usually does not produce a qualitative change in the results with samples that have a large number of bacteria, such as samples from pretreatment sites, samples taken after therapy will tend to have relatively few microorganisms. A loss of viability in these samples may dramatically change the results, producing samples that are reported as negative but may actually have had pathogens present.

The other microbial testing service available at present uses DNA probe technology and has been made commercially available (Biotechnica, Boston). DNA probe analysis is inherently more sensitive than culturing and if properly carried out should produce consistently more reliable results than culture for transported samples. Comparisons of DNA probe results to culture by experienced oral anaerobe laboratories have demonstrated great reliability for the system. A major limitation of DNA probe technology may in fact be its exceptional ability to detect very low levels of pathogens, a technical capability referred to as *sensitivity*. Most previous associations between microbial findings and clinical results have involved cultural microbiology studies in which low levels of pathogens were probably not detected. DNA probe analysis may therefore give positive readings in situations in which the level of pathogen is actually too low to be clinically relevant. Current studies are attempting to resolve this dilemma, but at present the great sensitivity of DNA probes may actually complicate interpretation of the laboratory results.

New systems using nucleic acid probes, such as DNA probes, or antibody probes for specific microorganisms, are currently being tested and evaluated for their ability to provide clinically relevant information when used in a private practice environment. Although the technology is outstanding and very promising, its actual relevance to patient therapy is not yet clear.

ANTIBIOTIC SUSCEPTIBILITY

One of the major reasons for performing microbial evaluations with periodontal patients may be to select appropriate antibiotics. This can currently best be accomplished by culturing the bacteria and testing antibiotic susceptibility. This procedure with anaerobes, especially from samples with many different bacterial species, is both expensive and complicated to interpret. Although most subgingival bacteria will be susceptible to penicillin and tetracycline derivatives, this does not necessarily mean that those are the most effective agents for therapy. Clinical use of specific antibiotics often produces results that are not predicted based purely on in vitro susceptibility testing. Susceptibility testing is, however, effective and essential to selection of therapy in patients who may show antibiotic resistance or evidence of refractory disease.

If a patient has had multiple exposures to tetracycline derivatives or exposure to multiple antibiotics within the past 2 years, antibiotic resistance may present a problem during therapy. These patients should be evaluated for antibiotic susceptibility by means of culture and susceptibility studies.

PRACTICAL USES OF MICROBIAL INFORMATION TODAY

Suggestions for treatment have been derived from the literature, consultation with experienced practitioners, and from unpublished laboratory and clinical experience of the authors. Each dentist is, of course, ultimately and singly responsible for evaluating and selecting therapy for a patient based on the unique factors observed in each individual case. Our current recommendation for use of microbial tests is limited to situations in which the information appears to substantially improve results over the use of clinical information alone. The incorporation of this information into practice is closely linked to the diagnostic scheme described in chapter 5 and reviewed below.

1. If the initial clinical evaluation of a patient with no complicating systemic factors results in a presumptive diagnosis of **chronic adult periodontitis,** there does not currently appear to be an indication for the use of microbial tests.

2. If the initial clinical examination produces a presumptive diagnosis of one of the other forms of periodontitis, microbial tests appear to offer benefits in selecting therapy and / or in monitoring treatment as follows:

   a) If the presumptive diagnosis is **localized juvenile periodontitis:** treatment response appears to differ depending upon whether *A. actinomycetemcomitans* is found with or without *P. gingivalis* or *P. intermedia.* Successful treatment is indicated by both a favorable clinical response and a failure to detect *A. actinomycetemcomitans* 4 to 6 weeks after completing systemic antibiotics.

      i. *A. actinomycetemcomitans* **without** *P. gingivalis* or *P. intermedia:* treat with systemic tetracyclines, scaling and root planing, and rinses with chlorhexidine. See chapter 8 for details.

      ii. *A. actinomycetemcomitans* **with** either *P. gingivalis* or *P. intermedia:* systemic tetracycline, periodontal surgery, and rinses with chlorhexidine.

   b) If the presumptive diagnosis is **prepubertal periodontitis:** due to side effects with various antibiotics in children of this age, chemical therapy is generally limited to penicillin derivatives such as amoxicillin or Augmentin. Microbial tests on these children generally reveal *A. actinomycetemcomitans, Capnocytophaga sputigena,* or *P. intermedia.* Treatment with systemic penicillin derivatives plus scaling and root planing and plaque control, including chlorhexidine rinses, should be continued until the above suspected pathogens are eliminated.

   c) If the presumptive diagnosis is **rapidly progressive periodontitis:** a variety of microorganisms may be found in such cases, but generally one or more of the following suspected pathogens are found: *A. actinomycetemcomitans, B. forsythus, Eikenella corrodens, P. gingivalis, P. intermedia, Wolinella recta.* Patients who have a history of rapidly progressive periodontitis and a history of multiple antibiotic exposure, especially to tetracycline derivatives, should be evaluated for other pathogens, including some of the intestinal pathogens. Patients with rapidly progres-

sive periodontitis have been treated successfully using both tetracycline derivatives and the combination of amoxicillin plus metronidazole with chlorhexidine rinses. Our experience with both of these approaches has produced variable results (see chapter 6 for the management of these cases). Treatment success requires evidence of not only clinical improvement but of the elimination of suspected pathogens. Our experience with some of these patients suggests that elimination of the pathogens identified initially may be accompanied by reemergence of a new pathogen and continued disease progression. These patients must be monitored closely, and strong consideration should be given to the possibility of antibiotic resistance.

3. All patients sampled initially should be reassessed at the clinical reevaluation following initial therapy and again every 3 to 6 months during supportive periodontal therapy (SPT).

4. As discussed in chapter 5, some patients initially given a presumptive diagnosis of chronic adult periodontitis do not respond predictably to initial periodontal therapy. For these "refractory" patients, microbial samples should be taken at the clinical reevaluation following initial therapy and antibiotics should be selected as if the patient had rapidly progressive periodontitis.

5. During the SPT phase of therapy the prognosis of some patients will be identified as being unstable or questionable (see chapter 5 for more complete discussion of these

cases). Such patients may be classified as having refractory periodontitis, and questionable sites should be sampled microbiologically. Systemic or local antimicrobial therapy should be targeted as with rapidly progressive periodontitis.

6. As indicated above, for all patients treated with systemic antibiotics, chlorhexidine rinses twice daily and good plaque control appear to be essential for both good clinical and good microbial outcomes. The chlorhexidine therapy is continued for a full 4 to 6 weeks from the initiation of systemic or local antimicrobial therapy.

7. Local delivery of antibiotics may represent an alternative or additional therapy in selected patients (see below).

MICROBIAL EVALUATIONS IN PRIVATE PRACTICE

For a 3-year time period we have evaluated the role of microbial information in the therapy of patients in private periodontal offices throughout the United States. Clinical and microbial information was collected from patients with refractory and rapidly progressive periodontitis from 21 private practices. Microbial samples were collected and transported to experienced oral microbiology laboratories for evaluation. The details of the first patients have been reported.[4] Although the data are still in an early stage of evaluation, the following conclusions appear to be valid and reasonable:

1. Clinical and microbial information can be used to describe distinct patterns of disease among adult periodontitis patients.
2. These distinctions were not evident when patients were analyzed by microbial findings alone or clinical findings alone.
3. The different patterns of disease appear to respond differently to periodontal therapy.

These studies suggest that given a more comprehensive evaluation of patients incorporating microbial and clinical findings, we have the potential to provide a true infectious diseases approach to periodontitis in which specific disease patterns are treated differently for more predictable outcomes. Many of the suggestions outlined in this chapter are based on observations from this ongoing evaluation.

LOCAL DELIVERY OF ANTIMICROBIALS

The availability of local delivery devices for sustained release of antimicrobial agents may dramatically change therapy for some patients and may dramatically alter our recommendations for microbial analyses, especially in patients with chronic adult and refractory periodontitis. In a private practice environment, local delivery of tetracycline (Actisite) in periodontal maintenance patients with individual sites nonresponsive to local conventional therapy was significantly and clinically more effective than scaling and root planing alone for up to 6 months after therapy. Most important perhaps is that this therapeutic approach had a selective benefit in reducing *P. gingivalis*. For as yet unexplained reasons, it was less effective in the reduction of *P. intermedia* or *A. actinomycetemcomitans*. These findings again demonstrate that results with patients in a clinical setting may differ dramatically from what one expects based on laboratory susceptibility of microorganisms to a specific antibiotic. The extremely powerful and selective effect of this local delivery device against *P. gingivalis* and the relationship of elimination of that microorganism to good clinical outcomes suggest that microbial testing may assist in the selection of sites for the optimal use of this local delivery device.

CLINICAL APPLICATION

Advances in diagnosis and microbial analysis have had a profound impact on periodontal therapy. Until recently, many of the diseases now recognized were not named or categorized, thus limiting successful approaches to treatment. This section covers the tests currently used in the author's practice and provides information on when and where these approaches are used. In addition, specific material on how to use these tests for greatest effect is presented. Our knowledge is changing rapidly; therefore, the reader is advised to keep abreast of current trends as well as the specific applications of microbial analysis. An intimate knowledge of the literature is helpful to remain current.

RECOMMENDATIONS FOR MICROBIAL ANALYSIS

Microbial analysis is recommended for those cases that defy traditional approaches, or those that fall outside the parameters of disease seen in the majority of periodontal patients. In this book, periodontal problems have been divided into two broad categories: all types of gingivitis are grouped with chronic adult periodontitis in the first group, while other, more aggressive forms of periodontitis fall into the second group. This second group benefits mostly from microbial analysis.

At present there are two timeframes that seem appropriate for microbial analysis: (1) during the initial diagnosis for patients with aggressive periodontitis lesions, and (2) following completion of traditional forms of periodontal therapy for those patients who now fall into the category of refractory periodontitis. After a diagnosis of an aggressive type of periodontitis or refractory periodontitis is made, microbial analysis is suggested. At present there are two ways to determine bacterial populations: by culturing live microbes and by analyzing DNA strands (see page 32). Culturing live bacteria combined with antibiotic susceptibility testing is currently the preferred method. This approach is considered superior because it allows the clinician to identify specific bacterial strains and also to determine which antibiotics will be most successful in combating the microbes identified.

STEPS FOR SUCCESSFUL MICROBIAL SAMPLING

Successful sampling involves several specific steps. First, the area to be sampled is isolated with cotton rolls, then any visible supragingival plaque is removed with a sterile instrument. Next, a sample of the subgingival flora is taken with a second sterile instrument (a curet specific for the site is suggested), and carried to a container of transport medium. Care should be taken to ensure that the transport medium has not passed the time when it will successfully sustain the bacteria (further information can be found in chapter 1). Many laboratories incorporate an indicator that changes colors when the medium has expired. The clinician should ensure that the transfer from the periodontal pocket to the transport medium is done in a manner to reduce or eliminate exposure to air and the possibility of contaminating the sample. When small amounts of plaque are present, the placement of three sterile paper points (10 seconds each) can often gather more bacteria than the curet. Same day or overnight transfer to the laboratory is the next critical step. It is best to sample late in the day if overnight transfer is necessary. For those occasional times when morning sampling is needed, refrigeration (not freezing) prior to transfer is suggested (Figs 2-1a to d).

Laboratories often take several weeks to return results. This fact should be taken into consideration when scheduling the patient for therapy.

Proper site selection is important since only a few sites (usually two) are sampled per patient. A typical site would be the pocket deemed most active by the clinician. Sites are selected in the following order of importance:

1. Sites that have recent loss of attachment
2. Sites that have suppuration
3. Sites with the deepest pocket probing depth
4. Sites that bleed upon probing
5. Sites that have gingival color changes suggesting underlying inflammation

Once the results are returned from the laboratory, the patient is scheduled for thorough subgingival scaling and root planing, either closed or open. Although no hard and fast rules exist at present, clinical experience has shown that for patients who have not had root planing for some time, an average

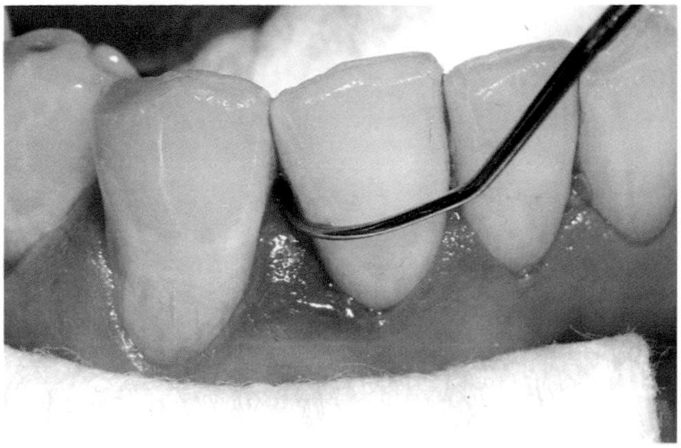

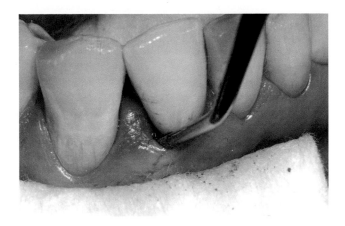

Fig 2-1a   The area to be sampled is isolated with cotton rolls and any supragingival plaque is removed with a sterile instrument.

Fig 2-1b   A second sterile instrument (a curet) is taken to the depth of the pocket, then drawn coronally to remove the bacterial sample.

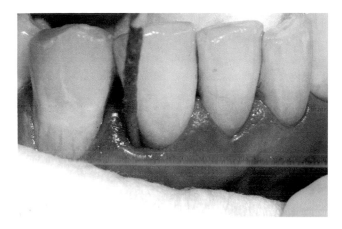

Fig 2-1c   In areas where little bacterial material can be produced with a curet, sterile paper points are used. Three separate points placed in the pocket for 10 seconds each are recommended.

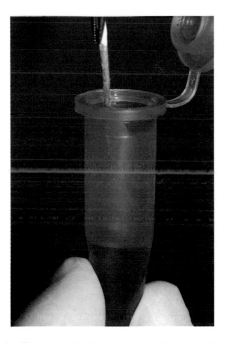

Fig 2-1d   The sample is placed in the transfer medium for delivery to the laboratory.

of over 10 minutes per tooth is required to produce the desired clinical result. (Such experience is based on treatment by an experienced periodontist; other practitioners with less experience may take considerably longer.) In instances where the patient has been in an ongoing program of supportive periodontal treatment (SPT), the time needed to provide a biologically acceptable root surface may be reduced.

Prior to scaling and root planing, the appropriate antibiotic(s) is (are) administered. Twice daily rinses with chlorhexidine are started within 24 hours following therapy. The antibiotics are continued for 10 to 21 days, depending on the antibiotic, and the mouthrinses for 1 month. Microbial sampling is repeated periodically during SPT.

This form of combined treatment has provided significant clinical improvement in the vast majority of cases of aggressive periodontitis. This includes some cases where previously extreme efforts on the part of the patient and the clinician had provided unsatisfactory results. It is puzzling and a bit disquieting that when repeat samples of clinically successful cases are performed, traces of the bacteria initially thought to be responsible for the tissue breakdown are sometimes still present. It is hoped that ongoing studies will bring further knowledge about this group of patients.

QUICK REVIEW

- This chapter describes general principles and limitations of the use of microbial testing in periodontal therapy in private practices.
- Although some of these limitations are great and our understanding is currently limited, there appear to be some important uses of this technology in private practice today.
- In spite of the complications, the current data are sufficiently strong to indicate that this approach has a high probability of providing important information to patient therapy.
- Our current challenge is to properly use this information and technology to better deliver care to our patients.

REFERENCES

1. Newman MG, Socransky SS, Savitt ED, Propas DA, Crawford A: Studies of the microbiology of periodontosis. *J Periodontol* 1976;47:373-379.
2. Socransky SS, Haffajee AD: Microbiological risk factors for destructive periodontal diseases. In: Bader JD, ed. *Risk Assessment in Dentistry.* Chapel Hill, NC: University of North Carolina Dental Ecology, 1990.
3. Beck JD, Koch GG, Rozier RG, Tudor GE: Prevalence and risk indicators for periodontal attachment loss in a population of older community-dwelling blacks and whites. *J Periodontol* 1990;61:521-528.
4. Kornman KS, Newman MG, Alvarado R, Flemmig TF, Nachnani S, Tumbusch J: Clinical and microbiological patterns of patients with adult and refractory periodontitis. I. Clinical. *J Periodontol* 1991 (in press).

Imaging Techniques for the Periodontium

by Marjorie Jeffcoat

INTRODUCTION TO DIAGNOSTIC IMAGING

At present, clinicians rely on a limited number of major tools for the diagnosis of periodontal disease; these include the patient history, visual inspection, periodontal probing, and radiographic examination (see chapter 1). The proper use and interpretation of these readily available diagnostic modalities requires a clear understanding of their respective limitations and capabilities. This principle becomes even more important for the prescription and interpretation of more advanced imaging methods such as digital radiology, computed tomography, magnetic resonance imaging, and nuclear medicine techniques. This chapter presents the range of imaging techniques that have potential use for the diagnosis of periodontal diseases. The underlying principles, advantages, and limitations of each imaging method are discussed in relation to their clinical utility.

PRESCRIPTION OF THE IMAGING EXAMINATION

The use of diagnostic imaging in making diagnoses presents new opportunities and challenges for the dentist. However, it must be stressed that an image never makes a diagnosis, the dentist does. The image simply provides information regarding the calcified tissues, soft tissues, or their metabolism that is not accessible to the unaided human eye. Only clinical correlation among the history, clinical signs, laboratory tests, and the results of the imaging examination(s) will result in a well-considered, accurate diagnosis.

The availability of more than one imaging modality places new responsibilities on the dentist. All imaging examinations are prescription items. They should never be prescribed by rote or by policy; rather, a careful assessment of the patient, including an examination by the responsible practitioner, should be performed before such tests are ordered.

In order to select an examination, the clinician must first define the question to be answered. Common questions include: (1) has bone loss progressed since the last examination; (2) is the disc displaced in a patient with temporomandibular joint pain; and (3) is there sufficient space above the mandibular canal to place a root form implant? The choice of an imaging modality is strikingly different for each of these questions. Also, it is difficult or impossible to answer these questions on the basis of clinical observation alone. At all times, clinicians should be guided by the principle of using the least invasive test with the lowest risk that is likely to answer the question.

TRANSMISSION RADIOGRAPHY

Transmission radiographs, including periapical and bite-wing films, are currently the mainstay of radiographic imaging for dental diagnosis. Modern equipment and film have greatly reduced the radiation exposure associated with dental radiographs. However, the selection of radiographic projections, number of films, speed of film, and settings on the x-ray source are all under the control of the practitioner. Proper selection will increase the likelihood of obtaining the required diagnostic information while limiting the risk to the patient due to radiation exposure.

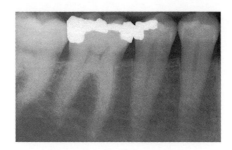 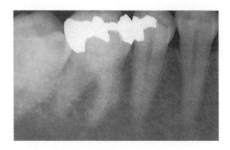

Fig 3-1a (above left) *Well-angulated periapical film. Note the height of the alveolar crest and the location of the cusp tips at approximately the same level.*

Fig 3-1b (above right) *Poorly angulated periapical film of the same tooth shown in Fig 3-1a. Note the cusp tips appear at different heights and bone appears above the cementoenamel junction.*

Selecting the Radiographic Projection

Various radiographic projections have been designed to increase the likelihood of obtaining different types of information.[1] Clearly, although radiographs are prescription items, it is incumbent on the practitioner to make the most of the diagnostic potential of any radiographic view. Transmission radiographs are limited by their very nature. They are two-dimensional representations of the three-dimensional alveolar bone, tooth, and soft tissue. This two-dimensional mapping is highly susceptible to angulation error induced when the dental technician positions the films and the x-ray tube head to expose the film.

The periapical view has been designed to minimize distortion of the bone-to-root relationship while imaging the root apex (Fig 3-1a). This view is most important when the dentist is attempting to answer questions about the root apex, or when bone loss is extremely severe. Traditional periapical films are susceptible to operator error, especially in the maxillary molar region. The resultant film may therefore show a distorted bone-tooth relationship, which manifests as foreshortening or elongation (Fig 3-1b). Clearly,

this kind of distortion makes it difficult to assess bone height along the tooth root. The dentist may assess the quality of the periapical film by examining the cusp tips of the posterior teeth. Buccal and lingual cusp tips should be imaged at approximately the same level. When cusp tips appear at different levels, the film probably was misangulated, which will also distort the apparent location of the bone height along the root surface. It is this misangulation that results in the radiographic phenomenon of "growing or losing bone" for the patient.

Techniques are readily available to minimize this source of distortion in the dental office. First, a long cone should always be used: the relatively parallel rays will minimize distortion of the image that would be caused by a divergence of the beam between the bone and teeth and the film. Second, the use of paralleling positioning devices helps the technician to standardize the relationship between film, object, and x-ray source. Such devices reduce operator error and can aid in reducing radiation exposure by minimizing retakes due to mis-

angulation. Furthermore, the usefulness of the image for diagnosis may be improved because the dentist is more sure of the validity of the relationship between the bone and the tooth root.

Other views are also useful for periodontal diagnosis. In fact, the bite-wing is often the forgotten radiograph in periodontal diagnosis. Bite-wing radiographs are taken with the x-ray beam perpendicular to the bone and the tooth root, thus there is minimal distortion of the location of the bone height along the tooth root.[2] A disadvantage of the conventional bite-wing film is that a limited view of the osseous crest is available, so even moderate bone loss due to periodontitis may preclude its usefulness as a diagnostic image. More recently, vertical bite-wing films have been taken with the long axis of the film placed vertically in the mouth in either anterior or posterior sites. The resultant film (Fig 3-1c) shows considerably more bone and can be used to assess bone height in patients with moderate to severe bone loss. Radiation dose is reduced because several maxillary and mandibular teeth are viewed

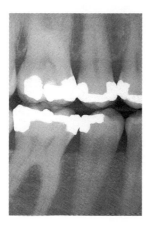

Fig 3-1c *Vertical bite-wing view of the same tooth. The alveolar crest is readily visible for both maxillary and mandibular teeth. Because the x-rays are perpendicular to the crest, bone height is accurately represented.*

in one image. The bone height is generally imaged very accurately along the root surface due to the ease of directing the x-ray beam perpendicular to the tooth either by eye or using a specially designed vertical bite-wing positioning device. Of course, the bite-wing film, either horizontal or vertical, does not image the root apex. The dentist must judge whether it is in the best interest of the patient to do so.

Other radiographic views should always be considered when other questions need to be answered. For example, the Water's view is suitable for imaging the sinuses, and the panoramic radiograph (although not a transmission radiograph in the usual sense) is useful for gaining a global view, including, for example, the location of impacted third molars. Note, however, that panoramic radiography does not provide sufficient detail concerning bone height to permit a comprehensive diagnosis using the imaging modality alone.

Selecting Film Type and X-Ray Setting

Film type and settings of the x-ray machine should not be selected by rote either.[3] All of these, like the selection of the projection, should focus on the question to be answered. Dental film for intraoral use is presently available in two speeds: Ultraspeed (D), and Ektaspeed (E). These two film speeds have replaced slower films available in the past. Essentially, the difference between the two films is the grain size in the emulsion. The larger the grain size, the less detail in the image but the faster the exposure. Therefore, D speed film provides somewhat more detail, on a microscopic level, but does so by using twice the radiation dose of E speed films. Most studies comparing the ability of dentists to diagnose lesions using D or E speed film have failed to show any difference in the diagnostic efficacy of the two films in conventional dental practice.[4]

In the future, all radiographic examinations may not even rely on film. Manufacturers are beginning to develop and market direct digital imaging systems. This means the x-rays strike an intraoral electronic imaging device similar to a miniaturized video camera. The radiographic image is displayed on a monitor and may be printed using a specially adapted printer. Major advantages of this technique include the elimination of film processing and the reduction of the radiation dose relative to conventional radiographs taken with film.

X-ray machine settings are also important because they influence the image quality and radiation dose. Dental radiographs are generally taken at either low kVp (65 to 70 kVp) or high kVp (90 kVp). The kilovoltage of the x-ray beam is related to the energy of the beam. In practical terms, this means that lower kilovoltage x-rays are more likely to be absorbed in the tissues, resulting in a radiographic image with a dark background and high contrast. These films are especially useful to the dentist who is trying to answer questions that need a high-contrast image, for example when trying to determine if the file is at the apex in a root canal treatment procedure. Higher kVp x-rays, on the other hand, are less likely to be absorbed in the tissues; the result is less radiation dose to the patient and a lower-contrast image that shows more shades of gray. Such a radiograph would be most useful when trying to answer a question such as whether there is a small change in the crestal bone in a periodontitis patient.

Detecting Osseous Changes Between Radiographic Examinations

All radiographic methods simply image the existing anatomy of the teeth and supporting tissue. Radiographs do not indicate the rate or presence of active bone or attachment loss, nor do they indicate whether past episodes of destruction and healing have occurred. To do so, the clinician must compare two or more carefully exposed radiographs taken at different examinations.

Most assessment of bone loss in clinical practice today is achieved by visual comparison of the radiographs. The radiograph contains so much information that it is difficult for the human eye to detect small changes in bone support in the presence of a busy background containing the teeth and cortical and trabecular bone. Studies have shown that a 30% to 50% change in bone mineral is needed to be visible even to the experienced clinician using interpretative radiography.

Several methods have been developed to allow measurement of bone height on serial radiographs. The simplest method involves measuring the distance from the CEJ to the alveolar crest.[2] Of course, this method is limited both by the geometry of the film and the ability of the clinician to detect the alveolar crest. Methods have been developed that, in part, correct for errors in angulation.[5,6] Bone loss may be expressed as a percentage of the root length to partially correct for errors due to foreshortening or elongation. This method, like the direct measurement method, is also limited by the ability of the clinician to accurately detect the alveolar crest. Nonetheless, such methods have substantial sensitivity in experienced hands. Changes in bone height as small as 0.1 mm may be detected.

Techniques have been developed that enhance our ability to "see" small changes over time in the bone. These include digital subtraction radiography[7-10] and computer-assisted densitometric image analysis methodology (often abbreviated as CADIA).[11] Digital radiography is especially useful in detecting small changes in hard tissues that occur between examinations. In brief, the purpose of digital subtraction radiography is to subtract all unchanging structures from a set of two films displaying only the area of change. In practical terms, for periodontal defects this will mean subtraction of the teeth, cortical bone, and trabecular pattern, leaving only the bone gain or loss standing out against a neutral gray background.

The technique first involves simplifying the information in the radiograph to a form that can be understood by a computer. The computer will then analyze and display the information; this process is called digitization. Essentially, the digitization process converts the analog (nearly continuous gray level information), contained in the transmission radiograph, to discrete numbers that are proportional to the brightness of the radiograph at a particular location.

In order to digitize a radiograph, a "picture" is usually taken of the radiograph using a sensitive black and white video camera. The computer's digitizer automatically superimposes a grid over the radiograph and converts the gray level of the radiograph within each box of the grid to a number from zero (black) to 255 (white). The fineness of the grid will determine the spatial resolution of the digitized image. Generally, at least a 512 by 480 picture element (pixel) grid is used. It is very important to realize that the digitization process per se does not increase the information content of the transmission radiograph. On the contrary, information content is decreased, but it is put into a form that a computer can use so as to aid the dentist in detecting changes in bone not visible to the unaided eye.

An example of the utility of subtraction radiography in enhancing the appearance of radiographic changes is schematically represented in Fig 3-2. Careful examination reveals that there is a difference between panel A and panel B; a square has been added to panel B. In panel C, all structures present in panel A have been subtracted from panel B, leaving only the area of change (the square) against a neutral gray background. In actual use, the computer subtracts the gray value at each picture element location of the first radiograph from the second radiograph. Wherever no change occurs, the subtraction results in zero. In digital subtraction radiography, the image after subtraction is usually offset to obtain a gray background and to ease the eye. By convention, areas of bone gain are shown as light and areas of bone loss are shown as dark. In computer-aided densitometric image analysis, the images are not always displayed but the numeric values after subtraction in areas of interest are analyzed to detect osseous changes. Figure 3-3 is a clinical example of digital subtraction radiography. The dark areas (highlighted by arrows) indicate bone loss that was not perceptible on the original radiographs.

Use of subtraction radiography or CADIA presupposes that the radiographs are taken with similar contrast, density, and angulation. Thus, exquisite attention to detail is critical when exposing radiographs for use in digital radiographic techniques. Fortunately, the computer can aid in the correction of errors. Computer algorithms have been developed that can correct for variations in radiograph image density[12] and contrast (Fig 3-4). Standardization of

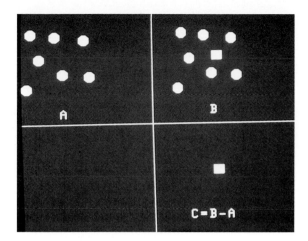

Fig 3-2 *Schematic representation of digital subtraction radiology. Panels A and B represent two radiographs taken at different examinations. All features that have not changed (ie, the hexagons) are subtracted, resulting in a subtraction image (panel C), displaying only the area of change (ie, the square) against a neutral gray background.*

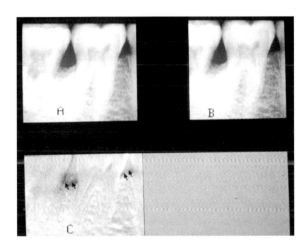

Fig 3-3 *Subtraction radiography. (A) Radiograph taken at visit one. (B) Radiograph taken at visit two. It is difficult to determine if bone loss has occurred. The subtraction image (C) shows clear dark areas (arrows), which indicate interproximal crestal and subcrestal bone loss.*

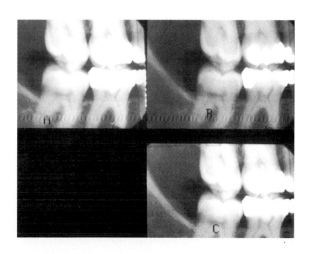

Fig 3-4 *Correction of image contrast and density. A and B, two radiographs of the same teeth, show different contrast and density. Computer software takes the information in B and displays it with the brightness and contrast of the radiograph in A. The image in panel C is the result of this process.*

image geometry may be achieved using a stent[8] to stabilize the relationship between the teeth, film, and x-ray source. Alternatively, the relationship between the x-ray source and the teeth may be stabilized using a cephalostat[9] and the computer can be used to correct image distortion caused by film placement.[6] An example of computer correction of image distortion due to film placement is seen in Fig 3-5.

Subtraction radiography is most useful in determining whether bone has been lost or gained between periodontal examinations or whether the bone around dental implants is stable. Color coding the subtraction images improves the ability of the novice clinician to detect bone loss or gain.[13] In the color images, bone gain appears as shades of green and bone loss as shades of red. Figures 3-6 and 3-7 show examples of color subtraction images. Furthermore, the location of bony change may be more readily visualized by superimposing the area of change on the original radiograph (Fig 3-8). This technique can be important because the teeth are nearly invisible in the ideal subtraction image. The clinician often needs to find out where the bone has been lost.

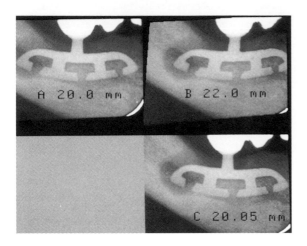

Fig 3-5 *Correction of planar angulation errors. A and B are two radiographs of the same area taken with different planar angulation. Note the difference in the length of the implants. Computer software takes the information in B and displays it with the geometry of the radiograph in A. The image in panel C is the result.*

The usefulness of subtraction radiology as a research tool can be extended by incorporating a reference wedge in the original radiographic image. Software presently under development will allow quantification of actual milligrams of bone loss or gain.

Digital subtraction radiology is presently in use in several clinical centers. This technique has been shown to be valuable in assessing the natural history of periodontal disease as well as in determining the efficacy of proposed new treatment modalities.

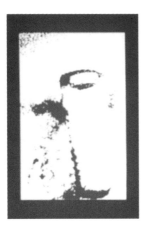

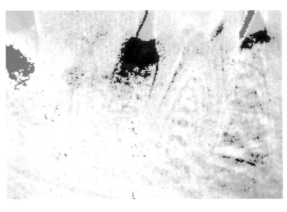

Fig 3-6 *Color-coded subtraction radiograph showing bone loss around a failing implant. Bone loss into the threads of the implant is shown in red.*

Fig 3-7 *Color-coded subtraction radiograph simultaneously showing bone gain (green) in the region of a demineralized bone graft and bone loss (red) in other interproximal regions.*

COMPUTED TOMOGRAPHY

Computed tomography (CT) is a specialized radiographic technique that allows visualization of planes or slices of interest.[14] Unlike conventional tomography, which blurs all structures not in the plane of interest, computed tomography actually removes the structures not in the plane of interest, resulting in an image with a clear visualization of the slice through the organ(s) under study.

To accomplish this, multiple exposures are taken using known geometry around the area of interest. Specialized hardware, known as the CT scanner, is used to accomplish this. Software is then used to reconstruct each plane or slice of interest. The quality of the image depends on hardware, software, and technical factors. It is important that the hardware and software be capable of producing an image with sufficient resolution to answer the clinician's question. Since CT equipment is expensive and the procedure carries a relatively high radiation burden for the patient, its use should be reserved for questions that cannot be an-

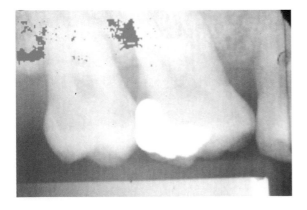

Fig 3-8 *Color-coded subtraction radiograph superimposed on the original radiograph. Note the bone gain (green) in the base of the defect.*

swered via clinical examination and/or conventional transmission radiography. For example, CT would be appropriate when determining how much space is available above the mandibular canal to receive a dental implant[15,16] or whether there is a space-occupying lesion in the maxillofacial region.[17]

The specific use of CT images is covered in chapter 20. Interpretation of images does, however, require some understanding of the potential sources of error.[14] Image artifacts may be caused by patient movement during multiple exposures, volume averaging effects, beam hardening effects, and high-density effects. Two of these are especially important to oral and maxillofacial CT imaging. High density restorative materials such as gold or titanium implants will virtually stop the x-rays and limit the ability of the CT software to accurately reconstruct the image. Volume averaging errors can result in a CT image that does not "look like" the original. This error occurs because the CT image is made up of multiple volume elements (voxels). The length, width, and depth of the elements depend on the hardware and software, but each voxel will have only a single gray level assigned to it. The error that can be induced by this is shown in Fig 3-9. A dental implant occupies only a small portion of a volume element. However, when the CT software calculates the gray level of that voxel, the entire voxel will be influenced by the presence of the implant in a portion of the volume element. The result is an image with an implant that is longer than its actual size.

It is very important that the dentist work closely with an expert CT radiologist. The question to be answered by the CT scan must be clearly posed so that the radiolo-gist can select the resolution appropriate to the task. Also, the radiologist can elect to use specialized software best suited to dental applications, such as that designed to account for the curvature of the mandible so that the slices are perpendicular to the mandible (Fig 3-10). This is most important when applying CT to preimplant diagnostics. Further image processing can result not only in the display of slices through the mandible but in a three-dimensional display of the maxilla or mandible (Fig 3-11) (for further information see chapter 20).

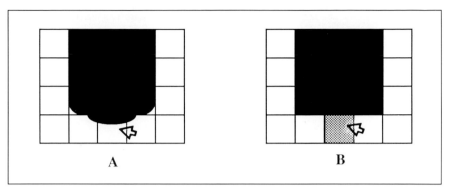

Fig 3-9 Schematic representation of volume-averaging error in CT. For simplicity, a dental implant is shown in two dimensions. Each box within the grid represents a volume element. The voxel denoted by the arrow is partially occupied by the implant. Since the CT scanner assigns a single gray value to each volume element, the gray level of the entire voxel in the scanned image will reflect the presence of the implant in a portion of its volume. Thus the implant represented in panel A will appear to have a different size and shape on the CT scan as represented in panel B.

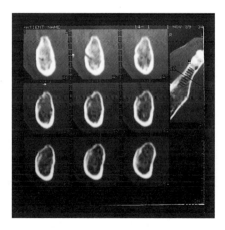

Fig 3-10 CT scans using software designed to account for the curvature of the mandible. Note multiple slices through the mandible provide a clear view of the mandibular canal. (Courtesy of Columbia Scientific.)

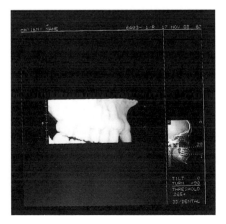

Fig 3-11 Three-dimensional reconstruction of the maxilla from a CT scan. (Courtesy of Columbia Scientific.)

MAGNETIC RESONANCE IMAGING

Magnetic resonance imaging (MRI) is fundamentally different from the other imaging techniques described in this chapter.[18] MRI does not use ionizing radiation. Unlike conventional radiographic techniques, the hard tissues, bone, and teeth are not strongly imaged in MRI. The strength of MRI is therefore its ability to image soft tissue.

To acquire an MRI image the patient is placed in a strong magnetic field. The protons of the hydrogen nuclei of the water within the tissues precess (rotate like a spinning top) about the direction of the magnetic field. Resonance frequency energy is applied and then removed. The response of the nuclei to the resonance frequency stimulation is observed in a receiver coil. Three parameters, called $T1$ (the spin lattice relaxation time), $T2$ (the spin-spin relaxation time), and p (nuclear magnetic volume density) describe the MRI signal.

These technical terms are not easily conceptualized by the average clinician accustomed to radiographic images based on the attenuation of an x-ray beam by hard tissue. However, the clinician should realize that the MRI scanning parameters are set to maximize image quality for viewing protons or water. Mathematical algorithms then reconstruct slices or planar images of the MRI appearance of the organs of interest.

Based on these principles it is not surprising to find that alveolar bone is only weakly imaged, whereas soft tissue, such as salivary glands, dental pulp, and the disc of the temporomandibular joint, may be easily observed if the correct scanning parameters are used. Therefore, at present MRI is not well suited to answering questions about alveolar bone support. Recent reports do, however, indicate that MRI has a role in answering questions such as whether the meniscus of the TMJ is displaced (Fig 3-12).[19,20]

The advantages of using MRI to answer appropriate questions is clear. It is noninvasive and we are presently unaware of significant biological risks. MRI imaging is, however, expensive, requires considerable scan time for high resolution images, and may be claustrophobic for the patient. MRI is prone to some of the same errors as CT, including motion and volume-averaging artifacts. Most important, however, are the large artifacts produced due to metal in the field under examination. The presence of dental restorations or implants can, in certain circumstances, render the MRI image uninterpretable. MRI is a rapidly evolving field and its usefulness to dental applications is under investigation. Like CT, the involvement of the radiologist is a key factor in the production of clinically meaningful images that will answer the clinicians' questions.

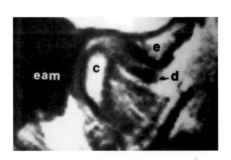

Fig 3-12 *Magnetic resonance image of the temporomandibular joint in the closed position. There is anterior disc displacement. The anteriorly displaced disc (d, arrow) is shown as a black structure located below the articular eminence (e) and anterior to the condyle (c). (Courtesy of Dr P. L. Sadowsky.)*

NUCLEAR MEDICINE BONE SCANS

Nuclear medicine is the branch of radiology that uses radiolabeled pharmaceuticals that are specifically intended to image particular organs or detect specific disease processes. The radiopharmaceutical is, in effect, a magic bullet that is taken up selectively by the organ or tissue of interest. Radiopharmaceuticals are routinely used to image the brain, bone, kidneys, heart, bone marrow, liver, spleen, and lungs.

For the diagnosis of periodontal disease, bone scans have been used to detect sites of active bone loss.[21,22] The radiopharmaceutical is a technetium-labeled disphosphonate called 99m-Tc-methylene diphosphonate. The diphosphonate moiety is the bone seeker that is adsorbed onto the forming front of bone that occurs either during bone apposition or behind the bone resorption. The radiolabel, technetium, is a synthetic element with a 6-hour physical half-life. The biological half-life of the radiopharmaceutical is 3 hours.

The bone scan does not image the anatomy of the area of interest. Rather, it detects alterations in bony metabolism that may occur prior to radiographically detectable changes. It is also important to note that these changes are not specific to a particular disease. Therefore, the bone scan must be used in conjunction with clinical findings and radiographs in order to make an accurate diagnosis.

To perform a bone scan, the radiopharmaceutical is injected intravenously. Following a period to allow for bony uptake of the agent, uptake is either imaged using a gamma camera or measured using specially designed detectors for intraoral use. Areas of active bone loss appear as hot spots in the image (Fig 3-13). Studies have shown that the sensitivity and specificity of this technique in prognosticating alveolar bone loss due to periodontitis subsequently determined radiographically is over 90%.[22]

Bone scans are best used to determine whether a patient has active sites of bone loss and could benefit from an experimental treatment, or to determine whether a patient who is to undergo a bone marrow transplant has sites of active periodontal disease or occult disease that need immediate attention.

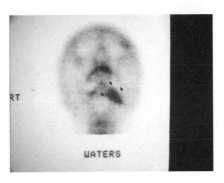

Fig 3-13 *Modified Water's view of a bone scan of a patient with a site of active bone loss due to periodontitis in the mandible. Areas of active bone loss appear as red areas. Note that the teeth are not imaged in a bone scan.*

SUMMARY

The world of imaging for dentists has greatly widened in the past decade. No longer are we restricted to the transmission radiographs that can be easily taken in the office. The new imaging methodologies present both opportunities and challenges to the practitioner. Information previously unattainable by noninvasive means can now be gathered. No longer will every patient receive the same diagnostic examination; instead, the prescription of the diagnostic examinations must be individualized to each patient's needs. Clearly, the end result of better diagnosis should be early intervention and better treatment of dental diseases.

QUICK REVIEW

I. Transmission radiography
Purpose: to obtain a two-dimensional view of the anatomy of the teeth, alveolar bone, and surrounding structures.
Method: x-rays are attenuated by the oral structures. Transmitted x-rays expose the film.
- Selection of kVp: low kVp-higher contrast and radiation dose; high kVp = lower contrast, more shades of gray, lower radiation dose.
- Selection of projection: periapical views are most useful to visualize apex and bone-tooth relationships when there is moderate or severe bone loss.
- Bite-wing views are most useful to visualize caries and bone-tooth relationships when there is mild to moderate bone loss. Less susceptible to angulation artifact.

Applications: best suited to viewing calcified structures.

II. Subtraction radiography
Purpose: to enhance visualization of bone loss or gain that has occurred between radiographic examinations not detectable by eye.
Method: standardized radiographs are entered into an image processing computer. Specialized software is used to subtract all unchanging structures from the pairs of radiographs. Areas of bone loss or gain are displayed.
Image enhancement: pseudocolor or lesion detection software is used to color code areas of bone loss and gain.
Applications: longitudinal assessment of bone loss or gain around teeth and dental implants.

III. Computed tomography
Purpose: to allow visualization of two-dimensional slices or three-dimensional reconstructions of organs or regions of interest.

Method: multiple exposures taken using known geometry around the area of interest. Specialized software used to reconstruct the slices or a three-dimensional view of the organ.
Applications: detection of space-occupying lesions, assessment of anatomy for pre-implant diagnosis, assessment of the three-dimensional shape of the maxilla or mandible.

IV. Magnetic resonance imaging
Purpose: to use a magnetic field to produce an image that is related to the protons or water in organs. Soft tissue is more strongly imaged than calcified tissue.
Method: after the patient is placed in a strong magnetic field, resonance frequency energy is applied and then removed. The response of the nuclei is observed in a receiver coil, and specialized software is used to generate an image. No ionizing radiation is used.
Applications: imaging of soft tissues including space-occupying lesions and the location of the TMJ discs.

V. Nuclear medicine bone scans
Purpose: to visualize the location of areas of altered bone metabolism.
Method: a radiolabeled pharmaceutical (99m-Tc-methylene-diphosphonate) is injected intravenously. Following a waiting period for uptake and clearance from the blood and soft tissue, emitted radioactivity is imaged using a gamma camera. Areas of altered bone metabolism appear as dark or "hot" spots in the image.
Applications: to detect areas of altered bone metabolism due to active bone loss. The method is most useful for clinical trials or for medical or dental conditions (such as bone marrow transplantation) that require immediate disclosure of possible occult infections.

REFERENCES

1. Goaz PW, White SC: *Oral Radiology: Principles and Interpretation.* St Louis: CV Mosby Co; 1987:113-120.

2. Hausmann E, Allen K, Christersson L, Genco R: Effect of x-ray beam vertical angulation on radiographic alveolar crest level measurement. *J Periodont Res* 1989;24:8-19.

3. Goaz PW, White SC: *Oral Radiology: Principles and Interpretation.* St Louis: CV Mosby Co; 1987:97-112.

4. Kaffe I, Littner MM, Kuspet ME: Densitometric evaluation of intraoral x-ray films: Ektaspeed versus Ultraspeed. *Oral Surg* 1984;57:338-342.

5. Schei O, Waerhaug J, Lovdal A, Arno A: Alveolar bone loss as related to oral hygiene and age. *J Periodontol* 1959;30:7-16.

6. Jeffcoat MK, Jeffcoat RL, Williams RC: A new method for the comparison of bone loss measurements on non-standardized radiographs. *J Periodont Res* 1984;19:434-440.

7. Webber RL, Ruttimann UE, Grondhal HG: X-ray image subtraction as a basis for assessment of periodontal changes. *J Periodont Res* 1982;17:509-511.

8. McHenry K, Hausmann E, Wikesjö U, Dunford R, Lyon-Bottenfield E, Christersson L: Methodological aspects and quantitative adjuncts to computerized subtraction radiography. *J Periodont Res* 1987;22:125-132.

9. Jeffcoat MK, Reddy MS, Webber RL, et al: Extraoral control of geometry for digital subtraction radiography. *J Periodontol* 1987;22:396-402.

10. Vos MH, Janssen PT, van Aken J, Heethar RM: Quantitative measurement of periodontal bone changes by digital subtraction. *J Periodont Res* 1986;21:583-591.

11. Bragger U, Pasquali L, Rylander H, Carnes D, Kornman KS: Computer-assisted densitometric image analysis in periodontal radiography. A methodological study. *J Clin Periodontol* 1988;15:27-37.

12. Ruttimann UE, Webber RL, Schmidt E: A robust digital method for film contrast correction in subtraction radiography. *J Periodont Res* 1986;21:486-495.

13. Reddy MS, Bruch JM, Jeffcoat MK, Williams RC: Contrast enhancement as an aid to interpretation in digital subtraction radiology. *Oral Surg Oral Med Oral Radiol* (in press).

14. Coulam CM, Erickson JJ: Image considerations in computed tomography. In: Coulam CM, Erickson JJ, Rollo RD, James AE Jr, eds. *The Physical Basis of Medical Imaging.* New York: Appleton-Century-Crofts, 1981.

15. Berman CL: Osseointegration. Complications, prevention, recognition, treatment. *Dent Clin North Am* 1989;33:635-663.

16. Schwarz MS, Rothman SL, Chafetz N, Rhodes M: Computed tomography in dental implantation surgery *Dent Clin North Am* 1989;33:555-597.

17. Ohba T, Yang RC, Chen CY, et al: Application of computed tomography and scintigraphy in the diagnosis of lesions of the maxillofacial region. *Dentomaxilofac Radiol* 1982;11: 81-87.

18. Partain CL, Price RR, Erickson JJ, Patton JA, Coulam CM, James AE Jr: Nuclear magnetic resonance imaging. In: Coulam CM, Erickson JJ, Rollo RD, James AE Jr, eds. *The Physical Basis of Medical Imaging.* New York: Appleton-Century-Crofts, 1981.

19. Katzberg RW, Schenck J, Roberts D, et al: Magnetic resonance imaging of the temporomandibular joint meniscus. *Oral Surg Oral Med Oral Pathol* 1985;59:332-335.

20. Schach RT, Sadowsky PL: Clinical experience with magnetic resonance imaging in internal derangements of the TMJ. *Angle Orthod* 1988;58:21-32.

21. Jeffcoat MK, Williams RC, Reddy MS, English R, Goldhaber P: Flurbiprofen treatment of human periodontitis: Effect on alveolar bone height and metabolism. *J Periodont Res* 1988; 23:381-385.

22. Jeffcoat MK, Capilouto ML: Problems in risk assessment in periodontal disease-use of clinical indicators. In: Bader JD, ed. *Risk Assessment in Dentistry.* Chapel Hill, NC: University of North Carolina Dental Ecology; 1990:109-113.

Periodontal Disease Activity

CURRENT CONCEPTS by Ray C. Williams

CLINICAL APPLICATION by Wayne B. Kaldahl / Kenneth L. Kalkwarf

CURRENT CONCEPTS
The need for better diagnosis of
    periodontal disease
New diagnostic tests
Detection of specific bacteria in
    the periodontal pocket

CLINICAL APPLICATION
Gingivitis
Periodontitis
Probing depth and clinical attach-
    ment level
Gingival bleeding

Gingival suppuration
Supragingival plaque
Radiographic changes
Tooth mobility change
Microbiological monitoring
Crevicular evaluation
Occlusal trauma
Dental implants

QUICK REVIEW

REFERENCES

CURRENT CONCEPTS

INTRODUCTION

For decades the dental profession thought that once periodontal disease initiated in an individual, it would slowly but continuously progress over time if treatment were not instituted. A number of epidemiological surveys in the 1960s and 1970s lent support to this concept, because they linked increasing age with increasing severity of periodontal destruction.[1-3] Thus it was inferred that over time, an individual would continuously experience destruction of the attachment structures until teeth were lost. However, even during this era, practitioners were noting that individual patients with periodontal pockets,

radiographic loss of alveolar bone, and gingival inflammation might not necessarily have progression of periodontal disease of all teeth in the absence of periodontal treatment. Similarly, patients maintained on a regular regimen of supportive care following periodontal treatment might suddenly have an episode of attachment loss around one or several teeth, then followed by another period of remission. Observations such as these suggested periods of remission and exacerbation of disease progression that was not uniform for all teeth in a patient, or for all patients.

Several landmark studies of the early 1970s began to alter the long-held concept of continuous disease progression.[4,5] During this

era, investigators were placing a renewed research emphasis on finding the specific bacteria responsible for disease causation and for linking host responses such as lymphocyte blastogenesis with periodontal disease progression. Thus, periodontal researchers sought, in their studies of the bacterial etiology and the host responses important in disease progression, to study patients who were actually losing attachment structures at the time of study. In this way the bacteriologic and host response data would be more appropriately linked to "active" periodontal disease destruction.

Socransky, Goodson, and co-workers,[4-7] in a study of the bacterial etiology of human periodontal disease, tried to relate the predominant cultivable flora of a tooth to the actual course of disease of the tooth. Probing attachment level changes over time were used to designate a tooth as "actively" or "not actively" losing attachment between two examination intervals. Thus the cultivable flora of a tooth could be associated with "active" disease progression, or disease in remission or arrested or healthy sites.

These investigators reported that in their patient population, periodontal disease progressed by recurrent acute episodes. They also reported that in some individuals, rates of attachment loss were faster than those seen using the concept of slowly progressing disease. Alternatively, they found sites in patients that progressed much slower (or not at all) than would have been expected based on the radiographic and clinical history of previous disease progression.[4-7] This research group, as well as others, made a compelling argument against the concept of continuously progressing disease and called for research that would clarify the true nature of periodontal disease progression. In addition, it became readily apparent that a major effort needed to be instituted into new ways to diagnose periodontal diseases. In this way clinicians and research

workers could better prevent disease, treat "active" disease, and more accurately relate etiologic and host factor research findings to disease initiation and progression.[8]

THE NEED FOR BETTER DIAGNOSIS OF PERIODONTAL DISEASE

In the last 8 years a major research effort has been instituted into examining the true nature of periodontal disease "activity" and new ways to diagnose the different periodontal diseases and their "active" progression. The profession has begun to speak about "risk" for periodontal disease and "risk factors" that may predispose an individual to disease initiation and progression.[9,10] At the same time, innovative researchers have pursued several new areas of diagnosis. Although new diagnostic tests hold promise, only a few are yet tried enough to be useful in the day-to-day practice of dentistry. Still, there is much promise in this area and the likelihood that this decade will see innovative diagnostic tests in periodontics is excellent. It is hoped that improved diagnosis of periodontal disease will better:

1. Differentiate periodontal diseases
2. Identify disease initiation and progression
3. Identify persons and teeth that are susceptible to disease initiation and progression
4. Monitor the response to treatment

The current diagnosis of periodontal disease relies on several indicators that have long been used in dentistry. At examination, the gingival tissues are assessed for inflammation based on redness, swelling, bleeding to probing, and exudate (see also chapter 1). The loss of attachment structures is assessed by measuring periodontal pocket depths and probing attachment loss from a fixed reference such as the cementoenamel junction, and the extent and severity of radiographic alveolar bone loss is determined. Figure 4-1a is a simple diagram of periodontal disease examination. At the time of examination (time zero), the periodontal examination determines a history of past tissue destruction. Clinical and radiographic data reflect historical disease occurrence. Subsequently, a specific amount of time (for example, 3 months) must pass and the examination be repeated. Only then can a determination of

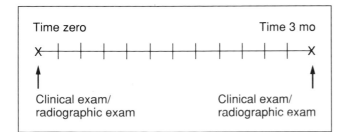

Fig 4-1a *Diagram of the time in months (12 weeks) that it theoretically would take to determine active periodontal disease using conventional clinical and radiographic techniques.*

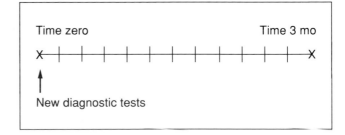

Fig 4-1b *Diagram of the information new diagnostic tests may provide at time zero about periodontal disease activity.*

disease "activity" be made based on changes from time zero, or the absence of change. It may take several months to determine radiographically that there has or has not been further loss of alveolar bone. Similarly, it may take weeks or several months to determine, with probing, whether or not there has been further loss of attachment. Thus the question arises, are there new diagnostic tests that at time zero, or very soon thereafter, will provide information at the time of examination about the actual nature of periodontal disease activity (Fig 4-1b)? Would it be possible using constituents of crevicular fluid or peripheral blood, for example, to detect at time zero an individual patient or specific teeth in a patient experiencing active periodontal tissue destruction, or highly susceptible to future active periodontal tissue destruction?

NEW DIAGNOSTIC TESTS

Several new diagnostic tests appear to hold considerable promise in their application for determining periodontal disease activity and susceptibility.[9-11] Likely other tests will be forthcoming in the near future. This chapter examines some of the new diagnostic tests that have promise in the immediate future (see also chapter 3 for more detail on imaging techniques). Table 4-1 lists six general categories of new diagnostic tests.

Radiographic Techniques

The use of radiographs to determine disease "activity" requires that two radiographs of a tooth be separated in time in order to detect change or lack of change in the bony architecture around the tooth. With conventional dental

TABLE 4-1 *New diagnostic tests to determine periodontal disease activity*

Radiographic techniques
Controlled-force, standardized periodontal probes
Nuclear medicine techniques
Markers in peripheral blood:
  • Neutrophil functional profile
  • Circulating antibody to plaque bacteria
  • Monocyte responsiveness to LPS
Crevicular fluid contents:
  • Products of host immunity
  • Products of tissue breakdown
  • Products of host cells
  • Products of bacteria
Detection of specific periodontal pocket bacteria:
  • Culturing techniques
  • DNA probes
  • Antibody techniques
  • BANA hydrolysis

radiographs, it may take several months to be able to visually detect bone loss on the radiograph. Thus, improved radiographic techniques are needed to detect small losses or gains of alveolar bone in a dental radiograph in a short period of time, allowing the clinician in a few weeks, with two radiographs, to determine that a particular site is losing alveolar bone.[12] Various reports[13-16] suggest that *subtraction radiography* techniques are useful indicators of periodontal disease activity.

Subtraction radiography requires that the two radiographs be alike except for the alveolar bone that has been lost or gained in the time interval between the two images. Several advances suggest that the ability to accomplish this may be applicable to clinical practice in the future. Jeffcoat and co-workers[15] have simplified the ability to take geometrically standardized radiographs that no longer require oral stents. In addition, the development of the image-processing microcomputer has made the application of sub-

traction radiography to dental problems more convenient. A video camera is used to input the radiographs into the computer. The computer is then used to locate and highlight areas of change. Promising data suggest that bone loss may be detected (1) when only 1% to 5% of the mineral is lost; (2) where there is as little as 0.5 mm of bone loss along the tooth root; or (3) when there is less than 1 mm^3 of bone loss.[12] Recently, pseudocolor image enhancement has been used to further enhance the ability to detect small changes between two radiographs.[17] Figure 4-2 is an example of pseudocolor enhancement of experimental bone loss in an in vitro study of subtraction radiography. Figure 4-3 illustrates the shortened amount of time required for detecting radiographic changes in alveolar bone density and height when subtraction radiography is used. In this example, two films taken 4 weeks apart could theoretically indicate loss of alveolar bone. This would allow the dentist to determine periodontal disease activity of a tooth in a 4-week period.

Nuclear Medicine Techniques

Radiographic techniques are capable of detecting changes in bony osseous architecture only after they have occurred. There has therefore been much interest in developing ways to detect changes in bone metabolism around a tooth long before the change (bone loss or bone gain) would show up on a radiograph. In the mid 1970s, Goldhaber and co-workers began to examine the possibility that nuclear medicine techniques for the study of alveolar bone metabolism might be applicable to the bone resorption of periodontitis. Nuclear medicine

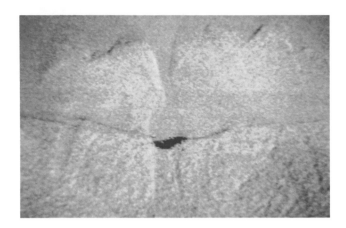

Fig 4-2 *Pseudocolor-enhanced subtraction radiography. In this simulation a small amount of bone loss between two radiographs is easily noted and measured with pseudocolor enhancement. (Courtesy of Dr Jean Bruch.)*

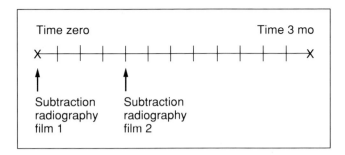

Fig 4-3 *Diagram of the possibility that two radiographs taken 4 weeks apart and analyzed with subtraction techniques can determine bone loss. This would be much sooner than the 3 to 6 months that might be necessary with a conventional dental radiograph.*

techniques, termed *bone scanning,* use a radiolabeled bone-seeking radiopharmaceutical. The label 99m-technetium is a short-lived element with a 6-hour physical half-life. Technetium is characterized by its ability to complex with carrier agents and create tissue-specific radiopharmaceuticals. For bone studies, the technetium label is complexed with tin and a diphosphonate moiety, giving the radiopharmaceutical its bone-seeking quality. To examine bone, the bone-seeking radiopharmaceutical is injected intravenously, and a waiting period of 2 hours is required for clearance from the blood and soft tissue and for uptake by the bone. In general, the bone-seeking radiopharmaceutical is taken up in the calcifying front of forming bone. Since bone resorption is usually coupled with formation behind the resorbing front, nuclear medicine is used to detect alterations in bone metabolism in diseases of bone resorption as well as bone formation.

Because periodontal disease is a disease of bone resorption, it seemed logical to study whether a measurement of bone-seeking radiopharmaceutical uptake (BSRU) would be indicative of bone loss occurring at the time of examination. Kaplan and co-workers[18] reported that the alveolar bone in beagles with moderate to advanced periodontitis had a six times greater BSRU of technetium than dogs with no alveolar bone loss. This finding indicated that bone scanning technology was applicable to the bone loss of periodontitis. These investigators then designed a miniaturized hand-held radiation detector that could measure the uptake of bone-seeking radiopharmaceuticals around individual teeth and tooth sites (Fig 4-4).[19] Jeffcoat and co-workers[20] examined the usefulness of BSRU in diagnosing periodontal disease activity. A single measurement of BSRU around a tooth correlated well with the radiographic loss of bone of that tooth over the subsequent 2 years (Fig 4-5). A tooth with a high BSRU at time zero lost significant bone radiographically, whereas a tooth with a low BSRU lost little bone. Subsequently, beagle dogs being studied longitudinally for the ef-

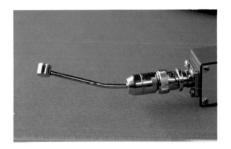

Fig 4-4 *Hand-held detector for measuring bone-seeking radiopharmaceutical uptake around individual tooth sites.*

fect of tetracycline or nonsteroidal anti-inflammatory drugs on slowing periodontal disease progression were used to further assess the ability of bone-seeking pharmaceuticals to indicate "active" periodontal disease. The ability of the uptake around a tooth at time zero to indicate whether that tooth was "actively" or "not actively" losing bone as measured 6 months later with a radiograph revealed that a single measurement of BSRU around a tooth could indicate activity with an accuracy of 83.5%.[21]

Recently, the use of nuclear medicine techniques for deter-

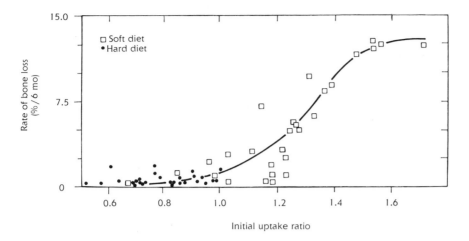

Fig 4-5 *Correlation of the amount of bone-seeking radiopharmaceutical uptake around a tooth and the rate of bone loss of that tooth measured radiographically in beagles. When the initial BSRU was high, the radiographic bone loss 6 months later was also high. (Courtesy of Dr M. Jeffcoat.)*

mining disease activity has been demonstrated in humans. Twelve patients with advanced periodontitis were studied. The ability of a single nuclear medicine exam to indicate which teeth were actively losing alveolar bone radiographically was tested. The findings indicated a highly significant association between high BSRU around a tooth and active bone loss, as measured radiographically, with an accuracy of 79%.[22]

Overall, the progress made in using nuclear medicine techniques for determining periodontal disease activity is promising, but nuclear medicine is not yet applicable to clinical practice. Nonetheless, its usefulness in research applications seems excellent.

Controlled-Force, Standardized Probes

Just as two radiographs separated by time are necessary to determine periodontal bone loss, probing attachment level must also be separated in time to detect changes. Given the error inherent in conventional periodontal probing, for many years investigators have sought a more precise method for measuring attachment level changes. In this way small changes in attachment occurring over a shorter period of time might be detected and used to indicate periodontal disease activity.

Conventional probing measurements are influenced by probing force, probe size and shape, angulation of the probe, and the degree of gingival inflammation.[11] Several automated probes developed in the last 5 years have been designed to overcome some of these areas of error, and they appear to hold considerable promise for allowing the detection of small attachment level changes. The Florida Probe was developed on the assumption that constant probing force, precise electronic measurement, and the use of an occlusal stent as a probe tip guide and fixed reference would greatly reduce measurement error in comparison to the conventional probe. Gibbs and co-workers[23] reported that the Florida Probe detected a loss of attachment level of less than 1 mm change with a certainty of 99%.

An automated probe has been developed that can record the cementoenamel junction, thus providing for the recording of a fixed reference point as well as probing pocket depths. An initial report indicated that the CEJ probe could determine attachment level with a repeatability of 0.2 mm in an in vitro study of odontotype mounted teeth.[24] Clearly, the automated, computerized periodontal probe holds promise as a new diagnostic test for periodontal disease activity. Since conventional probing requires that there be a change in probing attachment level of 2 to 3 mm before a site can be designated as actively losing attachment, the ability to detect much smaller changes accurately should mean that the time necessary between two sequential probings can be shortened. In Fig 4-1a, 3 months are required to detect an attachment level change of 2 to 3 mm with conventional probing. As illustrated in Fig 4-6, with the automated, computerized probe, an attachment level change of 0.2 mm is considered an accurate indication of active disease, and this change in attachment level of a tooth or site hypothetically might be detected in 4 weeks rather than in months.

Markers in Peripheral Blood

The possibility that the contents of circulating peripheral blood can be used to diagnose periodontal disease has been considered for several years. Research workers have examined elements such as white blood cells and circulating antibody levels to periodontal pathogens and have sought cor-

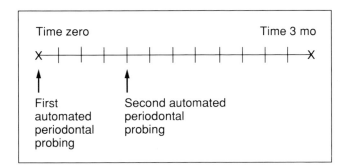

Fig 4-6 *Diagram of the possibility that two probing attachment level measurements taken 4 weeks apart with an automated probe can determine loss of attachment, which is much sooner than conventional probing.*

relations of these components with periodontal disease activity. Although the usefulness of peripheral blood has promise, much research is needed to amplify and clarify how this area of diagnosis may best be used. It is generally believed that disease susceptibility and progression occur on a site basis, and thus markers of disease activity that can identify teeth and tooth sites are preferred. Still, individuals at risk for active periodontal disease need to be identified, and peripheral blood may provide an excellent tool to aid in this diagnosis.[9-11]

The measurement of three constituents of peripheral blood has demonstrated promise for diagnosis. These constituents are PMN function, circulating antibody level, and monocyte responsiveness to bacterial lipopolysaccharide. The landmark studies by Lavine et al,[25] Cianciola et al,[26] and Clark et al[27] established an essential role for the neutrophil in the pathogenesis of periodontal disease. Defects in neutrophil function such as chemotaxis and/or phagocytosis have been clearly associated with some severe forms of periodontal disease such as localized and generalized juvenile periodontitis, rapidly progressive periodontitis, and prepubertal periodontitis. In addition, systemic diseases such as Down's syndrome, agranulocytosis, Papillon-Lefevre syndrome, type I diabetes mellitus, and cyclic neutropenia

have neutrophil abnormalities and more severe periodontal disease. It has also been proposed that transient neutrophil abnormalities in adults may lead to periods of increased disease activity.[28]

It seems likely that measuring peripheral blood neutrophil function should be a way to identify individuals at risk for active periodontal disease progression. This is already done on a limited basis in research patients, but because laboratory assessment of neutrophil chemotaxis and phagocytosis is expensive and time-consuming, this diagnostic test may not yet be applicable to practice. The finding that neutrophil disorders in localized juvenile periodontitis such as chemotactic receptors are genetically based suggests that genetic markers may be identified that would allow individuals at risk for active periodontal destruction to be more easily identified.[28]

For many years it has been recognized that circulating peripheral blood contains antibody titers to periodontal pocket bacteria. A number of investigators have reported that elevation in serum antibody to plaque bacteria is associated with increasing severity of periodontal disease. Much of the early work examined periodontal disease in cross-sectional studies; more recently, investigators have tried to correlate elevated serum antibody levels to specific bacteria with episodes of periodontal dis-

ease activity.[11] It is not yet clear whether elevated serum antibody levels signify protection of an individual against a pathogen, and thus disease inactivity, or whether this is a host response associated with active periodontal destruction.

Ebersole and co-workers[29] have been conducting a large longitudinal study of periodontal disease progression in adults. They have sought correlations between clinical, immunologic, and microbiologic features of patients and the actual activity of periodontal progression. Their findings, although incomplete, suggest that most patients with periodontal disease exhibit significantly elevated antibody responses to suspected periodontal pathogens. In one report of 13 patients, 80% of the bacterial samples from "actively" progressing sites had detectable levels of bacteria to which the patient had an elevated systemic antibody response. Thus, in this study systemic antibody measurements were a reflection of host response to an infection associated with an episode of active periodontal disease progression. The true relationship of elevated serum antibody levels to disease activity, although still unclear, holds promise as a new diagnostic test in periodontics.

Garrison and Nichols[30] have reported an interesting test for examining susceptibility or resistance to periodontal disease based on a possible altered host response examining monocyte responsiveness. They hypothesized that susceptibility to periodontal destruction could be related to an increased host response to gram-negative bacteria as reflected in a study of the lipopolysaccharide of endotoxin. In an initial study, patients with generalized severe adult periodontal disease were compared to six patients "resistant" to periodontal disease. Patients who were classified as susceptible to periodontitis demonstrated a two- to threefold greater responsiveness of blood monocytes to lipopolysaccharide (as measured by prostaglandin E_2 release) than did patients classified as resistant. Susceptible patients with severe disease had a greater monocyte responsiveness, regardless of what stages of treatment or maintenance they were in. This interesting study needs to be extended, but it represents a possible simple test for determining a patient's susceptibility to active periodontal disease, which may have a genetic basis.

Constituents of Crevicular Fluid

Gingival crevicular fluid flow and the components of crevicular fluid have been studied in relation to periodontal disease since the 1960s. The progress made in this area is noteworthy, and there is now very reasonable expectation that crevicular fluid can be useful in diagnosing periodontal disease activity. Crevicular fluid can be obtained easily with minimal intervention or discomfort in a patient. Second, because periodontal disease is considered site specific, individual tooth sites can be easily studied using crevicular fluid samples. Also, many constituents of crevicular fluid can be measured — some of these at chairside in the dental office.

The research into the usefulness of crevicular fluid for diagnosing periodontal disease activity has recently been reviewed,[9,11,31] and four constituents appear to be quite promising. The assumption by investigators in the field is that certain products of microbial plaque or products of the host have elevated crevicular fluid levels that can indicate or predict active periodontal destruction. Table 4-2 lists several categories of products that may be measured in crevicular fluid for correlations with periodontal disease activity.

Prostaglandins and Interleukins Offenbacher and co-workers[32] demonstrated that crevicular fluid prostaglandin E_2 levels can predict active periodontal disease progression. The metabolites of arachidonic acid such as the prostaglandins have for many years been highly implicated in the inflammation of gingivitis and in particular the bone loss of periodontitis. Offenbacher and co-workers studied 41 adult periodontitis patients over a 3-year period. Attachment level measurements and crevicular fluid PGE_2 levels around selected teeth were determined at 3-month intervals. Crevicular fluid PGE_2 levels were found to increase significantly before an episode of attachment loss at a specific site, reach a maximum level at sites with active destruction, and subside after treatment of a site. The sensitivity and specificity of the test were excellent with a predictive value of active disease of 0.92 to 0.95. As easier techniques for detecting prostaglandins in crevicular fluid become available, this constituent of crevicular fluid may be a good in-office indicator of disease activity. Using a similar concept, it has recently been proposed that interleukins hold promise in diagnosing active periodontal disease.[33]

Aspartate aminotransferase Two products of tissue breakdown, aspartate aminotransferase and glycosaminoglycans, also appear to be useful in indicating periodontal disease activity. Chambers and co-workers[34] proposed that during active phases of periodontal tissue destruction, aspartate aminotransferase (AST) might be released into crevicular fluid. In a study of five beagle dogs, they reported a marked increase in crevicular fluid AST levels 2 weeks after ligation of

TABLE 4-2 *Crevicular fluid components for diagnosing periodontal disease activity*

| | PRODUCTS OF | | |
HOST CELLS	HOST IMMUNITY	TISSUE BREAKDOWN	MICROBIAL PLAQUE
Enzymes:	Antibodies	Collagens	Endotoxin
— lysozyme	Complement	Proteoglycans and hyaluronic acid	Enzymes
— acid and alkaline phosphatases	Interleukins		End products
— β-galactosidase		Electrolytes	
— β-glucuronidase	Arachidonic acid		
— arylsulfatase	Metabolites	Aspartate amino-transferase	
Lactoferrin		Glycosaminogly-cans	

teeth to induce periodontal tissue destruction. Since AST levels increased at the same time that tissue destruction was previously reported to occur in the beagle, AST was likely related to disease activity. Persson and co-workers[35,36] greatly extended this observation to a clinical trial of 16 patients with gingivitis and 25 patients with previously treated periodontitis. They reported a significant correlation between elevated crevicular fluid AST levels and periodontal inflammation as well as attachment loss. A multicenter study to confirm and extend the usefulness of crevicular fluid AST levels as indicators of periodontal disease activity is being completed, and the data are very promising.

Glycosaminoglycans The extracellular ground substance of connective tissue contains a complex mixture of polysaccharides linked to specific proteins, termed glycosaminoglycans. As bone and connective tissue are destroyed in periodontal disease, the glycosaminoglycans are released into crevicular fluid. Last and co-workers[37] have reported that a sulfated glycosaminoglycan, chondroitin-4-sulfate, was found in crevicular fluid of patients with untreated advanced periodontitis. Since chondroitin-4-sulfate is prominent in bone, its detection in gingival crevicular fluid may prove to be a sensitive indicator of periodontal alveolar bone destruction. After surgery or after chlorhexidine irrigation of pockets, the chondroitin-4-sulfate was no longer detected, suggesting that with therapy and thus disease remission, this constituent was not present. Longitudinal studies in more patients will be necessary to confirm the exact role of this constituent of gingival crevicular fluid in indicating periodontal disease activity.

PMN Enzymes Lamster and co-workers[38] have examined the relationship of crevicular fluid levels of two PMN enzymes, β-glucuronidase and arylsulfatase, as well as the cytoplasmic enzyme lactate dehydrogenase, to periodontal disease activity. As cells are destroyed during periodontal disease progression, the release of these enzymes should be associated with the loss of attachment structures. Presently, β-glucuronidase appears to offer the most promise as an indicator of periodontal disease progression. Lamster reported that patients who had a generalized form of disease activity, as well as individual tooth sites found to be undergoing destruction, had a significantly elevated level of crevicular fluid β-glucuronidase.

DETECTION OF SPECIFIC BACTERIA IN THE PERIODONTAL POCKET

Since the early 1970s, a major effort has been ongoing to determine which specific bacteria or groups of bacteria are the primary etiologic agents causing the different types of periodontal diseases. Of the more than 300 types of bacteria that can inhabit a person, only a few of these may be responsible for active periodontal disease progression; thus, there has been a long-held hope that identification of these etiologic bacteria at a tooth site would be indicative of active periodontal disease.[11] Currently, some innovative and rapid tests are available to detect specific bacteria within a pocket. Researchers must now confirm what the presence of these bacteria means in terms of actual periodontal disease progression.

Over the years, investigators,

using primarily culturing techniques, have reported that specific bacteria such as *Porphyromonas (Bacteroides) gingivalis, Prevotella intermedia (Bacteroides intermedius), Actinobacillus actinomycetemcomitans, Wolinella recta, Peptostreptococcus micros, Bacteroides forsythus, Treponema denticola, Eikenella corrodens,* and *Fusobacterium nucleatum* are repeatedly cultured at sites of periodontal tissue destruction and can often be associated with active periodontal disease progression.[39] How then might these organisms be easily identified and what does their presence mean in terms of actual periodontal disease activity? Some of the tests for specific bacteria include (in addition to direct culturing) DNA or RNA probes and antibody and enzyme markers.

Selective Media Culturing

The use of selective media fosters the growth of the microorganism to be studied while suppressing growth of all other organisms. This eliminates the time-consuming task of sorting out which bacteria were in the sample by culturing and classification methods. One example of selective media culturing is described in the work of Mandell and Socransky,[40] who developed a malachite green/bacitracin media for the selective growth of *A. actinomycetemcomitans*. Although the use of selective media requires that the microorganisms be viably sampled, diluted, and dispersed, this culturing method of identifying specific bacteria has promise.

DNA Probes

The use of DNA probes to detect specific bacteria at a site has been developed considerably, and probes are available for detecting *A. actinomycetemcomitans, P. gingivalis,* and *P. intermedia.* DNA probes can detect specific sequences of nucleic acids to identify bacterial species. A DNA library for testing plaque samples is created from pure cultures by enzyme digestion of bacterial DNA and by radiolabeling fragments of single strands that are representative of individual species. Plaque samples from patients are mailed to a laboratory for analysis. Samples are enzymatically digested and their fragmented single strands are attached to a nitrocellulose filter to which are attached the complementary labeled single strands from the DNA library. The linked strands are exposed to autoradiographic plates to determine the extent of hybridization. This method is rapid, can detect 10^3 organisms, and is not dependent on cell viability.[11,41] The ability to detect a wide range of periodontal pathogens should now be available. The next step is to study the presence of these bacteria for their indication of risk or active disease.

Immunologic Assays

Immunologic assays to rapidly detect bacteria have been developed that use specific antibodies to bacterial antigens. These techniques include flow cytometry, enzyme-linked immunosorbent assays (ELISA), and immunofluorescent microscopy. Zambon and co-workers[42] reported a rapid identification of *P. gingivalis* with indirect immunofluorescent techniques. Antiserum or antibody were prepared to *P. gingivalis,* and bacterial samples were taken from the periodontal pocket, diluted, placed on a glass slide, and fixed. The slide was then incubated with antibodies to *P. gingivalis* followed by incubating antiserum to IgG, which was conjugated to fluorescein. Under an ultraviolet light microscope, bacterial cells that were *P. gingivalis* in the sample fluoresced green and could be easily detected and counted.

Loesche and co-workers[43] have developed a rapid diagnostic test for detecting *T. denticola, P. gingivalis,* and *B. forsythus* in dental plaque samples. These three bacteria possess an enzyme that can hydrolyze the synthetic trypsin substrate, N-benzoyl-DL-arginine-2-naphthylamide (BANA), forming a color reaction with Evans black dye. This simple color reaction indicates the presence or absence of one or more of these organisms. In a multicenter trial of the BANA test, 702 plaque samples were examined in 119 patients. The ability of the BANA test to accurately detect *T. denticola* or *P. gingivalis* was confirmed by immunologic assay (ELISA). The BANA test was positive in sites that had periodontitis. Of interest was the finding that some clinically healthy sites also had a positive BANA test. It is not yet clear what this finding means in terms of disease activity, but longitudinal studies are underway to determine the ability of the BANA test to indicate disease activity or signal teeth or patients at risk for active disease.

SUMMARY

The diagnosis of periodontal disease activity is being greatly facilitated by new diagnostic tests in dentistry. The ability to detect teeth and individuals who are at risk for active disease or who are experiencing active disease should allow new prevention and treatment strategies.

CLINICAL APPLICATION

The previous section of this chapter demonstrates that clinicians are on the threshold of being able to identify active disease sites and predict future breakdown with greatly improved sophistication and accuracy. Today, diagnosis and treatment determinations in dental practice rely primarily on the examination techniques and clinical parameters that have been used for years. However, the clinical judgment necessary to interpret this information and relate it to disease activity and impending destruction has been greatly enhanced by information obtained from recent research.

Examination methodology and respective clinical parameters have been discussed in chapter 1. Most traditional periodontal examination procedures measure only the results of past periodontal destruction (increased probing depth, loss of clinical probing attachment, gingival recession, alveolar bone loss as viewed in radiographs, tooth mobility, furcation invasion, etc). Recent additions to the diagnostic armamentarium focus on identification of disease activity. This section discusses the role of clinical determinations currently used in clinical practice to evaluate periodontal pathosis, disease activity, or impending clinical attachment loss.

GINGIVITIS

Gingivitis is, by definition, inflammation of the gingiva.[44] Historically, this term has been reserved for clinical situations involving sites with no previous loss of periodontal attachment. Today, the diagnosis of gingivitis also includes inflamed gingival sites that have had prior loss of attachment but are presently not undergoing attachment destruction.

Areas of active gingivitis are easy to clinically identify. They have one or more of the signs and symptoms of inflammation: redness, bleeding upon provocation, increased crevicular fluid flow, swelling, or tenderness (Figs 4-7a to d). Gingivitis is most often associated solely with the presence of bacterial plaque and subsides when the bacteria are removed.

Several factors may have a bearing on the clinical management of gingivitis. These factors may be systemic (patient age, infections, hormones, endocrine disturbances, medications, stress) or local (restorative margins, prosthetic appliances, mouth breathing). Therapy for gingivitis must focus on removal of bacteria and adjustment or correction of modify-

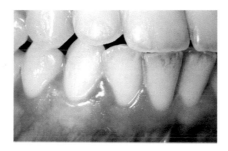

Fig 4-7a *Gingivitis lesion with edematous papillae particularly noticeable between the mandibular lateral incisor and canine.*

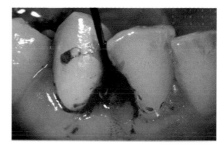

Fig 4-7c *The papilla bleeds very easily upon probing.*

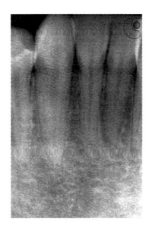

Fig 4-7b *Radiograph of area demonstrating no alveolar bone loss.*

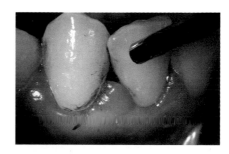

Fig 4-7d *There is a decreased amount of collagen content in the papilla, therefore a blast of air retracts the papilla, exposing subgingival calculus on the dental interproximal surfaces.*

ing factors, when possible. Clinical judgment must enter into not only the choice of the therapeutic method to treat gingivitis but also the degree of aggressiveness needed.

The active state of one type of gingivitis, necrotizing ulcerated gingivitis, is unmistakable. There is a characteristic necrosis and associated necrotic membrane, usually involving the tip of the gingival papillae, a foul odor, pain, and significant bleeding following provocation. There is no clinical question as to the need for rapid intervention.

PERIODONTITIS

By definition, periodontitis is the inflammation of the supporting tissues of the teeth with progressively destructive change leading to loss of supporting bone and periodontal ligament.[44] Periodontitis may be subdivided into multiple subcategories dependent upon age of onset, rapidity of progression, and response to traditional mechanical therapy.[45] The quandary for the clinician is the determination of whether an inflamed site indicates nonadvancing gingivitis or destructive periodontitis that will result in further loss of attachment. This decision process has a vast impact on the clinical practice of periodontics as to appropriateness and timing of therapy. Within clinical practice we must constantly address the question: when is a periodontal site undergoing active destruction of attachment?

The following clinical evaluations are used to qualitate and quantitate clinical parameters in an attempt to identify destructive disease.

PROBING DEPTH AND CLINICAL ATTACHMENT LEVEL

One purpose of initial and subsequent periodontal clinical examinations is to longitudinally record the patient's periodontal status. Active periodontitis has occurred if there has been a longitudinal loss of clinical probing attachment between examinations. Because of the limitations inherent in the periodontal probe (outlined in the earlier part of this chapter) there is always uncertainty regarding the magnitude of change necessary to allow one to reliably say that true destruction has occurred and the change is not a measurement error or a manifestation of probe penetration due to increased inflammation. Many clinical studies have used a threshold of ≥2 or 3 mm of probing attachment loss to denote true destruction of periodontal attachment. This threshold has been deemed appropriate in ensuring that identified "breakdown sites" are true positives and uphold the particular study's criteria. However, if one were to use this high threshold of change to monitor patients in clinical practice, many active sites would go undetected (false negatives). On the other hand, if a lower threshold of ≥1 mm is used, there may be many sites classified as being active that are really measurement errors (false positives). But because initial treatment for a suspected active site usually consists of locally delivered nonsurgical periodontal therapy, for which the morbidity is very low, it ultimately seems appropriate to potentially overtreat by using the lower threshold of ≥1 mm change so that one does not overlook true active sites. If there is not an appropriate response to nonsurgical

treatment, more aggressive periodontal therapies are indicated.

Recently, automated periodontal probes have been developed in an attempt to standardize the taking and recording of probing depth and probing attachment levels. These probes eliminate variables such as probing force and errors in reading the probe. It has been shown in some situations that reproducibility of measurement by these probes may be at a level much less than 1.0 mm.[23] The clinician must remember, however, that this degree of sensitivity may be measuring reversible alterations in the collagen of the attachment region. While automated probes are a necessary component of controlled clinical trials that must identify initial change, their role in clinical practice is primarily one of convenience, potential time savings, and the opportunity to avoid human errors in reading and recording measurements.

The clinician must constantly keep in mind that sites that exhibit negative longitudinal measurement change can only be classified as having experienced past activity and may or may not be presently undergoing active destruction.

GINGIVAL BLEEDING

Clinical studies have enumerated several methods of assessing gingival bleeding and have correlated their relationships to active periodontitis or impending periodontal attachment loss. Within the limitations of these studies, gingival bleeding at a site during a single examination or longitudinally at multiple visits has been shown to be either nonpredictive or an extremely weak predictor of progressive periodontitis.[7,46-52]

Gingival bleeding denotes the presence of inflammation and, when making clinical decisions, must be considered in the light of other clinical parameters. One can assume that, of the several bleeding sites a patient may exhibit, only a few are undergoing active destruction of periodontal attachment.

Absence of bleeding upon probing is implicated to be related to a high predictability of health with no breakdown occurring.[48,49] Treatment philosophy based upon this information leads the clinician to not treat non-bleeding sites.

GINGIVAL SUPPURATION

The presence of gingival suppuration has been related histologically to a more severe state of inflammation and the presence of more PMNs.[53] A few clinical studies have assessed the presence of gingival suppuration and its relation to active or impending attachment loss at a specific site. Suppuration has been shown to be a weak predictor of active periodontal destruction, but better than bleeding.[7,49-52] Suppurating sites should be considered more likely to be active and therefore

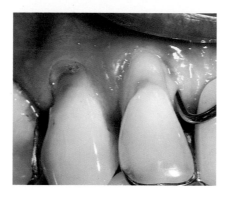

Fig 4-8 *Suppuration exudes from a deep pocket on the mesial aspect of the lateral incisor in conjunction with periodontal probing.*

should be treated aggressively (Fig 4-8).

It is recognized that there is variance in the chemical and bacteriological makeup of what is clinically called "suppuration." As detailed on page 29, current research endeavors may soon allow the clinician to assess the biochemical factors of "suppuration" and gingival crevicular fluid as indicators of periodontal destruction.

SUPRAGINGIVAL PLAQUE

Clinical studies have assessed the relationship of the presence of supragingival plaque at a site to at-

tachment destruction at the same site. The presence of plaque noted at a specific site either once or several times longitudinally is a poor predictor of periodontal destruction at that site.[7,47,50-52] The total amount of plaque in a mouth has also been assessed and related to periodontitis activity. Patients with more generalized plaque exhibit more attachment destruction over time.[54]

Active periodontitis at a specific site cannot be assessed by the presence or absence of plaque at that site. However, evaluation of the patient's overall plaque control is important in identifying individuals who are more likely to have future destruction. Likewise, it is generally valuable to continually reinforce plaque control.

RADIOGRAPHIC CHANGES

Conventional radiographs have many limitations in periodontal assessment. They, like probing, record historical changes (Figs 4-9a and b). Loss of clinical attachment has been compared to the respective crestal changes noted on radiographs over time. The attachment measurement changes preceded changes in the

Figs 4-9a and b *This 37-year-old man was undergoing regular supportive periodontal treatment every 3 months. These two vertical bitewing radiographs taken 1 year apart demonstrate increased bone loss on the distal surface of the maxillary first premolar and the mesial surface of the maxillary second premolar. The probing attachment levels for each site demonstrated 2 mm of loss during this period of time.*

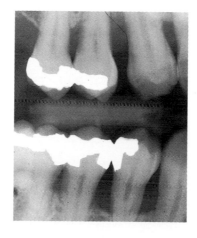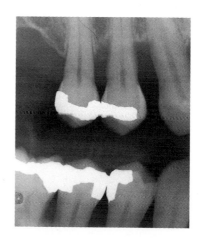

crestal height by approximately 6 months.[55] Therefore, conventional radiographs are not particularly helpful in identifying present or future disease activity.

Use of sensitive radiographic evaluative methods such as Computer Assisted Density Image Analysis (CADIA) will potentially allow the identification of very early and small amounts of attachment loss. However, due to the level of technical control necessary[56] and the inherent problems of high sensitivity, resulting in a high number of false positive observations, these techniques may not be clinically applicable procedures.

TOOTH MOBILITY CHANGE

A mobile tooth may be the result of lost alveolar bone support from a past episode of periodontitis. It also may be from other events or pathology (eg, pulpal disease, occlusal traumatism, orthodontics). When there is an increase in mobility over a specific time period, it may be caused by further loss of periodontal attachment. However, an increase in mobility, particularly during a relatively short time interval, is likely to indicate the presence of another etiologic event that should be considered in the differential diagnosis. The recent introduction of the Periotest allows the clinician to measure relative change in the damping constant of the periodontal ligament. While a modification in the damping constant may be indicative of reduced periodontal support, the clinician must be aware that other alterations (eg, systemic collagen modifications, increased width of the periodontal ligament from occlusal traumatism, etc) may also offer it.

MICROBIOLOGICAL MONITORING

Much recent research has been devoted to the microbiological assessment of periodontitis lesions, backed by a great commercial push. Yet, there are many unknowns, limitations, and unanswered methodological questions about routine use of microbial analysis in the management of periodontal patients.[57] In evaluating a patient who has symptoms indicative of chronic adult periodontitis, the clinician must ask several questions prior to the use of microbial evaluation: *(1)* When to evaluate?; *(2)* Where to evaluate?; *(3)* How to evaluate?; and most importantly, *(4)* What impact will the information have upon treatment decisions? When these questions are answered, the usual conclusion is that the time, effort, and cost of the procedure are out of proportion with the relatively small amount of information that is important for decision making.

There are two clinical situations where microbiological assessment may be helpful. First, patients with localized juvenile periodontitis who are not responding well to therapy should be monitored for the presence of *A. actinomycetemcomitans (Aa)* (see chapter 2). The presence of *Aa* requires that the therapist proceed with more aggressive therapy until *Aa* is eradicated. If there is a recurrence of inflammation and / or a subsequent loss of clinical attachment, monitoring for a reinfection of *Aa* is appropriate. Second, microbial analysis of isolated sites refractory to traditional periodontal therapy may be helpful. A vast number of organisms or combinations of organisms have been implicated in refractory periodontitis[58,59]; therefore, microbiological culturing and susceptibility to antibiotics

should be performed in the active sites. Microbial approaches that only assess the presence of selected pathogens may miss important causative agents and not provide the necessary guidance for appropriate antibiotic therapy. Microbiological assessment for refractory periodontitis should not only identify the infective pathogens and assist in selecting the antibiotic therapy, it should also monitor therapeutic outcomes.

The refractory periodontitis patient is clinically unique and requires special monitoring attention. It is important that the clinician recognize the differences between refractory periodontitis and periodontitis that is in relapse or recurrence. The latter responds favorably to conventional retreatment procedures and possible alterations in the supportive periodontal treatment frequency. This category includes patients who have not remained compliant either with their personal plaque control or professional supportive periodontal treatment or who have other contributing etiological factors that have yet to be identified or controlled.

CREVICULAR EVALUATION

Numerous techniques are now available in evaluating biological turnover of tissues adjacent to the gingival crevice or measuring crevicular temperature change, enzyme activity, or levels of immune components. Unfortunately, in the trials that evaluated these techniques, the researchers had no choice but to use change in probing attachment level as the "gold-standard" of disease progression. The use of this standard has not allowed us to determine whether crevicular evaluation techniques have the ability to predict the eventual onset of clinically relative periodontal breakdown. While these tests may be a valuable adjunct to clinical diagnosis in the future, results from these tests at the present time do not provide a basis for therapy decisions.

OCCLUSAL TRAUMA

Occlusal trauma is defined as an injury to the attachment apparatus (especially the alveolar bone, periodontal ligament, and cementum) as a result of excessive occlusal forces.[44] The symptoms of active occlusal trauma include increasing mobility, widened periodontal ligament space, sensitivity to percussion, and occasionally cold sensitivity. When present, appropriate therapy is warranted to eliminate the occlusal trauma.

DENTAL IMPLANTS

The involvement of the same clinical parameters for determining the activity of a periodontitis lesion applies to determining whether there is activity around a dental implant. However, more emphasis must be placed on radiographic changes and the presence of mobility. Radiographically, one must be concerned not only with crestal bone loss, but also with any radiolucency development around the implant. (It must be remembered that there is normally an initial slight crestal bone loss associated with implant placement that quickly stabilizes.) If an implant exhibits mobility, it is indicative of a breakdown activity. Appropriate intervening therapy is necessary as outlined in chapter 21.

SUMMARY

Today's clinician must rely extensively upon his / her clinical judgment to decide whether a site presently has active disease or is at risk for attachment loss. An assessment of the individual patient's susceptibility, as well as the local site susceptibility, is necessary. Patient susceptibility can be ascertained from an evaluation of past periodontal destruction in relationship to age. Evaluation of a 30-year-old patient with multiple areas of significant attachment loss requires that the clinician be more suspicious of an enhanced possibility for subsequent breakdown and consider more aggressive therapy than he / she would for a 70-year-old with minor loss of attachment. Likewise, certain systemic situations predispose patients to periodontitis (eg, diabetes, HIV infection, stress, family history) and require consideration in diagnosis and treatment decisions. Identification of local factors that have been shown to contribute to periodontitis will earmark local areas that are potentially more susceptible to periodontitis (eg, subgingival restoration overhangs and margins, anatomical factors such as furcations and grooves). When clinical parameters of past disease are present in patients who are more susceptible to periodontitis or are associated with susceptible site locations, the clinician has to be suspicious of active destruction. Appropriate periodontal treatment is warranted in these situations. Research has demonstrated that people can successfully maintain their teeth with periodontal treatment and the necessary intervening therapy over time when there is a recurrence of disease activity.

QUICK REVIEW   PERIODONTAL DISEASE ACTIVITY

I. Determining periodontal disease activity
  • To determine disease activity:
    — two dental radiographs of a tooth must be separated by several months
    — two attachment level measurements of a tooth must be separated by several months
  • Subtraction radiography can detect loss of bone on a radiograph in a few weeks.
  • Controlled-force, automated probes can detect loss of attachment in a few weeks.
  • Nuclear medicine techniques indicate active alveolar bone resorption at the time of examination.
  • Peripheral blood components, crevicular fluid components, and rapid tests for detecting certain bacteria can be measured to indicate active periodontal destruction.

II. Clinical uses
  • Clinical determination of active periodontal attachment loss or impending destruction may be based on the following parameters:
    — negative change in probing depth and / or probing attachment level
    — negative change in radiographic bone height
    — presence of gingival suppuration (limited)
    — poor patient plaque control
    — increasing tooth mobility
    — lack of bleeding upon probing
    — microbiological identification
    — clinical judgment using composite from clinical examination

REFERENCES

1. Scherp H: Current concepts in periodontal research: Epidemiological contributions. *J Am Dent Assoc* 1964; 68:667-675.
2. Russell AL: Epidemiology of periodontal disease. *Int Dent J* 1967;17:282-296.
3. Löe H, Anerud A, Boysen H, Smith M: The natural history of periodontal disease in man. The rate of periodontal destruction before 40 years of age. *J Periodontol* 1978;49:607-620.
4. Socransky SS, Haffajee AD, Goodson JM, Lindhe J: New concepts of destructive periodontal disease. *J Clin Periodontol* 1984;11:21-32.
5. Goodson JM, Tanner ACR, Haffajee AD, Sornberger GC, Socransky SS: Patterns of progression and regression of advanced destructive periodontal disease. *J Clin Periodontol* 1982;9:472-481.
6. Haffajee AD, Socransky SS, Ebersole JL, Smith DJ: Clinical, microbiological and immunological features associated with the treatment of active periodontosis lesions. *J Clin Periodontol* 1984;11:600-618.
7. Haffajee AD, Socransky SS, Goodson JM: Clinical parameters as predictors of destructive periodontal disease activity. *J Clin Periodontol* 1983;10: 257-265.
8. Polson AM, Goodson JM: Periodontal diagnosis — current status and future needs. *J Periodontol* 1985;56:25-34.
9. Fine DH, Mandel ID: Indicators of periodontal disease activity: An evaluation. *J Clin Periodontol* 1986;13:533-546.
10. Johnson NW: Detection of high-risk groups and individuals for periodontal diseases. *Int Dent J* 1989;39:33-47.
11. Caton JG: Periodontal diagnosis and diagnostic aids. In: *Proceedings of the World Workshop in Clinical Periodontics.* Chicago: American Academy of Periodontology; 1989: I-1 to I-22.
12. Jeffcoat MK: Future directions in measurement of periodontal diseases. In: Genco RJ, Goldman HM, Cohen DW eds. *Contemporary Periodontics.* St Louis: CV Mosby Co; 1990: 690-695.
13. Grondahl HG, Grondahl K, Webber RL: A digital subtraction technique for dental radiography. *Oral Surg* 1983; 55:96-102.
14. Bragger U, Pasquali L, Rylander H, Carnes D, Kornman K: Computer assisted densitometric image analysis in periodontal radiography. A methodological study. *J Clin Periodontol* 1988;15:27-37.
15. Jeffcoat MK, Reddy MS, Webber RL, et al: Extraoral control of geometry for digital subtraction radiography. *J Periodontol* 1987;22:396-402.
16. Hausmann E, Dunford R, Christersson L, Allen K, Wikesjo U: Crestal alveolar bone change in patients with periodontitis as observed by subtraction radiography: an overview. *Adv Dent Res* 1988;2:378-381.
17. Reddy MS, Bruch JM, Jeffcoat MK, Williams RC:Pseudocolor image enhancement in digital subtraction radiography. *J Periodontol* (Submitted).
18. Kaplan ML, Garcia DA, Goldhaber P, et al: Uptake of 99m Tce-Sn-EHDP in beagles with advanced periodontal disease. *Calcif Tissue Res* 1975;19:91-98.
19. Kaplan ML, Jeffcoat MK, Goldhaber P: Semiconductor probe measurements in beagle dogs with periodontal disease. *J Dent Res* 1978;57:340-344.

20. Jeffcoat MK, Kaplan ML, Goldhaber P: Predicting alveolar bone loss in beagles using bone-seeking radiopharmaceutical uptake. *J Dent Res* 1980;59:844-848.

21. Jeffcoat MK, Williams RC, Kaplan ML, Goldhaber P: Nuclear medicine techniques for the detection of active alveolar bone loss. *Adv Dent Res* 1987;1:80-84.

22. Jeffcoat MK, Williams RC, Holman BL, et al: Detection of active alveolar bone destruction in human periodontal disease by analysis of radiopharmaceutical uptake after a single injection of 99m-Tc-methylene diphosphonate. *J Periodont Res* 1986;21:677-684.

23. Gibbs CH, Hirschfeld JW, Lee JG, Low SB, Magnusson I, Thousand RR, Yernen P, Clark HB: Description and clinical evaluation of a new computerized periodontal probe — The Florida Probe. *J Clin Periodontol* 1988;15:137-144.

24. Jeffcoat MK, Jeffcoat RL, Jens SC, Captain K: A new periodontal probe with automated cemento-enamel junction detection. *J Clin Periodontol* 1986;13:276-280.

25. Lavine W, Stolman J, Maderazo E, Ward P, Cogen R: Defective neutrophil chemotaxis in patients with early onset periodontitis. *J Dent Res* 1976;55B:603 (Abstract).

26. Cianciola LJ, Genco RJ, Patters MR, McKenna J, Van Oss CJ: Defective polymorphonuclear leukocyte function in a human periodontal disease. *Nature* 1977;265:445-447.

27. Clark RA, Page RC, Wilde G: Defective neutrophil chemotaxis in juvenile periodontitis. *Infect Immun* 1977;18:694-700.

28. Genco RJ, Van Dyke TE, Levine MJ, Nelson KD, Wilson ME: Molecular factors influencing neutrophil defects in periodontal disease. *J Dent Res* 1986;65:1379-1391.

29. Ebersole JL, Frey DE, Taubman MA, Haffajee AD, Socransky SS: Dynamics of systemic antibody responses in periodontal disease. *J Periodont Res* 1987;22:184-186.

30. Garrison SW, Nichols FC: LPS-elicited secretory responses in monocytes: Altered release of PGE$_2$ but not IL-IB in patients with adult periodontitis. *J Periodont Res* 1989;24:88-95.

31. Curtis MA, Gillett IR, Griffiths GS, et al: Detection of high-risk groups and individuals for periodontal disease: Laboratory markers from analysis of gingival crevicular fluid. *J Clin Periodontol* 1989;16:1-11.

32. Offenbacher S, Odle BM, Van Dyke TE: The use of crevicular fluid prostaglandin E$_2$ levels as a predictor of periodontal attachment loss. *J Periodont Res* 1986;21:101-112.

33. Honig J, Rordorf-Adam C, Siegmund C, et al: Increased interleukin-1 beta concentration in gingival tissue from periodontitis patients. *J Periodont Res* 1989;24:362-367.

34. Chambers DA, Crawford JM, Mukherjee S, Cohen RL: Aspartate aminotransferase increases in crevicular fluid during experimental periodontitis in beagle dogs. *J Periodontol* 1984;55:526–530.

35. Persson GR, DeRouen TA, Page RC: Relationship between levels of aspartate aminotransferase in gingival crevicular fluid and gingival inflammation. *J Periodont Res* 1990;25:17-24.

36. Persson GR, DeRouen TA, Page RC: Relationship between gingival crevicular fluid levels of aspartate aminotransferase and active tissue destruction in treated chronic periodontitis patients. *J Periodont Res* 1990;25:81–87.

37. Last KS, Stanbury JB, Embery G: Glycosaminoglycans in human gingival crevicular fluid as indicators of active periodontal disease. *Arch Oral Biol* 1985;30:275-281.

38. Lamster IB, Oshrain RL, Harper DS, et al: Enzyme activity in crevicular fluid for detection and prediction of clinical attachment loss in patients with chronic adult periodontitis. *J Periodontol* 1988;59:516-523.

39. Genco RJ, Zambon JJ, Christersson LA: The origin of periodontal infections. *Adv Dent Res* 1988;2:245-259.

40. Mandell RL, Socransky SS: A selective medium for *Actinobacillus actinomycetemcomitans* and the incidence of the organism in juvenile periodontitis. *J Periodontol* 1981;52:593.

41. Savitt ED, Strzempko MN, Vaccaro KK, et al: Comparison of cultural methods and DNA probe analyses for the detection of *A.a, P. gingivalis,* and *B. intermedius* in subgingival plaque samples. *J Periodontol* 1988;59:431-438.

42. Zambon JJ, Reynolds HS, Chen P, Genco RJ: Rapid identification of periodontal pathogens in subgingival dental plaque. Comparison of indirect immunofluorescence microscopy with bacterial cultures for detection of *Bacteroides gingivalis*. *J Periodontol* 1985;56:32-40.

43. Loesche WJ, Bretz W, Lopatin D, et al: Multi-center clinical evaluation of a chairside method for detecting certain periodontopathic bacteria in periodontal disease. *J Periodontol* 1990;61:189-196.

44. American Academy of Periodontology: *Glossary of Periodontic Terms.* Chicago: American Academy of Periodontology, 1986.

45. American Academy of Periodontology: *Proceedings of the World Workshop in Clinical Periodontics.* Chicago: American Academy of Periodontology; 1989:23.

46. Harley A, Floyd P, Watts T: Monitoring untreated periodontal disease. *J Clin Periodontol* 1987;14:221-225.

47. Listgarten MA, Levin S: Positive correlation between the proportions of subgingival spirochetes and motile bacteria and susceptibility of human subjects to periodontal deterioration. *J Clin Periodontol* 1981;8:122-138.

48. Lang NP, Joss A, Orsanic T, Gusberti FA, Siegrist BE: Bleeding on probing. A predictor for the progression of periodontal disease? *J Clin Periodontol* 1986;13:590-596.

49. Chaves ES, Caffesse RG, Stults DL: Diagnostic discrimination of bleeding and exudate during maintenance periodontal therapy. *J Dent Res* 1986;65:227 (Abstr. no. 522).

50. Badersten A, et al: Scores of plaque, bleeding, suppuration and probing depth to predict probing attachment loss. 5 years of observation following nonsurgical periodontal therapy. *J Clin Periodontol* 1990;17:102-107.

51. Claffey N, Nylund K, Kiger R, et al: Diagnostic predictability of scores of plaque, bleeding, suppuration and probing depth for probing attachment loss. 3½ years of observation following initial periodontal therapy. *J Clin Periodontol* 1990;17:108-114.

52. Kaldahl WB, Kalkwarf KL, Patil KD, Molvar MP: Relationship of gingival bleeding, gingival suppuration and supragingival plaque to attachment loss. *J Periodontol* 1990;61:347-351.

53. Passo SA, Reinhardt RA, DuBois LM, Cohen DM: Histological characteristics associated with suppurating periodontal pockets. *J Periodontol* 1988;59:731-740.

54. Lindhe J, Westfel E, Nyman S, Socransky SS, Haffajee AD: Long-term effects of surgical/non-surgical treatment of periodontal disease. *J Clin Periodontol* 1984;11:448-458.

55. Goodson JM, Haffajee AD, Socransky SS: The relationship between attachment level loss and alveolar bone loss. *J Clin Periodontol* 1984;11:348-359.

56. Hausmann E: A contemporary perspective on techniques for the clinical assessment of alveolar bone. *J Periodontol* 1990;61:149-156.

57. American Academy of Periodontology: *Proceedings of the World Workshop in Clinical Periodontics.* Chicago: American Academy of Periodontology; 1989:1-11, 27-29, 32.

58. Haffajee AD, Socransky SS, Dzink JL, Taubman MA, Ebersole JL: Clinical microbiological and immunological features of subjects with refractory periodontal disease. *J Clin Periodontol* 1988;15:390-398.

59. Slots J, Rams TC, Listgarten MA: Yeasts, enteric rods and pseudomonades in the subgingival flora of severe adult periodontitis. *Oral Microbiol Immunol* 1988;3:47.

Diagnosis of Periodontal Diseases and Conditions Using a Traditional Approach

by Thomas G. Wilson, Jr / Kenneth S. Kornman / Michael G. Newman

---

Overview
Gingivitis
Periodontitis
Gingival recession
Peri-implantitis

QUICK REVIEW

REFERENCES

OVERVIEW

Our approach to diagnosing periodontal diseases has changed over time and will continue to evolve. Several distinct forms of periodontal diseases have been described in the last few years.[1] For the purposes of this text, these diseases will be separated into six groups based on practical approaches to the treatment of these diseases.

Group I: chronic form of gingivitis and adult periodontitis. The chronic forms of these diseases may be caused by host defense or a nonspecific infection. Therapy is covered in chapters 8 to 12.

Group II: other, less commonly seen forms of gingivitis. Therapy for these problems is covered in this chapter.

Group III: more "aggressive" forms of periodontitis. In these more aggressive diseases, combinations of a few species of

bacteria may be the primary extrinsic etiologic factors. Therapy is covered in chapter 6.

Group IV: periodontitis associated with systemic diseases.

Group V: the condition termed *gingival recession*. Treatment methods are found in chapter 15.

Group VI: inflammation around dental implants, currently termed *peri-implantitis*. Therapy is covered in chapter 21.

The watchwords here are caution and study, because our knowledge is growing rapidly.

GROUP I: CHRONIC GINGIVITIS AND CHRONIC ADULT PERIODONTITIS

For insurance reporting purposes, periodontal diseases were at one time separated into four classes according to amount of attachment

loss; this classification is helpful in formulating treatment plans for patients with chronic gingivitis and chronic adult periodontitis.[2] For instance, a Class I case is gingivitis (1- to 3-mm pocket probing depths with signs of disease activity). Class II and higher are cases of periodontitis. In this text, Class II patients will be assumed to have pocket probing depths ranging from 4 to 5 mm with no furcation invasions and to be associated with signs of disease activity (Table 5-1). Cases will be called Class III if early furcation involvement is found associated with 5- to 6-mm pocket probing depths and signs of disease activity. More advanced problems (pocket probing depths of 7 mm or greater) are termed Class IV cases. It is also assumed that tooth mobility and fremitus usually increase as the class number increases.

TABLE 5-1 *Classification of chronic periodontal diseases*

CLASS	TYPE	SIGNS OF DISEASE ACTIVITY	FURCATION INVASION	POCKET PROBING
I	Gingivitis	Yes	No	1–3 mm
II	Mild periodontitis	Yes	No	4–5 mm
III	Moderate periodontitis	Yes	Yes	5–6 mm
IV	Advanced periodontitis	Yes	Yes	≥7 mm

Chronic Gingivitis

Patients with probing depths of 3 mm or less and signs of disease activity have gingivitis. This condition is often associated with reddened, edematous tissue. At present several forms of this disease are recognized, as described on the following pages.

Chronic gingivitis (Figs 5-1a to c)

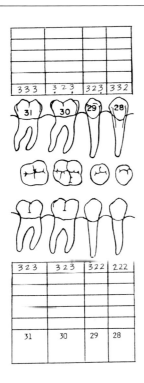

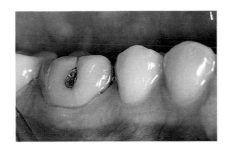

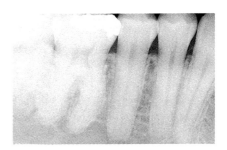

Clinical presentation
- Most common form of periodontal disease
- Pocket probing depths range from 1 to 3 mm
- Bleeding upon probing, suppuration, or other signs of active disease
- Plaque and calculus usually present

- Precedes periodontitis but does not always lead to periodontitis
- Is reversible

Radiographic presentation
- No bone loss is seen

Periodontitis

Patients with periodontitis usually have pocket probing depths of 4 mm or greater when the gingival margin is at or near the cementoenamel junction. Bleeding upon probing or suppuration is often found. It should also be noted that patients previously treated for periodontitis whose tissues have been stable for some time may see a reactivation of their problem. The patient's status would then be reflected by combining the previous amount of attachment loss with the "new" loss, to reflect the present status of the periodontium. At present there are six categories of this disease, as discussed on the following pages.

Mild chronic adult (Class II) periodontitis (Figs 5-2a to c)

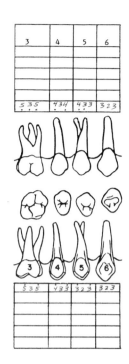

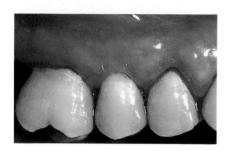

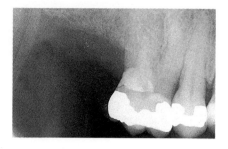

Clinical presentation
- 4- to 5-mm pocket probing depths
- Minimal or no furcation invasion
- Bleeding upon probing, suppuration, or other signs of active disease present

- May see fremitus or early bidigital tooth mobility

Radiographic presentation
No bone loss is apparent on the radiograph of the area shown in the clinical photograph

Chronic Adult Forms of Periodontitis

This is the type of periodontitis most commonly encountered in the average clinical practice. It progresses slowly, and recent studies suggest that the progression may occur in bursts of attachment loss.[3] It is usually associated with accumulation of supragingival and subgingival bacterial plaque where the patient does not (or cannot) clean. Calculus is present in varying degrees but is usually a clinical feature. In this text, chronic adult periodontitis is divided by degree of bony destruction. Patients with 4- to 5-mm pocket probing depths and minimal or no furcation invasion are said to be Class II. Patients with 5- to 6-mm pocket probing depths and early to moderate furcation invasions are considered Class III (moderate). Severe disease (Class IV) is seen when pocket probing depths are 7 mm or above or when through-and-through furcation invasions are seen. All of these definitions assume that the gingival tissues approximate the cementoenamel junction and that root length is normal.

Moderate chronic adult (Class III) periodontitis
(Figs 5-3a to c)

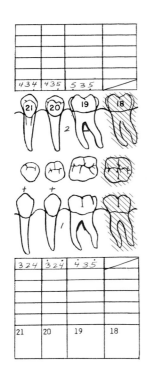

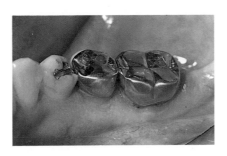

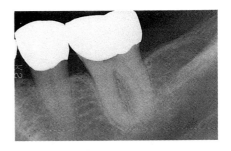

Clinical presentation
- 5- to 6-mm pocket probing depths
- Early to moderate furcation invasion
- Bleeding, suppuration, or other signs of disease activity present
- Often see fremitus or bidigital tooth mobility

Radiographic presentation
A radiograph of the area in the clinical photograph, showing minimal apparent bony destruction

Severe chronic adult (Class IV) periodontitis
(Figs 5-4a to c)

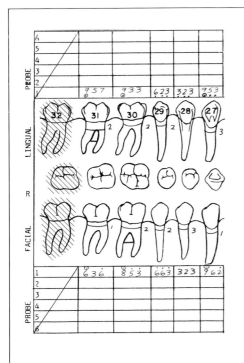

Clinical presentation
- 7-mm pocket probing depths or greater
- Furcation invasion ranging from early to through-and-through
- Bleeding upon probing, suppuration, or other signs of disease activity present
- Usually fremitus and bidigital tooth mobility

Radiographic presentation
Severe bone loss is seen on this radiograph of the area shown in the clinical photograph

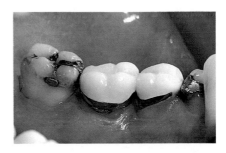

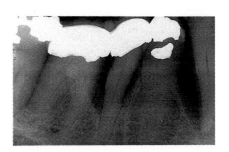

GROUP II: NONCOMMON TYPES OF GINGIVITIS

Acute necrotizing ulcerative gingivitis (ANUG)

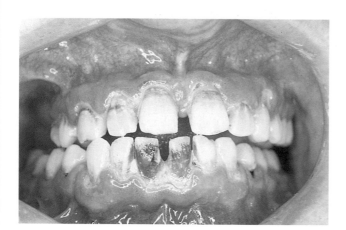

Otherwise systemically healthy (Vincent's) (Fig 5-5)

Clinical presentation
- Accompanied by pain, gingival bleeding, and halitosis
- Spirochetes invade the soft tissues
- Repeated episodes may lead to bone loss
- Therapy consists of gentle debridement by the dental professional on several consecutive days while encouraging the patient toward improved personal oral hygiene

---

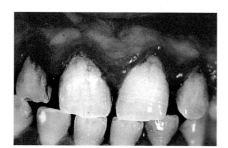

HIV-gingivitis in a 28-year-old man.

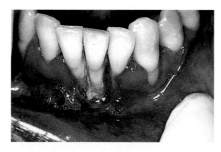

HIV-periodontitis. Rapid localized bone destruction occurred in a few weeks' time.

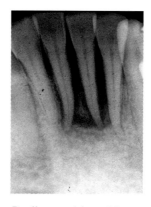

Radiographic evidence of extensive localized osseous destruction associated with HIV-periodontitis.

AIDS-associated gingivitis/ periodontitis (Figs 5-6a to c)

Clinical presentation
- Occurs in patients who have contracted the HIV virus
- Severe marginal inflammation of the gingival tissues is seen
- With gingivitis, patients are often unaware that they are seropositive for the HIV virus
- Periodontitis can often progress rapidly
- Local cleaning alone may be effective. Adjunctive chemical agents such as povidone-iodine and chlorhexidine have been used successfully in combination with local scaling and root planing (see chapter 8)

(Illustrations courtesy of Dr Terry Rees.)

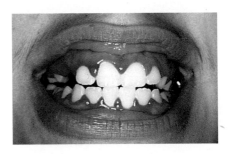

Pubertal gingivitis in an 11-year-old girl.

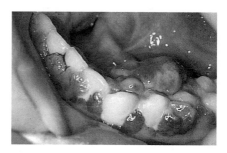

Severe pregnancy gingivitis with pregnancy tumor evident on left lingual incisor.

Steroid hormone–influenced gingivitis
(Figs 5-7a and b)

- Presents during natural or induced hormonal change
- Has been reported in pregnancy, a few days prior to menstruation, during puberty, and in some women on oral contraceptives for extended periods of time
- Has been associated with an increase in specific bacteria (eg, *Prevotella [Bacteroides] intermedia*)
- Although hormone influenced gingivitis is reversible, hormonal changes in a patient with untreated or unstable periodontitis may induce substantial loss of attachment
- Treatment in most instances consists of local debridement, scaling and root planing and improved plaque control techniques. Surgical correction is sometimes necessary in severe cases

(Illustrations courtesy of Dr Terry Rees.)

Medication-influenced gingival overgrowth (hyperplasia) (Figs 5-8a and b)

Hyperplasia is the increase in size of an organ or its parts. It is characterized by an increase in the numbers of cellular elements and does not serve a functional purpose.[4]

There are three commonly used medications that cause most of these overgrowths. They are phenytoin (Dilantin, Parke-Davis and other manufacturers), cyclosporine (Sandimmune, Sandoz), and nifedipine (Adalat, Miles; Procardia, Pfizer). In general, the better the patient's oral hygiene, the less the problem. For an excellent review see Butler et al.[5]

Clinical presentation
- Overgrowth is often interproximal
- Oral hygiene is difficult

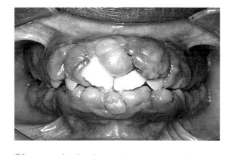

Phenytoin-induced overgrowth.

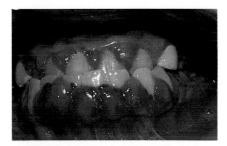

Cyclosporine-induced overgrowth.

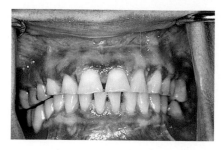

Localized atrophic and erosive gingival lesions in erosive lichen planus.

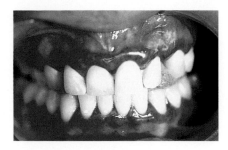

Generalized atrophic gingivitis common in benign mucous membrane pemphigoid.

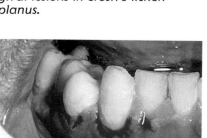

Irregular gingival erosions in pemphigus vulgaris.

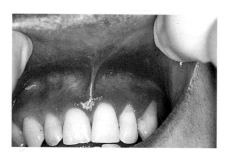

Hypersensitivity reaction to a tartar-control toothpaste.

Desquamative gingivitis
(Figs 5-9a to d)

- Dermatoses:
  — erosive lichen planus
  — phemphigoid
  — pemphigus
- Allergic reactions
- After diagnosis, treatment of a dermatosis must often be coordinated with the patient's physician. Topical and / or systemic corticosteroids are frequently administered. Allergic reactions are treated by discontinuing use of the causative material

(Illustrations courtesy of Dr Terry Rees.)

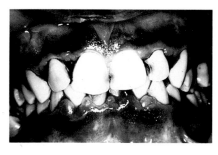

Spontaneous gingival bleeding in a patient suffering from idiopathic thrombocytopenic purpura.

Other causes of gingivitis (Figs 5-10a to c)

- Blood disorders
- Nutritional deficiencies
- Tumors
- Genetics
- Mouthbreathing
- Bacterial and viral infection
- Oral treatment is often palliative while underlying systemic disorders are being managed. Oral debridement and meticulous oral hygiene are initiated when possible. Surgical correction is usually necessary for tumors or hyperplastic gingival enlargements

(Illustrations courtesy of Dr Terry Rees.)

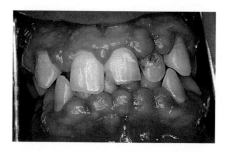

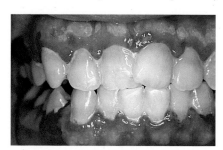

(left) *Gingival hyperplasia resulting from inadequate plaque control in a patient who is a chronic mouth breather.*

(right) *Generalized gingivitis and vesiculation associated with primary herpetic gingivostomatitis.*

GROUP III: AGGRESSIVE FORMS OF PERIODONTITIS

This group contains lesions often characterized by rapid loss of attachment, therefore "aggressive" periodontitis.

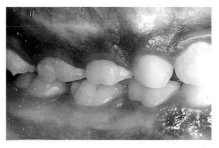

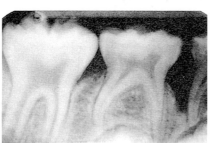

Prepubertal periodontitis

This form of periodontitis is usually seen after the eruption of the primary teeth. There are two forms: generalized and localized.

Localized prepubertal (Figs 5-11a and b)

Clinical presentation
- Little or no inflammation of gingiva
- Usually amenable to standard periodontal therapy with appropriate antibiotics

Radiographic presentation
A radiograph of the area seen in the clinical photograph shows bone loss localized to the distal of the primary first molar

Generalized prepubertal (Figs 5-12a and b)

Clinical presentation
- Extreme gingival inflammation
- Rapid bony destruction
- Often accompanied by severe functional defects of neutrophils and monocytes
- Otitis media and upper respiratory infections are also often found
- In some cases the more severe lesions are refractory to antibiotics[6]

Radiographic presentation
Generalized bone loss is evident on radiographs

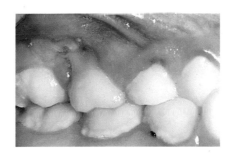

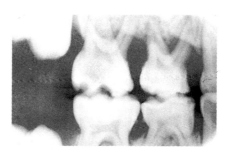

(Illustrations courtesy of Dr Jayne Delaney.)

Localized juvenile periodontitis (Figs 5-13a to c)

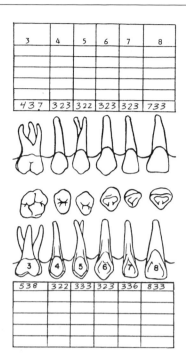

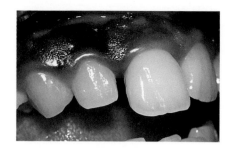

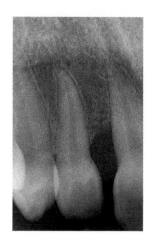

Clinical presentation
- Occurs around puberty
- Usually localized to molars and incisors
- Minimal inflammation and plaque
- Often associated with a systemic host defense defect

Radiographic presentation
Note bone loss localized to the distal of the maxillary central incisor

Generalized juvenile periodontitis (Figs 5-14a to c)

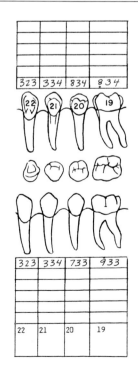

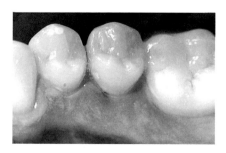

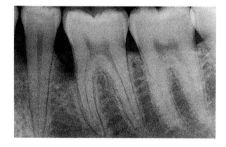

Clinical presentation
- Occurs around puberty
- Generalized bone loss
- Minimal inflammation and plaque
- Often associated with a systemic host defense defect

Radiographic presentation
Despite the clinically healthy appearance of the gingiva seen in the clinical photograph, severe bony destruction around premolars and molars can be seen in the accompanying radiograph

Rapidly progressive periodontitis (Figs 5-15a to d)

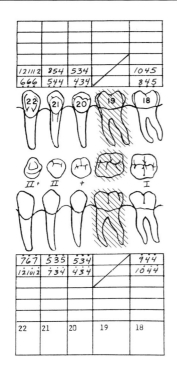

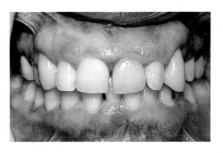

Clinical presentation
- Seen from puberty to approximately age 35
- Characterized by periods of severe gingival inflammation, edema, and rapid bone loss
- Frequently seen in conjunction with malaise, depression, and lowered immune competency

This radiograph was taken 6 months after the one above and shows the bony deterioration seen despite closed subgingival root planing and splinting.

Radiographic presentation
A radiograph of the patient at the initial visit.

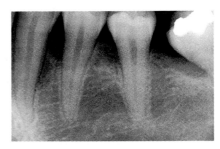

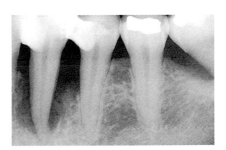

Refractory periodontitis
(Figs 5-16a to c)

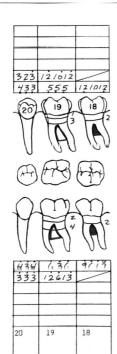

Clinical presentation
- Attachment loss seen after initially effective traditional periodontal therapy
- Patient's oral hygiene is usually better than average
- May be a single disease or several diseases

Radiographic presentation
Initial radiograph of a 45-year-old woman with no known systemic diseases

This radiograph was taken 9 months after the one above.

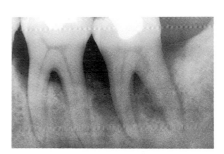

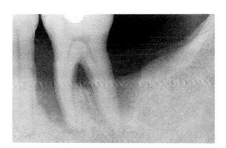

Gingival recession (Figs 5-17a to c)

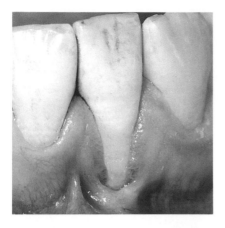

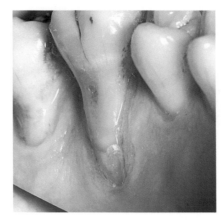

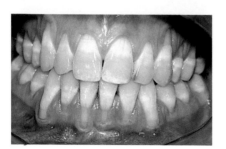

Clinical presentation
- May be localized or generalized
  - facial (buccal)
  - lingual (palatal)
- True periodontal pockets are not always present
- Often associated with local anatomical variations, including bony fenestrations or dehiscences and inadequate bands of attached gingiva

GROUP IV: PERIODONTITIS ASSOCIATED WITH SYSTEMIC DISEASES AND CONDITIONS

A number of systemic problems have been implicated in contributing to periodontal breakdown. They include: HIV-related periodontitis; that associated with insulin-dependent diabetes; nutritional deficiencies such as scurvy; stress; Papillon-LeFevre syndrome; Down's syndrome; and others.

GROUP V: GINGIVAL RECESSION

These patients can exhibit gingival recession secondary to an anatomical problem or as a result of a disease process.

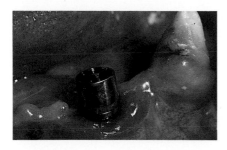

Gingivitis seen around an implant cylinder.

Peri-implantitis (Figs 5-18a to d)

Clinical presentation

- Often accompanied by bleeding upon probing or other signs of disease activity

- Probing depths are increased from baseline

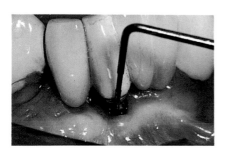

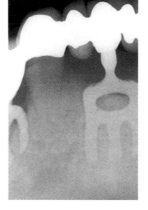

Bone loss seen clinically and radiographically around a fibro-osseous implant.

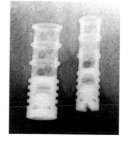

Bone loss seen on radiographs around osseointegrated implants.

GROUP VI: PERI-IMPLANTITIS

The soft and hard tissues surrounding implants can be affected by inflammatory lesions. As a rule, this problem is more prevalent around fibro-osseous implants than around osseointegrated fixtures. Early evidence suggests that the microflora around failing implants mimics that around teeth with periodontitis.[7-9]

QUICK REVIEW

Periodontal diseases and conditions can be grouped into six categories.

Group I: most periodontal patients fall into this group
— chronic gingivitis
— chronic adult periodontitis

Group II: other forms of gingivitis
— acute necrotizing ulcerative (ANUG)
  otherwise systemically healthy (Vincent's)
  AIDS-associated (may progress to periodontitis)
— steroid hormone-influenced
— medication-influenced gingival overgrowth
— desquamative gingivitis
— other causes

Group III: aggressive forms of periodontitis
— prepubertal periodontitis
  localized
  generalized
— localized juvenile periodontitis

— generalized juvenile periodontitis
— rapidly progressive periodontitis
— refractory periodontitis

Group IV: periodontitis associated with systemic diseases or conditions
Examples include:
— HIV-related
— diabetes (Type 1)
— nutritional deficiencies (scurvy, etc)
— stress
— Papillon-LeFevre syndrome
— Down's syndrome

Group V: gingival recession
— localized
— generalized

Group VI: peri-implantitis — soft and hard tissue breakdown seen around dental implants

---

REFERENCES

1. Kornman KS, Newman MG, Alvarado R, Flemmig TF, Nachnani S, Tumbusch J: Clinical and microbiological patterns of patients with adult and refractory periodontitis. I. Clinical. *J Periodontol* 1991; (in press).

2. American Academy of Periodontology: *Current Procedural Terminology for Periodontics.* 5th ed. Chicago: American Academy of Periodontology, 1988.

3. Goodson JM, Tanner ACR, Haffajee AD, Sornberger GC, Socransky SS: Patterns of progression and regression of advanced destructive periodontal disease. *J Clin Periodontol* 1982;9:472.

4. Grant DA, Stern IB, Everett FG: *Periodontics in the Tradition of Orban and Gottleib.* St Louis: CV Mosby Co, 1979.

5. Butler RT, Kalkwarf KL, Kaldahl WB: Drug-induced gingival hyperplasia: Phenytoin, cyclosporine, and nifedipine. *J Am Dent Assoc* 1987;114:56.

6. Page RC, Bowen T, Altman L, Vandersteen E, Ochs H, Mackenzie P, Osterberg S, Engel LD, Williams BL: Prepubertal periodontitis. I. Definition of a clinical disease entity. *J Periodontol* 1983;54:257.

7. Lekholm U, Ericsson I, Adell R, Slots J: The condition of the soft tissues at tooth and fixture abutments supporting fixed bridges. A microbiological and histological study. *J Clin Periodontol* 1986;13:558.

8. Mombelli A, Van Oosten MAC, Schurch E Jr, Lang NP: The microbiota associated with successful or failing osseointegrated titanium implants. *Oral Microbiol Immunol* 1987;2:145.

9. Becker W, Becker BE, Newman MG, Nyman S: Clinical and microbiologic findings that may contribute to dental implant failure. *Int J Oral Maxillofac Implants* 1990;5:31.

Treatment Planning for Patients With Inflammatory Periodontal Diseases

by Kenneth S. Kornman / Thomas G. Wilson, Jr

Overview of the treatment planning process

Treatment planning for chronic gingivitis and chronic adult periodontitis

Treatment planning for aggressive periodontitis

QUICK REVIEW

REFERENCES

OVERVIEW OF THE TREATMENT PLANNING PROCESS

Practical diagnostic systems should assist the practitioner by guiding the plan for therapy and by indicating the expected prognosis following therapy. This chapter describes an approach to treatment planning that is based on evidence suggesting that chronic gingivitis and chronic adult periodontitis will respond predictably to therapy directed at reducing the bacterial challenge and that other forms of the disease are less predictable in their response to that approach to therapy. This system focuses the evaluation and diagnostic process to "screen" for cases that are less likely to be chronic gingivitis and chronic adult periodontitis. The goal is early identification of patients who may require or benefit from therapeutic approaches other than those routinely used for these chronic diseases. It is assumed that some of these cases of periodontitis, if not identified early, will be identified, after great frustration on the part of the practitioner and patient, as "refractory."

Our approach to treatment planning builds on the diagnostic process established in chapter 5. The process includes the establishment of a *presumptive diagnosis* based on clinical findings; this diagnosis is used to guide initial therapy. The *final diagnosis* is the result of the clinical findings and observations of how the patient responds to initial therapy; it guides later therapy and assists in the assessment of prognosis for the case.

Before a presumptive diagnosis can be made, the following must be considered:

1. It must be determined whether the patient is healthy, or has gingivitis or periodontitis. These distinctions are based on the clinician's interpretation of the findings from the clinical examination. (Details of the clinical examination process are given in chapter 1.) "Health" describes a patient with no clinical or radiographic evidence of current or previous loss of connective tissue attachment or supporting bone, no bleeding on probing, and no signs of gingival inflammation or other signs of disease activity. This definition intentionally excludes patients who have been successfully treated and are currently healthy but have a past history of periodontitis. This exclusion is based on the knowledge that such patients have a demonstrated susceptibility to periodontitis if the bacterial challenge is present, whereas healthy and previously nondiseased patients are either unchallenged or nonsusceptible. Recent studies of disease progression have shown that the greatest predictor of future progression is a previous history of periodontitis.

2. Most patients who show signs of gingivitis but not periodontitis have chronic gingivitis. In such patients the host is effectively controlling the bacterial challenge at that time, so there is minimal to no loss of bone or connective tissue. The process by which the host controls the challenge of course produces inflammation, which may set the stage for development of periodontitis or may be an esthetic problem for the patient. Management of chronic gingivitis is presented in chapter 8. Some forms of gingivitis may be the result of dermatologic conditions or alterations in the host defenses. If the gingivitis is related to a dermatologic condition, it is most likely a manifestation of a connective tissue or immunologic disorder. These conditions therefore do not respond predictably to conventional periodontal therapy directed at reducing the bacterial challenge. Many times, however, these conditions are overlayed by chronic gingivitis — the result of poor plaque control due to discomfort of the involved gingiva. Reducing the bacterial challenge will usually aid resolution of the condition by subsequent reduction of the overlying chronic gingivitis. Treatment of gingivitis related to a dermatologic condition should begin with conventional therapy for chronic gingivitis as described in chapter 8. After the chronic gingivitis is under control it is possible to better assess other treatment needs to assist in the control of the dermatologic condition.

Other forms of gingivitis, such as hormonal or HIV gingivitis, are actually chronic gingivitis in which the patient's threshold for disease has been lowered due to an altered host response and/or altered bacterial challenge. Such cases therefore may respond less predictably to conventional ther-

apy or may require more specific therapies.

3. If there are signs of periodontitis, it must be determined if it is most likely chronic adult periodontitis or one of the more aggressive forms of periodontitis, and a presumptive diagnosis can then be assigned. For a graphic summary, see Figs 6-1 to 6-3.

Presumptive Diagnosis: Chronic Adult Periodontitis
(Figs 6-2 and 6-3)

Chronic adult periodontitis is seen in individuals 35 years or older in whom plaque and calculus accumulations are consistent with clinical evidence of loss of attachment and bone. Although the rate of disease progression has been greatly discussed in recent years, the net destruction over time is such that the disease appears to be slowly progressing. Specific findings relative to severity of destruction as indicated by probing depths, furcation involvement, and mobility are discussed in chapter 5.

It should be noted that if past destruction is "severe" (Type IV), the patient is currently, or has previously been, less able to control the microbial challenge, as evidenced by extreme destruction. Although current knowledge indicates that these patients should be given a presumptive diagnosis of chronic adult periodontitis, they may very well exhibit a different response to therapy as noted on page 92.

Since most chronic adult periodontitis patients respond well and predictably to current conventional periodontal therapy, patients should usually receive initial therapy involving approaches known to reduce the microbial challenge. Surgical therapy should follow as indicated if

the reevaluation confirms the presumptive diagnosis of chronic adult periodontitis. This therapy is outlined on pages 148 to 176.

Presumptive Diagnosis: Aggressive Periodontitis
(Fig 6-3)

Patients in whom the disease severity is extreme or in whom the disease progression is rapid are not "managing" the bacterial challenge as seen in the case of chronic adult periodontitis. The term "aggressive periodontitis" merely indicates that the disease has most likely progressed in a manner that was more rapid than the net rate of loss seen in chronic adult periodontitis. Such situations are most commonly the result of inadequate host defenses, but occasionally they are caused by an unusual bacterial challenge. Patients with inadequate host defenses do not respond predictably to conventional periodontal therapy; instead, they require efforts to improve the host status if possible (as with diabetes) or require more rigorous bacterial control.

The altered host status frequently interferes with the patient's response to periodontal surgery, and surgery may therefore not be indicated in these patients until the active infectious process is under control.

Accepted diagnostic categories for the aggressive forms, as shown below and described in detail in chapter 5, are not well defined except for prepubertal and localized juvenile periodontitis.

Accepted diagnostic categories for aggressive periodontitis:
- Early onset periodontitis —
    Prepubertal periodontitis: generalized; localized
    Localized juvenile periodontitis

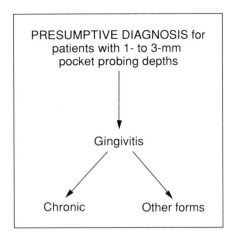

Fig 6-1 Presumptive diagnosis —
gingivitis.

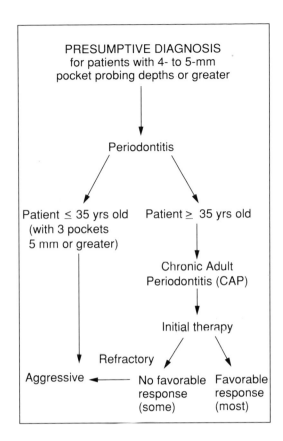

Fig 6-2 Presumptive diagnosis —
periodontitis.

Fig 6-3 Therapy
based on presump-
tive diagnosis.

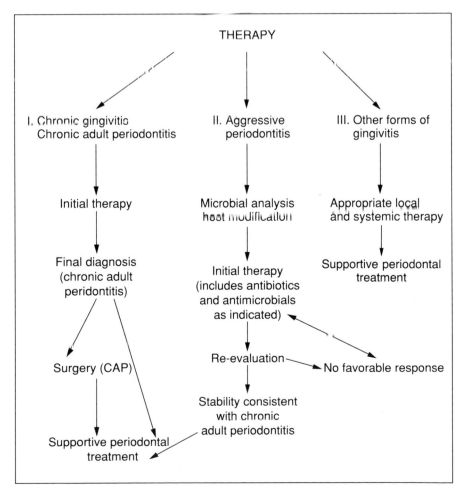

Generalized juvenile perio-
dontitis
Rapidly progressive perio-
dontitis
• Periodontitis associated with sys-
temic disease —
Diabetes
HIV
Others
• Refractory periodontitis

The goal of therapy in aggressive cases is to halt the bacterial
process and convert the case to a
more favorable balance between
the bacteria and the host, so that
conventional therapy may be
more predictably applied.

Initial therapy is modified in
these cases to attempt to control
systemic factors that may influence treatment response and to
achieve more definitive control of
the bacterial challenge.

The guidelines for surgical therapy in aggressive cases are very
different from those in chronic
adult periodontitis. Therapy for
aggressive periodontitis is outlined on pages 93 to 95.

TREATMENT PLANNING FOR CHRONIC GINGIVITIS AND CHRONIC ADULT PERIODONTITIS

Chronic gingivitis and chronic
periodontitis appear as slowly
progressing diseases that are associated with bacterial plaques.
The approach outlined below can
be used to treat patients originally
diagnosed with one of these
chronic diseases or patients who
were first diagnosed with other,
more aggressive periodontal
problems that converted to a
chronic state. With this latter
group, the traditional approaches
outlined in this section can be
used once the microorganism(s)
and/or host factors associated

with these more aggressive problems have been reduced or eliminated. The clinician must first
gather the information discussed
in chapter 1 in order to make an
adequate diagnosis; then an appropriate treatment plan can be
formulated. It is very helpful to
gather records of the patient's
past history of compliance to
health care suggestions (and especially to suggestions by dental
professionals) since compliance to
oral hygiene and supportive periodontal therapy are essential to
the long-term success of periodontal problems.

These two chronic inflammatory periodontal diseases represent the vast majority of periodontal problems seen in the average periodontal practice. Their
treatment can be divided into two
stages: *active therapy* and *supportive periodontal treatment*
(SPT). Active therapy can be further subdivided into *initial* and
surgical therapy. SPT was formerly called maintenance therapy. The outline of therapy used
in this chapter for these chronic
problems was introduced in the
1960s[1] but with certain modifications it is still very relevant. Figure
6-4 shows a schematic diagram of
this approach, and an outline is
found in Fig 6-5.

Initial Therapy

Initial therapy begins after the initial examination has been completed, a diagnosis has been
made, and a treatment plan has
been accepted by the patient. The
first step in initial therapy should
be a review of the patient's oral
hygiene. This is usually followed
by scaling and, where attachment
loss has occurred, root planing.
In most Class I and Class II cases,
these procedures eliminate the local factors well enough to be the
only form of periodontal therapy

needed prior to SPT. Only occasionally is surgery needed in these
cases, and this is usually to correct
some gingival deformity. The goal
of initial therapy is to remove
enough local irritants to stop the
progression of attachment loss
and to encourage the patient to
comply to suggested oral hygiene
and SPT so that the stability created by the active therapy can be
maintained. In many Class III and
most Class IV cases, the goal of removing all of the tooth-borne
subgingival accretions will not be
met using closed scaling and root
planing.[2-5] The studies cited show
that in pockets deeper than 5 mm,
the odds are about even that some
subgingival bacterial plaque and
calculus will remain despite as
much as 30 minutes of subgingival
scaling and root planing on a single tooth. The more advanced the
bone loss, the less the chance of
removing these deposits.

After a short healing period
(usually 30 days), data are again
collected (see "Reevaluation," below). If signs of disease activity are
still found around a tooth with
fremitus or a tooth mobility of one
and a half (I+) (see page 30) is
found, then occlusal adjustment
should be performed on that
tooth. The adjustment should remove detrimental occlusal interferences and eliminate fremitus. In
addition, it will often eliminate or
ameliorate thermal sensitivity and
discomfort experienced after subsequent surgery. In those instances where hypermobility, increasing tooth mobility or fremitus
still exist after occlusal adjustment,
habit appliances, splinting, or in
some cases, both are often warranted. In cases of advanced mobility, procedures designed to reduce this parameter can be performed at the same time that
closed subgingival scaling and
root planing is done.

The initial stage of therapy is

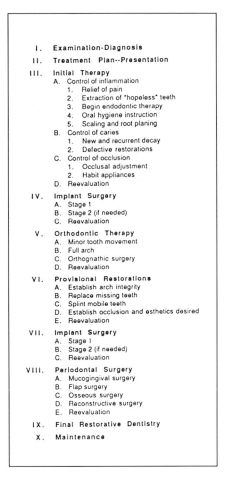

I. Examination-Diagnosis
II. Treatment Plan--Presentation
III. Initial Therapy
   A. Control of inflammation
      1. Relief of pain
      2. Extraction of "hopeless" teeth
      3. Begin endodontic therapy
      4. Oral hygiene instruction
      5. Scaling and root planing
   B. Control of caries
      1. New and recurrent decay
      2. Defective restorations
   C. Control of occlusion
      1. Occlusal adjustment
      2. Habit appliances
   D. Reevaluation
IV. Implant Surgery
   A. Stage 1
   B. Stage 2 (if needed)
   C. Reevaluation
V. Orthodontic Therapy
   A. Minor tooth movement
   B. Full arch
   C. Orthognathic surgery
   D. Reevaluation
VI. Provisional Restorations
   A. Establish arch integrity
   B. Replace missing teeth
   C. Splint mobile teeth
   D. Establish occlusion and esthetics desired
   E. Reevaluation
VII. Implant Surgery
   A. Stage 1
   B. Stage 2 (if needed)
   C. Reevaluation
VIII. Periodontal Surgery
   A. Mucogingival surgery
   B. Flap surgery
   C. Osseous surgery
   D. Reconstructive surgery
   E. Reevaluation
IX. Final Restorative Dentistry
X. Maintenance

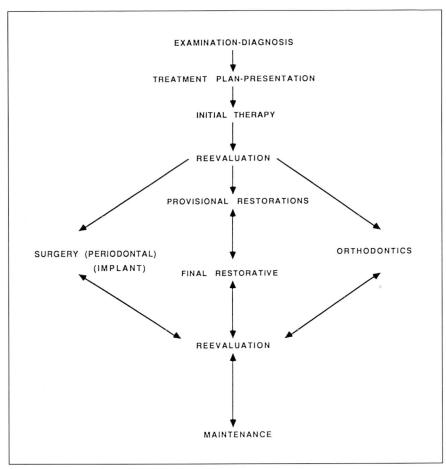

Figs 6-4 and 6-5 *Outline of typical therapy for the patient with chronic adult periodontitis.*

often an ideal time to place dental implants. For example, if the treatment plan calls for one- or two-stage implants, then stage one surgery can be performed at the same time that subgingival scaling and root planing are done. If periodontal surgery is subsequently indicated, it can be performed when the implants are uncovered or placed into furcation.

Surgical Therapy

Although some deeper lesions can be controlled with closed scaling and root planing, deeper probing depths often require surgery. Surgery in Class III and IV cases offers the following advantages:

1. Less treatment time for the patient

2. Increased visualization of the root surface for more effective scaling and root planing and root detoxification

3. The chance to perform pocket reduction surgery

4. In cases of advanced disease, the opportunity to regenerate lost tissues

5. The ability to more accurately determine prognosis by visualizing root anatomy

6. Improved access for oral hygiene by the patient

7. Easier access for root planing during SPT

However, not all Class III and IV patients may be candidates for surgery. To be a candidate, the patient should be in good enough physical health to undergo surgery, the teeth must be stable enough to allow a comfortable healing period, and the patient would optimally be a good complier to suggested oral hygiene or SPT or both. In most cases, they should also *(1)* have had adequate closed subgingival scaling and root planing to prevent unneeded surgery or to prepare the tissues for surgery, *(2)* have pocket probing depths of 5 mm or greater, and *(3)* show signs of active disease. The decision to perform surgery is made by both the therapist and the patient and is made after adequate informed consent.

At present, because of our lack of accuracy in deciding when the disease process is active, overtreatment and undertreatment probably occur. Once we are better able to establish disease activity, it may be possible to treat more accurately and more selectively.

Once the decision is made to go ahead with surgery, the therapist must decide (again with the patient's consent) which form (or forms) of surgery will be best for the patient. There are two major categories of surgery for inflammatory periodontal diseases: resective and regenerative.

Resective Surgical Procedures There is a great debate concerning the most effective means to reduce pocket probing depths associated with shallow interdental osseous craters. These craters are the most commonly found bony defect associated with periodontitis[6] and usually manifest clinically as interproximal probing depths ranging from 5 to 6 mm. In those cases where other surgical criteria are met and where the gingival tissues are close to the cementoenamel junction on posterior teeth with normal root lengths, pocket reduction is most predictably performed using positive architecture osseous surgery[7-9] (see chapter 10). This procedure can also be used to lengthen clinical crowns to enhance restorative procedures or esthetics.

Regenerative Surgical Procedures In pocket probing depths associated with bony lesions deeper than 2 mm, regenerative procedures are indicated. These procedures are especially helpful in deep furcation invasions and in large, deep bony pockets. In such cases, bone removal might endanger the long-term prognosis for the tooth.

The four basic approaches to regeneration are (1) the flap operation, (2) the flap operation combined with hard tissue grafting, (3) the flap operation combined with guided tissue regeneration, and finally (4) combinations of the last two procedures. Each of these procedures is accompanied by mechanical debridement of the roots of the teeth and often with biomodification of the root surface (see chapter 11).

The goal of these procedures is regeneration or reattachment. This latter state is characterized by a reunion of connective tissue with a root surface that has previously been deprived of its periodontal ligament.[10]

Compliance and Its Effect on Treatment Planning

Chronic inflammatory diseases by definition are not curable. Patients with these problems require continuous monitoring of their periodontal status and oral hygiene and often require frequent SPT to maintain attachment levels. This means that patient compliance to professional suggestions is of the utmost importance in containing these diseases. Unfortunately, most patients have been shown not to comply to either suggested oral hygiene[11] or SPT.[12]

An Approach to Therapy

Treatment planning is relatively simple for Class III and IV patients who are either optimal or poor compliers to both suggested oral hygiene and SPT. For optimal compliers, all that is necessary is to perform the procedure that removes the supragingival and subgingival etiologic factors most expeditiously and economically (in deeper pocket probing depths this is usually surgery). For noncompliers to oral hygiene and SPT, closed supragingival and subgingival scaling and root planing should be provided since this group's problems worsen after surgery. Problems do, however, arise when choosing the appropriate therapy for the large group of patients who fall between these two extremes. There are no clear answers for these patients, but the following approach can often prove successful.

For those patients who clean well but do not comply to suggested SPT, surgery can be beneficial, but the patients must be informed that periodic professional assessment and SPT will enhance their chances of retaining their dentitions. Patients with less-than-optimal oral hygiene can still have surgery and, if they remain compliant to suggested SPT, their periodontiums often remain stable.[13]

For erratic compliers to oral hygiene and SPT, the choice of therapy becomes even more problematic. These patients often need more advanced care than complete compliers and also benefit from frequent positive reinforcement concerning their dental needs. They will often need occlusal therapy and splinting. Surgery for these patients should be directed toward reducing pocket probing depths to facilitate oral hygiene efforts.

Reevaluation of Chronic Adult Periodontitis

The initial phase of therapy is intended to begin the therapeutic objectives of reducing and controlling the bacterial challenge. Reevaluation allows the practitioner an opportunity to assess how the patient has responded to the therapy and to identify additional therapeutic needs. Although experienced practitioners often identify areas requiring surgical intervention on the basis of the initial examination, the reevaluation is essential to the recognition of atypical response patterns prior to embarking on a therapeutic approach that produces a less-than-optimal outcome. *In the treatment planning process described in this chapter, reevaluation is the means of confirming or modifying the presumptive diagnosis.* Until more specific diagnostic tools are available, clinical response to scaling, root planing, and plaque control provides a practical approach of grouping patients and selecting therapy for the most predictable clinical outcomes.

Expected Reevaluation Findings

1. At sites on *single-rooted teeth* that initially had 4 to 5 mm probing depths:
   * A decrease in probing depths of 1 to 2 mm
   * Elimination of or substantial reduction in signs of disease activity
2. Rationale:
   * Single-rooted teeth with shallow to moderate pocket depths are accessible for scaling and root planing and plaque control. It is therefore possible to accurately assess the quality of therapy and the patient's response to therapy with minimal complicating factors. Such assessments cannot be made in sites with furcation involvement or deeper pocket probing depths. Accessible sites in a patient with chronic adult periodontitis will show a good response to local therapy.

3. A failure to get the expected response in accessible sites may indicate:
   * Inadequate scaling and root planing
   * Inadequate home care
   * A more aggressive disease pattern
4. If the expected response in accessible sites is not achieved, rule out:
   * Inadequate scaling and root planing
   * Inadequate home care
5. Assign a final diagnosis of aggressive periodontitis if the expected response is not achieved in spite of adequate scaling and root planing and home care.
6. If the expected response in accessible sites is achieved:
   * Assign a final diagnosis of chronic adult periodontitis
   * Plan further treatment as necessary for remaining sites with evidence of disease

If a case presents initially as severe adult periodontitis, there is an increased likelihood that the patient is currently, or has previously been, less able to control the microbial challenge, as evidenced by extreme destruction. These patients should be given a presumptive diagnosis of chronic adult periodontitis but may very well have an altered ability to cope with the microbial challenge. The therapist should be especially attuned to reevaluation results following initial therapy. If the patient does not respond predictably during the first phases of therapy, the case of periodontitis should be reclassified as aggressive. This approach will hopefully allow the early identification of some cases that may have a greater likelihood of becoming "refractory" if taken through complete conventional therapy.

TREATMENT PLANNING FOR AGGRESSIVE PERIODONTITIS

Early Onset Types of Periodontitis

Prepubertal Periodontitis Little information is currently available relative to the treatment of prepubertal periodontitis. Most reports indicate that the generalized form of this disease occurs in children with severe and often complex defects in host defenses, most usually monocytes and polymorphonuclear neutrophil leukocytes (PMNs). As a result, these patients usually have other systemic manifestations of their host defect such as severe skin and / or respiratory infections. Such patients require extensive medical workups with the goal of therapy being to limit systemic infection and disease in the hope that the host will mature through puberty with a more competent defense system. Preliminary reports of systemic therapy with granulocyte-colony stimulating factor (G-CSF) have been very promising in controlling not only the systemic complications but also the severe periodontal disease in these children. Local therapy for generalized prepubertal periodontitis includes scaling and root planing and plaque control, plus selected extractions of severely involved primary teeth and administration of antibiotics as an adjunct to therapy. The antibiotics most commonly used in such cases are amoxicillin and Augmentin.®

Localized prepubertal periodontitis is thought to result from a less severe host response defect than that seen in the generalized form. As a result, patients with this disease are less likely to have complicated systemic involvement. Periodontal therapy again includes scaling and root planing and plaque control, with selected extractions and the use of systemic antibiotics as indicated. For all prepubertal cases, close monitoring and frequent supportive periodontal treatment (SPT) are essential. The goal of therapy with prepubertal cases is to control the infection in the primary dentition in the hopes of limiting its expansion into the permanent dentition.

Localized Juvenile Periodontitis Treatment of localized juvenile periodontitis (LJP) has been very well defined in recent years and the essential elements for success now appear to be clear. Since the primary microorganism in these cases is *Actinobacillus actinomycetemcomitans,* which is not a heavy plaque or calculus former, conventional therapy directed at removing plaque and calculus has had little success. Depending upon the preferences of the practitioner and the patient, two general approaches to successful therapy in LJP cases are possible: treatment with and treatment without microbial information.

Treatment With Microbial Information In this approach, pretreatment microbial samples are taken. DNA probe analysis appears to be optimal in these cases.

If microbial analysis reveals *A. actinomycetemcomitans* with no black-pigmented *Bacteroides,* the patient may be treated with closed scaling and root planing plus 100 mg of doxycycline twice daily for 21 days. The patient should be reevaluated clinically and microbiologically 4 to 6 weeks after completion of antibiotic therapy. Chlorhexidine rinses twice daily should be initiated with the start of antibiotics and continued for 6 weeks. If at reev-

aluation the patient is deemed stable clinically and microbiologically, SPT may be instituted or regenerative therapy may be considered. If reevaluation shows continued clinical signs of disease or persistent levels of *A. actinomycetemcomitans,* the patient should be treated by surgical access plus a second course of systemic doxycycline.

If the initial microbiological analysis shows *A. actinomycetemcomitans* plus one of the black-pigmented *Bacteroides* such as *Porphyromonas(Bacteroides)gingivalis* or *Prevotella intermedia (Bacteroides intermedius),* then surgery plus doxycycline is indicated as the first phase of therapy.

LJP cases appear to have great potential for regeneration. However, regeneration should be considered only when the microbial challenge has been adequately controlled.

Treatment Without Microbial Information If clinical and radiographic findings are consistent with LJP, then the clinician can assume that microorganisms present will be sensitive to a member of the tetracycline family of antibiotics. In such cases surgery is carried out in conjunction with the regimen of antibiotics and antimicrobials described above. SPT follows and can be accompanied by DNA probes or microbiologic monitoring if clinical or radiographic signs of the disease recur.

Generalized Juvenile Periodontitis Generalized juvenile periodontitis (GJP) is a confusing term frequently used synonymously with *rapidly progressive periodontitis.* A true case of GJP is one in which lesions originate as LJP but where defects in the host immune system ultimately prevent localization of the lesions. Patients with GJP therefore show symptoms of LJP that later spread

into the premolar region. In these cases *A. actinomycetemcomitans* is usually present, but other suspected pathogens may be involved. Microbial analysis is recommended before therapy and at each reevaluation until clinical and radiographic stability have been achieved. The goal of therapy is elimination of the suspected pathogens, which requires systemic antibiotics. Contrary to the approach recommended for LJP, surgery is not advisable until there are clinical and microbial signs of periodontal stability.

Rapidly Progressive Periodontitis Rapidly progressive periodontitis (RPP) is most likely a collection of several different conditions that may show various microbial and host problems as well as various responses to therapy. Microbial analysis is recommended before therapy and at each evaluation until stability has been achieved. Careful consideration should be given to the possibility of undiagnosed systemic disease that may be compromising the host response in these patients. The goal of therapy should be to strengthen the host, if possible, by means of controlling systemic disease; rest; good nutrition; stress reduction; and elimination of suspected pathogens. Therapy generally includes systemic antibiotics. Surgery should not be considered until clinical and microbial stability have been achieved.

Refractory Periodontitis Refractory periodontitis (RP) is one of the most difficult situations faced by today's practitioners. Since this term encompasses multiple conditions, it is important to group patients routinely referred to as "refractory." For instance, localized deep sites or sites with furcation involvement frequently show disease progression over time even though all other sites in the mouth are stable during SPT. Patients with such sites do not have refractory periodontitis but instead exhibit nonresponsive sites in chronic adult periodontitis. The lack of response in such sites is most likely due to an inability to deliver conventional therapy successfully in very deep sites and in furcation areas. The term refractory periodontitis should therefore most properly be reserved for patients showing disease progression even in sites with mild to moderate previous disease and minimal furcation involvement. This progression is seen in spite of good conventional therapy and regular supportive periodontal therapy. Treatment of refractory periodontitis should follow the same approach and protocols as described for rapidly progressive periodontitis.

It should be clear that aggressive types of periodontitis pose substantial risk to the patient and provide substantial frustration for the practitioner. Cases of aggressive periodontitis may be most appropriately dealt with by specialists who have a particular interest and experience in managing them. Extensive studies of progress in this area should provide additional insights that may facilitate more predictable management of these cases.

Reevaluation of Aggressive Periodontitis Cases

Reevaluation of all cases classified as aggressive periodontitis should follow the same clinical protocols as described for reevaluation of cases of chronic adult periodontitis. In addition, microbial analysis is recommended since it is currently assumed that more rigorous microbial control is essential to stability. Once control has been achieved, patients with aggressive periodontitis may be treated as if they had chronic disease. Our experience indicates that with the exception of LJP, the aggressive forms of periodontal disease frequently do not benefit by and may actually be worsened by surgical approaches instituted before a chronic state of stability is achieved.

QUICK REVIEW

I. Make a diagnosis
Health:
- No signs of current or past periodontal disease

Gingivitis:
- Most cases will be chronic gingivitis: traditional approaches to reducing bacterial insult (see pages 103 to 123).
- Other forms of gingivitis (see pages 78 to 80).

Periodontitis:
- Most cases will be chronic adult periodontitis: traditional approaches to reducing bacterial insult (see pages 124 to 194).
- Aggressive forms of periodontitis (see pages 2-3 to 2-5).

II. Treatment planning for chronic gingivitis and chronic adult periodontitis

Initial therapy:
- Begins after initial examination, diagnosis, and acceptance of treatment plan by the patient.
- By definition this therapy is nonsurgical.
- A general outline is as follows:
  - modification, where appropriate, of personal oral hygiene
  - removal of subgingival and supra gingival deposits with closed scaling and root planing
  - reevaluation in approximately 30 days
  - therapy to eliminate occlusal trauma, when appropriate
  - reevaluation:
    (1) surgery where appropriate, followed by SPT
    (2) SPT if surgery is not performed

Quick Review continues on page 96.

QUICK REVIEW
(continued)

- Nonsurgical therapy is most often successful for Class I and II cases.
- This stage is an appropriate time to place dental implants (one and two stage).

Surgical therapy:

- Many Class III and most Class IV cases will benefit from surgery.
- To achieve the maximum efficacy from these procedures, the patient should have:
  — adequate physical condition
  — stable teeth
  — adequate compliance to oral hygiene and / or SPT
  — had previous closed subgingival scaling and root planing
  — at least 5 mm pocket probing depths that show signs of active disease
- There are two basic types of surgery:
  — resective: this works best in most Class III cases
  — regenerative: this works best in some Class III and most Class IV cases
- Second stage implant surgery can be combined with periodontal surgery.

III. Compliance

- Most patients do not comply to professional suggestions.
- Those who do not comply to either suggested personal oral hygiene or SPT are not surgical candidates.

Treatment planning approach based on compliance and any alternative to the traditional approach:

- For patients with optimal oral hygiene or complete compliance to suggested SPT, simply remove tooth-borne accretions in the simplest way possible. Note that this often means surgery. SPT follows this care.
- For noncompliers to oral hygiene and SPT, remove as much of the supragingival and subgingival plaque and calculus as possible using nonsurgical means, then suggest that the patient be monitored at appropriate SPT intervals.
- For erratic compliers to personal oral hygiene and SPT, surgery is often beneficial for those meeting the other surgical criteria.

IV. Treatment planning for aggressive periodontitis

Early types of onset periodontitis:

- *Prepubertal periodontitis:*
  — generalized: local and systemic therapy
  — localized: local and possibly systemic therapy
- *Localized juvenile periodontitis:* clinician may opt to treat surgically or nonsurgically with or without microbial sampling or DNA probes.
- *Generalized juvenile periodontitis:* probably continuation of LJP; microbial monitoring is suggested.
- *Rapidly progressive periodontitis:* microbial monitoring suggested.

Periodontitis associated with systemic disease:

- Diabetes (see chapter 17)
- HIV (see chapter 5)

Adult onset / refractory periodontitis: follows well-delivered traditional therapy; microbial monitoring is suggested.

REFERENCES

1. Corn H, Marks MH: Strategic extraction in periodontal therapy. *Dent Clin North Am* 1969;13:817.

2. Stambaugh RV, Dragoo M, Smith DM, Carasal L: The limits of subgingival scaling. *Int J Periodont Rest Dent* 1981;1:30.

3. Waerhaug J: Healing of the dento-epithelial junction following subgingival plaque control. II. As observed on extracted teeth. *J Periodontol* 1978;49:119-134.

4. Caffesse RG, Sweeney PL, Smith BA: Scaling and root planing with and without periodontal flap surgery. *J Clin Periodontol* 1986;13(13):205.

5. Brayer WK, Mellonig JT, Dunlap RM, Marinak KW, Carson RE: Scaling and root planing effectiveness: The effect of root surface access and operator experience. *J Periodontol* 1989;60:67-72.

6. Saari JT, Hurt WC, Biggs NL: Periodontal bony defects on the dry skull. *J Periodontol* 1968;39:278.

7. Everett FG, Waerhaug J, Widman A: Leonard Widman: Surgical treatment of pyorrhea alveolaris. *J Periodontol* 1971;42:571.

8. Schluger S: Osseous resection — a basic principle in periodontal surgery. *Oral Surg* 1949;2:316.

9. Ochsenbein C, Ross S: A re-evaluation of osseous surgery. *Dent Clin North Am* 1969;13:87.

10. American Academy of Periodontology: *Current Procedural Terminology for Periodontics.* Chicago: American Academy of Periodontology, 1986.

11. Johansson L, Oster B, Hamp S: Evaluation of cause related periodontal therapy and compliance with maintenance care recommendations. *J Clin Periodontol* 1984;11:689.

12. Wilson TG, Glover ME, Schoen J, Baus C, Jacobs T: Compliance with maintenance therapy in a private periodontal practice. *J Periodontol* 1984; 55:468.

13. Shick RA: Maintenance phase of periodontal therapy. *J Periodontol* 1981;52:576.

The Referral Process

by Richard D. Wilson

Introduction	Responsibilities of a referring dentist
Selection of a periodontist	

INTRODUCTION

The referral process is an integral component of all three aspects of clinical periodontics: diagnosis, therapy, and supportive periodontal therapy (maintenance). Decisions regarding patient care often include seeking the help of another dentist. This may involve merely advice and counsel or an actual referral of the patient for treatment. The tradition of referring the patient is well established in dentistry, is a reflection of the caring practitioner, and has substantially elevated the level of oral health care.

Decisions to refer patients are influenced by a number of disparate factors. These include egos, competition, varying levels of competence, personal ethics, and the potential of litigation. Such factors influence specialists and general dentists alike. Therapeutically speaking, the prognosis of the treatment being offered by the general dentist and its degree of success also affects the referral decision. If careful and thorough root planing and scaling in the office of the general dentist does not arrest the active signs of periodontal disease, surgical intervention should be considered in probing pocket depths of 5 mm or greater.

The decision to treat surgically or to refer is not only influenced by the above factors, but also by the general dentist's abilities, confidence level, and preferences and by patient attitude. Patient welfare must be the practitioner's primary concern.

SELECTION OF A PERIODONTIST

Many general dentists select a periodontist the way many patients select a general dentist: by what others say and by location. "Personality" of a specialist — a vague, all-encompassing term usually meaning whether he / she is likeable — is important in creating rapport with both patient and referring dentist. Although never mutually exclusive, a dynamic personality does not ensure competence. With good reason, patients express a preference for a conveniently located specialist. However, these two factors, personality and location, should be secondary to the quality of a periodontist's care. It may require a number of referred patients as well as personal conferences with the periodontist before the general dentist decides to sustain a referral relationship. Other factors in this relationship affect patient care and professional compatibility:

1. What happens to referred patients? Do they get "lost?" Is the referring dentist constantly informed of patient progress, postponed or interrupted treatment, or of problems that have developed during treatment? Are patients returned to the referring dentist? Are patients referred on to others without consultation with the original therapist?

2. Does the periodontist consult frequently about care of the patient? Are all referred patients, regardless of the individuality of problem, funneled into the same duplicatable therapy? Does the periodontist seek the opinion of the referring dentist? Is there a mutuality in consultation as treatment plans are developed?

3. How do referred patients react? Do they complain of pain? Of staff indifference? Or of the periodontist's haste or lack of time to discuss patient inquiries?

4. What is the quality of care that is received at the periodontist's office? Is there adequate attached gingiva remaining surrounding teeth that are to receive intracrevicular restorations? Does gingival retraction reveal retained calculus? Do pockets still bleed? With time, do many patients demonstrate multiple recurrent disease sites?

RESPONSIBILITIES OF A REFERRING DENTIST

Once the decision to refer is made by the general dentist, the process should proceed with equal concern for the same communication and quality of care that is expected of the periodontist. During the referral consultation, the patient should be informed of the benefits of the treatment to be presented by the specialist. If the periodontist and general dentist so agree, a candid review of risks, options, and disadvantages of treatment should take place to aid the patient and his/her decision.

Only one specialist's name should be given to the patient. A transfer of confidence is most helpful to the specialist, and this is difficult if three or four names are casually given by the referring dentist. In these cases, the patient usually will then seek the advice of others, often resulting in a selection not in keeping with the referring dentist's wishes or needs.

Prior to the referral, the general dentist should review what additional treatment he/she is anticipating after the periodontist has completed treatment. A fee quotation, probably estimated, is very appropriate here. The periodontist should not only be aware of the fee but should also have participated in planning the postperiodontal treatment. Just as the periodontist should not dictate treatment to the referring dentist, so should the referring dentist not "lock" the periodontist into a specific treatment. Final decisions should be developed mutually and then mutually presented to the patient as agreed upon therapy.

Recent periapical radiographs of high quality are imperative and must precede the patient to the periodontist's office. The patient should be informed that the periodontist may take additional films as necessary. The periodontist is legally and morally obligated to examine the patient's entire dentition. Even if the patient is referred for treatment for one site only, that patient should be told to expect a complete and thorough full-mouth examination by the periodontist.

The periodontist should be informed of the patient's past dental history, either as it took place in the referring dentist's office or in a predecessor's office. The periodontist may not be able to support the general dentist's previous care (or suggested future treatment) unless good communication takes place.

Periodontal treatment may involve some discomfort, possibly occasional and unexpected episodes of hemorrhage or postsurgical tooth sensitivity. Patients may complain to their referring dentists. Just as the referring dentist expects support from the periodontist, so should these patient concerns be overcome by strong supporting comments by the referring dentist.

The timing of a referral may be fundamental to treatment success. Delay in a referral could change a treatable situation into a hopeless one. It is a rare 7-mm pocket that wasn't 4 or 5 mm at one time. Timely inclusion of a specialist in therapy may preserve a patient's confidence as well as a patient's dentition.

The periodontist and the general dentist must establish a therapeutic understanding on patient care. If the general dentist has a strong preference to implement initial root planing and scaling in his/her office, the periodontist should help shape these skills. If the general dentist needs guidance as to the timing of a referral for surgery, the periodontist might consider offering such counsel without prejudice. Difficult decisions regarding referral to other specialists, how to deal with recurrent periodontal disease or caries, and how to confront the sharing of supportive periodontal treatment (SPT; formerly called maintenance) should be addressed early on in a referral relationship.

The SPT dilemma is one of divisive controversy. In some cases of periodontal disease that are difficult to manage, the periodontist's office should be solely responsible for ongoing support of periodontal care. Clearly, these cases compel appropriate communication with the referring dentist. In most instances, however, the sharing of patient care is best, but only if the quality of the SPT is comparable. Patients who receive an hour of thorough root planing and scaling in one office may not be satisfied with a 20-minute recall visit in another office. Fees may also impact on patient preference. Patients may request to be maintained in one office only. Practitioners should do everything possible to resist these preferences and should attempt to keep patients on a mutual care basis.

Just as the general dentist should expect quality care from the periodontist, so the periodontist should expect quality care from the general dentist. Quality of care may be the most damaging factor in disrupting a referral relationship.

The termination of a referral relationship should always be accompanied by an explanation. Frequently, a specialist is bewildered by a general dentist's abrupt withdrawal from referring patients. If a correctable problem exists, the specialist should know about it and take steps to correct it.

Lastly, both the periodontist and the referring dentist should be willing to work together to moderate fees and therapy with those patients who are well-motivated but may not be financially competent. In many cases these patients will eventually be able to complete proper, more sophisticated therapy. As always, patients must be informed of the risks involved.

PART II

Therapy for Chronic Gingivitis and Chronic Adult Periodontitis

How to Use Chapters 8 Through 12

The following five chapters comprise a different approach to treatment for patients with chronic periodontal diseases. Traditional approaches detailed various surgical and nonsurgical procedures, but often the reader was left with the mechanical skill but without the knowledge of where that skill was best applied. Our approach first assumes that the clinician has made a proper diagnosis. It is therefore suggested that if you have not become intimately familiar with those chapters dealing with diagnosis, that you do so before trying to apply the information found in the following pages.

Proper use of chapters 8 to 12 requires that the clinician has already determined that the patient most likely has one of the chronic periodontal diseases (see chapter 5).

Although pocket probing depths alone do not dictate therapy, the severity of past disease does indicate the patient's ability to handle the microbial challenge and does suggest therapeutic approaches that are most likely to adhere to the therapeutic principle of reducing the microbial load and maintaining a reduced microbial challenge.

This section is grouped by diagnosis and chapters are meant to be followed in order. Chapter 8 on chronic gingivitis deals with patients who have 1- to 3-mm pocket probing depths (Class I) and bleeding on probing; this material deals primarily with oral hygiene.

Mild chronic adult periodontitis (4- to 5-mm probing depths with minimal or no gingival recession and no furcation invasion) is dealt with first by oral hygiene then with closed subgingival scaling and root planing (Class II). The subject of personal oral hygiene is not covered in this chapter in detail, but the reader is referred back to the chapter on gingivitis. These first two chapters compose what can also be termed *initial* or *basic periodontal therapy*.

Moderate chronic adult periodontitis includes those patients who have been taught oral hygiene and who have had adequate closed subgingival scaling and root planing but who at reevaluation after initial therapy still have minimal or no recession associated with 5- to 6-mm probing depths (usually with bone loss in furcations), and signs of active disease (moderate adult {chronic} periodontitis — Class III). Regenerative procedures are suggested for patients who have had initial therapy and who have residual probing depths of 7 mm or more with signs suggestive of active disease (Class IV patients).

This section closes with a chapter on supportive periodontal treatment, formerly termed maintenance, which is an integral part of periodontal therapy.

Chronic Gingivitis

CURRENT CONCEPTS by Bjorn Steffensen

CLINICAL APPLICATION by John S. Sottosanti

CURRENT CONCEPTS
Definition of chronic gingivitis
Epidemiology of chronic gingivitis
Etiology of gingivitis
Histopathology of gingivitis
Progression of chronic gingivitis to periodontitis
Rationale for prevention and treatment of chronic gingivitis
Prevention and treatment modalities

CLINICAL APPLICATION
Treatment goal
Examination

Patient consultation
Plaque control
Manual personal oral hygiene
Mechanical appliances
Chemical plaque control
Appointment management
Calculus removal
Posttreatment evaluation

QUICK REVIEW

REFERENCES

C U R R E N T   C O N C E P T S

DEFINITION OF CHRONIC GINGIVITIS

The term *gingivitis* has been defined as inflammation of the marginal gingiva.[1] Specifically, *chronic* indicates that the inflammatory disease state may be present for an extended period of time. Several types of gingivitis have been recognized, such as plaque-associated, acute necrotizing ulcerative, hormonal, drug-induced, and desquamative gingivitis (Table 8-1). This chapter focuses on plaque-associated chronic gingivitis.

The clinical signs of inflammation in the gingival tissues reflect the classical signs of inflammation: rubor (redness), tumor (swelling), calor (warmth), and dolor (pain). Although these signs may be readily apparent to the dentist or dental hygienist, the threshold for discomfort experienced by patients with chronic gingivitis is commonly not reached. This chronic inflammation is therefore often not discovered by the individual or is tolerated well over an extended period of time.

Gingivitis is ubiquitous in most populations, reaching prevalences of around 90%. To address the potential impact of this disease, the following discussion includes the epidemiology, etiology, pathogenesis, risk of progression to periodontitis, and rationale for treatment. Also included are approaches to intervention based on current knowledge about the disease process.

EPIDEMIOLOGY OF CHRONIC GINGIVITIS

The epidemiology of gingivitis is important when the potential risks for progression of gingivitis to periodontitis are determined and when decisions are made related to the allotment of resources for treatment and prevention. Unfortunately, a major constraint in evaluating and comparing existing data on gingivitis is the lack of agreement regarding diagnosis criteria between studies.[2] However, sufficient data are available

TABLE 8-1 *Classification of gingivitis*

Chronic gingivitis	Longstanding; plaque-associated
Acute necrotizing ulcerative gingivitis	
1. Otherwise systemically healthy	Vincent's
2. AIDS-associated gingivitis	Unique clinical appearance
Steroid hormone-influenced gingivitis	Puberty; pregnancy; birth control medication; steroids
Medication-influenced gingival overgrowth	Phenytoin; cyclosporin; nifedipine
Desquamative gingivitis	
1. Dermatoses	Erosive lichen planus; pemphigoid; pemphigus
2. Allergic reactions	
Other causes of gingivitis	Blood disorders; nutritional deficiencies; tumors; genetics; mouthbreathing; bacterial or viral infections

to distinguish general trends for the distribution of gingivitis.

Gingivitis can be found in early childhood and apparently affects a high number of children. Thus, in spite of considerable variation between studies, the prevalence of gingivitis has been reported to be as high as 36% and 64% among 3- and 5-year-old Swedish children, respectively.[3] From studies in several countries, there are good indications that the prevalence and severity of gingivitis among children increase with age to reach a peak prevalence of 90% around the age of 11.[4-6] As children enter adolescence the prevalence begins to decline, a trend

that continues through the age of 17.[6]

Epidemiologic studies of gingivitis in adult persons, conducted several decades apart, have suggested that the prevalence of gingivitis increases between the ages of 20 and 70 years.[4,7] In the age group over 30 years, as many as 95% of examined persons presented with clinical signs of plaque-associated gingivitis. In comparison, when the most recent national survey of oral health in the United States[8] used bleeding on probing as an indicator of gingival inflammation, it was observed that 44% of the examined persons between the ages of 18 and 64 years had sites with bleeding on probing. Approximately 5% of the studied sites bled on examination. This variation between the studies also demonstrates that varying measures of disease may provide different estimates of gingival inflammation in a population. While this United States survey found little change with age, a Danish population study observed an increase in the proportion of teeth with at least one bleeding site from the ages of 16 to 19 years through the ages of 65 to 81 years.[9]

Inflammatory conditions in the gingival tissues such as chronic gingivitis cannot be considered compatible with oral health. For this reason there is ample concern that chronic gingivitis is widespread in the general population.

ETIOLOGY OF GINGIVITIS

Microbiology

Gingival inflammation has been associated with the presence of "tartar" and deposits on the teeth for centuries,[10] but it was not until the late 1950s and early 1960s that

the role of plaque in the etiology of chronic gingivitis became more clearly understood. It was then demonstrated that roughness of tooth surfaces or gold foil, when placed in contact with gingival tissues, would lead to gingival inflammation only if bacteria were concurrently present on these surfaces.[11,12] Studies performed in germ-free animals supported the role of bacteria as a primary etiologic factor in the development of gingival inflammation; dental calculus that formed in those animals was not associated with gingival inflammation until bacterial plaque was introduced into the ecological system.[13,14]

Shortly thereafter, in 1965, Löe and co-workers presented the results of experimental gingivitis studies in humans.[15,16] Dental students who initially had healthy gingiva abstained from all oral hygiene procedures; bacterial plaque was allowed to accumulate. Clinical signs of gingival inflammation developed after 10 to 14 days of plaque accumulation on the teeth. Characteristic shifts in the microbiota were also noted over time. The composition changed from one consisting predominantly of gram-positive cocci and rods towards one with a significantly higher proportion of gram-negative fusiforms, filaments, and eventually spirochetes as the gingival inflammation developed. Of great significance was the finding that upon reinstitution of plaque-removing measures, the signs of inflammation were reversed and the return to a healthy gingival condition was assured.[17] These studies demonstrated beyond a doubt that plaque was to be considered the main etiologic agent as well as the point of focus in prevention and treatment of chronic gingivitis.

In these studies of "experimental gingivitis," the focus had been on the presence and amount of plaque; the results therefore created the basis for the *nonspecific plaque hypothesis,* which emphasized that the number of microorganisms was the major factor of importance. It has since become clear that certain microorganisms in the plaque are present at significantly higher levels in specific periodontal disease processes and that some bacteria apparently possess greater potential for producing tissue inflammation than others. The hypothesis that select microorganisms may be responsible for the disease processes was termed the *specific plaque hypothesis,* and it was proposed that the disease processes could be controlled by the use of antibiotics to specifically eliminate select pathogenic bacteria.[18]

Studies of the microbiota during the transition from a state of health to gingivitis have assisted in clarifying the roles of certain microorganisms in this process. First, during the increase in plaque mass and thickness, members of the gram positive genera *Actinomyces* and *Streptococcus,* which also are associated with plaque of healthy sites, predominate in the supragingival plaque. As experimental gingivitis develops, there is a shift towards an *Actinomyces-*dominated plaque along with increases in the subgingival flora of gram-negative species including *Fusobacterium nucleatum, Veillonella parvula,* and *Treponema.*[19-22] In chronic or long-standing gingivitis, 25% of the bacteria may be gram-negative and include large filaments members of *Fusobacterium, Veillonella, Campylobacter,* and *Prevotella intermedia (Bacteroides intermedius).*[22-24] It is significant to note that gingivitis with bleeding was associated with *Actinomyces viscosus* and pigmenting *Bacteroides,* which are also found in sites

of periodontal disease.[21] Thus, there are good indications of sequential progression of species during the development of gingivitis rather than just an increase in the number of microorganisms.

In spite of strong correlations between specific bacteria and gingival inflammation, these associations may be parallel temporal phenomena rather than causative relationships. For example, early efforts to eliminate selected components of the microbiota were not successful in preventing experimental gingivitis development.[25] Current concepts suggest that gingival inflammation develops when selected bacterial species accumulate in undisturbed and maturing plaque. Therapy should therefore focus on interfering with plaque maturation to prevent gingivitis. This may be accomplished successfully by regular mechanical cleaning at least every 48 hours.[26] Another approach to disturb the maturation may be the selective inhibition of *Actinomyces* species which appear to be essential for later stages of plaque development. Recent studies of the effects of oral irrigation in gingivitis have raised interesting questions as well.[27-29] Irrigation with water alone reduced gingival inflammation without changes in the clinical plaque score or the microbial composition of the plaque. One may speculate that the irrigation diluted or removed microbially derived agents capable of invoking inflammation in the gingival tissues.

In spite of a better understanding of the role of microorganisms in chronic gingivitis, a scientific basis for intercepting the development of gingival inflammation by targeting specific microorganisms has not yet emerged. Therefore, in preventing and treating chronic gingivitis in the majority

of patients, we currently have to rely on a nonspecific model aiming for regular plaque removal and elimination of plaque-retaining factors.

Contributing Factors

The influence of local factors has been reviewed previously in detail.[30] A few select conditions of some controversy will be discussed in this section, including tooth malalignment, width of the attached and keratinized gingiva, and faulty restorations.

The position or malalignment of teeth has been assigned various degrees of importance to plaque accumulation and thereby gingival inflammation. In the wake of various study approaches that yielded contradictory results, it was demonstrated that the effect of malalignment is influenced by the general degree of plaque control in the patient.[31] Thus, in categories of patients with either perfect or very poor oral hygiene levels, the plaque accumulation around a malaligned tooth was found to be affected very little. In contrast, among patients with a medium degree of plaque control, malalignment could be isolated as an important contributory factor to local plaque accumulation and gingival inflammation.

Another localized phenomenon of controversy has been whether the amount of keratinized and attached gingiva provides increased resistance to gingival inflammation. Most studies contain results for teeth without restorations. For example, it was shown in animal studies by histological evaluation that a gingival area supported by loosely attached mucosa had no higher susceptibility to plaque-induced inflammation, and the size of the inflammatory cell infiltrate was similar to that seen in areas with a wide band of supporting keratinized and attached gingiva.[32,33] Controlled longitudinal clinical trials in humans have not been able to show that a certain minimum width of the attached and keratinized gingiva is critical to development or progression of gingival inflammation.[34,35]

Quite recently, new data again have stressed the importance of careful restorative procedures that extend subgingivally.[36] It was demonstrated that around clinically perfect margins there were only minor tissue changes and the microbiota reflected gingival health. In contrast, when restorations with overhanging, subgingival margins were inserted at the same sites, gingival inflammation developed and a subgingival microbiota evolved that had increased proportions of anaerobic gram-negative microorganisms and also contained black-pigmenting *Bacteroides* species. These findings clearly illustrate the importance of avoiding restorations or other types of prosthodontic devices that promote local plaque accumulation and maturation and thereby jeopardize gingival health.

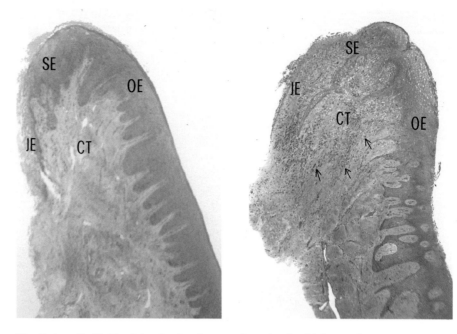

Fig 8-1a (left) *The histologic picture of a gingival biopsy from an area that has been maintained at optimal clinical health for 4 months. The junctional epithelium* (JE) *is well defined and distinct in its structure from sulcular* (SE) *and oral epithelium* (OE). *In the connective tissue* (CT), *practically-no inflammatory cells are detectable.*

Fig 8-1b (right) *After 4 months of gingival inflammation, note that the appearance of a histologic section of gingiva is characterized by inflammatory alterations. Such changes from health include the presence of an infiltrate by inflammatory cells* (small arrows) *that extends deeply into the connective tissue* (CT). *In addition, changes in the structure of the junctional* (JE) *and sulcular* (SE) *epithelium are common along with vascular proliferation. (Figures 8-1a and b courtesy of Dr N. P. Lang.)*

HISTOPATHOLOGY OF GINGIVITIS

The histological characteristics of chronic gingivitis have been studied in animals as well as humans (Figs 8-1a and b). Page and Schroeder[37] in 1976 presented a classification for the pathogenesis of gingivitis that categorized the histopathological events into three sequential stages: initial lesion, early lesion, and established lesion of gingival inflammation.

Initial Lesion

According to Page and Schroe-der's classification, the earliest stage of gingival inflammation is the *initial lesion*, which occurs within 4 days of the beginning of plaque accumulation. At this time no clinical signs of inflammation are detectable. However, within the tissues the host response to the bacterial accumulation and the challenge from the toxic microbial by-products presents itself as an acute inflammatory reaction.[37,38] At this stage the inflammatory cells are mainly neutrophilic granulocytes and macrophages that accumulate in the coronal portion of the connective tissue. Although present at all stages of the gingival inflammation, the neutrophils become less prominent in later stages when the levels of other inflammatory cell types increase. These neutrophilic granulocytes may be contributory to the loss of collagen, which is already observed in the connective tissue at this early point in time.[39] There is increased vascularity, and the intercellular spaces widen between the junctional epithelial cells and maintain the junction between gingiva and tooth. From the subepithelial vascular plexus there is increased fluid penetration and migration of polymorphonuclear leukocytes (PMNs) into the gingival sulcus. This exudate is known as the *gingival crevicular fluid.*

Although not yet a reliable indicator of disease activity, increases in fluid flow as well as certain inflammatory mediators and enzymes have been shown to be associated with gingival inflammation.[40,41]

Early Lesion

Uninterrupted plaque accumulation will promote progression to the next stage of inflammation, termed the *early lesion*. It evolves after approximately 7 days of plaque accumulation and may then persist for extended periods of time.[42] The alterations are still located just beneath the junctional epithelium and lymphocytes become the major inflammatory cell type (about 75%), along with macrophages.[43] The vascular changes are more pronounced and the changes of the connective tissue component now include lysis of paravascular connective tissue and degenerative changes of fibroblasts.[37] In the infiltrated area, the destruction of collagen may reach 60% to 70%.[43] When exposing clinically healthy gingiva to undisturbed plaque accumulation in humans, the histopathological events characteristic of the early lesion have been observed to develop after 3 weeks[44] and to persist for as long as 6 months.[37,46]

Established Lesion

The final stage of the reversible inflammatory changes is termed the *established lesion*. Inflammation of this character may evolve with the passage of variable periods of time and can then persist for months or years without progression to periodontitis. The area of inflammation is further extended, and plasma cells and B-lymphocytes become the predominant cells of the infiltrate. In addition, the junctional and pocket epithelia are highly infiltrated by PMNs,[46] and cells from the junctional epithelium form rete pegs as they proliferate into the underlying degenerating subepithelial connective tissue. The attachment to the tooth of this ulcerated epithelium may be lost, and a sulcus lined by pocket epithelium may form.[47]

While the stages described above accurately reflect the histology of developing gingivitis, great variations may be seen in the transitions. Also, it is important to note that as inflammatory alterations in the tissues advance on a histological level, the classical signs of inflammation, including redness, swelling, and bleeding on probing, become detectable in the clinic, and the diagnosis of gingivitis can be attained.

PROGRESSION OF CHRONIC GINGIVITIS TO PERIODONTITIS

Until recently, it was a widely accepted concept that gingivitis, if left untreated, over time would lead to destructive periodontitis.[48] The periodontal destruction would then progress over the years at a relatively constant rate. However, recent studies have radically altered this perception of the periodontal disease process. Current evidence strongly indicates that the chance of periodontal destructions developing in a site with gingival inflammation is less than previously believed, and that at least some of the destructive disease events occur in short episodes, or "bursts." Of particular interest has been the great difference in the prevalence of gingivitis and destructive periodontitis that has been observed in the adult population. The prevalence of gingivitis in some studies has approached 90% of the examined persons, but only about 10% of the individuals exhibited signs of advanced periodontitis.[4,8,49] Such results have been shown in populations with a poor oral hygiene, severe gingivitis, and very limited access to oral health care[49,50] as well as in populations with a better level of oral hygiene and access to dental services.[4,51] The risk of developing periodontitis of milder severity is higher. This is illustrated by the recent United States survey from 1985 to 1986, which found the prevalence of persons with at least one site of attachment loss of 4 mm or over to be 24%.[8]

In clinical studies, periodontal changes can be monitored over time in greater detail than in epidemiological surveys. When a group of 61 adult persons with varying severity of gingivitis but no periodontitis was followed during a 3-year time period without treatment, the incidence of conversions of chronic gingivitis to periodontitis was very low.[52] This study illustrates that over a relatively short time, compared to life-long exposure, very few gingivitis sites will present clinically measurable loss of periodontium by conventional diagnostic methods (see chapter 4).

The principle that periodontitis does not always develop at sites of gingivitis has been supported by results from long-term experimental studies of dogs.[38,53] As a result of plaque accumulation by soft diet, in the absence of oral hygiene measures, local periodontal lesions and bone loss were experimentally provoked. However, from the results of these investigations it became clear that there were great variations in disease susceptibility between the animals. Some of the dogs did not develop periodontitis at any sites of gingivitis. In other studies of dogs in the age range of 8 to 14 years and characterized by large amounts of plaque deposits, calculus, and chronic gingivitis, around 20% of the animals presented no signs of periodontal breakdown during examination.[38]

Histologically, there is evidence from such animal models that in a periodontium with long-standing gingivitis there will be episodes of acute inflammation in localized areas. At these sites there is ulceration of the junctional epithelium and infiltration by neutrophils as well as increased osteoclast activity. The active periods are then followed by longer quiescent periods.[54,55]

The results of clinical studies in humans have demonstrated also that attachment loss at individual sites tends to occur in episodic "bursts" of disease activity.[56-58] It was determined that a low frequency of recorded sites (2% to 6%) showed clinical breakdown during a 1-year period. These data were derived from a combination of gingivitis and periodontitis sites in patients with past experience of periodontitis and may therefore be an overestimate of the risk of progression for patients with gingivitis only. However, the results are in agreement with the previously described studies of disease progression patterns in other models and therefore bear clear implications to the relationship between gingival inflammation and progression to destructive periodontal disease.

Thus, current knowledge indicates that although gingivitis is widespread in the populations, only a small number of these gingivitis sites in a limited number of susceptible persons will develop into periodontitis with loss of attachment. The mechanism of attachment loss is most probably one of episodic bursts of acute inflammatory activity at select sites. One may speculate that determinants for such localized disease activity may be unbalanced alterations in the pathogenicity of the plaque, the host response, and local factors.

RATIONALE FOR PREVENTION AND TREATMENT OF CHRONIC GINGIVITIS

When considering the need for prevention and treatment of gingivitis, an important factor to consider is the cost-benefit ratio as this relates to the economical, functional, and personal well-being of the individual, as well as to the population as a whole. For the professional who is confronted daily with chronic gingivitis in the individual patient, two questions arise. Can chronic gingivitis be prevented and treated effectively? And, what are the benefits of such efforts?

Several studies have evaluated the effects of various periodontal procedures over time in controlling the periodontal health status. In a unique approach, the effects of prophylactic measures were evaluated among large groups of Swedish persons.[59,60] Groups of 209 schoolchildren ages 7 to 14 years and 375 adults received individual oral hygiene instructions and regular frequent prophylaxes by dental hygienists. After study periods of 2 years for the children and 3 years for the adults, the periodontal status was carefully reevaluated. The children generally had very limited plaque accumu-lation on their teeth and only negligible signs of gingivitis. The adults who followed the program adopted improved oral hygiene habits and had only negligible signs of gingivitis and no new periodontal attachment loss. This status was clearly better than that of a control group, which, in spite of regular dental care, had gingivitis, continued loss of periodontium, and new carious lesions.

Comparable results of preventive periodontal approaches have been shown among such differing groups as factory workers in Norway, young Californian employees, and US Air Force students, during study periods of 3 to 5 years.[61-63] On the basis of these reports it may be concluded that the combination of regular and thorough self care by individuals and preventive professional therapy does lead to improved gingival health, decreased attachment loss, and maintenance of the natural dentition. From an economical aspect, over time the initial added expenses to preventive programs may well be converted to substantial gains from savings on otherwise needed complex treatment procedures such as tooth replacements. Based on existing data, a recent United States governmental task force strongly emphasized the value of preventive measures in managing gingivitis and periodontitis.[64]

In the context of a population approach and the previously described limited risk of disease progression, if frequent dental visits for periodontal management are prescribed for all persons, we may be overtreating a proportion of the population who are at low risk. But while it might therefore be best to only direct efforts towards persons at risk, unfortunately at this time risk profiles for identifying such persons of susceptibility are not available. However, it is known from closely monitored patients in clinical studies with prior history of at least mild to moderate periodontitis as an indicator of susceptibility, that the periodontal disease process will progress if left untreated.[57]

Today it still remains a major problem that there is no easy, reliable method of isolating periodontal sites with disease activity from stable sites. One very interesting line of research has correlated bleeding on probing to the risk for progressing periodontal attachment loss. Although not highly accurate as a predictive tool, there is considerable promise in this method of managing periodontal patients.[65]

Once a patient has been identified as susceptible, has undergone quality care, and is under careful maintenance, the prognosis for long-term periodontal health is good. It is known from longitudinal studies of posttreatment maintenance therapy that repeated prophylaxis to control gingival inflammation at regular intervals will greatly delay or prevent reemergence of active disease in the patient.[66]

In conclusion, on a population basis, we should make it a top priority to develop diagnostics that identify persons at risk for periodontal disease or sites of disease activity. Currently, in the absence of such reliable diagnostic indicators, treatment should be based on a preventive approach. It is now known that controlled oral hygiene in combination with professional prophylaxes at regular intervals is effective in preventing transition from gingivitis to periodontitis. In persons with chronic gingivitis, the care should focus on behavioral modification, motivation of the patient, and elimination of local factors important to plaque retention.

PREVENTION AND TREATMENT MODALITIES

Oral Hygiene Control

As described above, gingival inflammation can be controlled in both adults and children who follow intensive supportive periodontal treatment programs provided by dental hygienists.[59,60] The challenge, however, is to achieve such a level of patient motivation for optimal oral health that the responsibility for thorough oral hygiene can be transferred successfully from the practitioner to the patient.

Methods for motivation and patient instruction have been researched; scientifically based theories that are now available should be integrated into daily practice.[67,68] It is known that individualized and specifically designed oral hygiene interventions may be required to improve oral hygiene behavior, skills, and attitudes. For example, some people may accept and respond well to repeated instructions, but others may react with resistance to this approach and demand greater personal responsibility.[61,62,69]

To involve the patient in a process leading to greater self-interest and personal responsibility, self-instruction programs have yielded encouraging long-term improvements in achieving oral cleanliness and gingival health.[59,70,71] Success in such patient motivation and instruction also relies on active feedback mechanisms, which may be built into self-instructional programs.[71] The oral hygiene therapist should be available to the patient for counseling and demonstrations and should develop a good understanding of personality characteristics, and should develop an individualized schedule for re-evaluation and feedback.[67,72]

Researchers have realized that improvements in oral hygiene levels do not depend so much on toothbrush designs or specific methods as they do upon the performance and motivation by the person using any of the methods.[72] Although no specific toothbrush design appears to be universally superior in plaque removal, it has been recognized that soft, rounded-end bristles may be less damaging to the gingival tissues.[73] Toothbrushing may be effective in removing plaque on buccal and lingual surfaces, but it will not reach interdental plaque. For this reason a series of other oral hygiene devices are available, including dental floss or tape, interdental brushes, and toothpicks.[72] The oral hygiene therapist should carefully analyze the needs and manual dexterity of each individual patient and then develop an optimal oral hygiene regimen with the patient.

Plaque and Plaque-retaining Factors

The professional who is responsible for the care of a patient should assure that all "plaque-traps," including insufficient restoration contours or margins, are eliminated. Also, in the treatment planning phase, prosthetic devices that interfere with optimal plaque control by infringing on the dentogingival region with clasps should be evaluated and, whenever possible, avoided or replaced. This is important to prevent gingival inflammation which, on a longer-term basis, can create permanent loss of periodontal support.[74-76]

To establish optimal conditions for oral hygiene control and patient motivation, all calculus deposits should be removed. This may be done manually with hand instruments such as scalers and curets or with ultrasonic devices. The procedure may be time-consuming by both approaches. Ultrasonic devices tend to leave rougher surfaces following instrumentation, but comparisons of the two methods have not shown any significant differences in the clinical response.[77]

Traditionally, prophylaxis has included the removal of extrinsic tooth stains. This part of treatment may not have any significant effect in preventing periodontal breakdown, but from cultural and societal expectations, and possibly motivational benefits, it appears that polishing hardly can be avoided.[78] When applying surface-abrasive pumices for polishing, it is recommended that these contain fluorides to compensate for the abrasive effects on the enamel.[79] Rather than polishing all tooth surfaces at each appointment, it is appropriate to "selectively polish" only those surfaces that have plaque or staining.

In spite of prior concerns, there now appears to be sufficient evidence that the air-powered abrasive devices are acceptable methods for stain removal. The injuries to gingival tissues are minor and reversible, and the systemic introduction of salts is not significant.[80,81] Care is, however, recommended to prevent loss of tooth structure when working in the vicinity of exposed root surfaces.[82]

Mouthrinses

Generally, the use of chemotherapeutic products for controlling gingivitis among patients without a history of periodontitis is not indicated. However, for special patient groups who are unable to maintain oral plaque control, such products may be beneficial when used as adjuncts to regular plaque control procedures. This may include persons with impaired manual dexterity, systemically compromised individuals, or patients during postsurgical care.[83-86]

Among the increasing number of products available today, those based on chlorhexidine gluconate are superior.[83,84,87] This ingredient has been shown to be effective in supragingival plaque control and in reducing gingival inflammation when used in mouthrinses, gels, or delivered by irrigation devices.[88-91] It is important to note that while the use of chlorhexidine rinses may result in a beneficial change in the microbial composition, this change is a temporary phenomenon. Once the rinse is discontinued, the microbial profile will revert to one similar to the original.[92] In addition, a reduction in sensitivity to chlorhexidine among certain bacterial species was temporary and diminished after cessation of the rinses.[93]

Certain side effects associated with chlorhexidine products may limit their use. These effects include varying degrees of brownish staining of the teeth, tongue, and restorations.[86] Also, a few patients have reported some mucosal irritation and changes in taste sensation.[90,94]

The beneficial results obtained in short-term clinical studies have also been seen after long-term use of chlorhexidine. Reduction in plaque and gingivitis scores, as well as reduced gingival bleeding were demonstrated after 2 years of oral rinses among medical and dental students[95] and after 6 months of rinses among schoolchildren[96] or adults.[88] It is important that medical parameters, including blood counts, urinalysis, and sedimentation rate, were not affected after such extended periods of use.[97] However, staining was also a prominent side effect of long-term use. A reduction in the concentration of the rinse might provide less staining but presumably also less efficacy. Overall, long-term use of chlorhexidine may also be considered safe and efficacious, and particularly useful for such patient groups that are characterized by less resistance to bacterial plaque accumulation. These include patients with systemic conditions, the physically or mentally handicapped, and others with increased susceptibility to periodontal disease.[90]

Other Products

Among other oral chemotherapeutic rinses are those based on essential oils. One of these contains several essential oils in addition to a substantial proportion of alcohol. Another product is available as an oral rinse or dentifrice. The active ingredient, sanguinarine, is an alkaloid extract from the plant *Sanguinaria canadensis*.

Both of these products have been shown to be associated with some reduction in plaque accumulation and gingival inflammation and appear to have less side effects than chlorhexidine-based products for use over extended periods.[83] Comparative studies, however, have generally shown that the effects of these other products are less than those of chlorhexidine.[83,87]

Finally, an additional oral hygiene product is the anticalculus, or "tartar-controlling" agent. Based on soluble pyrophosphatase to interfere with calculus formation, this agent, by delivery through dentifrices, may be helpful for controlling plaque-retaining factors and thus maintaining gingival health.[98]

CLINICAL APPLICATION

TREATMENT GOAL

Successful therapy involves the establishment of:

1. A plaque-free dentition
2. Return of physiologic contour
3. Cessation of bleeding
4. Reduction of edema
5. Return of oral comfort

EXAMINATION

Visual inspection of the teeth and gingival tissues may tell the clinician about the patient's:

1. Level of oral hygiene skills
2. Dental "intelligence quotient"
3. Degree of manual dexterity
4. Degree of motivation
5. Level of self-esteem

The clinician should note and record the amount of:

1. Food debris (Fig 8-2)
2. Noncalcified plaque (Fig 8-3)
3. Calcified plaque (Fig 8-4)
4. Color changes (Fig 8-3)

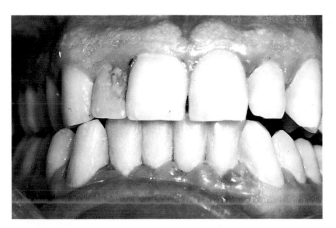

Fig 8-2 Food debris. *Most often this is a minor problem that can be corrected easily, but it indicates a potentially serious situation. The patient may simply be ignorant of proper oral hygiene measures or may be unaware of proper etiquette regarding visits to a health care practitioner. Occasionally this lack of basic oral hygiene will alert the clinician to mental disturbances such as depression or senility. Often the condition may be related to physical impairments such as Parkinson's disease, severe arthritis, or disability caused by a stroke. Food debris is present upon initial examination. This patient has been receiving psychiatric treatment.*

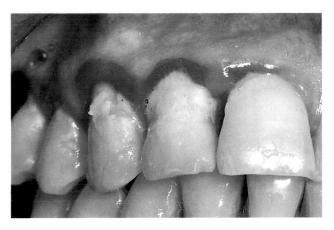

Fig 8-3 Noncalcified plaque. *Heavy plaque deposits will usually be visible to the naked eye. They may be heavy in all areas, indicating an absence of knowledge or motivation regarding plaque control standards. Or, they may be simply in localized areas, very often in difficult-to-reach places such as the lingual surfaces of mandibular molars and the distal surfaces of maxillary second molars. Heavy plaque associated with subjacent bleeding gingival tissues usually indicates longstanding accumulation. Heavy plaque without bleeding might indicate more food debris than actual bacterial accumulation, and the duration of its existence might be several days or less. In this patient, heavy plaque accumulation was responsible for an intense inflammatory response, as evidenced by the dramatic color change.*

Color. *The gingival tissue may be either red or magenta in color, indicating an inflammatory response related to a local irritant. When there is much color change and little or no visible plaque and calculus, one must be concerned about a possible systemic condition that is weakening the patient's immune response. Determine whether the number of local irritants is commensurate with the amount of inflammation. Increased levels of inflammation with little plaque and calculus may mean a more aggressive periodontal problem or may necessitate a medical consultation, whereas increased levels of plaque and calculus and moderate to severe inflammation may require no more than plaque control instruction and calculus removal.*

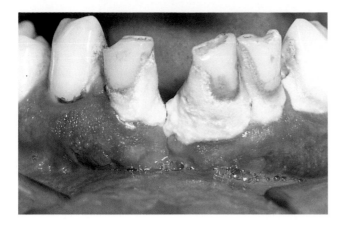

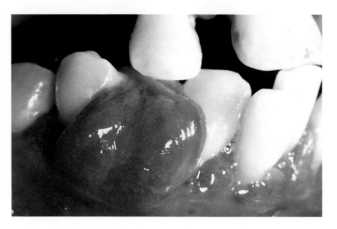

Fig 8-4 Calcified plaque (calculus). Heavy supragingival deposits may be the result of a long span of time passing since the patient's last dental scaling, poor plaque removal techniques, or a rapid calcification rate. A combined rapid calcification rate plus an overextended recall period resulted in this heavy accumulation of calculus in this patient.

Fig 8-5 Pregnancy. An increase in inflammation and even tumorlike growths are common in pregnant women. This may begin in the second month and continue to increase until the eighth month. Pregnancy is a time when intensive plaque control measures should be instituted, particularly because antibiotics and other medications should be minimized. Scaling, when necessary, should also be performed. This tumor grew to a very large size; scaling plus improved plaque control caused it to shrink. It was excised after delivery of the baby.

Medical History Review

A thorough review of the patient's medical condition should precede treatment. Some common conditions that will influence gingivitis are pregnancy, uncontrolled diabetes, and puberty (Figs 8-5 through 8-7).

Iatrogenic Dentistry Assessment

Iatrogenic factors can be assessed with the aid of explorers, radiographs, and mouth mirrors. Possible problem areas include crown contours, margins, width of embrasure spaces, and contacts. Corrective action should be taken when it is in the best interest of the patient.

Other Etiologic Factors

Crowding, mouth breathing, allergies, smoking, orthodontic appliances, and ill-fitting removable partial dentures may contribute to the severity of the gingivitis. Each situation needs to be reviewed individually. Whenever possible, the causative factors should be eliminated or at least reduced.

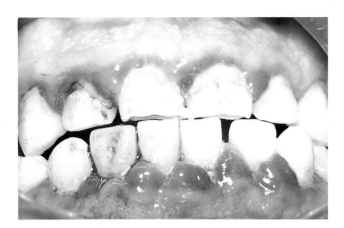

Fig 8-6 *Uncontrolled diabetes.* Patients suspected of having diabetes should be immediately referred to their physician for appropriate testing. Patients with controlled diabetes can have a normal tissue response and should be treated in the same way as nondiabetic persons, with the exception that the clinician should make sure that the usual dosages of insulin have been taken and the appropriate meals have been eaten. Morning appointments after breakfast are most ideal. In this patient the maxillary arch was scaled weeks earlier. Note the persistent inflammation of the maxillary gingiva and the violent tissue reaction of the unscaled mandibular arch.

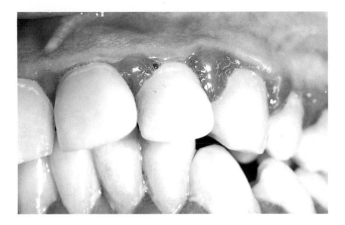

Fig 8-7 *Puberty.* Gingival tissues that are very inflamed, bleed easily, and are often hyperplastic may characterize the onset of puberty in some individuals with poor oral hygiene. Excellent oral hygiene may reduce or negate the hormonal influence in most of these individuals. The hyperplastic tissue response shown here is a reaction to local irritants. Shrinkage of the papillae and reduction of pocket depth is expected after plaque control and scaling.

Charting and Records

Chronic gingivitis patients do not exhibit loss of attachment, but edema and hyperplasia (Fig 8 7) often occur, causing an increase in pocket depth. Pocket depths should be measured in order to assess the results of therapy and also to provide baseline data should a progressive condition develop. The charting sheet should have space to record bleeding and exudate. Bleeding is noted as a red dot (Fig 8-8) and exudate as an "E" placed above or below the corresponding pocket depth score. Supragingival plaque and calculus are individually categorized as "light," "moderate," or "heavy." (See also chapter 1 for other approaches.)

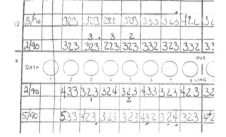

Fig 8-8 These are pocket chartings on the maxillary right quadrant done 3 months apart. The red dots represent pockets that bled with probing; no exudate was present. The red numbers above or below the pocket recordings represent millimeters of recession. The circles indicate where mobility would be recorded if it were present.

PATIENT CONSULTATION

A patient is informed that he or she has a "gum" infection that needs to be treated and that treatment consists of four parts:

1. One or more visits related to the control of the bacterial plaque that is infecting their gums
2. A dental scaling and polishing appointment
3. A reevaluation appointment to determine the level of disease control
4. A regular supportive periodontal treatment (SPT) to maintain the teeth and gums in a state of health

Some patients are reluctant to schedule a plaque control appointment if they believe they will simply be shown how to brush their teeth. They may feel that it is an insult to their intelligence and a waste of their time. For this reason it is important to make the following points:

1. The anatomy of their teeth and gums makes it difficult for them to remove the bacterial plaque.
2. They will be shown *new* techniques that will allow them to brush further under the gums and to clean better between the teeth. The word "new" must be emphasized.
3. If appropriate for their condition, there are mechanical appliances and mouthrinses that may be helpful. This will be determined after the type and location of their plaque is analyzed.
4. It is important to reduce the infection first so that during scaling there will be less bleeding and tenderness.

PLAQUE CONTROL

Psychological Aspects

Early in the appointment it is important that the therapist evaluate how the patient relates to the following.

Degree of Dental Phobia Unfortunately, many patients are not relaxed in the dental environment because of a traumatic prior experience. It is important to let these patients know that treatment will not be painful for them and that they are free at any time to express concerns. The dental history can include the following questions, which are helpful in determining whether or not dental phobia will be a factor in the patient's receptivity to treatment: "Have you ever had a bad dental experience?" followed by the words "yes" and "no" with a notation to circle one answer. "Do you have any concerns about dental treatment?" again followed by "yes" and "no" and then a place for "comments." If one or both of these questions is answered in the affirmative, patients should be invited to share whatever information they would like. They can then be reassured that their treatment should be a pleasant experience and given the reasons why.

Degree of Unfilled Dental Needs It is important to determine whether the patient is embarrassed over the poor condition of their oral cavity. Clinical findings may include untreated carious lesions, fractured teeth, unreplaced missing teeth, and lost fillings. It is also wise to determine the cause of such findings, whether due to dental phobia, financial problems, stress, depression, or fatigue. The clinician's approach should be one of compassion, empathy, and understanding.

Age Teenagers and young adults are the most difficult to motivate since oral hygiene is often not a priority. This age group is usually very concerned about relationships with the opposite sex, and a discussion of how materia alba, plaque, and gingivitis contribute to bad breath can be very motivating.

Low "Dental IQ" Many people come from cultural, ethnic, and social backgrounds where little value is placed on the preservation of the natural dentition. They often expect that complete dentures are inevitable. Showing them dentures and discussing their negative aspects combined with educating them about preventive dental care can be helpful.

Physical or Mental Disabilities The degree of dexterity, deformity, or malfunction will need to be assessed. In some instances, mechanical devices can be used to help overcome the problem. In other cases, a spouse or a caretaker may need to perform the functions for the patient and should be present at the plaque control appointment.

Personality Types A skilled plaque control therapist can recognize that different personalities respond best to different approaches. When teaching plaque control, four distinct personality types have been recognized. Obviously, there will be some overlap of traits in many individuals.

1. The "people" type: pleasant, wants to be liked, informal. The therapist should be patient, open, and minimize details unless asked.
2. The "analytical" type: formal, conservative, needs to understand the process, wants to do a thorough job. The best approach is to be organized and detailed.
3. The "in charge" type: businesslike, wants control. The therapist should provide definite answers, allow the patient options.
4. The "socialite" type: friendly, concerned with image, wants attention and approval. The best approach is to emphasize how skills can promote image; praise.

Level of Unfulfilled Needs Maslow described humankind's necessity to have basic needs met before being concerned about higher needs. For instance, a man feeling intense pain must have it relieved before he will be concerned about his appearance. Other basic needs are for food and shelter. People who are hungry and have nowhere to sleep are most likely unconcerned about bleeding gingiva. The therapist must determine what basic needs are not being met for a specific patient and interpret how this will affect his or her ability to receive dental treatment. Once basic needs are met and patients have reasonably high self-esteem, they will be concerned about the function and esthetics of their dentition.

Patient Education

It is important that patients understand their condition is a bacterial infection that is harmful to delicate tissues. If they showed the same amount of infection on the surface of their skin as they do in the oral cavity, they would most likely seek the help of a physician. Photographs, drawings, or models of teeth and plaque deposits may be shown to the patient to help explain the etiology. Some clinicians use a microscope or television monitor to show patients plaque samples from their mouth.

The concept of subgingival plaque and the need for its removal should be explained. A drawing done by the therapist or a pamphlet with printed depictions will often suffice. It may be helpful to compare subgingival plaque to the situation of dirt under the fingernail and how that needs to be scraped away.

Once it is established what plaque is and where it resides, the next issue is to describe the changes it can cause in the oral cavity. Bleeding, color changes, edema, bad taste, and bad breath

can be discussed in general before relating them to conditions in the patient's own oral cavity. Wherever possible, their disease condition is compared with the normal situation, using the healthy areas of the patient's oral cavity or photographs of normal tissues (Fig 8-9).

The possible progression of gingivitis into periodontitis should be discussed using a visual aid.

MANUAL PERSONAL ORAL HYGIENE

1. Seat patient in a dental chair and review oral condition.
2. Demonstrate color changes, bleeding, and edematous papillae.
3. Scrape visible plaque using a probe until it can easily be seen as a white mass at the end of the probe. When necessary, use a disclosing solution (Fig 8-10). **Note:** It is important to obtain the patient's permission before using a dye because they might have an important engagement after the dental appointment. **Helpful hint:** minimize residual stain by coating the patient's lips with petroleum jelly and applying the disclosing solution to the marginal and interproximal areas with a soaked cotton tip before having the patient rinse lightly.
4. Show patients the stained plaque and let them know that it extends under the gingiva and between the teeth further than they can see.
5. Tell them brushing under the gums and contoured dental flossing are the most important techniques for them to master.

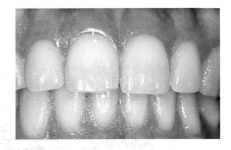

Fig 8-9 A photograph of teeth and gingiva in which there is no evidence of gingival inflammation. Note the pink color, the flat, pointed papillae, and the presence of stippling.

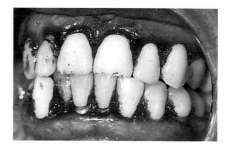

Fig 8-10 Disclosing solution has stained difficult-to-see plaque. Patients with reasonably good oral hygiene will stain mostly in the interproximal areas and, sometimes, adjacent to the marginal tissues. Check the lingual surfaces of the mandibular molars carefully since this is a very common place for residual plaque.

Brushing

A toothbrush should have a relatively small head (1 inch to 1¼ inch for adults, smaller for children) (Fig 8-11); soft nylon, multi-tufted, polished bristles (usually in three rows); and contra-angle heads if access is difficult.

Give patients a suitable new brush and ask them to demonstrate their technique first. Some will need only minor corrections. Others will need extensive counseling with considerable detail.

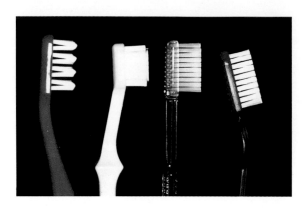

Fig 8-11 Four styles of brushes that are effective for the removal of plaque. (Left to right): rose colored brush has contra-angle bend away from the teeth, and bristles are in a "V" arrangement for interproximal penetration; yellow brush with contra-angle bend toward the teeth; blue brush made of translucent plastic without any bends; red brush is the same style as the blue brush, but with a bend made by the therapist to facilitate cleansing. Patients can easily learn to bend their brushes at home by running them under a stream of warm water or rubbing them vigorously between the thumb and finger.

Interdental Cleaning

Floss There is no one type of floss that is superior to other types in all situations. If the rules regarding the use of floss are too stringent, patients will be reluctant to floss at all. A lightly waxed, mint-flavored floss is tolerated quite well by most patients. It is important that the floss slip easily between the teeth and past restorative margins without tearing and becoming lodged in the interproximal spaces.

Most people who do not floss believe that it is too time-consuming and too difficult a skill for them to master. Many people who floss do it incorrectly and simply use it to remove food particles lodged between the teeth.

For those patients who say they do floss, hand them a container of floss and ask them to show you their technique. Many will tear off a short piece, often about 6 to 12 inches in length, wrap it around their index fingers, and attempt to floss. Explain to them that there is an easier way and proceed to demonstrate.

Tell the patients who are not flossing that there have been improvements in the techniques that will make it easier for them to do. These patients also need to understand that flossing is essential for cleaning under the gum and between the teeth, where most

disease is present. Toothpicks or rubber tips do not do the same thing.

Besides the basic brush and dental floss, many other useful aids are available (Fig 8-12). Some adult patients will need to use a floss holder because of dexterity problems, arthritis, or other reasons. Defer to this device only when absolutely necessary because these holders usually stretch the floss very tightly, preventing it from being wrapped around proximal tooth surfaces or being slipped subgingivally.

Children may find flossing easier if they start with a shorter piece of floss (about 12 inches), tie the ends together with a square knot forming a loop, grasp the loop with the third, fourth, and fifth fingers of each hand, and use the thumb and index fingers to guide the floss.

Interdental Brushes When teeth are spaced apart or the gingiva has receded to allow sufficient room, interdental brushes may be preferred for their ease of use and their ability to penetrate into concave root surfaces.

End-tuft Brushes These are brushes that only have bristles at the very end of the head (see Fig 8-12). Special areas, such as the distal surfaces of second molars, may require an end-tuft brush. These are also good for reaching difficult access areas when teeth are crowded.

Toothpicks and Interdental Cleaners Toothpicks can be broken and the pointed ends attached to the plastic handles, creating a wooden dental instrument excellent for penetrating into the

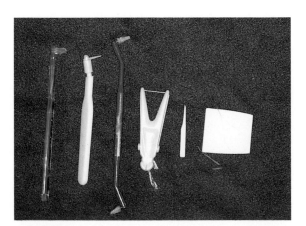

Fig 8-12 Additional useful plaque control aids include (left to right): end-tuft brush; toothpick in holder; double-ended interdental brush; floss holder; plastic interdental cleaner; loop floss threader for using under fixed bridgework.

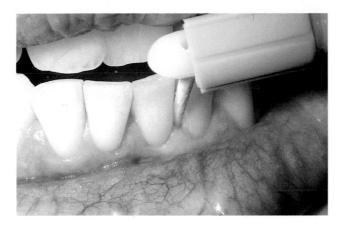

Fig 8-13 *The toothpick is tracing the gingival sulcus of a mandibular anterior tooth.*

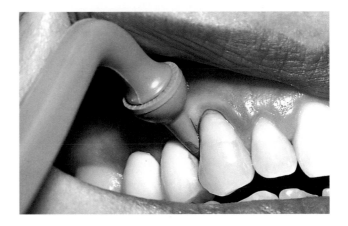

Fig 8-14 *The rubber tip is being used to apply pressure to an inflamed papilla. Note blanching of the tissue and the angle at which the tip is applied.*

deep grooves of teeth, as well as for cleaning at the gingival margin and slightly subgingivally on the facial and lingual surfaces (Fig 8-13). Before using, have the patient blunt the sharp tip by running it under warm water and then tapping it on a hard surface.

Wooden interdental cleaners can be useful for dislodging retained food particles from between the teeth. Because of their small size and packaging, they can be carried in purses and pockets and are useful when eating away from home. The wooden tip should be thoroughly moistened in the mouth to soften. The pointed end is inserted between the teeth and gently moved in and out.

Plastic interdental cleaners are similar to wooden ones and are made by a variety of manufacturers. Since they are usually quite thin, they have a better chance of some subgingival penetration. But because they are constructed of harder material, they are not as comfortable to use as the wooden instruments.

Rubber tip stimulators were once considered essential in the reduction of interproximal inflam-

mation. We now know that plaque removal is the primary method of controlling gingivitis. Stimulators are sometimes used to aid in plaque removal by applying contouring pressure to hyperplastic interdental papillae (Fig 8-14).

It is important to remember that when teeth are in close proximity and the papilla fills the interdental area, none of the interdental brushes, picks, or stimulators will penetrate the interproximal subgingival area as well as properly contoured dental floss. For this reason, proper brushing and flossing techniques are considered essential in the control of gingivitis.

MECHANICAL APPLIANCES

Recently, mechanical brushes combined with updated information on pulsating irrigation devices have given us new ammunition in the war against plaque and gingivitis.

Multiple Rotating Tuft Brushes

These brushes have separate tufts of very soft bristles that rotate individually. One brush has two rows with five tufts in each. The unique aspect of this brush is that although the tufts rotate very rapidly (a reported 4,200 times per minute), they reverse direction 46 times per minute, causing the bristles to extend outward toward the interproximal spaces and into the subgingival areas. Regular toothpaste is not usually recommended with this brush due to the possibilities of damage to the delicate gears in the head and abrasion of the gingiva.

Indications for recommendation of the Interplak brush are:

1. Persistent marginal plaque
2. Handicapped person
3. Poor manual dexterity
4. Parkinson patients
5. Orthodontic patients
6. Patients who prefer electric toothbrushes

Negative aspects are:

1. Large head
2. Need for a recharging stand to be carried when traveling
3. Abrasive grit clogs the gears
4. Claims of interproximal cleansing often discourage patients from using dental floss
5. Cost

The outstanding feature of this brush is the ease with which patients who have repeatedly been poor brushers with a manual brush can, in a very short time, improve their ability to remove plaque. It must be remembered that mechanical devices will eventually stop working. Patients who use these brushes should continue to be counseled in manual techniques so that plaque levels will not increase while the brush is being repaired or replaced.

Single Rotating Tuft Brushes

These brushes are based on the cleansing principles long used by the dental hygienist when performing prophylactic procedures with contra-angle handpieces and rubber polishing cups. One single tuft rotary brush has received the American Dental Association seal of approval and is gaining in popularity.

Indications for recommendation of the rotating single tuft brush are:

1. Soft bristles are kind to hard and soft dental tissues
2. Small head, which can reach into tight areas
3. Can be used with toothpaste for stain removal
4. Orthodontic, fixed bridge, and implant patients
5. Patients who travel frequently since charging is not necessary between each use

Contraindications for its use include:

1. Subtle changes in angles and directions may be difficult for handicapped patients with poor eye/hand coordination
2. Prolonged use of brush tips held against root surface with pressure and an abrasive toothpaste may cause abrasion
3. Patients unable to tolerate the tickling sensation
4. Failure to recommend flossing as an adjunctive procedure
5. Cost

The main benefit of this brush is to replace the need for multiple manual brushes for patients who would otherwise be told to use a regular toothbrush, an end-tuft brush, and an interproximal brush. It is relatively lightweight and very portable. Once again, patients need to know how to use the manual brushes for times when the mechanical device is not functioning.

Pulsating Irrigation

More than 20 years ago pulsating water irrigation was introduced. It was mostly used for dislodging food particles, particularly around fixed bridgework, but the procedure never became popular as a plaque control device. This is because plaque was not totally removed from tooth surfaces due to tenacious pellicle attachment. Also, occasionally periodontal patients developed abscesses because root planing with concomitant calculus removal was not performed before the irrigation procedures were started.

A greater understanding of the microbiology and pathogenesis of gingivitis has brought renewed interest in the ability of pulsating irrigation to reduce not only plaque, but also gingivitis. Water irrigation is now believed to:

1. Produce physical changes in adherent dental plaque masses, resulting in the death of the organisms or at least rendering them nonpathogenic
2. Produce qualitative changes in plaque, in particular, reducing motile bacterial forms
3. Considerably reduce the occurrence of gingivitis with plain water and gain an enhanced reduction with the addition of chemical agents

The following types of patients should be placed on powered, pulsating irrigation in addition to brushing and flossing:

1. Those with many food retentive areas (eg, pontics, diastemata, and orthodontic appliances)
2. Those with persistent gingivitis even after manual plaque control has been mastered to the extent of the patient's ability
3. Those who particularly enjoy this device because of the feeling of cleanliness they derive from it

CHEMICAL PLAQUE CONTROL

Patients are intrigued by the application of topical agents that can aid them in their war against plaque. Because plaque buildup is constant and relentless, patients are often willing to spend considerable sums of money, endure strong tastes, and, to a lesser degree, tolerate stains on the teeth caused by the agents.

Chlorhexidine

Chlorhexidine is a potent antiplaque agent available in Europe in a 0.2% concentration and in the United States in a 0.12% concentration (with a prescription).

Indications

1. As a treatment for gingivitis when conventional manual anddmechanicaltechniquesare insufficient
2. As the initial method of plaque control when plaque-induced gingivitis has resulted in extreme gingival sensitivity to touch

Side Effects

1. Slight, moderate, or severe brown stain on the teeth, tongue, and silicate and resin restorations. Some solutions are to only give chlorhexidine to patients who have minimum stain before usage; have patients avoid smoking, coffee, tea, and red wine; do not administer it to patients with bonded restorations or cracked or pitted enamel.
2. Prolonged bitter taste and transient impairment of taste perception. A solution is to tell patients in advance that they may experience a bitter taste, but that it usually diminishes in a few days.
3. Excessive supragingival calculus formation (due to the accumulation of large numbers of dead bacterial organisms attracting calcium ions). Some solutions are using a tartar-control toothpaste and brushing more frequently.

If the patient has minimal side effects after 2 weeks and is in need of continual adjunctive aid in the control of gingivitis, chlorhexi-dine usage can continue long term. If either cost, staining, taste, or calculus cause problems, chlorhexidine can be diluted with an equal amount of water; the patient should rinse twice a day with the diluted mixture. Although the effectiveness is decreased, there is still a considerable therapeutic benefit at the 0.06% concentration.

For patients who do not wish to use chlorhexidine long term, there are alternatives. An essential oil mouthrinse may be used. It is recommended that patients rinse with it for 30 seconds, morning and evening. It has been approved by the ADA for control of plaque and gingivitis. It is contraindicated for patients who cannot tolerate the taste, who experience a burning sensation, or who have high alcohol intake (it contains 26.9% alcohol). Since alcohol is responsible for most forms of oral and esophageal cancer, one should be concerned about adding additional alcohol to the delicate tissues of the oral cavity in high-risk patients.

Chemical Irrigation

Since pulsating water irrigation in itself reduces gingival inflammation, it follows that the addition of antibacterial agents to the pulsating water may increase this effect even when used in low concentrations.

APPOINTMENT MANAGEMENT

For patients who need minimal improvement in their plaque control, one visit from 30 to 60 minutes should be sufficient. Important feedback as to the patient's progress can be delivered at the scaling appointment. All dental needs, such as manual toothbrushes, floss, disclosing solution, and plastic dental mirror, should be provided for the patient to take home and begin using immediately.

It is very difficult for most patients to master more than two new oral hygiene techniques in one treatment session. For patients with very poor oral hygiene who need to begin with basic brushing and flossing techniques, it is best to schedule two sessions approximately 1 week apart. The second session can begin with an evaluation of what has been accomplished since the last appointment, and what further improvements can be made. Subsequently, new aids such as the end-tuft brush or the toothpick holder might be introduced. Another scenario of the second appointment might include a realization that the patient's manual brushing technique is not adequate and that a battery-powered mechanical brush is needed. Above all else, one should be flexible in teaching and motivating patients to higher levels of oral hygiene.

CALCULUS REMOVAL

The advantages of calculus removal are less bleeding, less discomfort, and less edema. It should be started two weeks after institution of plaque removal techniques.

Most patients with gingivitis can be scaled in one session of approximately 45 to 60 minutes. Occasionally, two or more sessions are needed, depending on the amount and tenacity of the calculus and the degree of stain.

Once scaling is complete, the patient should be appointed for a reevaluation session in 2 to 4 weeks, the amount of time needed for maximum healing to take place.

POSTTREATMENT EVALUATION

At the evaluation stage, pretreatment and posttreatment pocket chartings are compared. Plaque control is evaluated, and the patient is encouraged to continue the high level of achievement or to strive for improved levels of excellence. When necessary, additional instruction is given.

A determination is made regarding supportive periodontal treatment (SPT). SPT appointments will be every 6 months in mild cases of gingivitis. In more severe cases, SPT appointments should be scheduled every 3 to 4 months. If a chemical agent such as chlorhexidine is being used, the therapist should determine among the following to either *(1)* stop the agent and not replace it with another, *(2)* replace it with one that has fewer side effects for that individual, or is less costly if finances are a problem, or *(3)* continue the agent but vary its method of delivery (eg, use irrigation).

If the patient has not responded to treatment as expected, every attempt should be made to determine the cause. Some reasons might be patient noncompliance in controlling plaque, an underlying systemic problem, or the presence of subgingival calculus. Patient noncompliance might require one or more additional sessions of instruction and motivation, or the addition of different aids such as a mechanical toothbrush and / or a floss holder. Suspected systemic complications may necessitate a medical consultation. It may also be determined that additional scaling or root planing is necessary.

QUICK REVIEW

I. Epidemiology of chronic gingivitis
- Among children 3 to 5 years old, 36% to 64% show gingivitis.
- During early adolescence, the gingivitis prevalence reaches 90%.
- Among adults over age 30 years, 95% have some degree of gingivitis and 44% show bleeding on probing.

II. Progression of chronic gingivitis to periodontitis
- Gingivitis does not always progress to periodontitis.
- Transition from gingivitis to periodontitis appears to occur at individual sites during relatively short, episodic bursts.
- In the population, approximately 10% show areas with advanced periodontal lesions, while 25% have areas of slight or early signs of periodontitis.
- Some persons are more susceptible to developing periodontal lesions at sites of gingivitis than others. No reliable clinical or diagnostic tests are yet available to detect these persons except past history of periodontitis.

III. Rationale for prevention and treatment of chronic gingivitis
- Gingivitis can be avoided and progression to periodontitis generally prevented by optimal oral hygiene control and close supervision by the oral health professional.
- In the absence of clinical or diagnostic tests to identify persons "at risk" for periodontitis, care should rely on preventing a transition from gingivitis to periodontitis.
- Gingival inflammation does not reflect health and should be treated to assure overall personal health, wellness, and quality of life.

IV. Patient consultation (what to look for in the examination)
- Large amounts of plaque and calculus necessitate the institution of plaque control and scaling measures.
- Minimal amounts of plaque and calculus accompanied by gingivitis exhibiting dramatic color change and increased bleeding may necessitate a medical evaluation.

QUICK REVIEW
(continued)

- Pregnancy, uncontrolled diabetes, and puberty onset may result in severe gingivitis. Institute plaque control and scaling.
- Chart pockets and bleeding to compare to posttreatment results.

V. The psychology of plaque control
- It is important to find out why patients may be fearful of dental treatment and to allay those fears.
- Dental phobia, financial problems, stress, depression, and fatigue are common reasons for dental neglect. Compassion, empathy, and understanding are important responses in these situations.
- Teenagers and young singles often pay attention to the opposite sex and will be interested in ways to reduce bad breath.
- Low "dental IQ" needs to be overcome with education.
- Patients with physical or mental impairments may do better with mechanical toothbrushes and floss holders.
- Identification of personality types helps in knowing how to relate to and motivate different patients.
- Do not expect improved plaque control results when a patient has unfulfilled basic needs such as relief of pain, hunger, and anxiety.

VI. Gingivitis control
- The teaching of correct techniques and the motivation of the patient toward long-term compliance are the most important aspects. They include:
  - proper toothbrushing to remove marginal and subgingival plaque on the facial, palatal, and lingual tooth surfaces.
  - cleansing with floss and/or interproximal brushes to rid the interdental spaces of hard-to-remove plaque.
  - identification of the patient's personality type and modification of approach.
- Scale and polish the teeth to remove hard deposits and stain.
- Reevaluate the results of therapy and institute additional therapy as necessary.
- Place the patient into supportive periodontal treatment every 6 months for minor cases of gingivitis and every 3 to 4 months for serious cases.

VII. Chemical plaque control
- Chlorhexidine in a 0.12% concentration is a potent inhibitor of plaque. Its major side effect is a brown stain on the teeth.
- An essential oil mouthrinse at the time of writing is the only nonprescription mouthrinse having received the ADA seal of approval for control of plaque and gingivitis. It has a strong taste and is high in alcohol content.
- Pulsating water irrigation helps to control bleeding and gingivitis. The results may be enhanced by adding chemical agents such as chlorhexidine, essential oils, or sanguinarine to the water.

REFERENCES

1. American Academy of Periodontology: Glossary of Periodontic Terms. *J Periodontol* 1986;57(suppl).
2. Stamm JW: Epidemiology of gingivitis. *J Clin Periodontol* 1986;13:360-370.
3. Hugoson A, Koch G, Rylander H: Prevalence and distribution of gingivitis-periodontitis in children and adolescents. *Swed Dent J* 1981;5:91-103.
4. Hugoson A, Jordon T: Frequency distribution of individuals aged 20-70 years according to severity of periodontal disease. *Community Dent Oral Epidemiol* 1982;10:187-192.
5. Curilovic Z, Mazor Z, Berchtold H: Gingivitis in Zurich school children. A reexamination of 20 years. *Schweiz Monatsschr Zahnheilk* 1977;87:801-808.
6. Sutcliffe P: A longitudinal study of gingivitis and puberty. *J Periodont Res* 1972;7:52-58.
7. Marshall-Day CD, Stephens RG, Quigley LF Jr.: Periodontal disease: Prevalence and incidence. *J Periodontol* 1955;26:185-203.

8. National Institute of Dental Research: Oral health of United States adults. National findings. 1987;DHHS, PHS, NIH; NIH Pub. No. 87-2868.

9. Kirkegaard E, Borgnakke WS, Gronbaek L: *Survey of Oral Health of Danish Adults.* Aarhus, Denmark: Aarhus Odontologiske Boghandel, 1987.

10. Allen C: *The Operator for the Teeth.* New York: John White, 1965.

11. Waerhaug J: Effect of rough surfaces upon gingival tissue. *J Dent Res* 1956;35:323-325.

12. Waerhaug J: Observations on replanted teeth plated with gold foil. *Oral Surg Oral Med Oral Pathol* 1956;9:780-791.

13. Fitzgerald RJ, McDaniel EG: Dental calculus in the germ-free rat. *Arch Oral Biol* 1960;2:239-240.

14. Gibbons RJ, Berman KS, Knoetner P, Kapsimalis B: Dental caries and alveolar bone loss in gnotobiotic rats infected with capsule forming streptococci of human origin. *Arch Oral Biol* 1960;11:549-560.

15. Löe H, Theilade E, Jensen SB: Experimental gingivitis in man. *J Periodontol* 1965;36:177-187.

16. Theilade E, Wright WH, Jensen SB, Löe H: Experimental gingivitis in man. A longitudinal clinical and bacteriological investigation. *J Periodont Res* 1966;1:1-13.

17. Löe H, Schiott CR: The effect of mouthrinses and topical application of chlorhexidine on the development of dental plaque and gingivitis in man. *J Periodont Res* 1970;5:79-83.

18. Loesche WJ: Chemotherapy of dental plaque infections. *Oral Sci Rev* 1976;9:65-107.

19. Moore WE, Holdeman LV, Smibert RM, et al: Bacteriology of experimental gingivitis in young adult humans. *Infect Immun* 1982;38:651-667.

20. Syed SA, Loesche WJ: Bacteriology of human experimental gingivitis: Effect of plaque age. *Infect Immun* 1978; 21:821.

21. Loesche WJ, Syed SA: Bacteriology of human experimental gingivitis: Effect of plaque and gingivitis score. *Infect Immun* 1978;21:830.

22. Listgarten MA, Mayo HE, Tremblay R: Development of dental plaque on epoxy resin crowns in man. A light and electron microscopic study. *J Periodontol* 1975;46:10.

23. White D, Mayrand D: Association of oral *Bacteroides* with gingivitis and adult periodontitis. *J Periodont Res* 1981;16:259.

24. van Palenstein Helderman WH: Total viable count and differential count of *Vibrio (Campylobacter) sputorum, Fusobacterium nucleatum, Selenomonas sputigena, Bacteroides ochracea,* and *Veillonella* in the inflamed and noninflamed human gingival crevice. *J Periodont Res* 1975;10: 294.

25. Löe H, Theilade E, Borglum Jensen S, Schiott CR: Experimental gingivitis in man. III. The influence of antibiotics on gingival plaque development. *J Periodont Res* 1967;2:282-289.

26. Lang NP, Cumming BR, Löe H: Toothbrushing frequency as it relates to plaque development and gingival health. *J Periodontol* 1973;44:396-405.

27. Flemmig TF, Newman MG, Doherty FM, et al: Supragingival irrigation with 0.06% chlorhexidine in naturally occurring gingivitis. I. 6 months clinical observation. *J Periodontol* 1990;61:112-117.

28. Newman MG, Flemmig TF, Nachnani S, et al: Irrigation with 0.06% chlorhexidine in naturally occurring gingivitis. II. 6 months microbiological observation. *J Periodontol* 1990; 61:427-433.

29. Brownstein CN, Briggs SD, Schweitzer KL, et al: Irrigation with chlorhexidine to resolve naturally occurring gingivitis. A methodologic study. *J Clin Periodontol* 1990;17:588-593.

30. Pennell B, Keagle JG: Predisposing factors in the etiology of chronic inflammatory periodontal disease. *J Periodontol* 1977;48:517-532.

31. Ainamo J: Relationship between malalignment of teeth and periodontal disease. *Scand J Dent Res* 1972; 80:104-110.

32. Wennstrom J, Lindhe J: Plaque-induced gingival inflammation in the absence of attached gingiva in dogs. *J Clin Periodontol* 1983;10:266-276.

33. Wennstrom J, Lindhe J, Nyman S: The role of keratinized gingiva in plaque-associated gingivitis in dogs. *J Clin Periodontol* 1982;9:75-85.

34. Dorfman HS, Kenedy JD, Bird WC: Longitudinal evaluation of free autogenous gingival grafts. A four year report. *J Periodontol* 1982;53:349-352.

35. Hall WB: Gingival augmentation/mucogingival surgery. In: *Proceedings of the World Workshop in Clinical Periodontics.* Chicago: American Academy of Periodontology; 1989:VII-1—VII-15.

36. Lang NP, Kiel RA, Anderhalden K: Clinical and microbiological effects of subgingival restorations with overhanging or clinically perfect margins. *J Clin Periodontol* 1983;10:563-578.

37. Page RC, Schroeder HE: Pathogenesis of inflammatory periodontal disease. A summary of current work. *Lab Invest* 1976;34:235.

38. Page RC, Schroeder HE: *Periodontitis in Man and Other Animals. A Comparative Review.* Basel, Switzerland: S. Karger, 1982.

39. Attstrom R, Schroeder HE: Effect of experimental neutropenia on initial gingivitis in dogs. *Scand J Dent Res* 1979;87:7-23.

40. Fine DH, Mandel ID: Indicators of periodontal disease activity: An evaluation. *J Clin Periodontol* 1986;13:533-546.

41. Cimasoni G (ed): *Crevicular Fluid Updated.* Basel, Switzerland: S. Karger, 1983.

42. Payne WA, Page RC, Ogilvie AL, Hall WB: Histopathologic features of the initial and early stages of experimental gingivitis in man. *J Periodont Res* 1975;10(2):51-64.

43. Schroeder HE, Munzel-Pedrazzoli S, Page RC: Correlated morphometric and biochemical analysis of gingival tissue in early chronic gingivitis in man. *Arch Oral Biol* 1973;18:899-923.

44. Brecx MC, Schlegel K, Gehr P, Lang NP: Comparison between histological and clinical parameters during experimental gingivitis. *J Periodont Res* 1987;22:50-57.

45. Brecx M, Frohlicher I, Gehr P, Lang NP: Stereological observations on long-term experimental gingivitis in man. *J Clin Periodontol* 1988;15:621-627.

46. Seymour GJ, Greenspan JS: The phenotypic characterization of lymphocyte subpopulations in established human periodontal disease. *J Periodont Res* 1979;14:39-46.

47. Schroeder HE, Attstrom R: *Pocket Formation: A Hypothesis.* London: Academic Press, Inc, 1980.

48. Greene JC: Oral hygiene and periodontal disease. *Am J Publ Health* 1963;53:913-922.

49. Löe H, Anerud A, Boysen H, Morrison E: Natural history of periodontal disease in man. Rapid, moderate, and no loss of attachment in Sri Lankan laborers 14 to 46 years of age. *J Clin Periodontol* 1986;13:431-445.

50. Ismail AI, Eklund SA, Burt BA, Calderone JJ: Prevalence of deep periodontal pockets in New Mexico adults age 27 to 74 years. *J Publ Health Dent* 1986;46:199-206.

51. Beck JD, Lainson PA, Field HM, Hawkins BF: Risk factors for various levels of periodontal disease and treatment needs in Iowa. *Community Dent Oral Epidemiol* 1984;12:17-22.

52. Listgarten MA, Schifter CC, Laster L: 3-year longitudinal study of the periodontal status of an adult population with gingivitis. *J Clin Periodontol* 1985;12:225-238.

53. Lindhe J, Hamp SE, Löe H: Experimental periodontitis in the beagle dog. *Int Dent J* 1973;23:432-437.

54. Garant PR, Cho MI: Histopathogenesis of spontaneous periodontal disease in conventional rats. I. Histometric and histologic study. *J Periodont Res* 1979;14:297-309.

55. Garant PR: Light and electron microscopic observation of osteoclastic alveolar bone resorption in rats monoinfected by *Actinomyces naeslundii. J Periodontol* 1976;47:717-723.

56. Socransky SS, Haffajee AD, Goodson JM, Lindhe J: New concepts of destructive periodontal disease. *J Clin*

Periodontol 1984;11:21-32.

57. Lindhe J, Haffajee AD, Socransky SS: Progression of periodontal disease in adult subjects in the absence of periodontal therapy. *J Clin Periodontol* 1983;10:433-442.

58. Goodson JM, Tanner ACR, Haffajee AD, Sornberger GC, Socransky SS: Patterns of progression and regression of advanced destructive periodontal disease. *J Clin Periodontol* 1982;9:472-481.

59. Axelsson P, Lindhe J: Effect of controlled oral hygiene procedures on caries and periodontal disease in adults. *J Clin Periodontol* 1978; 5:133-151.

60. Lindhe J, Axelsson P: The effect of controlled oral hygiene and topical fluoride application on caries and gingivitis in Swedish school children. *Community Dent Oral Epidemiol* 1973;1:9-16.

61. Suomi JD, Greene JC, Vermillion JR, Doyle J, Chang J, Leatherwood EC: The effect of controlled oral hygiene procedures on the progression of periodontal disease in adults: Results after third and final year. *J Periodontol* 1971;42:152.

62. Lightner LM, O'Leary TJ, Drake RB, Crump PP, Allen MF: Preventive periodontic treatment procedures: Results over 46 months. *J Periodontol* 1971;42:555.

63. Lovdal A, Arno A, Schei O, Waerhaug J: Combined effect of subgingival scaling and controlled oral hygiene on the incidence of gingivitis. *Acta Odontol Scand* 1961;19:537.

64. United States Preventive Services Task Force: *Guide to Clinical Preventive Services.* (Prepublication copy). Washington, DC, The Task Force, 1989.

65. Lang NP, Joss A, Orsanic T, Gusberti FA, Siegrist BE: Bleeding on probing. A predictor for the progression of periodontal disease? *J Clin Periodontol* 1986;13:590-596.

66. Knowles JW, Burgett FG, Nissle RR, Shick RA, Morrison EC, Ramfjord SP: Results of periodontal treatment related to pocket depth and attachment level. Eight years. *J Periodontol* 1979;50:225-233.

67. Glavind L: Means and methods in oral hygiene instruction of adults. A review. Thesis. *Tandlaegebladet* 1990;94:213-246.

68. Kiyak HA, Mulligan K: Behavioral research related to oral hygiene practices. In: Kleinman DV, Löe H, eds. *Dental Plaque Control Measures and Oral Hygiene Practices.* Oxford: IRL Press, 1986.

69. Glavind L: Effect of monthly professional mechanical tooth cleaning on periodontal health in adults. *J Clin Periodontol* 1977;4:100-106.

70. Glavind L, Zeuner E, Attstrom R: Oral cleanliness and gingival health following oral hygiene instruction by self-educational programs. *J Clin Periodontol* 1984;11:262-273.

71. Glavind L, Zeuner E, Attstrom R: Oral hygiene instruction of adults by means of a self-instructional manual. *J Clin Periodontol* 1981;8:165-176.

72. Frandsen A: Mechanical oral hygiene practices. In: Kleinman DV, Löe H, eds. *Dental Plaque Control Measures and Oral Hygiene Practices.* Oxford: IRL Press, 1986.

73. Breitenmoser J, Morman W, Mühlemann H: Damaging effects of tooth brush bristle end form on gingiva. *J Periodontol* 1979;70:212.

74. Lang NP, Kaarup-Hansen D, Joss A, et al: The significance of overhanging filling margins for the health status of interdental periodontal tissues of young adults. *Schwei Monatsschr Zahnmed* 1988;98:725-730.

75. Ramfjord SP, Ash MM Jr: *Periodontal Considerations in Restorative Dentistry.* Philadelphia: WB Saunders Co; 1979: chap 26.

76. Valderhaug J, Birkeland JM: Periodontal conditions in patients 5 years following insertion of fixed prostheses. Pocket depth and loss of attachment. *J Oral Rehabil* 1976;3:237.

77. Badersten A, Nilveus R, Egelberg J: Effect of nonsurgical periodontal therapy. I. Moderately advanced periodontitis. *J Clin Periodontol* 1981;8:57-72.

78. Sheiham A: The prevention and control of periodontal disease. University of Illinois. International Conference on Research in the Biology of Periodontal Disease. 1977:309-376.

79. Tinanoff N, Wei SH, Parkins FM: Effect of a pumice prophylaxis on fluoride uptake in tooth enamel. *J Am Dent Assoc* 1974;88:384-389.

80. Snyder JA, McVay JT, Brown FH, et al: The effect of air abrasive polishing on blood pH and electrolyte concentrations in healthy Mongrel dogs. *J Periodontol* 1990;61:81-86.

81. Mishkin DJ, Engler WO, Javed T, et al: A clinical comparison of the effect on the gingiva of the Prophy-Jet and the rubber cup and paste techniques. *J Periodontol* 1986;57:151-154.

82. Galloway SE, Pashley DH: Rate of removal of root structure by the use of the Prophy-Jet device. *J Periodontol* 1987;58:464-469.

83. Bral M, Brownstein CN: Antimicrobial agents in the prevention and treatment of periodontal disease. *Dent Clin North Am* 1988;32:217.

84. Listgarten MA: The Role of Dental Plaque in Gingivitis and Periodontitis: Mouthrinses In the Treatment and Prevention of Gingivitis. Proceedings of a Symposium, 11 December 1987. *J Clin Periodontol* 1988;15:485-530.

85. Kornman KS: Antimicrobial agents. In: Kleinman D, Löe H, eds. *Dental Plaque Control Measures and Oral Hygiene Practices.* Oxford: IRL Press, 1986.

86. Greenstein G, Berman C, Jaffin R: Chlorhexidine. An adjunct to periodontal therapy. *J Periodontol* 1986;57:370.

87. Siegrist BE, Gusberti FA, Brecx MC, et al: Efficacy of supervised rinsing with chlorhexidine digluconate in comparison to phenolic and plant alkaloid compounds. *J Periodont Res* 1986;21 (suppl 16):60-73.

88. Grossman E, Reiter G, Sturzenberger OP, et al: Six-month study of the effects of a chlorhexidine mouthrinse on gingivitis in adults. *J Periodont Res* 1986;21(suppl 16):33.

89. Lie T, Enersen M: Effects of chlorhexidine gel in a group of maintenance-care with poor oral hygiene. *J Periodontol* 1986;57:364.

90. Lang NP, Brecx MC: Chlorhexidine digluconate — An agent for chemical plaque control and prevention of gingival inflammation. *J Periodont Res* 1986;21(suppl 16):74-89.

91. Löe H, Schiott CR: The effect of suppression of the oral microflora upon the development of dental plaque and gingivitis. In: McHugh WD, ed. *Dental Plaque.* Edinburgh: E & S Livingstone, 1970.

92. Briner WW, Grossman E, Buckner RY, et al: Effect of chlorhexidine gluconate mouthrinse on plaque bacteria. *J Periodont Res* 1986;21(suppl 16):44-52.

93. Briner WW, Grossman E, Buckner RY, Rebitski GF, Sox TE, Setser RE, Ebert ML: Assessment of susceptibility of plaque bacteria to chlorhexidine after six months' oral use. *J Periodont Res* 1986;21(suppl 16):53-56.

94. Flotra L, Gjermo P, Rolla G, Waerhaug J: Side effects of chlorhexidine mouthwashes. *Scand J Dent Res* 1971; 79:119-125.

95. Löe H, Schiott CR, Glavind L, Karring T: Two years oral use of chlorhexidine in man. I. General design and clinical effects. *J Periodont Res* 1976;11:135-144.

96. Lang NP, Hotz P, Graf H, Geering H, Saxer UP, Sturzenberger OP, Meckel AH: Effects of supervised chlorhexidine mouthrinses in children. A longitudinal clinical trial. *J Periodont Res* 1982;17:101-111.

97. Schiott CR, Löe H, Briner WH: Two year oral use of chlorhexidine in man. IV. Effect on various medical parameters. *J Periodont Res* 1976;11:158-164.

98. McFall WT Jr: Supportive treatment. In: *Proceedings of the World Workshop in Clinical Periodontics.* Chicago: American Academy of Periodontology; 1989:IX-1—IX-23.

Mild Chronic Adult Periodontitis

CURRENT CONCEPTS by Bengt G. Rosling

CLINICAL APPLICATION by Michael K. McGuire

C U R R E N T   C O N C E P T S

TRADITIONAL APPROACHES TO TREATING PERIODONTITIS

Russel's[1] introduction of pocket depth measurement in the Periodontal Index resulted in a clinical approach to mild chronic adult periodontitis that primarily aimed at pocket elimination. However, a greater dimension to clinical periodontology and periodontal research was presented when indices reflecting the degree of oral hygiene were introduced.[2,3] Russel[4] stated that the amount of bacterial plaque and calculus, together with the age of an individual, might explain up to 90% of the periodontal disease found in groups of individuals. Data from epidemiologic research therefore resulted in a clinical approach that was mainly focused on removing plaque and calculus in combination with eliminating periodontal pockets by surgical intervention.

A further development that had a great impact on clinical periodontology occurred when the correlation between bacterial plaque and gingival inflammation was established at the time the Gingival Index system was presented by Löe and Silness.[5] The interpretation of these findings, together with experimental, epidemiologic, and clinical data, resulted in clinical concepts that stressed the importance of removing the main local irritants: supragingival and subgingival dental plaque and calculus. Hence, the elimination of the periodontal pocket (which is recognized as the niche for accumulating subgingival plaque) became a logical rationale for periodontal surgery. As a consequence, the main goal of periodontal therapy—to eliminate the total subgingival plaque mass and create an anatomy in the dentogingival region to facilitate further control of the disease by supragingival plaque control — was accepted.[6-9]

Periodontal therapy directed toward removing unspecific local factors, that is, "cause-related therapy" combined with proper supportive periodontal treatment (maintenance), has been demonstrated to be effective in the treatment of most periodontal diseases. Reports from longitudinal clinical studies have demonstrated that periodontal treatment modalities aimed at removal of supragingival and subgingival plaque result in substantial improvement of clinical disease symptoms (eg, reduction of probing pocket depths, increased or stabilized probing attachment level, and decreased degree and frequency of gingival inflammation).[6-14] Results of several of these studies indicate that the choice of treatment modality is not as important as complete removal of the subgingival plaque mass and proper preparation of the root surfaces for healing accompanied by a high standard of posttreatment plaque control.[7-9,15,16]

Results from recent research in oral microbiology have led to increased understanding of the importance of the specific composition of the supragingival and subgingival microbiota in the development of inflammatory periodontal diseases.[17-19] The recognition of specific microorganisms associated with various forms of severe (aggressive) periodontal disease opens the possibility for the use of specific microbiology in evaluating therapy and in devising more specifically oriented antimicrobial approaches to periodontal therapy.[20-22]

Because access to most of the infecting organisms in periodontal diseases can be accomplished through the orifice of the periodontal pocket, mechanical debridement of the plaque-infected root surfaces logically has been suggested as the first choice of therapy. And combining this treatment with the application of antimicrobial agents locally in the periodontal pocket may represent an important alternative for managing the periodontopathic microflora to supplement mechanical debridement of the root surfaces.[21,23,24] The use of antimicrobial agents, administered systemically or topically, may give additional clinically significant benefit over mechanical subgingival debridement alone. However, a certain risk for uncontrolled adverse reactions and bacterial drug resistance must be considered.[25]

The topical use of antimicrobial agents with low toxicity and a broad antimicrobial spectrum may be important in enhancing the effects of mechanical subgingival debridement.[23,26,27] Furthermore, by applying chemical agents topically, a relatively low total dose can be administered while achieving high concentrations at the site of infection. Delivery of the chemotherapeutic agent into the subgingival periodontal lesions, however, is difficult and likely is best accomplished when professionally applied as a part of open surgical treatment. Although the use of antimicrobial agents in the treatment of periodontal diseases may be promising, it is important to stress that results from recent clinical studies seem to indicate that traditional subgingival scaling and supragingival plaque control procedures, when performed adequately, may be optimal in the treatment of most initial lesions.

TREATMENT OF MILD CHRONIC ADULT PERIODONTITIS

Convincing evidence of the central role of microorganisms in the etiology of gingivitis and periodontitis has been presented.[18,28,29] Since periodontal diseases are primarily infectious, in general, early diagnosis and "cause-related" therapy are considered the main principles in treatment and may well be the key to successful results in the overall clinical management of periodontal diseases.

Although modulation of the host response, as with flurbiprofen, theoretically may be one way of controlling periodontal diseases, elimination of bacterial dental plaque and/or bacterial retention factors may be for the foreseeable future the only practical way to arrest progressive breakdown of the periodontal tissues in the vast majority of patients.[6,8,9,12,30-33]

The effectiveness of mechanical supragingival plaque control to prevent and resolve existing gingival inflammation was documented by Löe et al,[34] Nyman et al,[7] and Axelsson and Lindhe.[35] On the other hand, supragingival plaque control alone has been demonstrated to have only limited effect in arresting the progressive course of periodontitis.[23,36,37] Thus, optimal periodontal therapy must always consist of a combination of supragingival and subgingival plaque control procedures.

Traditional periodontal scaling and root planing carried out without supplemental periodontal surgery has been demonstrated to be one practical way to arrest periodontal tissue breakdown.[14,38-40] Tagge et al[36] and Hughes and Caffesse[41] demonstrated clinical improvement in gingivitis and periodontal pocket depths following subgingival mechanical debridement of mild periodontitis lesions. Badersten et al[14] studied the effect of nonsurgical periodontal therapy on moderately advanced periodontitis lesions and confirmed that scaling and root planing performed using either ultrasonic or traditional hand instruments resulted in marked improvement in gingival inflammation, a significant reduction in probing pocket depths, and a gain in probing attachment level in early periodontitis lesions. However, Waerhaug[42] showed that optimal subgingival debridement may be difficult in periodontal pockets of depths exceeding 3 to 5 mm. Thus, mechanical debridement needs to be combined with surgical procedures to improve accessibility to the infected root surfaces.[12,33,43,44] On the other hand, there is overwhelming documentation in the literature supporting the clinical value of supragingival and subgingival scaling as a powerful basic therapy in the treatment of mild chronic adult periodontitis.

Adjunctive Antimicrobial Agents

The above review indicates that most current treatment procedures are directed toward eliminating the total plaque mass — subgingivally as well as supragingivally. Recent data, however, suggest that there is a close association between certain specific microorganisms and various forms of periodontal disease.[17] *Porphyromonas gingivalis (Bacteroides gingivalis)* has been implicated in many cases of rapidly advancing adult periodontitis,[45] and *Actinobacillus actinomycetemcomitans* has been implicated in localized juvenile periodontitis.[46] In addi-

tion, *Capnocytophaga* species have been associated with periodontitis in juvenile diabetics,[47] and *Prevotella intermedius (Bacteroides intermedius)* has been associated with acute necrotizing ulcerative gingivitis.[48,49] Of course, other organisms may also play a role in the pathogenesis of certain forms of human periodontal disease (see chapter 2).[50,51]

Based on the concept of specificity of bacterial infection in periodontal diseases, it should be possible to use appropriate **systemic antimicrobial agents** to supplement mechanical debridement in the management of periodontal disease. However, Listgarten et al[52] suggested that systemic tetracycline therapy had only a minor additional effect on the periodontal microflora and clinical healing as compared to scaling and root planing alone. Other studies, however, have indicated that systemic antimicrobial therapy may be useful in the treatment of chronic adult periodontitis.[25,53-55]

Because access to most infectious agents in periodontal disease can be accomplished through the orifice of the periodontal lesion, **topical application of antibacterial agents** would also be a possibility in the management of periodontopathogenic infections. During the last decades an increasing interest in topical application of antimicrobial agents to supplement mechanical debridement of periodontal lesions has been directed towards a few chemical agents. Topical use of chlorhexidine digluconate as a mouthrinse will substantially diminish gingival inflammation.[56-60] Although the effect of chlorhexidine on established periodontitis appears limited when delivered supragingivally,[61] it has demonstrated promising results when delivered subgingivally.[62,63] Ultimately, however, Garrett[64]

was unable to show any difference in clinical or microbiological parameters between periodontal lesions scaled and root planed compared to those also irrigated with 0.2% chlorhexidine or tetracycline solutions.

Other agents with expected antimicrobial activity (including stannous fluoride,[65] hydrogen peroxide,[66] iodine,[23,67] and tetracycline[68]) have also been evaluated for topical use in periodontal treatment. Positive as well as negative results have been reported with these agents. In order to minimize the risk of any adverse effects, antimicrobial agents with low toxicity and a broad antimicrobial spectrum should be used. Also, the optimal concentration, the duration of the drug exposition, and bacteriostatic or bacteriocidal properties are important pharmacological properties to observe.[69]

An important question to address is to what extent bacterial resistance will occur. So far, no bacterial resistance has been demonstrated against any type of iodine solutions. Topical irrigation of 0.05% povidone-iodine solution at the site of instrumentation has been demonstrated to enhance the effect of subgingival scaling.[23,24] Povidone-iodine solution was selected because of its well-known broad antimicrobial spectrum. Iodine in alcoholic solution may cause allergic and/or toxic reactions, but when combined with povidone or other similar protein molecules, this serious adverse effect disappears without diminishing the broad antibacterial effect of the iodine.

Iodine does not demonstrate any type of resistance but is effective against all vegetative forms of microorganisms and most viruses as well. Thus, the risk for superinfection may be limited. On the other hand, iodine is a strong oxidant and is irreversibly bound to proteins, which may obstruct the antibacterial effect. In order to overcome this negative effect, it is important to extend the time of exposure and deliver the antibacterial solution at the site of infection at the same time as most of the protein debris (dental plaque and exudate) is mechanically washed away.

A system with such potential has been created by using an ultrasonic scaling instrument. By exchanging the water in the cooling system for 0.05% povidone-iodine-water solution, the cooling property will still remain at the same time that an antibacterial agent is added. The antibacterial solution is irrigated into the site of infection where the working piece of the ultrasonic instrument will decrease the amount of dental plaque mechanically. At the same time, the iodine solution will reduce the number of remaining microorganisms. Results from clinical tests[23,24] seem to justify the use of topical application of povidone-iodine solution to enhance the antibacterial effect of ultrasonic scaling. It should be emphasized that the results reported up to now are from controlled clinical trials with close monitoring of all procedures and of patient compliance. Field trials, with large number of subjects and less continuous monitoring and control, which would be more comparable to a dental practice setting, will be necessary to establish the optimal treatment approach.

Finally, it is important to stress that the pharmacokinetic properties of different chemical agents may exhibit great differences. Thus, H_2O_2 may be inactivated by katalase producing microorganisms such as A. actinomycetemcomitans. This means that irrigation with H_2O_2 may have limited effect in A.a. positive lesions.

Management of Periodontal Diseases as Infectious Diseases

Porphyromonas gingivalis (Bacteroides gingivalis) and *A. actinomycetemcomitans* have been reported to be regular and prominent members of the subgingival flora in periodontal lesions of chronic adult and localized juvenile periodontitis. Thus, it may be possible to use these microorganisms as indicators of success or failure of treatment.[23,24] Even though the use of specific microbiology seems to be promising, it is important to stress that this may be of minor importance in the treatment of mild chronic adult periodontitis. So far, no scientific data support the possibility of using these bacterial indicators as predictors of the outcome of periodontal therapy in daily clinical practice. However, the combination of measurements of traditional clinical parameters, gingival inflammation, and probing depth, in combination with monitoring specific microorganisms, may be used to identify patients at risk after treatment.

Presently, the emphasis in clinical periodontology is principally directed towards three major goals: *(1)* treatment of the disease, *(2)* reconstruction of lost tooth support, and *(3)* supportive measures to maintain periodontal health.

Because periodontal diseases are primarily of infectious nature, the treatment modality principally must include an anti-infectious approach.

The importance of nonspecific plaque control measures performed by mechanical debridement, including various forms of surgical and nonsurgical periodontal therapy, has been well documented in clinical studies over the years.[6,12,14,29,43,44,70-73] Results from these studies clearly indicate that the progressive course of periodontal disease can be arrested or essentially retarded regardless of the technique used for subgingival instrumentation. Furthermore, these studies confirm that gingival inflammation and further progression of periodontal breakdown will be prevented when periodontal therapy is combined with optimal supervised supportive treatment (SPT).

The potential of nonsurgical periodontal therapy (that is, traditional supragingival and subgingival scaling alone) to resolve even advanced periodontitis lesions also has been well documented in clinical trials.[13,14,23] However, the healing pattern following nonsurgical therapy is suggested to be a gradual process over an extensive period of time primarily related to the result of plaque removal. Thus, the initial severity of the disease, the tooth type, the anatomy, and the skill of the operator will all be important factors to consider. Furthermore, results from numerous long-term evaluations of periodontal therapy have suggested that an appropriate supportive periodontal treatment regimen to prevent reinfection is as important as the regimen used to eliminate the periodontal infection.

A decrease in probing pocket depths seems to be strictly related to the degree of plaque control. In addition, the trauma from the technique used for subgingival debridement seems to be an important factor to consider for the outcome of gain in probing attachment level. It is important to stress, however, that the effect of the trauma as the result of traditional subgingival scaling is limited to a minor loss of supporting tissues at the time of instrumentation. Thus, this change has to be defined as an isolated phenomenon that will never cause progressive loss of attachment. On the other hand, it is important to stress the importance of avoiding repeated subgingival scaling with too-close intervals. Subgingival scaling should only be performed in areas showing disease symptoms.[13,23,74]

Supragingival Plaque Control

Even though the central role of dental plaque in the etiology and pathogenesis of periodontal disease is unquestionable, the effect of supragingival plaque control alone on the healing response of periodontal tissues in established periodontitis is limited.[23,37,74,75] Thus it is important to stress that supragingival plaque control per se cannot prevent disease progression in already established periodontitis. On the other hand, it is possible to achieve a limited decrease in probing depth principally as a result of reduction in inflammatory edema. It is also important to stress that it is possible to achieve a low plaque score independent of the level of initial probing depth. The decisive role of supragingival plaque control for the long-term result of periodontal therapy is unquestionable.[7-9,14]

The importance of removal of subgingival plaque and calculus in combination with optimal supragingival plaque control has been documented in several clinical studies. Thus, Badersten and coworkers[14,74,75] studied the effect of oral hygiene instructions and nonsurgical subgingival scaling with hand as well as ultrasonic instruments. It was concluded that, independent of the technique used for subgingival scaling, it was possible to achieve the following clinical pattern:

- Decreased frequency and degree of gingival bleeding
- Reduced probing pocket depth, mainly because of gingival recession
- Clinical improvements during the first 4 to 6 months
- Increased degree of gingival retraction and gain in probing attachment level with initial probing depth
- Loss in probing attachment level in lesions with initially shallow probing depth (1 to 3 mm)
- An 80% to 90% reduction in the occurrence of periodontal lesions

Repeated subgingival scaling during active therapy appears not to be an absolute necessity provided that complete cleaning of the root surface is achieved at one single session. There was no difference in clinical results between ultrasonic and hand-instrument scaling.

SCALING TECHNIQUE

The scaling procedure constitutes the principal instrumentation of crown and root surfaces aimed at eliminating dental plaque and plaque-retention factors:

- Removal of supragingival and subgingival soft and hard debris from the tooth surfaces
- Root planing (ie, removal of root cementum and irregularities of the root surface, including removal of some dentin, to create a hard and smooth root surface)
- Removal of restorative overhangs as well as other plaque retention factors or remodeling of otherwise adequate restorations
- Polishing of teeth and restorations

Supragingival scaling is easiest to perform because direct observation of the tooth surfaces is possible. Subgingival scaling, however, can be performed either as a surgical or a nonsurgical procedure. Nonsurgical scaling involves traditional scaling by hand instruments and/or ultrasonic instruments without reflecting the marginal gingival tissues surgically, thus resulting in incomplete observation of the subgingival located plaque accumulation. To facilitate direct observation and better accessibility of the subgingival area, reflection of the marginal gingival tissue by using different surgical techniques has been accepted.

The surgical technique may also be used to obtain regeneration of periodontal tissues in severe cases of chronic adult periodontitis.

The treatment of mild chronic adult periodontitis is usually best treated by using a nonsurgical technique. Good tactility sense may compensate for incomplete observation of the root surface during the treatment.

The right instrument for scaling (ie, curet and/or scaler) must be applied in order to cut the root cementum and/or dentin of the root. Furthermore, foreign body material such as calculus should be cut away from the root surface. This means that the scaling procedure should result in the formation of chips (Fig 9-1).[76]

Root Planing

A long-standing periodontal lesion contains dental plaque and subgingival calculus in close contact with the tooth substance. Small irregularities caused by resorption of the root cementum is a constant finding, thus resulting in firm retention of plaque and calculus to the root surface, which constitutes the main reason for the

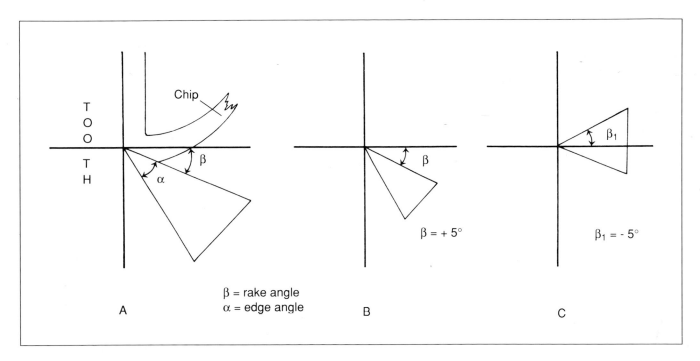

Fig 9-1 (A) *The scaling procedure should result in the formation of chips. To facilitate the scaling procedure, the edge of the instrument should be applied with a rake angle of about ±5 degrees. A working angle of this magnitude will result in optimal cutting even with low pressure on the instrument. (B) Increased angulation of the instrument will increase the risk for "chopping" strokes, resulting in nicks and/or scratches on the root surface. (C) Increase of a negative cutting angle will reduce the cutting effect of the instrument at a constant force. A sharp edge facilitates an optimal result.*

root planing procedure. Of course, the scaling procedure per se also may lead to scratches and irregularities, which should be eliminated by root planing to diminish plaque retention. By using a negative cutting angulation, the cutting effect is diminished and the possibility of achieving a smooth surface is increased. All scaling and root planing should also include polishing of the tooth substance, followed by fluoride application.

The instrument should be sharpened repeatedly and regularly during the scaling and root planing session to secure an optimal result.

Initial periodontal lesions in multirooted teeth often demand treatment of furcations. Odontoplasty, that is, grinding to diminish and widen the furcation opening to facilitate optimal plaque control by toothbrushing and prevent further destruction, constitutes an important part of the treatment in cases of mild periodontitis.

In the light of the result of well-documented clinical trials during the last decade, it is obvious that the basic periodontal therapy always should include traditional scaling and root planing procedures combined with individualized plaque control measures repeated regularly according to needs. An acceptable and realistic level of plaque control may be visible plaque not exceeding 15% to 20% of the tooth surfaces.

REINFORCED BASIC PERIODONTAL THERAPY

To support the posttreatment supragingival plaque control in patients having difficulties with the mechanical plaque control program, it is possible to use a 0.05% to 0.2% solution of chlorhexidine as a mouthrinse for a short time. However, long-term use of chlorhexidine should never be an acceptable solution for plaque control because of the risk for adverse effects such as discoloration of the teeth, changes in taste, and effects on the mucous membranes.

CLINICAL APPLICATION

OBJECTIVE OF THERAPY

The periodontal literature is replete with studies demonstrating that scaling and root planing are generally effective in controlling periodontal disease when probing pocket depths do not exceed 4 mm in depth.[42,77,78] These data would suggest that scaling and root planing with effective plaque control should be the treatment of choice for patients with early adult periodontitis. And, in fact, the literature does demonstrate that mild chronic adult periodontitis is usually successfully treated by scaling and root planing combined with effective plaque control (Figs 9-2a and b).[43,79,80]

The goal of treatment should be to render the roots biologically compatible with soft tissue by eliminating calculus and altered cementum and by reducing periodontal pathogenic microorganisms. Therapy should also address environmental factors affecting bacterial colonization such as root surface irregularities, defective restorations, tooth malposition, and occlusion, as well as the patient's ability to perform effective oral hygiene. The product of these efforts should resolve the inflammation, decrease probing pocket depth and increase attachment level.

The treatment discussed in this chapter can be performed by the general practitioner, depending on his / her skills and interests.

PREOPERATIVE EVALUATION

The sequence of treatment for patients with mild chronic adult periodontitis can and should be adapted to the patient's individual needs. The following paragraphs, however, will provide a treatment outline appropriate for most patients.

The first part of any evaluation begins with a review of the patient's medical history. One needs to ascertain contraindications to dental treatment or need for premedication prior to therapy.

ORAL HYGIENE INSTRUCTIONS, EDUCATION, AND MOTIVATION

It is best to begin patient education and oral hygiene instructions before scaling and root planing. The initial examination should have been an educational experience for the patient; if it was not, the patient should explore the mouth with a mirror as the practitioner points out signs of the disease such as edema, bleeding, purulence, and recession. It is also helpful if the practitioner has discovered what has motivated the patient to seek treatment and connect those wants to the dental needs demonstrated in the examination. The clinician should also try to discover what fears, real or imagined, the patient brings to treatment. These fears are best confronted and resolved before starting therapy. The patient's expectations of the therapy should also be explored to make sure they are realistic.

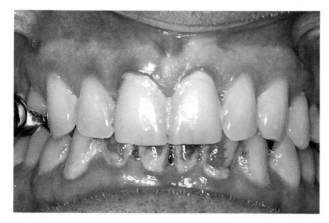

Fig 9-2a A patient with large amounts of plaque and calculus, resulting in mild chronic adult periodontitis.

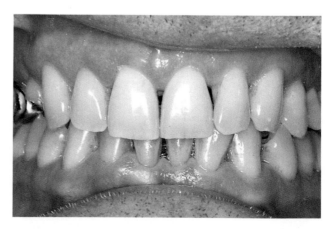

Fig 9-2b The same patient following scaling, root planing, and oral hygiene instruction. Note the resolution of the inflammation.

The importance of effective personal oral hygiene and its relationship to the success of treatment should also be discussed before therapy. The control of bacterial plaque is essential for long-term successful treatment.[31] An oral hygiene instructional visit may be best scheduled as a separate appointment prior to any scaling and root planing. During this visit, the patient can be introduced to disclosing tablets and proper brushing and flossing techniques. Plaque and its relationship to the disease can be discussed, but the clinician must remember that motivation is more important than information. At the next appointment, before beginning scaling and root planing, one should ask the patient the differences seen in the mouth following implementation of the new oral hygiene techniques. For example, does the patient notice less bleeding and swelling or better breath? The patient must establish what can be done and take responsibility for the disease. If oral hygiene instructions are given for the first time as part of the scaling and root planing appointment, it is likely that the patient will assume that all of the changes that he/she notes after the appointment are due to the scaling and not to any of the patient's own efforts. This line of thought breeds dependency and over the long run is counterproductive.

PATIENT AND OPERATOR PROTECTION

For protection of the operator and the patient, proper aseptic technique should be followed. Instruments should be sterilized and appropriate barrier techniques used. The clinician should wear eye protection, mask, and gloves. Having

the patient rinse with chlorhexidine for 30 seconds prior to treatment reduces the spread of microorganisms by atomization during therapy.[81] The clinician should explain to the patient what the scaling and root planing appointment will include, answer any questions, and secure the patient's informed consent. In general, there is very little patient risk associated with this treatment and the benefits are many. By eliminating the inflammation associated with periodontitis, the patient should notice less bleeding and swelling of the gingiva and improvement in both sense of taste and odor of breath.

SCHEDULING THE APPOINTMENT

Insufficient time is frequently allocated for scaling and root planing. It is not uncommon in a research setting for an operator to spend up to 30 minutes instrumenting one surface of one tooth, but in clinical practice one could easily take 45 minutes to an hour to scale and root plane an average quadrant. To minimize patient and operator fatigue, scaling and root planing can be performed a quadrant at a time or half of the mouth at a time. It is best not to scale and root plane any more teeth than you can complete in one appointment because resolution of tissue inflammation may prevent the operator from negotiating deep pockets at subsequent visits. The procedure should be performed systematically (not skipping around) to ensure that all areas are instrumented. Systematic use of individual instruments is also important. Using one instrument on all surfaces where it is applicable before moving on to the next instrument minimizes instru-

ment transfer and makes efficient use of time.

BASIC STROKES

Exploratory Strokes

Two basic strokes are used during root instrumentation: exploratory and working. Exploratory strokes provide information regarding the root surface. The information is usually gained by the use of an explorer, but scalers and curets can also be used with light strokes to identify areas that require further work. Exploratory strokes are the only strokes in which the same amount of pressure is used on both the push and pull aspects. This light pressure is usually directed in a vertical, oblique, or horizontal fashion (Fig 9-3). The periodontal probe is typically not thought of as an explorer, but with experience one can use it to explore the root surface for deposits and surface irregularities as well as to ascertain pocket depths (Fig 9-4). There are limitations, however, to the straight periodontal probe. Explorers with a curved tip (Fig 9-5) provide better access into root depressions and furcations (Fig 9-6).

Prior to beginning treatment, a fine explorer is used to examine the periodontal pockets to be instrumented. The information gained from this exploration combined with a review of the periodontal chart and radiographs will allow the operator to establish the topography of the pockets, root morphology, tissue tone, root surface deposits, and patient sensitivity. This exploration will assist in determining which areas will require more time for scaling and root planing, help in instrument selection, and determine the need for local anesthesia. Local

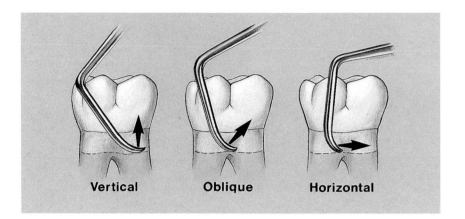

Fig 9-3 *Exploration of the root surface is usually accomplished with a vertical, oblique, or horizontal motion.*

Vertical   **Oblique**   **Horizontal**

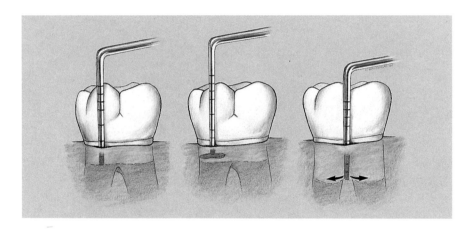

Fig 9-4 *Subgingival exploration with a periodontal probe. The probe is capable of determining probing depth as well as detecting root surface deposits and root topography.*

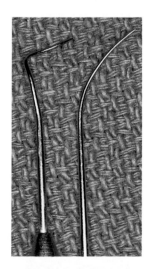

Fig 9-5 *The curved tip of the no. 2 explorer and EXS-3A explorer allow exploration of difficult-to-reach areas.*

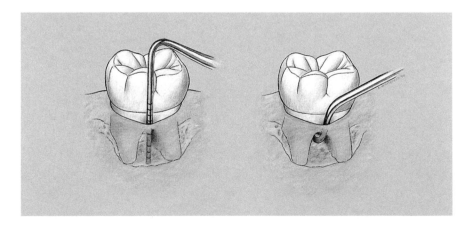

Fig 9-6 *The periodontal probe can provide useful information on root surface topography, but the furcation probe is necessary to totally explore a furcation.*

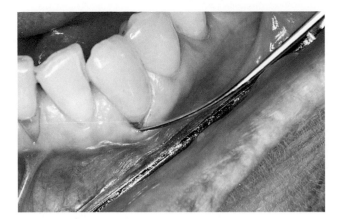

Fig 9-7a *A large piece of calculus can be seen on the root surface of the canine through the translucent gingiva. Its presence is confirmed by an explorer.*

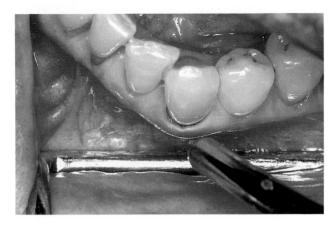

Fig 9-7b *The deposit can be visualized by directing a stream of air from the air water syringe directly into the sulcus.*

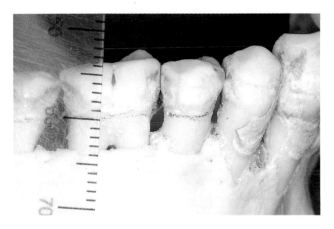

Fig 9-8 *Furcations can be encountered as little as 3 mm from the CEJ. This photograph of a dry skull demonstrates a grade II furcation involvement approximately 3 mm from the CEJ.*

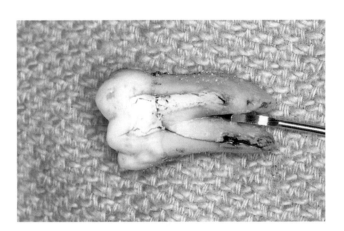

Fig 9-9 *Note the relationship between the size of the furcation opening and the blade of a Gracey curet.*

anesthesia will often be necessary, but its use will depend on the skill of the operator and patient tolerance.

Studies evaluating the effectiveness of scaling and root planing consistently demonstrate that the most difficult areas to instrument effectively are furcations, grooves, abnormalities, concavities, and at the cementoenamel junction.[42,78,82] Because of the ob-

vious difficulty in debriding these areas adequately, they should be explored carefully before moving onto another area. These explorations require a keenly developed tactile sensitivity. Figures 9-7a and b show commonly used methods to evaluate the root surface prior to instrumentation.

Furcation involvement can be a problem even in the patient with early periodontitis with attach-

ment loss of only 2 to 4 mm. Gher and Vernino[83] demonstrated that furcations frequently occur at as little as 3 mm from the cementoenamel junction (Fig 9-8). Bower[84] reported that 50% of the furcation openings he examined were smaller than the smallest curet blade available (Fig 9-9). This means that even when there is adequate access to the furcation, there may not be instruments

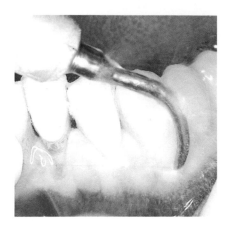

Fig 9-10 *Ultrasonic devices are extremely effective for gross debridement. Here the tip of the ultrasonic can be seen removing the large deposits of calculus discovered facial to the canine (see Fig 9-7).*

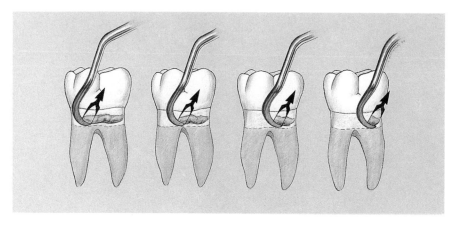

Fig 9-11 *It is inefficient and sometimes impossible to remove large root surface deposits with a single stroke. In gross scaling it is best to engage only a portion of the deposit at a time. This type of sectional scaling ensures that the entire deposit will be removed. Here four strokes are required.*

available to adequately debride the furcation. These facts should encourage the practitioner to aggressively treat patients with early periodontitis before 5 mm or more of attachment loss has occurred. At 5 mm or more, significant furcation involvement is often encountered, changing the prognosis dramatically.

Working Strokes

Once a plan of action has been established, one usually begins with gross scaling. Root surface debridement is usually accomplished with what is called a working stroke. This type of stroke provides constant lateral pressure of the instrument against the root surface. The lateral pressure is applied only on the pull strokes. The two types of working strokes used are the scaling stroke and the root planing stroke.

Scaling The literature is not clear as to whether hand instruments or ultrasonic devices are superior in terms of scaling.[85,86] Traditionally, both supragingival and subgingival gross debridement are accomplished by manual, ultrasonic, or combination techniques (Fig 9-10). Supragingival plaque and calculus removal is beneficial,[87] but one should limit the amount of supragingival root planing because it does not contribute to the success of therapy and leads to root surface sensitivity. Not only should gross scaling be performed in a systematic fashion from tooth to tooth, it should also be performed section by section on the actual root surface deposit (Fig 9-11). Each scaling stroke should overlap the previous one to ensure complete removal of deposits. Scaling should not be thought of as a shaving process in which layers are removed. Shaving often leaves a smooth layer of burnished calculus, difficult to distinguish from the root surface. Instead, all calculus should be removed with strong deliberate working strokes (Figs 9-12a and b). One should not hesitate, how-

ever, to repeat these strokes until the tooth surface has been adequately scaled.

Ultrasonic scalers have traditionally played an important role in gross scaling. Holbrook and Low[88] have suggested customizing tip design for ultrasonic scalers to permit more efficient scaling. These tips are then used with ultrasonic instruments that can have their frequency, amplitude, and water flow manually adjusted to ensure that the tip energy is kept at the minimal level to accomplish a given clinical task. These customized inserts permit access to areas that are very difficult to instrument adequately. At least one study has shown ultrasonic instrumentation to be more effective than hand scaling in grade II and III furcations.[89]

Root Planing Definitive root planing begins at the completion of scaling. Although it is academically beneficial to separate scaling from root planing, they are in reality tied one to another. The

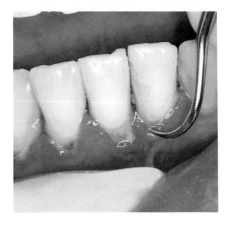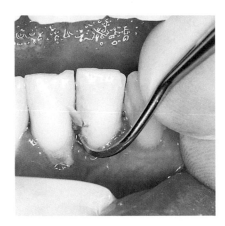

Figs 9-12a and b *The proper use of a scaler during gross debridement. Note that the entire portion of the calculus being instrumented is removed with a deliberate working stroke.*

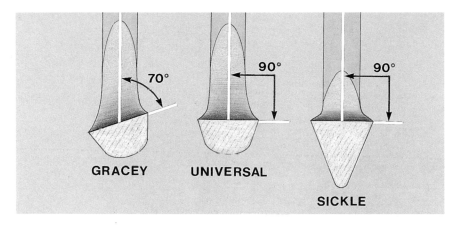

Fig 9-13 *Note the relationship of the blade to the shank on the Gracey curet, universal curet, and sickle scaler.*

two procedures fall along a continuum with scaling at the beginning and root planing near the end. Many instruments have been developed to plane the root, including but not limited to, curets, chisels, hoes, and files. Curets are generally the instrument of choice in root planing, primarily because their shape and size promote tactile sensitivity and provide the best access to difficult areas.

There are two broad categories of curets: universal and limited utility. The universal curets can be used on a number of surfaces of teeth and on different teeth. Examples of these curets are the Columbia 4R 4L or 13-14. Limited-utility curets such as the Gracey curets can be used only on particular surfaces of specific teeth. The major difference between the two types of curets is the angle that the curet blade makes with the shank of the instrument (Fig 9-13). Past experience with the instrument and the specific area being instrumented will generally dictate which curet will be used. Once

chosen, the manner in which the curet is used will determine its effectiveness.

Typically, the curet is held so that the working edge of the blade forms a 60- to 80-degree angle with the root surface. Under light pressure the curet is worked under the gingival margin while the instrument is kept in light contact with the root or calculus. Often, in order to allow the curet to pass over the calculus, the blade must be closed toward the tooth surface at or near an angle of zero degrees. The instrument continues along the root surface until soft tissue resistance is felt, indicating the depth of the pocket. Once at the base of the defect, the angle of the blade is reestablished and the deposit is removed through a deliberate working or power stroke (Fig 9-14). During instrumentation with a curet, it is often useful to vary the force of the stroke from the power stroke to exploratory strokes. These lighter exploratory strokes allow the clinician to determine where more work is needed.

Just as in scaling, root planing strokes should be overlapped. Root surfaces are generally concave or convex, and it is important to try to remove all deposits and altered root cementum. The direction of the stroke will vary depending on the tooth anatomy, design of the instrument, topography of the defect, and access. Most strokes are directed apicocoronally (vertically), but often it is necessary to make oblique, horizontal, and circumferential strokes to engage the interproximal concavities, incipient furcation involvements, and cemento-enamel junction (Fig 9-15).

Definitive root planing begins once all detectable subgingival deposits have been removed (Fig 9-16). A more delicate stroke is generally used for smoothing and

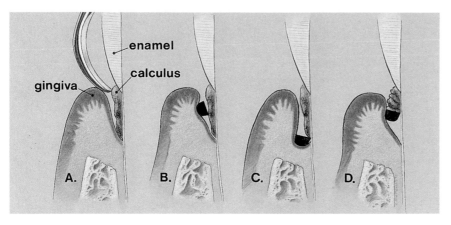

Fig 9-14 *Subgingival scaling. (A) The curet is inserted under the free gingival margin. (B) The curet is passed over the root surface and deposits by closing its angle to near zero degrees. (C) The base of the pocket is felt and the proper angulation of the blade is reestablished. (D) The deposit is removed through a deliberate working stroke.*

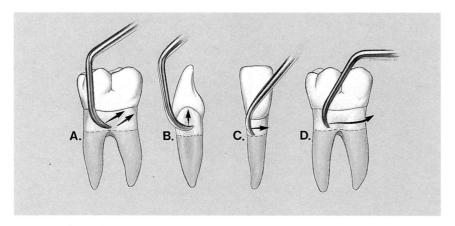

Fig 9-15 *Subgingival scaling or root planing strokes: (A) oblique, (B) vertical, (C) horizontal, and (D) circumferential.*

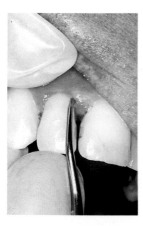

Fig 9-16 *Once subgingival debridement is complete, definitive root planing is begun.*

planing the root surface. The curets must be exquisitely sharp for root planing, and it is not uncommon to use a completely different set of curets for root planing than were used for subgingival scaling. As before, it is important to use overlapping strokes to ensure that all of the pathologically exposed root surface has been instrumented. It may take many strokes to render the root glassy smooth and hard, prior to moving on to another area.

It is often difficult to evaluate when the root has been planed enough. It is best to dry the field, blow air into the sulcus for direct vision when possible, and explore the root surface with a fine explorer. Fiberoptics may be useful and transillumination of the root is sometimes productive. Surgical telescopic glasses are often beneficial as they allow the operator to visually detect root surface imperfections not visible to the naked eye.

Determining the endpoint of scaling and root planing demonstrates the difficulty of translating the results of research to clinical practice. Research projects have clearly demonstrated that it is possible to scale and root plane pathologically exposed root surfaces, removing the endotoxins and rendering the root surface biologically compatible with the soft tissue.[90] These studies are able to determine their endpoints by very sophisticated measurements, yet we in clinical practice must continue to rely on crude and highly subjective methods such as exploring the root surfaces for roughness with an explorer. As crude as this measurement is, it has historically been effective. The ultimate test of the effectiveness of root instrumentation does not occur until 4 to 6 weeks after scaling when the soft tissue response to therapy is reevaluated. (This reevaluation visit is covered later in this chapter.)

CURETTAGE

Curettage is rarely part of the treatment for mild or moderate chronic adult periodontitis because studies have demonstrated no advantage to soft tissue curettage as part of scaling and root planing.[91] Only sulci exhibiting disease should be instrumented. Scaling and root planing of healthy sulci is unnecessary and can actually promote attachment loss.[77,92]

The importance of sharp instruments cannot be overemphasized. It is difficult to sharpen instruments effectively and many resources are available to provide guidance. Instruments should be sharpened prior to use and while performing scaling and root planing. To make this possible, a sterile sharpening stone should be kept on the tray.

CORONAL POLISHING AND POSTOPERATIVE INSTRUCTIONS

Once scaling and root planing is complete, the defect should be irrigated to remove fragments of calculus, shavings of cementum, and other debris. The supragingival portions of the tooth are generally polished with a handpiece and rubber cup or with an air-powder device. Oral hygiene instructions should be reviewed and particular attention should be given to areas that will be difficult for the patient to maintain. Patients should be told that they may experience some soreness in the scaled areas. Over-the-counter analgesics should be adequate for postoperative pain relief.

POST-SCALING ORAL HYGIENE INSTRUCTIONS

It is often useful to reappoint the patient for an oral hygiene instructional visit approximately 2 weeks after the scaling and root planing is completed. The patient should be asked if he/she is experiencing difficulty in performing any oral hygiene procedures he/she has been asked to do. This oral hygiene appointment can be particularly effective in demonstrating where the patient is having difficulty with home care. It can be explained to the patient that all plaque was removed at the previous visit; therefore, any plaque found today has accumulated since the last appointment, demonstrating areas the patient finds difficult to clean. Time should be spent developing effective ways to clean the areas that are difficult to maintain. Often, areas that a patient may tell you he/she has difficulty with may not be the same areas your examination reveals to be problematic. Positive reinforcement of properly performed home care is extremely important. One should point out as many areas as possible where the patient is effective with home care procedures. Some record of home care effectiveness or a plaque score should be recorded, and the types of home care devices given to the patient should be documented.

REEVALUATION

The next appointment typically takes place 4 to 8 weeks after completion of the scaling and root planing.[93] Although the primary function of the reevaluation visit is to determine the effectiveness of the scaling and root planing, it is also appropriate to review home care proficiency. Areas that are not responding as expected can be reinstrumented. Sometimes residual root surface deposits will be apparent due to tissue resolution. Probing depth should be recharted, and bleeding on probing, purulence, and tissue tone should be recorded. All inflammation, bleeding on probing, and purulence should be eliminated. Depending on the preoperative tissue tone, a reduction of probing depth from 1 to 2 mm would be expected.

The reevaluation appointment may reveal other problems requiring special considerations. For example, gingival hyperplasia or interproximal cratering may require a gingivectomy or gingivoplasty to create an environment more conducive to maintenance care (see chapter 12). Plaque retentive or biologically incompatible dental restorations should be replaced and other local factors that could make supportive periodontal treatment difficult should be corrected.

One should expect to resolve mild chronic adult periodontitis with the procedures mentioned up to this point. If the expected results are not achieved (ie, bleeding on probing not eliminated and probing depth not reduced by 1 to 2 mm), then one might consider referral of the patient to a periodontist for more advanced treatment. It is unlikely that performing any more of the same procedures will improve the results. At this time, it would be appropriate to assume that the initial diagnosis of early adult periodontitis was incorrect, and the therapist might consider microbial culture and sensitivity testing and the use of appropriate antibiotics. One also must consider the possibility that the patient could be dealing with a host containment defect. If the expected results are not achieved, then the patient should be referred for more specialized care and not continue to be treated for mild chronic adult periodontitis.

CHEMICAL PLAQUE CONTROL

Mild chronic adult periodontitis should respond well to scaling and root planing without chemotherapeutics. Their use may enhance tissue response but only minimally and for a short duration. Chemotherapeutics are not a substitute for diligent instrumentation even though they may mask (short-term) residual inflammation. Special mouthrinses and toothpastes have no effect on subgingival plaque even though they may suppress supragingival plaque formation.[92] At the present time, there are only two topical antimicrobials that have been shown to be effective at reducing supragingival plaque and gingivitis: chlorhexidine gluconate and phenolic compounds. The substantivity of chlorhexidine provides a sizable edge over the phenolic compounds, and, in fact, chlorhexidine is so superior to other topical antimicrobials that it is difficult to make a case for them.[94] While these topical antimicrobials may be useful occasionally as an adjunct in assisting patients with the control of supragingival plaque, none of them has ever been shown to be effective in treating periodontitis.[95]

ADJUNCTIVE ANTIBIOTICS

Studies have evaluated the efficacy of scaling and root planing with and without antibiotics.[52] It was demonstrated that the results from scaling and root planing with systemically administered antibiotics were not significantly better than results from scaling and root planing alone. Timed release and local delivery of antibiotics may offer promise in the treatment of aggressive forms of periodontitis. Compared to systemic administration, local delivery provides a significant increase in local concentration of the antibiotic with considerable reduction in the dose.[96] But in no way are antibiotics a substitute for effective scaling and root planing, and they are not indicated for the control of plaque and gingivitis because their potential adverse effects outweigh their therapeutic benefit. The value of adjunctive antibiotics in the treatment of mild chronic adult periodontitis has not been established.[97]

IRRIGATION

No irrigating agent has been shown to be effective for the treatment of adult periodontitis,[87] and the benefits of subgingival irrigation have not been clearly established. With chlorhexidine being found to be so effective in the control of supragingival plaque, a logical extrapolation would be its use in subgingival irrigation. Newman and co-workers[98,99] have recently demonstrated a positive effect on gingivitis by irrigating chlorhexidine following scaling and root planing. Other studies have evaluated this in periodontitis, and all of them have found that subgingival irrigation with chlorhexidine had little clinical value other than a short-term reduction in some bacteria.[100-103] Studies have evaluated many other irrigants, and it is difficult to translate the results from closed clinical trials to a private practice setting. Irrigants of any type generally are not needed in the treatment of mild chronic adult periodontitis because the disease responds so predictably to scaling and root planing alone.

SUPPORTIVE PERIODONTAL TREATMENT

After treatment is complete and the clinician is satisfied with the results, data (probing pocket depth, bleeding on probing, purulence, mobility) are collected to serve as a baseline for further evaluation and to provide the therapist with information to determine the most appropriate supportive periodontal treatment. Assuming appropriate response to therapy and adequate home care, one might initially place the average patient with mild chronic adult periodontitis on a 3-month recall. The actual length of this interval, however, should be customized for the patient's particular problems. Such factors as oral hygiene, anatomic considerations, restorative plans, and the patient's sensitivity to periodontal disease will ultimately determine the appropriate recall interval. This recall interval is shortened or lengthened as appropriate depending on how the patient responds.

The treatment of the patient with early adult periodontitis can be dramatic and often very gratifying. The therapist and the patient working together can predictably eliminate bleeding gums, improve breath, and enhance esthetics by eliminating soft tissue inflammation. The end result is a patient who appreciates not only the important part that periodontics plays in the overall healthcare program, but also the role he/she must assume in maintenance.

QUICK REVIEW

I. The concept of periodontal disease has evolved

- Therapy for mild chronic adult periodontitis is currently aimed at reducing or altering the makeup of bacteria and their products.
- Therefore, early diagnosis and treatment are important to stop disease progression.
- This early intervention usually involves improved oral hygiene on the part of the patient and closed subgingival scaling and root planing by the dental professional.
- At present, clinical parameters, not bacterial indicators, offer the preferred method for judging success.
- For long-term success, active therapy must be followed by supportive periodontal treatment (maintenance).

II. Treatment of the patient with mild chronic adult periodontitis (Instrumentation mentioned is appropriate, but the operator must develop his/her own technique.)

- Review medical history.
- Patient education and oral hygiene instruction:
  - demonstrate to the patient with a hand mirror plaque deposits, inflammation, bleeding pus, pockets, etc, and explain their relationship with periodontal disease
  - emphasize brushing and flossing technique:
    (1) Brush at dentogingival interface
    (2) Floss as deeply as possible
    (3) Inform patient of initial period of discomfort from this technique
- Two weeks later, patient returns for first scaling visit:
  - ask patient if he/she can tell any improvement in the mouth from the new oral hygiene technique; it is important to establish what the patient can accomplish himself/herself
  - discuss with patient his hopes, fears, and expectations regarding scaling and root planing

- explore periodontal pockets (Hu-Friedy EXD 11-12, EXS-3A, CH3, Nabers 2N furcation probes), review charting and radiographs, determine need for anesthetics
- gross scale (ultrasonics TFI-10)
- scaling and root planing (typically half of the mouth at a time):
  (1) Maxillary molars and premolars: Columbia 4R4L; Gracey 13-14 typically apicocoronal strokes on distal surfaces (if tissue is very inflamed, this instrument is useful with tip pointed into the sulcus with horizontal stroke); Gracey 11-12 mesial surfaces; Gracey 1-2 or Gracey 5-6 facial and lingual surfaces
  (2) Maxillary anterior teeth: Gracey 1-2 (good with horizontal strokes); (SH 6/7 effective for burnished subgingival calculus at CEJ)
  (3) Mandibular molars and premolars: Gracey 11-12; Gracey 13-14; Columbia 4R4L; S 107/108 Sickle (effective for subgingival flinty calculus); Gracey 1-2 or Gracey 5-6 for facial or lingual surfaces
  (4) Mandibular anterior teeth: SH 6/7; Gracey 13-14 (good angulation for access to lingual of mandibular anterior teeth); Gracey 1-2
  (5) Polish according to patient's specific needs: prophy jet; rotary cup with pumice; rotary cup with paste for composite resin or porcelain laminate veneers
  (6) Oral hygiene instructions especially as they relate to problem areas
- Oral hygiene instructions 2 weeks following completion of scaling and root planing; motivation is much more important than information.

Quick Review continues on page 140.

QUICK REVIEW
(continued)

MILD CHRONIC ADULT PERIODONTITIS

• Reevaluation to determine soft tissue response 4 to 6 weeks following scaling and root planing. Patient is placed on appropriate maintenance schedule if

therapy was successful or is referred for more specialized care if treatment was not effective.

REFERENCES

1. Russel AL: System of classification and scoring for prevalence surveys of periodontal disease. *J Dent Res* 1956;35:350-359.

2. Ramfjord SP: Indices for prevalence and incidence of periodontal disease. *J Periodontol* 1959;30:57-59.

3. Greene JC, Vermillion JR: Oral hygiene index: A method for classifying oral hygiene status. *J Am Dent Assoc* 1960;61:172-179.

4. Russel AL: International nutrition surveys: A summary of preliminary dental findings. *J Dent Res* 1963;42:233-244.

5. Löe H, Silness J: Periodontal disease in pregnancy. I. Prevalence and severity. *Acta Odontol Scand* 1963;21:532-551.

6. Ramfjord SP, Knowles JW, Nissle RR, Shick RA, Burgett FG: Longitudinal study of periodontal therapy. *J Periodontol* 1973;44:66-77.

7. Nyman S, Rosling B, Lindhe J: Effect of professional tooth cleaning on healing after periodontal surgery. *J Clin Periodontol* 1975;2:80.

8. Rosling B, Nyman S, Lindhe J: The effect of systematic plaque control on bony regeneration in infrabony pockets. *J Clin Periodontol* 1976;3:38.

9. Rosling B, Nyman S, Lindhe J, Jern B: The healing potential of the periodontal tissues following different techniques of periodontal surgery in plaque-free dentitions. A 2-year clinical study. *J Clin Periodontol* 1976;3:233.

10. Ramfjord SP, Knowles JW, Nissle RR, Burgett FG, Shick RA: Results following three modalities of periodontal therapy. *J Periodontol* 1975;46:522.

11. Isidor F: *Effect of Periodontal Surgery*. Thesis, Royal Dental College, Aarhus, Denmark, 1981.

12. Lindhe J, Westfelt E, Nyman S, Socransky SS, Heijl L, Bratthall G: Healing following surgical/non-surgical treatment of periodontal disease. A clinical study. *J Clin Periodontol* 1982;9:115-128.

13. Westfelt E, Bragd L, Socransky SS, Haffajee A, Nyman S, Lindhe J: Improved periodontal conditions following therapy. *J Clin Periodontol* 1985;12:283-293.

14. Badersten A, Nilvéus R, Egelberg J: Effect of nonsurgical periodontal therapy. I. Moderately advanced periodontitis. *J Clin Periodontol* 1981;8:57-72.

15. Ramfjord SP, Morrison EC, Burgett FG, Nissle RR, Schick RA, Zann GJ, Knowles JW: Oral hygiene and maintenance of periodontal support. *J Periodontol* 1982;53:26-30.

16. Lindhe J, Nyman S: Long-term maintenance of patients treated for advanced periodontal disease. *J Clin Periodontol* 1984;11:504-514.

17. Socransky SS: Microbiology of periodontal disease — Present status and future considerations. *J Periodontol* 1977;48:497-504.

18. Slots J: Subgingival microflora in periodontal disease. *J Clin Periodontol* 1979;6:351-382.

19. Slots J, Genco RJ: Black-pigmented *Bacteroides* species, *Capnocytophaga* species, and *Actinobacillus actinomycetemcomitans* in human periodontal disease: Virulence factors in colonization, survival, and tissue destruction. *J Dent Res* 1984;63:412-421.

20. Slots J, Rosling BG: Suppression of the periodontopathic microflora in localized juvenile periodontitis by systemic tetracycline. *J Clin Periodontol* 1983;10:465-486.

21. Christersson L, Slots J, Rosling B, Genco R: Microbiological and clinical effects of surgical treatment of localized juvenile periodontitis. *J Clin Periodontol* 1985;12:465-476.

22. Slots J, Emrich L, Genco RJ, Rosling BG: Relationship between some subgingival bacteria and periodontal pocket depth and gain or loss of periodontal attachment after treatment of adult periodontitis. *J Clin Periodontol* 1985;12:540-552.

23. Rosling B, Slots J, Webber RL, Chris-

tersson LA, Genco RJ: Microbiological and clinical effects of topical subgingival antimicrobial treatment on human periodontal disease. *J Clin Periodontol* 1983;10:487-514.

24. Rosling BG, Slots J, Christersson LA, Grondhal HG, Genco RJ: Topical antimicrobial therapy and diagnosis of subgingival bacteria in the management of inflammatory periodontal disease. *J Clin Periodontol* 1986;13:975-981.

25. Genco RJ: Antibiotics in the treatment of human periodontal diseases. *J Periodontol* 1981;52:545-558.

26. Goodson JM, Haffajee A, Socransky SS: Periodontal therapy by local delivery of tetracycline. *J Clin Periodontol* 1979;6:83-92.

27. Lindhe J, Heijl L, Goodson JM, Socransky SS: Local tetracycline delivery using hollow fiber devices in periodontal therapy. *J Clin Periodontol* 1979;6:141-149.

28. Hamp SE: *On the Development and Prevention of Periodontal Disease in the Beagle Dog*. Thesis, University of Gothenburg, Gothenburg, Sweden, 1973.

29. Lindhe J, Nyman S: The effect of plaque control and surgical pocket elimination on the establishment and maintenance of periodontal health. A longitudinal study of periodontal therapy in cases of advanced disease. *J Clin Periodontol* 1975;2:67-79.

30. Lövdal A, Arno A, Schei O, Waerhaug J: Combined effect of subgingival scaling and controlled oral hygiene on the incidence of gingivitis. *Acta Odontol Scand* 1961;19:537-555.

31. Suomi JD, Greene JC, Vermillion JR, Doyle J, Chang JJ, Leatherwood EC: The effect of controlled oral hygiene procedures on the progression of periodontal disease in adults: Results after third and final year. *J Periodontol* 1971;42:152-160.

32. Waerhaug J: Plaque control in the treatment of juvenile periodontitis. *J Clin Periodontol* 1977;4:29-40.

33. Lindhe J, Socransky SS, Nyman S, Haffajee A, Westfelt E: "Critical probing depths" in periodontal therapy. *J Clin Periodontol* 1982;9:323-336.

34. Löe H, Theilade E, Jensen SB: Experimental gingivitis in man. *J Periodontol* 1965;36:177-187.

35. Axelsson P, Lindhe J: Effect of controlled oral hygiene procedures on caries and periodontal disease in adults. *J Clin Periodontol* 1978;5:133-151.

36. Tagge DL, O'Leary TJ, El-Kafrawy AH: The clinical and histological response of periodontal pockets to root planing and oral hygiene. *J Periodontol* 1975;46:527-533.

37. Helldén LB, Listgarten MA, Lindhe J: The effect of tetracycline and/or scaling on human periodontal disease. *J Clin Periodontol* 1979;6:222-230.

38. Hartzell TB: The practical surgery of the root surface in pyorrhea. *Dental Cosmos* 1911;53:513-521.

39. Black GV: *A Work on Special Dental Pathology*. 1st ed. Chicago; Medico-Dental Publishing Co, 1915.

40. Waerhaug J, Arno A, Lövdal A: Dimension of instruments for removal of subgingival calculus. *J Periodontol* 1954;25:281-286.

41. Hughes TP, Caffesse RG: Gingival changes following scaling, root planing and oral hygiene. A biometric evaluation. *J Periodontol* 1978;49:245-252.

42. Waerhaug J: Healing of the dento-epithelial junction following subgingival plaque control. II. As observed on extracted teeth. *J Periodontol* 1978;49:119-134.

43. Knowles JW, Burgett FG, Nissle RR, Shick RA, Morrison EC, Ramfjord SP: Results of periodontal treatment related to pocket depth and attachment level. Eight years. *J Periodontol* 1979;50:225-233.

44. Pihlström BL, Ortiz-Campos C, McHugh RB: A randomized four-year study of periodontal therapy. *J Periodontol* 1981;52:227-242.

45. Slots J: Importance of black-pigmented *Bacteroides* in human periodontal disease. In: Genco RJ, Mergenhagen SE, eds. *Host Parasite Interactions in Periodontal Diseases*. Washington, DC: American Society for Microbiology, 1982; 27-45.

46. Slots J, Zambon JJ, Rosling BG, Reynolds HS, Christersson LA, Genco RJ: *Actinobacillus actinomycetemcomitans* in human periodontal disease. Association serology leukotoxicity, and treatment. *J Periodont Res* 1982;17:447-448.

47. Mashimo PA, Yamamoto Y, Slots J, Park BH, Genco RJ: The periodontal microflora of juvenile diabetics. Culture, immunofluorescence, and serum antibody studies. *J Periodontol* 1983;54:420-430.

48. Loesche WJ, Syed SA, Laughon BE, Stoll J: The bacteriology of acute necrotizing ulcerative gingivitis. *J Periodontol* 1982;53:223-230.

49. Chung CP, Nisengard RJ, Slots J, Genco RJ: Bacterial IgG and IgM antibody titers in acute necrotizing ulcerative gingivitis. *J Clin Periodontol* 1983;54:557-562.

50. Moore WEC, Holdeman LV, Smibert RM, Hash DE, Burmeister JA, Ranney RR: Bacteriology of severe periodontitis in young adult humans. *Infect Immun* 1982;38:1137-1148.

51. Tempro PJ, Slots J, Genco RJ: The relationship between oral *Haemophilus* and human periodontal disease. American Society for Microbiology. Annual Meeting of the American Society for Microbiology, 1983: Abstract No. I-150.

52. Listgarten MA, Lindhe J, Helldén L: Effect of tetracycline and/or scaling on human periodontal disease. Clinical, microbiological, and histological observations. *J Clin Periodontol* 1978;5:246-271.

53. Slots J, Mashimo P, Levine MJ, Genco RJ: Periodontal therapy in humans. I. Microbiological and clinical effects of a single course of periodontal scaling and root planing, and of adjunctive tetracycline therapy. *J Periodontol* 1979;50:495-509.

54. Loesche WJ, Syed SA, Morrison IC, Laughon B, Grossman NS: Treatment of periodontal infections due to anaerobic bacteria with short-term treatment with metronidazole. *J Clin Periodontol* 1981;8:29-44.

55. Lindhe J, Liljenberg B, Adielson B, Borjesson I: The effect of metronidazole therapy on human periodontal disease. *J Periodont Res* 1982;17:534-536.

56. Davies RM, Jensen SB, Schiött CR, Löe H: The effect of topical application of chlorhexidine on the bacterial colonization of the teeth and gingiva. *J Periodont Res* 1970;5:96-101.

57. Löe H, Schiött CR: The effect of suppression of the oral microflora upon the development of dental plaque and gingivitis. In: McHugh WD, ed. *Dental Plaque*. Edinburgh: E & S Livingstone; 1970: 247-255.

58. Löe H, Schiött CR: The effect of mouthrinses and topical application of chlorhexidine on the development of dental plaque and gingivitis in man. *J Periodont Res* 1970;5:79-83.

59. Löe H, Mandell M, Derry A, Schiött CR: The effect of mouthrinses and topical application of chlorhexidine on calculus formation in man. *J Periodont Res* 1971;6:312-314.

60. Löe H, Schiött CR, Glavind L, Karring T: Two years oral use of chlorhexidine in man. I. General design and clinical effects. *J Periodont Res* 1976;11:135-144.

61. Flötra L, Gjermo P, Rölla G, Waerhaug J: A 4-month study on the effect of chlorhexidine mouth washes on 50 soldiers. *Scand J Dent Res* 1972;80:10-17.

62. Cumming BR, Löe H: Optimal dosage and method of delivering chlorhexidine solutions for the inhibition of dental plaque. *J Periodont Res* 1973;8:57-62.

63. Soh LL, Newman HN, Strahan JD: Effects of subgingival chlorhexidine irrigation on periodontal inflammation. *J Clin Periodontol* 1982;9:66-74.

64. Garrett JS: Effects of nonsurgical periodontal therapy on periodontitis in humans: A review. *J Clin Periodontol* 1983;10:515-523.

65. Mazza JE, Newman MG, Sims TN: Clinical and antimicrobial effect of stannous fluoride on periodontitis. *J Clin Periodontol* 1981;8:203-212.

66. Wennström J, Lindhe J: Effect of hydrogen peroxide on developing plaque and gingivitis in man. *J Clin Periodontol* 1970;6:115-130.

67. Talbot ES: The treatment of interstitial gingivitis and pyorrhea alveolaris. *Dental Cosmos* 1915;57:485-491.

68. MacAlpine R, Magnusson I, Kiger R, Crigger M, Egelberg J: Antimicrobial irrigation of deep pockets to supplement nonsurgical periodontal therapy. *J Clin Periodontol* 1983;10:568-575.

69. Davies BD, Dulbecco R, Eisen HN, Ginsberg HS: *Microbiology*. 3rd ed. New York: Harper & Row Publishers, Inc, 1980.

70. Nyman S, Lindhe J, Lundgren D: The role of occlusion for the stability of fixed bridges in patients with reduced periodontal tissue support. *J Clin Periodontol* 1975;2:53.

71. Nyman S, Lindhe J, Rosling B: Periodontal surgery in plaque-infected dentitions. *J Clin Periodontol* 1977;4:240-249.

72. Axelsson P, Lindhe J: Effect of controlled oral hygiene procedures on caries and periodontal disease in adults. Results after 6 years. *J Clin Periodontol* 1981;8:239-248.

73. Axelsson P, Lindhe J: The significance of maintenance care in the treatment of periodontal disease. *J Clin Periodontol* 1981;8:281-294.

74. Badersten A, Nilvéus R, Egelberg J: Effect of nonsurgical periodontal therapy. II. Severely advanced periodontitis. *J Clin Periodontol* 1984;11:63-76.

75. Badersten A, Nilvéus R, Egelberg J: Effect of nonsurgical periodontal therapy. III. Single versus repeated instrumentation. *J Clin Periodontol* 1984;11:114-124.

76. Lindhe J: Orthogonal cutting of dentine. (A methodological study.) *Odontol Rev* 1964;15(suppl 8):5.

77. Pihlström BL, McHugh RB, Oliphant

TH, Ortiz-Campos C: Comparison of surgical and nonsurgical treatment of periodontal disease. A review of current studies and additional results after 6-1/2 years. *J Clin Periodontol* 1983;10:524-541.

78. Stambaugh RV, Dragoo M, Smith DM, Carasal L: The limits of subgingival scaling. *Int J Periodont Rest Dent* 1981;1(5):30-41.

79. Lindhe J, Westfel E, Nyman S, Socransky SS, Haffajee AD: Long-term effects of surgical/non-surgical treatment of periodontal disease. *J Clin Periodontol* 1984;11:448-458.

80. Ramfjord SP, Knowles JW, Morrison EC, Burgett FG, Nissle RR: Results of periodontal therapy related to tooth type. *J Periodontol* 1980;51:270.

81. Guest GF, Cottone JA: Personal protection: The first line of defense. *Texas Dent J* 1987;104(9):16-18.

82. Rabbani GM, Ash MM Jr, Caffesse RG: The effectiveness of subgingival scaling and root planing in calculus removal. *J Periodontol* 1981;52:119-123.

83. Gher ME, Vernino AR: Root morphology — Clinical significance in pathogenesis and treatment of periodontal disease. *J Am Dent Assoc* 1980;101:627-633.

84. Bower RC: Furcation morphology relative to periodontal treatment. Furcation entrance architecture. *J Periodontol* 1979;50:23-27.

85. American Academy of Periodontology: *Proceedings of the World Workshop in Clinical Periodontics.* Chicago: American Academy of Periodontology; 1989:II:1-20.

86. Walsh TF, Waite IM: A comparison of postsurgical healing following debridement by ultrasonic or hand instruments. *J Periodontol* 1978;49:201-205.

87. Ciancio SG, Genco RJ, Schallhorn RG, Goodsen JM: Non-surgical antibacterial approaches to periodontal treatment. *J Am Dent Assoc* 1988;116:22-32.

88. Holbrook TE, Low SB: Power-driven scaling and polishing instruments. In: Hardin J, ed. *Clark's Clinical Dentistry.* Philadelphia: JB Lippincott Co, 1989: 5-A, 1-24.

89. Leon LE, Vogel RI: A comparison of the effectiveness of hand scaling and ultrasonic debridement in furcations as evaluated by differential dark-field microscopy. *J Periodontol* 1987;58:86-94.

90. Jones WA, O'Leary TJ: The effectiveness of in vivo root planing in removing bacterial endotoxin from the roots of periodontally involved teeth. *J Periodontol* 1978;49:337-342.

91. Echeverria JJ, Caffesse RG: Effects of gingival curettage when performed one month after root instrumentation. A biometric evaluation. *J Clin Periodontol* 1983;10:277-286.

92. Ramfjord SP, Caffesse RG, Morrison EC, et al: Four modalities of periodontal treatment compared over five years. *J Clin Periodont Res* 1987;22:222-223.

93. Morrison EC, Ramfjord SP, Hill RW: Short-term effects of initial, nonsurgical periodontal treatment (hygienic phase). *J Clin Periodontol* 1980; 7:199-211.

94. Addy M: Chlorhexidine compared to other locally delivered antimicrobials. A short review. *J Clin Periodontol* 1986;13:957-964.

95. American Dental Association: *Council on Dental Therapeutics of the American Dental Association.* Chicago: American Dental Association; 1986:529-532.

96. Goodsen JM, Offenbacher S, Farr DH, Hogan PE: Periodontal disease treatment by local drug delivery. *J Periodontol* 1985;56:265-272.

97. van Palenstein Helderman WH: Is antibiotic therapy justified in the treatment of human chronic inflammatory periodontal disease? *J Clin Periodontol* 1986;13:932-938.

98. Flemmig TF, Newman MG, Doherty FM, et al: Supragingival irrigation with 0.06% chlorhexidine in naturally occurring gingivitis. I. 6 months clinical observation. *J Periodontol* 1990;61:112-117.

99. Newman MG, Flemmig TF, Nachnani S, et al: Irrigation with 0.06% chlorhexidine in naturally occurring gingivitis. II. 6 month microbiological observations. *J Periodontol* 1990; 61:427-433.

100. Haskel E, Esquenasi J, Yussim L: Effects of subgingival chlorhexidine irrigation in chronic moderate periodontitis. *J Periodontol* 1986; 57:305-310.

101. Lander PE, Newcomb GM, Seymour GJ, et al: The antimicrobial and clinical effects of a single subgingival irrigation of chlorhexidine in advanced periodontal lesions. *J Clin Periodontol* 1986;13:74-80.

102. Wennström JL, Heijl L, Dahlen G, Kerstin G: Periodic subgingival antimicrobial irrigation of periodontal pockets. I. Clinical observations. *J Clin Periodontol* 1987;14:541-550.

103. Wennström JL, Dahlen G, Grondahl K, et al: Periodic subgingival antimicrobial irrigation of periodontal pockets. II. Microbial and radiographic observations. *J Clin Periodontol* 1987;14:573-580.

Moderate Chronic Adult Periodontitis

O V E R V I E W by Kenneth L. Kalkwarf

C U R R E N T   C O N C E P T S by Erwin P. Barrington

C L I N I C A L   A P P L I C A T I O N by Dan M. Loughlin

O   V   E   R   V   I   E   W

During the past two decades, numerous research endeavors have supplied us with a wealth of information regarding the etiology of and therapy for chronic adult periodontitis. Some of the information presented is relatively straightforward and easily transferable to clinical practice. Other information appears to be contradictory and has created a somewhat confusing environment for the dental professional.

Prior to the 1970s, periodontal therapy was primarily aimed at surgical elimination of the defect created by the periodontitis and reduction of "pocket depth." Initial longitudinal clinical trials from the University of Michigan demonstrated that surgical reduction of probing depth was not absolutely necessary to halt the progression of disease as determined by measurement of mean probing attachment levels. These studies verified that surgical debridement with or without osseous resection, coupled with supportive periodontal therapy (maintenance), was capable of maintaining periodontal stability. Studies from the University of Minnesota later demonstrated that closed debridement, accomplished by root instrumentation without surgical flap reflection, was also capable of halting the progress of chronic adult periodontitis and stabilizing mean probing attachment levels when coupled with appropriate maintenance care.

The primary criticism of these original clinical trials was related to the statistical management of the data. Each study presented their conclusions based upon the comparison of mean data, which tends to mask the response of a small number of sites that respond differently from the majority of sites.

More recent data from the University of Nebraska have begun to address this concern and have demonstrated that certain types of sites, particularly those associated with furcations, do not respond as well as other sites, regardless of the type of surgical or nonsurgical debridement that is used as therapy.

It had been argued that surgical periodontal therapy provides a major advantage to nonsurgical approaches due to its ability to provide access and visualization for root instrumentation. This theory has been accentuated by a series of studies demonstrating the inability of scaling and root planing procedures to predictably remove all etiologic agents (plaque / calculus) from the root surface. Kepic and associates[1] have recently confirmed the preliminary findings of others and substantiated that the complete removal of calculus from periodontally diseased root surfaces is rare regardless of whether ultrasonics or hand instruments are used, and regardless of whether an open surgical or a closed nonsurgical approach is used. These data appear to be in conflict with results reported from the previously mentioned longitudinal

trials. If it is impossible to remove the etiologic factors for chronic adult periodontitis from the root surface, how is it possible to halt periodontitis as is evidenced by long-term stability of probing attachment? This dilemma is probably best explained by Robertson[2] when he states, "while total elimination of etiologic factors is the appropriate treatment goal, reduction of plaque and calculus below the threshold level that is acceptable to the host appears to control the infection process and improve the clinical signs of inflammation."

The stability of mean probing attachment levels, as shown in the longitudinal trials, indicates that root instrumentation by surgical and nonsurgical approaches is capable of reducing the level of etiologic agents below threshold levels at most sites in most individuals. Sites that do not respond like the mean are indicative of failure to reduce etiologic levels beneath the patient's threshold. Such failure may be a consequence of inadequate debride-

ment due to anatomical limitations (probing depth, root surface aberrations, grooves, or furcations) or due to an abnormally low patient threshold secondary to immunologic irregularities or other systemic complications.

Based on the compilation of this information, a rationale for the treatment of chronic adult periodontitis must be based upon debridement of the root surface associated with the periodontal defect. The initial approach to therapy should involve the type of debridement that can be rendered in the most expeditious and cost effective manner. Following adequate time for a healing response, an assessment should be completed. Those individuals, or sites within individuals, that do not respond favorably to therapy should be reexamined, including appropriate evaluation of local or systemic complications that may be influencing their response. Additional treatment should factor in the results of such reexamination.

CURRENT CONCEPTS

There are a variety of treatments for moderate chronic adult periodontitis that can be implemented with an acceptable degree of predictable success. By definition, moderate chronic adult periodontitis involves 5 to 6 mm of clinical probing depth with destruction of periodontal structures and noticeable loss of bone support, possibly accompanied by an increase in tooth mobility. There may be furcation involvement in multirooted teeth.[3] Probing depth varies with the position of the gingival margin. In most instances

probing depth closely correlates with the attachment loss. However, there are also instances where inflammatory enlargement of the tissue causes a deeper probing depth and instances where recession of the gingival margin causes a lesser probing depth. Radiographs generally show a corresponding loss of alveolar bone.[4] The pattern of bone loss will generally be horizontal, but in moderate periodontal disease vertical bone loss begins to appear.[5] For the purposes of this chapter it will be assumed that grade I or early

grade II furcations are also found in these cases and that closed subgingival scaling and root planing similar to that described in chapter 9 has been performed.

TREATMENT APPROACH TO MODERATE CHRONIC ADULT PERIODONTITIS

The purpose of treatment is to interrupt a sequence of destructive events called periodontitis. Treatment should be designed to stop the disease process and bring it under control. Personal oral hygiene is an integral part of all therapy and must be coordinated into the treatment plan.[6] In general, further treatment approaches involve either more closed scaling and root planing or a choice of several surgical therapies. Certainly, more than one treatment mode can be used in treating a patient.[3,6-9]

SCALING AND ROOT PLANING

Although scaling and root planing was covered in detail in chapter 9, scaling and root planing also extends into the treatment of moderate disease.

Four to six millimeters is about the depth limit that can be successfully negotiated with closed scaling and root planing. Several authors have reported that in pocket depths over 3 mm, removal of all calculus and plaque would be difficult, if not impossible. However, there are also several studies that support the finding that scaling and root planing is effective in moderate disease.[7-13]

The clinician must weigh all the factors of the case and the response of the patient in determining whether closed scaling and root planing will be effective.[14-16] For example, a patient with 4- to 6-mm probing depths and corresponding attachment loss, horizontal bone loss, no furcation problem, and soft edematous tissue certainly would be a better candidate for this approach than a patient with vertical bone loss, shallow two-wall interproximal bony craters, and furcation involvement and/or fibrous thick tissue. The crux of the decision must be related to the ability of

the clinician to cleanse and detoxify the diseased root surface.[15,16] Once the area is cleaned, it must be maintained.[17,18] Therefore, if adequate access can be obtained nonsurgically, scaling and root planing is the treatment of choice, but if root debridement cannot be accomplished with a closed approach, surgery is the treatment of choice.[14,15]

If a surgical approach is chosen, it should be site-specific. The anterior sextants can usually be treated quite successfully with closed scaling and root planing in cases of moderate disease. Posterior sextants with moderate disease generally require a surgical approach.[7,8,13,19]

If the anatomic divisions of the mouth were ranked according to their ability to respond favorably to closed scaling and root planing, the ranking would be as follows:

1. Maxillary and mandibular anterior teeth
2. Maxillary and mandibular premolars
3. Mandibular molars
4. Maxillary molars

It is certainly possible and in many cases desirable to plan a course of treatment that involves scaling and root planing in certain areas and surgery in other areas. The following concepts and therapeutic approaches apply clearly to patients with residual probing depths of 5 to 6 mm with inflammation following initial therapy. It is reasonable, however, for an experienced clinician to accurately identify sites at the initial examination that are most likely to require surgical intervention. The less experienced practitioner will be on firm ground if the major surgical decisions are reserved until the response to initial therapy is reevaluated. The more experienced practitioner may use "clin-

ical experience" to make such decisions at an earlier time in therapy. The clinical judgment that results from experience is a complex interpretation of multiple variables in a manner that can not currently be defined by tradiional clinical measurements.

SURGICAL APPROACH

The most common surgical approach to periodontal disease is the flap approach because it allows the therapist access to the underlying structures for visualization and thorough debridement and correction of any anatomic defects and deformities of the bony tissues and teeth.[15] The flap approach also permits repositioning of the tissue.

The flap approach gained its popularity because of dissatisfaction with the results of other treatment techniques such as closed scaling and root planing and gingivectomy techniques.[6,15,16,19,20] Also, the flap approach allows for preservation of gingival tissue, which then permits more rapid healing. Once the flap is raised, efforts can be concentrated on (1) removal of granulation tissue; (2) debridement and detoxification of the root surface; (3) correction of anatomic defects created by the periodontal disease process, either by bony recontouring or by regenerative procedures; and (4) correction of anatomic problems related to tooth structure (eg, odontoplasty).[15,16,20]

Modified Widman Flap

One of the original descriptions of a periodontal flap procedure was reported in 1918 by Leonard Widman.[21] A modification of this procedure was described and published by Ramfjord and Nissle in 1974,[22] and it is essentially an unrepositioned mucoperiosteal flap.

The purpose of the modified Widman flap is to gain access to the periodontal lesion and to enable removal of the infected soft tissue. The technique permits preservation of healthy tissue for healing. Elevation of flaps is kept to the minimum necessary for visualization of the lesion to be treated. In moderate chronic adult periodontitis, modified Widman flap elevation usually does not extend beyond the microgingival junction. There is no specific attempt to alter the bony architecture, except that it may be reduced and recontoured if it is necessary for flap adaptation and closure. There is no specific attempt at pocket elimination, but that event may occur through the healing process attendant to the technique.[22]

The technique's strongest point is that it offers visualization and access of the root surfaces. Debridement and detoxification can be carried out without the guess work involved in closed scaling and root planing. However, it is a technique-sensitive procedure with specific requirements for the incision, the reflection of tissue, and the closure of the tissue.[22]

The approach requires preservation of the interdental papillae in an attempt to obtain primary closure between the opposing labial and lingual papillae. Therein also lies a major weakness. That is, if the papillae are not closed, a defect will occur which then must heal by secondary intention. This leaves an interproximal gap, which acts as a trap for food debris and bacteria and requires close postoperative monitoring until healing is complete. When primary closure is not obtained, the healing process is delayed several weeks. If plaque control is not op-

timal during this time, there is a risk of starting the disease process over again.[22]

The modified Widman flap in its classic definition does not allow for definitive osseous recontouring except to effect better flap adaptation. Osteoplasty can be performed to reduce exostoses, ledges, and irregular contour so that the flap can be better fitted to the interproximal contour.[6] Osteoplasty is defined as the modification, reduction, and reshaping of defects and deformities in the bone surrounding the teeth. There is no conscious effort to remove supporting alveolar bone.[3,23]

The soft tissue portion of the flap may also be modified and trimmed in order to reduce tissue bulk and thus allow for better interproximal adaptation.

Because the technique is essentially an unrepositioned mucoperiosteal flap, it can also be used as a basic approach to other periodontal procedures, for example, open debridement necessitated by an isolated periodontal lesion such as a chronic periodontal abscess or root fracture.

In addition, because of the importance of the adaptation of the soft tissue to the root surfaces and the interproximal area, the modified Widman approach to incisions and flap management becomes an important and basic approach when using regenerative techniques.

Regenerative procedures are designed to reproduce or reconstitute a lost or injured part.[24] Whether they be autografts, allografts, guided tissue regeneration, or other types of epithelial exclusion procedures, regenerative techniques depend upon a close soft tissue adaptation to cover the defect and/or protect the graft material.

The result of the modified

Widman flap procedure is a resolution of the inflammatory process with shrinkage of the pocket and some gain of attachment. Specific amounts of gains of attachment are not predictable but are always there.[7,13,19,25]

The sulcular area heals with a long junctional epithelium. While this is considered to be a weakness by some practitioners, it has never been proven experimentally or clinically over any given period of time.[26]

Bone remodeling takes place as a by-product of this procedure.

In areas of intraosseous defects, bone regeneration has been reported within the alveolar housing of the alveolar defect. The amount of bone fill is unpredictable and depends upon the anatomy of the defect.[27-30]

Intraosseous or angular defects are classified by the number of osseous walls relating to the root surface of the affected tooth. They may have one, two, or three walls of bone. Most commonly the defects are combinations rather than pure isolates of one type only.[31] Because the three-wall infrabony pocket has the greatest number of osseous walls surrounding it, it is the best candidate from which to expect regeneration or bone fill. These surrounding bony walls act as a scaffolding for the regeneration of the alveolar bone. The more walls present, the greater the potential for reconstruction of the original alveolar bone.[5-27]

Based on several studies, there is almost always a net gain of attachment, which has helped to make the modified Widman flap a popular approach to treating moderate disease.[7-9,13,19,25] The major negative factors include deepened residual pocket probing depths, interproximal defects, and noncorrected bony problems.[8,9,22,23,25]

Long-term studies on the modified Widman flap have shown that results which are attained at the time of treatment can be maintained with proper compliance by the patient to supportive periodontal treatment (SPT).[17,18]

Apically Positioned Flaps With Osseous Surgery

Another approach to treating moderate chronic adult periodontitis can be aimed at maximum pocket reduction and pocket elimination. It involves a flap approach with the flap positioned at the bony crestal margin; this will tend to totally eliminate the periodontal pocket.[19,23,32,33]

An internal bevel incision is made at the gingival crest and a full thickness mucoperiosteal flap is raised. As with the other flap approaches, access to the infected tissues and teeth is secured and debridement is accomplished.

The use of the flap approach makes recontouring of the alveolar process a simple and straight forward procedure.[20,23,34] Osteoplasty and ostectomy are done to create contours that will be more harmonious with the gingival tissue. Bony ledges and ridges and irregular contours, all of which are by-products of the advancing disease process, can then be reduced or reshaped.[20,23,34]

One requirement of osseous recontouring is that there be adequate bone support available to ensure that proper recontouring techniques can be done without increasing the bone loss of the disease.[20] Certainly in moderate disease, there is adequate bone support. However, if the disease process has progressed too far, bony recontouring cannot be done without jeopardizing the prognosis of individual teeth or of the case (see chapter 11).

The coronal margin of the soft tissue is then positioned at the bony crest and sutured there. This results in an elimination of the pocket wall. This is the critical part of the technique. The contours of the gingival tissue must match with the contours of osseous tissue. If they do not, there is a chance that pocket elimination will be compromised.[20,23,34]

Advantages The strengths of this procedure are a predictable reduction of probing pocket depths; preservation of gingival tissue; control of tissue placement; facilitation of restorative dentistry by exposing tooth structure; and the obvious accessibility to bone, roots, furcations, subgingival caries, and anatomical defects.[35]

This technique for osseous recontouring has been a long time mainstay of periodontal therapy. Over the years it has come under critical review but has always emerged as an integral part of the periodontal armamentarium.[19,35]

This technique is an effective measure for reducing probing depths and maintaining attachment levels. The World Workshop in Clinical Periodontics determined that shallow probing depths permit effective plaque control measures by the therapist and the patient.[35]

Healing is generally noneventful and the surgical area will form a new dentogingival unit with sulcular depths similar to those in the nondiseased situation. Because the tissue is placed at the bony crest, there is no long junctional epithelium.

Disadvantages Some of the problems attendant to this technique include exposure of root surfaces that may be sensitive to thermal stimuli, the creation of an unesthetic result, and the possible iatrogenic loss of additional clinical attachment.[19,23,35]

SUPPORTIVE PERIODONTAL TREATMENT

No matter which approach is used to treat moderate periodontal disease, the success of the treatment will depend on the maintenance therapy rendered to and by the patient.[17,18,36,37] But this is, of course, true for all surgical and nonsurgical periodontal procedures.[38]

CLINICAL APPLICATION

MODERATE CHRONIC ADULT PERIODONTITIS DEFINED

Moderate chronic adult periodontitis can be defined as that stage involving 5 to 6 mm of clinical probing depth with 2 to 4 mm of attachment loss and possibly early to moderate furcation involvement. It may be associated with overlying swollen edematous or enlarged fibrotic soft tissue. This definition assumes normal root and oral anatomy and oral anatomic relationships.

RATIONALE FOR PROBING DEPTH REDUCTION THERAPY

The basic overall objective of dental therapy is to restore and maintain the health and function of the stomatognathic system and to restore or enhance esthetics as desired by the patient. The primary goal of periodontal therapy in this endeavor is the preservation of the attachment apparatus and, when appropriate, the selective enhancement of the quality and quantity of the attachment apparatus and esthetics. The majority of

therapeutic periodontal procedures are means to achieve these goals. Shallow probing depth per se is not the ultimate goal of periodontal therapy, as has so often been stated. However, establishing shallow probing depth is believed by many astute and conscientious clinicians to be a significant means in the long-term goal of preserving the attachment. In addition, a shallow probing depth is believed by many to be one of the most significant indicators of periodontal health and is significant in maintaining and monitoring health. However, based on scientific evidence, it cannot be irrefutably proven that decreased probing depth preserves the attachment level.

THERAPEUTIC MEANS TO ACHIEVE A SHALLOW PROBING DEPTH

A decrease in clinical probing depth can be achieved in one of three fundamental ways: increased resistance to probing, apical positioning of the free gingival margin, or coronal positioning of the attachment level. There are many therapeutic periodontal procedures available to accom-

plish this objective based on specific clinical criteria. Also, additional clinical procedures are available if significant probing depth reduction is not required by the therapist.

All periodontal defects should not be treated in the same manner. In the selection of the therapeutic procedure it is most significant that the clinician not make the patient fit a predetermined mode of therapy. Rather, the patient and his periodontal disease should be the determining factor in the choice of therapy. The therapist should select those procedures most appropriate for the given clinical circumstances and the desires and financial commitment of the patient.

It must be noted that some of these procedures may achieve decreased clinical probing depth not by altering the gingival margin apically or the attachment level coronally but by increasing the resistance to the apical placement of the periodontal probe. Decreasing the inflammatory cellular content and increasing the collagen content of the peri and apical sulcular tissues increases the resistance to apical probe placement.

Following are the surgical procedures used for the treatment of moderate chronic adult periodontitis.

EXTERNAL BEVELED GINGIVECTOMY AND GINGIVOPLASTY
(Figs 10-1 and 10-2)

The gingivectomy is primarily indicated in the presence of suprabony pockets in association with excessive thickness and width of gingiva following definitive initial therapy. It has limited application requiring careful clinical evaluation of disease, attachment level, anatomic considerations, and esthetics. Appropriately used it is an excellent procedure. The common clinical condition requiring a gingivectomy is that which is associated with phenytoin or idiopathic gingival hyperplasia. It is also of value in establishing symmetrical and esthetic gingival architecture, crown lengthening, elimination of soft tissue craters that may occur following ANUG, and some flap procedures. Adequate width of attached gingiva must remain following the procedure. Accurate evaluation of the osseous topography, crestal osseous margins, and attachment levels relative to the mucogingival junction is a must.

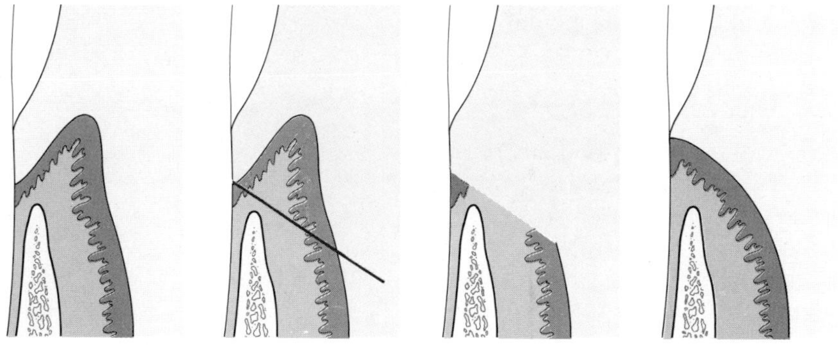

Fig 10-1 *Gingivectomy incision may be either coronal or apical to junctional epithelium.*

Technique

Anesthesia: administer block or infiltration as appropriate or preferred. Infiltration into marginal and papillary tissues with lidocaine and 1:100,000 epinephrine provides hemostasis and tissue rigidity to facilitate resection.

Mark probing depths: produce a series of bleeding points (Fig 10-2a) on the gingiva to be resected with a periodontal probe tip that represents the apical extent of the probing depth (Fig 10-2b) for the midfacial, midlingual, and interdental areas. This series of bleeding points (a dotted line) serves as a guide for the initial incision.

Indications

- Suprabony pockets
- Phenytoin-induced or idiopathic gingival hyperplasia
- Soft tissue craters post ANUG or flap procedures
- Crown lengthening
- Esthetic gingival architecture
- Symmetrical gingival architecture (eg, right and left maxillary anterior gingival contour and form)

Contraindications

- Inadequate attached gingiva
- Infrabony defects
- Esthetic compromise
- Acutely inflamed soft tissues
- Presence of thick bony ledges and exostosis
- An alternative, more effective procedure

Advantages

- Relatively easy procedure
- Access and visualization for root debridement
- Probing depth decrease
- Predictable morphology
- Esthetic result if appropriately done

Disadvantages

- Limited application
- Postoperative pain
- Slow healing
- Used inappropriately it may:
  — create inadequate attached gingiva
  — give unesthetic results
  — alter phonetics
  — expose bone

Incision: initiate in gingiva and direct coronally at a 45-degree angle to contact the tooth at the apical probing depth, level with the bleeding points (Fig 10-2b, incision A to B coronal to junctional epithelium or A′ to B′ apical to junctional epithelium). The incision usually starts at the distofacial or distolingual surface of the last tooth involved or may be blended in with a tuberosity or retromolar reduction. It is extended mesially using the bleeding points as a reference. This incision can be made on the facial surface with a 15 Bard Parker or the rounded heel of a Kirkland 15/16. The Kirkland must be used on the lingual and palatal surfaces to produce the necessary angulation. In the presence of very thick gingiva, a more acute angle is required. The interdental portion is completed with spear type knives such as the Orban 1 and 2. The angle of the initial incision and the interdental form may be further refined with diamond stones or a Kirkland 15/16 in a scraping motion.

Soft tissue, granulation tissue and tissue tag removal: remove excised tissue, granulation tissue and tissue tags with curets.

Root planing: thoroughly root plane to assure all subgingival calculus removal and smooth root surfaces.

Debridement: thoroughly evaluate soft tissue form and inspect root surfaces following wound irrigation and debridement.

Dressing: place periodontal surgical dressing of choice.

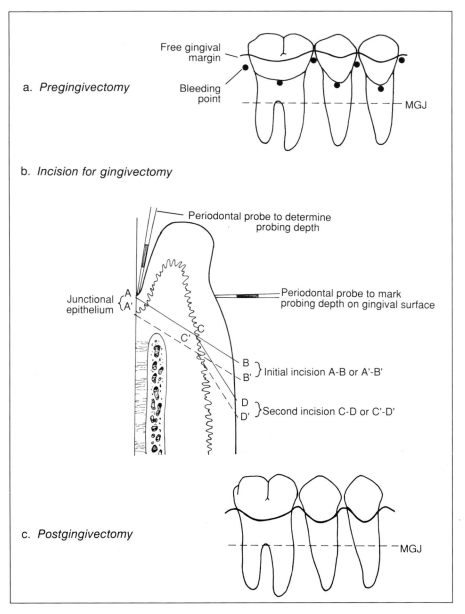

a. *Pregingivectomy*

Free gingival margin

Bleeding point

MGJ

b. *Incision for gingivectomy*

Periodontal probe to determine probing depth

Junctional epithelium

Periodontal probe to mark probing depth on gingival surface

A
A′

C′
C

B
B′ } Initial incision A-B or A′-B′

D
D′ } Second incision C-D or C′-D′

c. *Postgingivectomy*

MGJ

Fig 10-2a *Generalized hyperplastic gingiva, pseudo pockets, and no bone loss. Bleeding points represent probing depths and serve as a guide for the initial incision. (right) Normal physiological and esthetic gingival form and adequate attached gingiva.*

Fig 10-2b *Initial incision A-B or A′-B′ depends on operator's choice if significant to remove all junctional epithelium. This incision can be made with a 15 Bard Parker or a Kirkland 15/16. The second incision may become necessary to bevel the third gingiva, and can be made with diamond stones or a Kirkland 15/16 in a scraping motion.*

Fig 10-2c *Normal physiologic and esthetic gingival form and adequate attached gingiva.*

INTERNAL BEVELED GINGIVECTOMY

An internal beveled gingivectomy is basically an ENAP (see Fig 10-3) done in the presence of thick bulbous gingival tissues and suprabony pockets.

Technique

Refer to ENAP.

Advantages

- Gingival width is preserved
- Less postoperative pain, no exposed raw wound
- Surgical dressing not required
- Immediate plaque control possible

Disadvantages versus Gingivectomy/Gingivoplasty

- Technique is more difficult
- Ideal gingival architecture not easily achieved
- Possible papillary and marginal flap necrosis (associated with thinning thick tissue and compromising blood supply)
- Potential loss of attachment (associated with any flap elevation)

REPOSITIONED FLAPS

Repositioned flaps have been known by a number of different names and some entail slight technique modifications. There is the excisional new attachment procedure (ENAP), modified ENAP, flap curettage or open flap procedure, and the modified Widman/Ramfjord procedure.[39] Their primary objective is visualization and access for debridement of the root surfaces, osseous defects, and the soft tissue wall of the defect, and the establishment of a connective tissue or long junctional epithelial attachment. The existing width of gingiva is preserved. They also may create physiologic and esthetic soft tissue morphology.

Advantages

- More effective in single rooted teeth, particularly the maxillary anterior area where good flap adaptation to the entire root circumference may be possible
- Useful in the maxillary anterior region when there are esthetic concerns in the presence of significant probing depths and perhaps continued bleeding on probing following thorough root planing

Disadvantages

- Frequently a new connective tissue or long junctional epithelial attachment does not occur, especially in the posterior areas and in the presence of root concavities, interproximal infrabony defects, and furcations
- If there are thick bony margins and exostosis, good intimate flap adaptation is not always possible
- In the presence of infrabony defects, particularly in the interproximal areas, significant residual probing depth will remain
- Frequently heal with a soft tissue crater formation in the molar areas, which creates significant plaque control problems because the papilla does not heal or is very slow in healing to a normal interdental papilla formation
- Residual probing depths and soft tissue defects present significant maintenance problems and greater risk for future attachment loss

151

ENAP (EXCISIONAL NEW ATTACHMENT PROCEDURE) (Fig 10-3)

The ENAP is essentially subgingival curettage performed with a scalpel blade.

Technique

- Mark pocket
- Scallop internal beveled incision to the base of the pocket
- Remove all incised epithelium and granulation tissue
- Root plane
- Reposition and suture tissue to presurgical level
- Exert pressure with moistened gauze
- Apply dressing

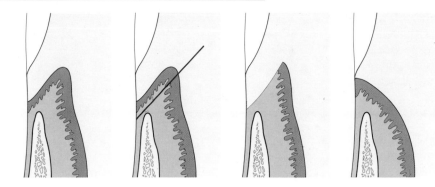

Fig 10-3 *Incision is directed at the junction of the epithelium and connective tissue attachment, preserving the coronal connective tissue attachment. Clinically the junction point of the epithelium and connective tissue is impossible to determine accurately.*

Indication

- Suprabony pockets in the presence of convex root surfaces, normal gingival form and width

Contraindications

- Inadequate keratinized gingiva
- Hyperplastic tissue
- Osseous defects
- Close root approximations
- Malposed teeth
- Developmental tooth defects
- Furcations

Advantages

- Removal of epithelial pocket lining, junctional epithelial attachment, and adjacent granulomatous tissues
- Improved visualization and access to the root surfaces
- Does not affect the bone
- Connective tissue attachment is left intact
- Minimal trauma to the gingiva
- Facilitates new attachment
- Minimal postoperative recession

Disadvantages

- Technically exacting to determine the apical extent of the epithelial attachment, the epithelial-connective tissue junction
- Limited application

MODIFIED ENAP (Fig 10-4)

The modified ENAP was developed due to the technical difficulties some operators had with maintaining their incisions within the soft tissue and directed to the apical extent of the epithelial attachment and coronal to the connective tissue attachment.

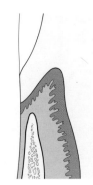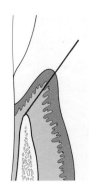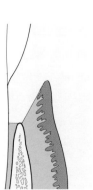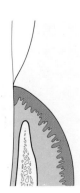

Fig 10-4 *Incision is directed to the alveolar crest, and the coronal connective tissue attachment is removed. Clinically easier to accomplish than standard ENAP.*

Technique (same as ENAP except)

- Incision directed at the alveolar crest
- Connective tissue, epithelial attachment, pocket epithelium, and granulation tissue are removed

Advantages versus ENAP

- Easier procedure
- Provides greater access
- Potential healing from the periodontal ligament (speculative)

Disadvantages versus ENAP

- Connective tissue attachment removal
- Loss of attachment

MODIFIED WIDMAN FLAP—RAMFJORD PROCEDURE (Figs 10-5 and 10-6)

The modified Widman flap—Ramfjord procedure and its modifications is perhaps the most universally used surgical periodontal procedure today for those clinicians who do not believe pocket elimination is necessary. It is adaptable to a variety of clinical circumstances.

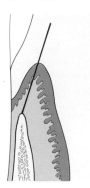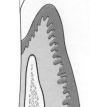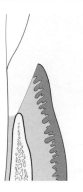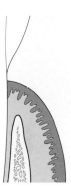

Fig 10-5

Technique (Fig 10-6)

- *Primary incision:* direct an internal bevel incision at the alveolar crest and parallel to the long axis of the tooth starting 0.5 to 1 mm or greater from the gingival margin. Only a minimal amount of interdental tissue is removed, producing an exaggerated scallop for primary closure faciolingually and intimate adaptation to the entire root circumference. A crevicular incision may be used when esthetics is of concern or minimal gingival width is present.
- *Flap elevation:* elevate a full-thickness flap, exposing 1 to 2 mm of alveolar bone for later access to the alveolar crest and root surfaces.
- *Second incision:* make an incision from the bottom of the pocket to the alveolar crest around the neck of each tooth.
- *Third incision:* pushing the facial and lingual flaps aside and

Advantages

- Access and visualization of the root surfaces
- Adaptation of healthy connective tissue to the root surfaces
- Better esthetics versus apically positioned flap
- Less potential root hypersensitivity versus apically positioned flap
- Preservation of gingival width

Disadvantages

- Postoperative soft tissue craters
- Residual probing depths in the presence of infrabony pockets
- New attachment is unpredictable
- Unstable junctional epithelial attachment long term

using a small Orban 1 and 2, make a horizontal incision along the alveolar crest, severing the supracrestal gingival fibers.
- Remove the severed supracrestal gingival tissues with sharp curets.
- Root plane all root surfaces exposed to the original pocket.

- Thoroughly debride and inspect.
- Possibly perform osteoplasty to facilitate flap adaptation.
- Adapt primary flap about the necks of the teeth and suture with interrupted sutures.
- Apply periodontal surgical dressing (variable).

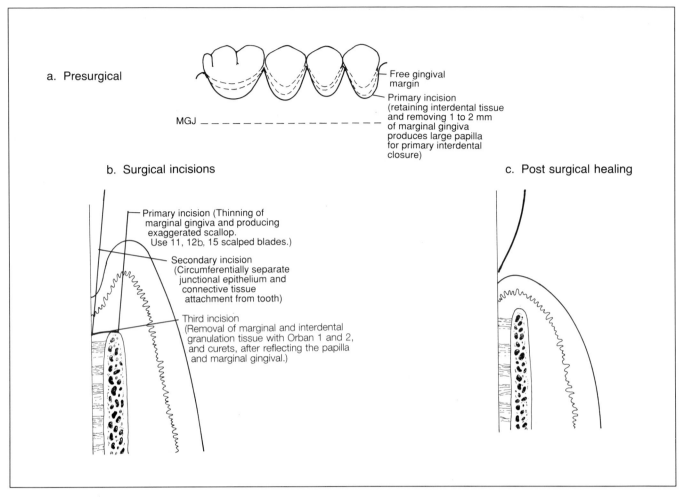

a. Presurgical

Free gingival margin

Primary incision (retaining interdental tissue and removing 1 to 2 mm of marginal gingiva produces large papilla for primary interdental closure)

MGJ

b. Surgical incisions

Primary incision (Thinning of marginal gingiva and producing exaggerated scallop. Use 11, 12b, 15 scalped blades.)

Secondary incision (Circumferentially separate junctional epithelium and connective tissue attachment from tooth)

Third incision (Removal of marginal and interdental granulation tissue with Orban 1 and 2, and curets, after reflecting the papilla and marginal gingival.)

c. Post surgical healing

Figs 10-6a to c *Modified Widman flap — Ramford procedure: Initial incision is directed to the alveolar crest. Second incision is directed via the sulcus to the PDL. Following conservative flap reflection, the third incision is directed from the alveolar crest to the tooth. The wedge of primarily granulomatous tissue is removed with curets.*

APICALLY POSITIONED FLAPS WITHOUT OSSEOUS RESECTION (Fig 10-7)

This is essentially the same procedure as the modified Widman procedure, with the exception that the marginal flap is apically positioned and sutured at or slightly coronal to the alveolar crest. This results in both an advantage and disadvantage compared to the modified Widman procedure: greater probing depth reduction but potentially unesthetic root exposure. Total or near total pocket elimination may be possible in areas of very thin radicular bone and narrow facio-

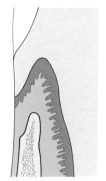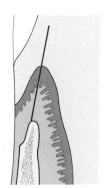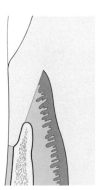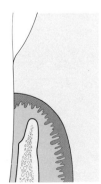

Fig 10-7 *Initial thinning incision is based on the width and thickness of the gingiva followed by a sulcular incision. Removal of the wedge of granulomatous tissue with a combination use of curets and/or a third incision.*

lingual jaw width with a horizontal pattern of bone loss. This occurs frequently in the mandibular incisor area but may also occur in other areas. This is one reason it is so important that the clinician is able to accurately evaluate the osseous morphology and predict future morphologic results with the various surgical procedures.

Advantage versus Modified Widman

• Potentially greater probing depth reduction

Disadvantages versus Modified Widman

• Potentially unesthetic root exposure
• Potentially greater root hypersensitivity
• Lack of flap adaptation in the presence of thick bony margins, exostosis and tori

---

APICALLY POSITIONED FLAPS WITH OSSEOUS RESECTION (Fig 10-8)

Any moderate-depth defects not resolvable by initial therapy, definitive root planing, orthodontics, gingivectomy, apical flap positioning without osseous resection, root amputations and hemisections, or regeneration are best treated with osseous resection if shallow probing depth rather than pocket maintenance is a desired therapeutic objective.

The ultimate goal of periodontal therapy is the total regeneration of lost attachment. This is not possible today on a predictable basis for the majority of presenting patients and defects. Considering the sum total of attachment loss of the average Class III and early Class IV patients who present with generalized horizontal bone loss associated with shallow to moderate grade II furcation invasions, generalized 1- to 2-mm posterior interdental crater formations, and some 1- to 2-mm hemisepta in the anterior and premolar regions, a very small area of attachment is regenerated versus the total area lost. This does not mean one should not attempt regeneration of the defects judged amenable to the regenerative procedures. Because the majority of the lost area of attachment can-

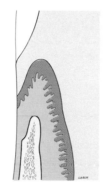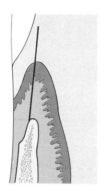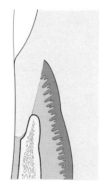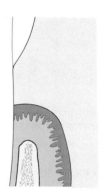

Fig 10-8 *Following an internal beveled incision, removal of granulomatous tissue, and osteoplasty and ostectomy, the flap is apically positioned just to cover the alveolar crest. Note resultant decreased probing depth (at the expense of increased root exposure, however).*

not be regenerated today, the clinician's next level of treatment is preventing any further attachment loss, and if this is not possible, significantly slowing the rate down to preserve the teeth for as long as possible.

Residual periodontal defects are nearly always blamed on poor plaque control by the patient or noncompliance with patient recall. Seldom is it acknowledged that perhaps a treatable defect was not eliminated in the first place. Even more significant is the removal of excessive alveolar bone proper, under the rationale of pocket elimination.

In order to have shallow sulcular depth, the alveolar bone and overlying gingiva must have the same morphologic form and be parallel with one another. Any disparity in form between the gingiva and underlying bone represents the areas of increased probing depth, assuming no extensive soft tissue attachment. In the presence of periodontal osseous defects, this can be achieved by either the addition of bone, regenerative procedures, or the subtraction of bone (osteoplasty-ostectomy) to achieve this morphologic form. As Ochsenbein and Ross[40] stated, to effect pocket

Indications for Osseous Resection Therapy (Infrabony Defects)

- Adequate attachment remaining once physiologic morphology established
- No esthetic limitations
- No anatomic limitations
- No root hypersensitivity limitations

Contraindications

- Inadequate remaining attachment
- Anatomic limitations
- Esthetic limitations
- Root hypersensitivity concerns
- Alternative, more effective therapy

Advantages

- Predictable results used appropriately
- Results are relatively immediate, no prolonged waiting to determine outcome

Disadvantages (Potentially, if Used Inappropriately)

- Attachment loss
- Unesthetic root exposure
- Hypersensitive roots

---

elimination in the presence of periodontal defects, an osseous morphology is established that the gingiva is going to assume following the postoperative and healing period. This is why it is so critical that one be knowledgeable of the anatomic determinants of gingival morphology. The gingiva will assume its morphologic form relative to local anatomic influences, primarily the teeth, with minimal effect from the underlying bone.

There are obvious and significant disadvantages with the resection procedures that are possible with any of the apical flap positioning and root instrumentation procedures. As will be described, esthetic compromise can be minimized by avoiding apical flap positioning in easily visualized areas such as the maxillary anterior area and sometimes the maxillary premolar region and using a lingual approach where applicable. The importance of individualized treatment cannot be overemphasized.

ART OF OSSEOUS RESECTION

The art of osseous resection is to remove a minimal amount of attachment while still establishing physiologic osseous morphology for eventual minimal sulcular depth. *With osseous resection, attachment is sacrificed, therefore the clinical result must justify that sacrifice of attachment.* One must carefully consider the amount of attachment removal from the involved teeth and adjacent teeth to establish a physiologic morphology. As Selipsky[41] noted, there is significantly less attachment removal than previously thought or visually judged. The majority of the attachment removal involves the midfacial and midradicular root surface, which accounts for a small area of the root circumference (Figs 10-9a and b).

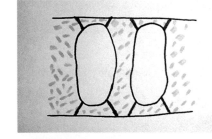

Fig 10-9a *Cross section of root illustrates the narrow facial and lingual radicular root surface and the broad proximal surface. The majority of alveolectomy, removal of alveolar bone proper, is primarily on the facial and lingual radicular areas between the noted line angle areas. This is a minimal area compared to the average interproximal attachment area.*

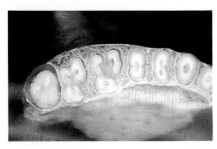

Fig 10-9b *Cross section of maxillae and teeth illustrates the broad area of attachment for the proximal root surface relative to the facial and lingual radicular surface.*

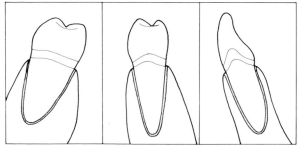

Figs 10-10a to c *Alveolar crest in health paralleling the CEJ and approximately 1.5 mm apical to the CEJ. The alveolar crest is peaked in the anterior, decreasing in the premolar area, and relatively flat in the molar area.*

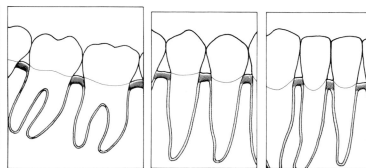

Figs 10-11a to c *The width of the alveolar crest is affected by the proximal crown contour: wide with bulbous proximal contours (eg, molar and premolars) and narrow with flat proximal contours (eg, mandibular incisors).*

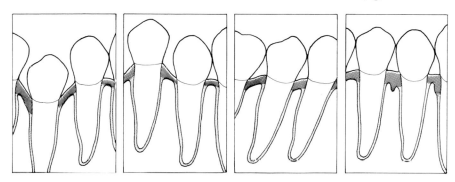

Figs 10-12a to c *The intrusion (left), extrusion (center), or tipping (right) of teeth alters the relationship of adjacent CEJs and thus the alveolar crest shape. However, the shape of the alveolar crest is still parallel to a line drawn between adjacent CEJs.*

Fig 10-13 *(far right) Osseous resorption of the interdental alveolar crest alters the alveolar crestal shape.*

Alveolar Process

The alveolar process is defined as that part of the maxilla and mandible that forms and supports the sockets of the teeth.[42] Orban further divides the alveolar process into the alveolar bone proper and the supporting alveolar bone. The alveolar bone proper consists of a thin lamella of bone that surrounds the root of the tooth and gives attachment to principal fibers of the periodontal ligament. The supporting bone surrounds the alveolar bone proper and supports the sockets. The term supporting bone is frequently used incorrectly in the periodontal literature when the term alveolar bone proper should be used.

Marginal bone contour. In health, the marginal bone contour follows the contour of the CEJ and about 1.5 mm apical to it (Figs 10-10a to c). In health, the morphology of the interdental bone and interdental crest is largely determined by the morphology of the teeth and their relationship to one another and the relationship of adjacent CEJs.[43] The interdental crest is parallel to a line drawn between adjacent CEJs (Figs 10-11a to c). Therefore, the shape of the alveolar crest can be altered with the extrusion (Fig 10-12b) or intrusion (Fig 10-12a) of an adjacent tooth, tipping (Fig 10-12c) of adjacent teeth, altered stage of eruption, or periodontal disease (Fig 10-13). With prominent convex proximal contours, the interdental width is wide. With flat proximal contours, the interdental width is narrow (assuming normal tooth alignment).

Teeth. One must clinically and radiographically evaluate the length and shape of the roots, the root trunk length or furcation level of molar teeth, the relationship of the teeth to each other, their position in the alveolus, and their axial inclination. These anatomic considerations must then be related to the defect location, defect severity, oral anatomic factors, and esthetics.

Gingival morphology. One must be knowledgeable of the anatomic factors determining gingival morphology when discussing pocket depth reduction by osseous resection. For shallow probing depth to exist, the alveolar bone and overlying gingiva must have the same morphologic form. When we alter the osseous form in the presence of periodontal osseous defects, we want to create a form that will be the same as the overlying gingiva following healing. When the gingiva is located at the CEJ, its form basically follows the CEJ of the teeth, assuming normal tooth alignment. However, when the gingiva is apically positioned, its morphology is not the same as it was at the CEJ. Therefore, we must be able to predict the eventual morphology of the gingiva in its new apical environment. It is that morphologic form that must be created in the bony tissue with our resective osseous therapy. The morphology of the gingiva is primarily due to the anatomic shape and position and relationship of the teeth to one another and in the alveolus and minimally on the underlying bone. Ochsenbein and Ross[40] stated that preoperatively the morphology of relatively healthy gingiva is the initial single best guide to use because it is a manifestation of the stated anatomic factors that determine the morphology. However, this guide must be used with caution; it can only serve as a general guide. It must be realized that with any significant apical positioning of the gingiva, its surrounding anatomic environment is going to be drastically changed. This may markedly alter the eventual gingival form from its original shape at the CEJ.

Scalloping. Scalloping may be defined as the difference in distance between the crest of the midfacial or lingual marginal bone or gingiva and the crest of the interdental bone or gingival papilla. Scalloping has been classified as flat, average, and pronounced as a general reference. No specific distance between the crest of the marginal gingiva and interdental papilla has ever been determined to indicate what is pronounced, average, or flat. This

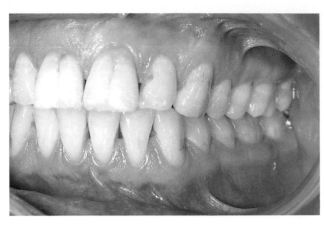

Fig 10-14
Relatively highly scalloped gingival margin in the anterior area gradually progresses to a relatively flat gingival margin in the molar area.

is a generalized clinical judgment used for communication. The degree of scalloping is quite variable among patients and variable within the same mouth. Generally, scalloping is greater in the anterior area, decreasing in the premolar area, and fairly flat in the molar areas (Fig 10-14). This assumes the gingival margin is at the CEJ, which is a significant consideration. As will be discussed, this generalized pattern may change with apical positioning of the gingiva. The significance of scalloping is that *with greater scalloping, a greater amount of marginal bone will have to be removed. With less scalloping less marginal bone will need to be removed.* These factors should be evaluated presurgically as much as possible when determining the therapeutic approach.

Surgical Access and Specific Flap Design

The design of the coronal incision for the facial and lingual surfaces of the mandible and the facial surface of the maxilla follows the same principles. An internal bevel incision is used, which is modified relative to gingival width and

thickness and esthetic considerations:

- For thick-narrow gingiva, thin with an inverse bevel incision but retain the entire width.
- For thick-wide gingiva, thin with an inverse bevel incision but possibly remove excess width if too wide for later objectives.
- For thin-narrow gingiva, no thinning, possibly use a sulcular incision and save the entire width.
- For thin-wide gingiva, no thinning, possibly use a sulcular incision and perhaps remove the excess width if too wide.

Adequate gingival width is retained based upon the future positioning of the gingival margin to assure adequate width of attached gingiva. If the gingival margin is to be placed at the CEJ for esthetic reasons, greater gingival width may be retained. The outline of the incision should also have an esthetic form. For example, if it involves the anterior teeth, the left and right outlines should be identical (see Figs 10-8a and b and 10-16a to e).

Fig 10-15a (left) *Hand instruments used for osseous resection: Ochsenbein 1, 2, 3, and 4; Loughlin's back action chisel; Rhodes chisel; Schluger file; Sugarman file; and Wedelstadt chisel.*

Fig 10-15b (right) *Rotary instruments used for osseous resection: burs no. 7009, no. 7004, no. 7903.*

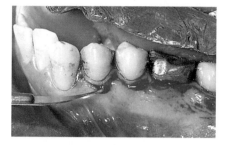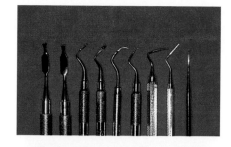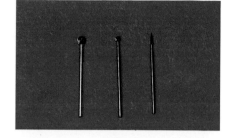

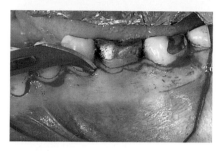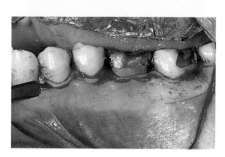

Fig 10-16 to c *Tracing a horizontally directed outline incision with a 12b followed by a vertical thinning incision with a 12b (Fig 10-16b) or 17 (Fig 10-16c) blade.*

Fig 10-16d (left) *The scalloped incision outline and retained cuff of tissues.*

Fig 10-16e (right) *The cuff of tissue that is removed with a Molt curet following a cervical incision with a 12b blade.*

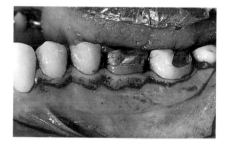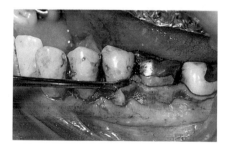

Palatal Flap Design

Unique Considerations in the Initial Incision
The palatal flap for osseous resective therapy presents unique design and handling concerns not present with non-osseous resection flap therapy or with the facial flap of the maxillary arch or the facial and lingual flaps of the mandibular arch. This is due to two primary reasons. First, the anatomy of the palatal soft tissues does not allow it to be freely positioned apically at a desired position once it has been elevated. Second, with osseous resection

(osteoplasty-ostectomy) the therapist is usually trying to achieve as much pocket depth reduction as possible within the limitations of the procedure. To achieve this postsurgical objective, the margin of the palatal flap will need to be placed at or slightly coronal to and have the same outline or form as the newly established alveolar crestal margin following the osseous resection surgical procedure. Because it cannot be freely positioned, it must be resected surgically and contoured to conform to the postosseous resection alveolar crestal level and form. To

achieve this, the clinician must be able to envision the postsurgery contour and form of the palatal alveolar crest and the anatomic factors that will affect the positioning of the soft tissue palatal flap margin. It is this outline form that must be scribed in the palatal soft tissues with the initial incision and not that parallel to the original gingival margin. If done incorrectly, additional soft tissue can be removed, which is difficult, but none can be added. Therefore, it is very important to be as accurate as possible in this initial incision.

Determining the location of the

future alveolar crestal margin and the point of the midradicular root surface at that position are very significant determinations prior to scribing the initial incisions. These factors will determine the future flap margin location and apex of the scallop. The mesiodistal alignment of the tooth must be taken into consideration. For example, one cannot assume the area of greatest curvature will be directly apical to the midpoint of the crown of the tooth. Mesiodistal tilting of the tooth will alter this. Clues to alteration could be the marginal ridge relationship of adjacent teeth, whether they are even or uneven. An uneven relationship would indicate mesial or distal tilting of the teeth. However, restorations and uneven wear could alter the original marginal ridge relationship, masking the existence of the tilting of the tooth. Therefore accurate radiographs of the area need to also be evaluated when considering palatal flap design in regards to mesial distal tilting of the tooth and width of the interdental space. The natural curve of Spee also affects the mesiodistal position, particularly for the second molars. The midradicular area of the second molar root surface is moved mesially with the normal curve of Spee.

Primary Palatal Flap Incision (Outline)
The basic incision outline will consist of a series of connecting Vs with their shape determined by the tip of the future interdental papilla and the future gingival margin location at the midradicular root surface. Apically, the mesiodistal interdental space becomes wider and the mesiodistal width of the root more narrow. This means the interdental papilla area will become wider and the radicular gingival contour more narrow with apical gingival

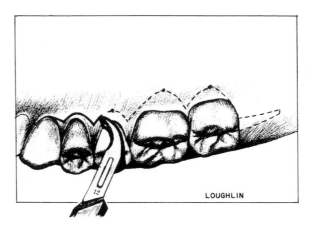
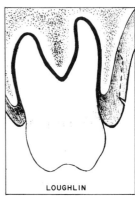

Fig 10-17a (left) *Tracing initial palatal incision with a 12b blade. Note bleeding points at midradicular gingival margin to serve as a guide.*

Fig 10-17b (right) *Proximal view showing initial, second, and third palatal incisions. The initial incision is 1 mm or greater in depth.*

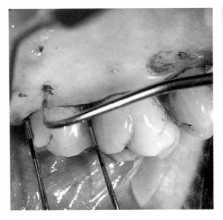
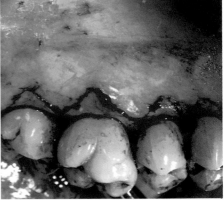

Figs 10-17c and d *Placing midradicular palatal bleeding points with a periodontal probe based on probing depths and anatomic factors serves as a guide for the initial incision.*

margin location. This future anatomic form should be determined prior to the initial incision. The outline and form of the initial incision should duplicate the future osseous contour about the roots following the osteoplasty/ostectomy procedures. Once the midradicular location of the palatal flap margin relative to the palatal surface of each tooth/root is determined, it is identified by placing a bleeding point (Figs 10-17a and c) with the tip of a periodontal probe. The primary incision is then made by a combination of push and pull strokes with a no. 12b or 15c blade connecting the tip of the future interdental papilla and the future midradicular point (Fig 10-17d). The depth of the initial incision should be a minimum of 1 mm but may extend deeper. The palatal flap outline incision is

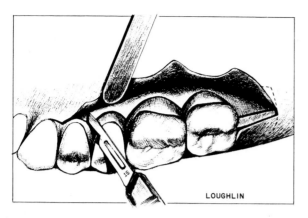
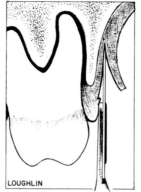

Figs 10-18a and b Palatal and proximal views of second palatal and retromolar incision with a 15 blade. Note long gradual taper of incision relative to palatal surface.

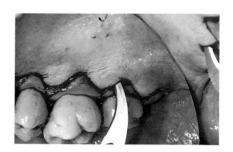

Fig 10-18c Second palatal incision with a 12b blade.

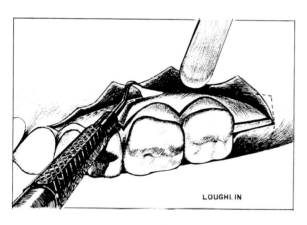
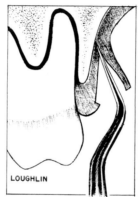

Figs 10-19a and b Third incision with a Kirkland 15 or 16 extending from the distal aspect of the retromolar incision to the anterior aspect of the flap and down to bone.

blended in with the retromolar outline incisions. Figure 10-17b demonstrates in cross section the first or flap outline incision, second or thinning incision and third incision or incision to bone.

Secondary Palatal Flap (Thinning) Incision Figure 10-10a demonstrates the second incision with the no. 15 blade to include the retromolar procedure while carefully retracting the already thinned portion of the flap so it will not inadvertently be incised by the cutting instrument. This secondary incision is the most difficult to make and will determine the thickness and flexibility of the flap and future adaptability to the underlying alveolus and teeth. The flatter the palatal form, the more

difficult this flap will be to thin. Nearly all palates are quite flat in the premolar area, especially in the area adjacent to the teeth. The incision generally parallels the surface of the palatal gingiva, gradually inclining toward the underlying alveolus. Instruments used to perform this incision may include the no. 12b and 15 blades, the Orban 1 and 2, and the Kirkland 15 and 16 gingivectomy knives. The most difficult area of this flap to thin is the papilla area due to its relationship to the teeth and the teeth obstructing the angulation of the various cutting instruments. Some operators will first thin the papilla with both a mesial and distal approach using a no. 12b blade (Fig 10-18c), while

others will manipulate the no. 15 blade to thin this area. Some operators will use an Orban 1 and 2 because it can be positioned to avoid the interference of the teeth and properly thin the papilla area. Once the papilla area is thinned the remaining portion of the secondary incision is usually best accomplished using a no. 15 blade. The marginal thickness of the flap is approximately 0.5 to 1 mm thick and then gradually increases in thickness as the flap tapers apically. If a feather edge margin is created, it will usually slough.

Figure 10-18b demonstrates the no. 15 blade having completed the secondary or thinning incision. The margin of the flap is approximately 1 mm thick. The incision follows the contour of the palate but gradually slopes toward the alveolus. This flap can be freely retracted to provide access for granulation tissue removal, root debridement, and osseous therapy. The form of this flap will depend on the degree of flatness or steepness of the palate and the degree of thickness or thinness of the palatal soft tissues.

Third Palatal Flap Incision (to Bone) Figures 10-19a and b demonstrate the placement and angulation of the Kirkland 15 or 16 in completing the third incision. The heel of a Kirkland 15 or 16 (Fig 10-19a) extends firmly to the underlying bone. This incision is carried all the way from the most terminal area of the retromolar wedge procedure to the most anterior extent of the palatal flap. The Kirkland 15 and 16 offer several advantages for this incision over other instruments. The Kirkland is a strong instrument, and firm, controlled pressure can be placed on it. Its angulation is well suited for this incision. The shank of the instrument is noncutting; therefore, it can be safely drawn along the base of the flap without the margin of the flap being cut, as can occur if a no. 15 blade is used for this step.

Intrasulcular Incision and Secondary Flap and Granulation Tissue Removal A no. 12b or 15 blade (Figs 10-20a and b) is used to separate the epithelial and connective tissue attachment from the tooth by placing the blade in the sulcus and extending it to the alveolar crest circumferentially about each tooth in the flap area. The collar of tissue, which should only be attached to the bony palate, is now removed. This is most efficiently done by using an Ochsenbein 2 (Figs 10-21a and b, 10-22a to c), starting from the most

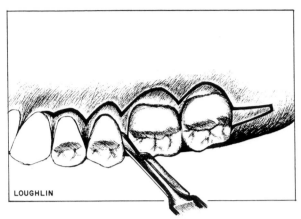
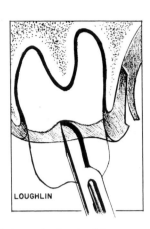

Figs 10-20a and b *Palatal and proximal views of the sulcular incision with a 15 blade (12b is also used).*

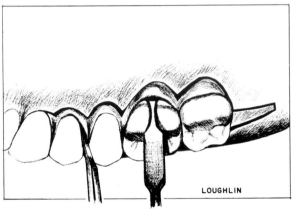
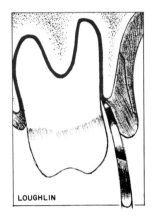

Figs 10-21a and b *Palatal and proximal views of Ochsenbein 2 removing the secondary flap and granulation tissue.*

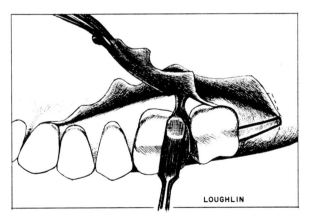
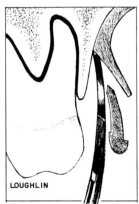

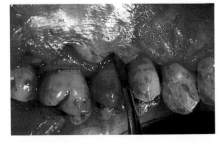

Figs 10-22a to c *Further removal of the secondary flap and granulation tissue, advancing from the anterior to the posterior.*

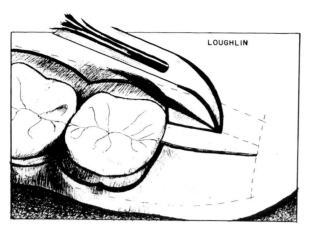
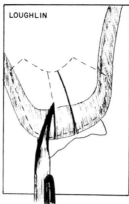

Figs 10-23a and b *12b blade tracing the initial retromolar incision about 1 to 2 mm in depth.*

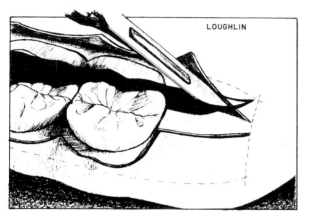
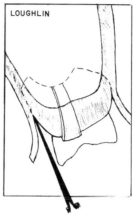

Figs 10-24a and b *Second incision with a 12b blade thinning the facial and palatal flaps to the distal extent of the tuberosity, then to the anterior extent of the flap.*

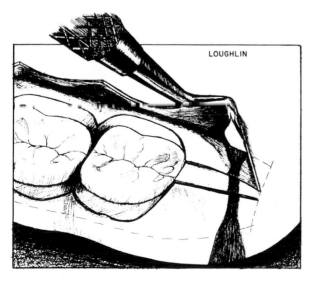
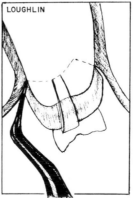

Figs 10-25a and b *Third incision with a Kirkland 15 and 16 extending from the posterior tuberosity to the anterior extent of the flap.*

anterior aspect of the flap, directing the chisel in the gingival sulcus, engaging the gingival tissue at the alveolar crest, and peeling it apically to the tertiary incision. This step is repeated along the palate going from anterior to posterior to include the undermined wedge of tissue from the retromolar procedure. Once enough tissue is elevated, it can be grasped with a small curved hemostat to elevate the wedge of tissue and provide better visualization for the placement of the Ochsenbein 2 and further elevation of the tissue wedge. Removal of this wedge of tissue by cutting with a gingivectomy knife leaves significantly more tissue tags than the cleaner result obtained by peeling the tissue out.

Retromolar Procedure

The retromolar procedure and incisions are extensions of the palatal and buccal flap incisions, joining at the hamular notch area using much the same approach as used with the palatal flap, and they are performed simultaneously.

First Retromolar (Outline) Incision The outline incision (Figs 10-23a and b) for the distal wedge is determined by many factors, including individual preference of the surgeon. The basic shape and size of the tuberosity are primary determining factors. The amount of keratinized mucosa, especially on the buccal aspect, as well as the degree of apical positioning of the buccal flap that may be required on the buccal aspect of the second molar, must be considered to assure primary closure of the retromolar area and yet not have excess tissue and overlapping flap margins. Sometimes it is necessary to place a vertical incision in the buccal flap at the approximate location of the distobuccal line angle of the second molar. With the vertical incisions placed, the buccal flap and buccal portion of the retromolar flap may be positioned independent of one another. It is preferable to make the palatal incision extending distally from approximately the distopalatal line angle of the second molar to the hamular notch area. This palatal location of the flap provides better access and visualization of the retromolar area, especially when trying to suture this area as opposed to trying to view this area from the buccal with the buccal cheek and advancing coronoid process with a wide-open mandible obstructing access and vision of this area. The palatal retromolar incision joins with the buccal retromolar incision at a common point approximately at the hamular notch area. Joining the buccal and palatal tuberosity incisions at a common point allows for postoperative primary flap closure and minimizes the potential for postoperative bleeding in this delicate and vascular tissue.

Second Retromolar (Thinning) Incision
Figures 10-24a and b, demonstrate the second or thinning incision using a no. 12b blade. Due to access considerations, the initial portion of this incision is usually done with a no. 12b blade, an Orban 1 or 2, or even a Kirkland 15 or 16. As with the secondary palatal incision, once the flap is partially dissected back, the remainder of the incision can usually be completed with a no. 15 blade. It is important this incision is extended well posteriorly and apically to provide for a flexible flap and to free the excessive underlying wedge of tissue. This incision is performed at the same time as the second palatal flap incision, extending from the most posterior aspect of the

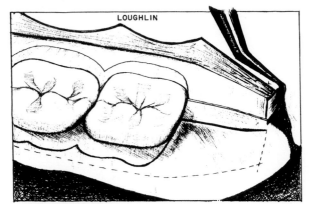
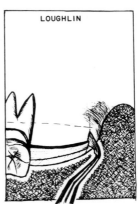

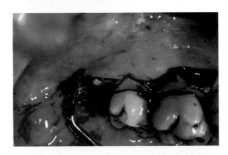

Figs 10-26a to c Kirkland 15 or 16 making the third incision at the distal extent of the tuberosity to bone. With the Kirkland, the blade can be angulated somewhat anterior to bone, avoiding the vascular loose tissue in the hamular notch area.

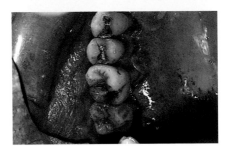

Fig 10-27 Usual posterior extent of the wedge.

retromolar area to the most anterior aspect of the palatal flap.

Third Retromolar Incision
Figures 10-25a and b demonstrate the placement of the Kirkland 15 or 16 for the third incision. Again, this incision is done in conjunction with the third palatal flap incision and extends from the most posterior aspect of the retromolar wedge to the anterior aspect of the palatal flap. It is important that this incision be extended fully to the posterior extent of the proposed wedge of tissue to be removed where it will join with the next incision.

Figures 10-26a and b demon-

strate the use of the Kirkland 15 or 16 in a continuation of the third incision about the terminal or posterior portion of the retromolar wedge. The Kirkland 15 or 16 blade is slipped under the undermined palatal and buccal flaps at the most posterior extent of the wedge and then used to incise anteriorly and apically to bone (Fig 10-26c). The Kirkland 15 and 16 have significant advantages over the straight-handled scalpel blade holder. Their shank allows the instrument to be angled in such a manner that the incision is directed from the most posterior aspect of the wedge at the terminal extent of the tuberosity, some-

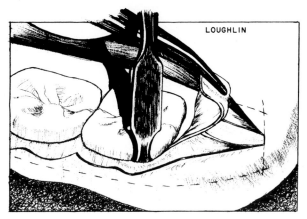

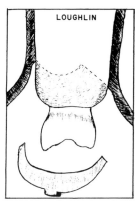

Figs 10-28a and b *Continued removal of the secondary flap and granulation tissue to include the retromolar wedge with an Ochsenbein 2 and hemostat.*

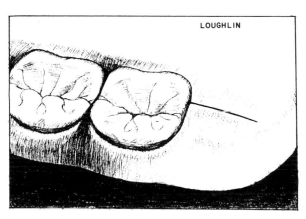

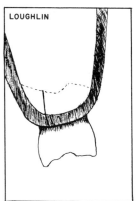

Figs 10-29a and b

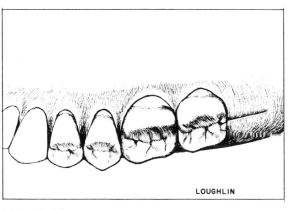

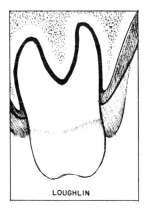

Figs 10-30a and b

what anteriorly, thus avoiding the hazardous and vascular areas posterior and superior to the tuberosity. The posterior extent of the wedge is usually more posterior than demonstrated in the drawing (Fig 10-27).

Removal of Distal Wedge Figures 10-28a and b demonstrate the use of the Ochsenbein 2 and small curved tip hemostat in the removal of the distal wedge of tissue and extending around to the buccal aspect of the second molar.

The Ochsenbein 2 is worked under the distal wedge, starting from the distal aspect of the second molar and working the entire wedge of tissue free. Sometimes limited oral opening and other access problems will require that the wedge be elevated by a lateral approach with a Molt 4 curet. Peeling this wedge of tissue free (versus cutting it off with a gingivectomy knife) leaves significantly fewer tissue tags, especially if there is an osseous defect on the distal surface of the second molar.

Final Closure Figures 10-29a and b and 10-30a and b demonstrate final closure of the palatal flap and retromolar areas.

TECHNIQUE OF OSSEOUS RESECTION

The osseous form that is to be established depends on the present base of the osseous defect becoming the crest or most coronal point of the interdental bony septum. The bone will be straight or flat mesiodistally. Faciolingually, the bone may be fairly flat or slope slightly apically or occasionally moderately to the facial and lingual, depending on the anatomic factors determining the area's gingival morphology. The base of the present defect must not be reduced. With the use of high-speed diamonds and burs, it is very easy to reduce the base of the defect apically. This leads to needless sacrifice of attachment.

The sequence of osseous pocket elimination is:

1. Elimination of bulk
2. Vertical grooving
3. Begin elimination of interproximal defects

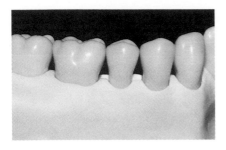

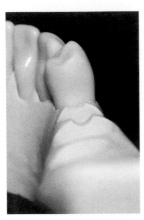

Figs 10-31a and b *Facial and proximal views of shallow interproximal crater located midfaciolingual.*

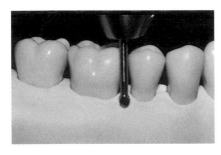

Fig 10-31c (above) *Facial view of 7009 bur representing bulk reduction step and vertical grooving.*

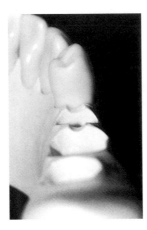

Fig 10-31d (right) *Proximal view following completion of bulk reduction and vertical grooving. Tooth aspect of the defect has not been affected.*

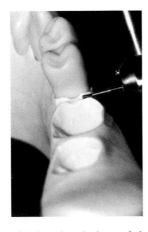

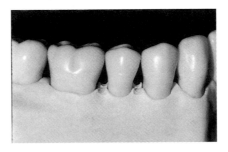

Fig 10-31e (left) *Proximal view of the initial reduction of the facial lip of the crater with a narrow finishing bur. This will be repeated for the lingual wall. Osteoplasty only is performed.*

Fig 10-31f (right) *Facial view following completion of the initial step in the reduction of the facial and lingual crater wall. Osteoplasty only, the entire tooth aspect of the defect still remains. Four peaks of bone now exist, one at each line angle area.*

a. Facial and lingual crater walls, hemisepta, walls of wide two wall and wide-shallow three wall defects, etc
b. Tooth aspect of the defect
4. Shaping of radicular bone — establish physiologic scallop
5. Final reshaping

Shallow Crater Located in the Midfaciolingual Region

Elimination of Bulk: Osteoplasty (Figs 10-31a to f) The extent of bony removal (osteoplasty) at this stage ranges from very extensive to none, depending on the existing osseous morphology. In the case of very thick osseous margins and some exostosis and tori formation in association with extensive osseous defects, bone removal will be very extensive. However, it is not unusual in the case of a thin periodontium associated with thin radicular bone and prominent root positions for this step to be very minimal or totally unnecessary, as would be any vertical grooving.

It is absolutely essential with the use of rotary instruments that copious amounts of irrigation be used. Gentle and effective flap retraction is essential. Large high-speed round burs in surgical length are the preferred instruments for this step. The no. 7009 twelve-bladed finishing bur is ideally suited for this step (see Fig 10-15b). It does not cut as roughly as the normal eight-bladed burs, and an experienced operator can safely thin bone closer to the teeth in the area that will be removed with the hand instruments in subsequent steps. The radicular bone in the area that will be removed in the scalloping procedure is thinned to facilitate the gentle use of the hand instruments.

It is emphasized that this procedure is strictly osteoplasty; no alveolar bone proper is removed. Excessive thinning of the radicular bone is contraindicated. The eventual marginal morphology is chisel edged as opposed to knife edged.

Vertical Grooving: Osteoplasty

(Figs 10-31c and d) Vertical grooving is used judiciously in the interdental and selective interradicular areas with furcation invasion to faciolingually narrow the interdental bone. This creates a relative root prominence leading to a more stable apical gingival margin and a narrow gingival papilla under the contact area. The groove is basically vertical. It is not beveled inward interdentally past the line angles or possibly the outer extent of the contact area. Its greatest use is where there are three or four teeth with relatively narrow mesiodistal embrasure width and sharply differing bone levels. A physiologic bony morphology can be created primarily with osteoplasty, thus minimizing the amount of ostectomy. Vertical grooving is used sparingly or not at all with a horizontally level bony morphology, especially when associated with prominent roots. The interdental area between the maxillary molars is usually avoided due to the possible exposure of the flared roots. All areas in which vertical grooving is used should be radiographically evaluated closely to note the interdental morphology and root locations. Vertical grooving is easily overdone with the use of high-speed burs.

Elimination of Interproximal Defect: Osteoplasty and Ostectomy

(Figs 10-31e and f) The initial reduction of the facial and lingual wall of the crater is usually done either with a narrow ta-

pered diamond or no. 7903 finishing bur, or a small round finishing bur sizes no. 7004 or no. 7006, depending on the interproximal width. There is much greater control and accurate reduction with the use of the long tapered bur or diamond than the round bur, especially for the neophyte. The facial and lingual walls are slowly and carefully reduced to the level of the base of the defect, establishing a flat form faciolingually. Coordinate this slope with the general angulation of the interdental bone relative to the defect location (facial or lingual) and the faciolingual inclination of the teeth. If the future gingival morphology of the area dictates a pointed papilla and scalloped radicular margin, the bony septum can now be gradually sloped apically, starting at the facial or lingual outer aspect of the contact area or the line angle, depending on the degree of pointed septum morphology and scalloping that is to be established.

All of this reduction is osteoplasty. In looking directly at the mesial or distal proximal surface (see Fig 10-31e), one would see a large peak of bone along the surface of the tooth approaching the line angles. The tooth aspect of the osseous defect has not been altered at all. If one were to stop now the original defect would still exist.

Clinicians who do not believe it is justifiable to sacrifice attachment (alveolar bone proper) to achieve additional probing depth reduction stop their osseous resection at this stage. This would be the approximate stopping point for those using a modified Widman procedure.

The Tooth Aspect of the Osseous Defect, Ostectomy (Removal of Alveolar Bone Proper)

(Figs 10-32 and 10-33) This is carefully

done with hand instruments so as not to damage the root surface (see Fig 10-15a). A variety of hand instruments have been adapted for this procedure. The Ochsenbein chisels are modified Chandler bone chisels. The sides have been modified to permit the instrument to reach further interproximally and to have a side cutting action (Figs 10-32a and b). The Rhodes 33 and 34 and Loughlin 1 and 2 are back-action scalers (modified Tracy scalers). The L 1 and 2 (Fig 10-32c) is designed with a greater angle to the shaft, permitting its use in the posterior as opposed to the Rhodes 33 and 34 (Fig 10-32d). Also, the blade edge is longer and more angulated, permitting it to reach further interproximally. The Rhodes 33 and 34 has a better angle for use on the midpalatal root surfaces. The Ochsenbein 1 end cutting is very effective for the anterior mesiofacial and distofacial and the posterior mesiofacial areas. The side cutting may be used for distofacial areas in the posterior region.

The mesiolingual aspect of the mandibular premolars may be easily ditched with the Ochsenbein 1 due to the necessary angle at which it is applied, reaching over the mandibular incisors. The Ochsenbein 2 actually will cut at a more perpendicular angle to the root in these areas. The mesiolingual and distolingual surfaces of the mandibular incisors are best contoured with the Loughlin 1 and Loughlin 2 and possibly the Rhodes 33 and 34. Many areas of the maxilla are best treated with the Ochsenbein 2. The mesiofacial distofacial mesiolingual and distolingual surfaces of the entire maxilla may be treated with the Ochsenbein 2, with the exception possibly of the distolingual areas of the first and second molars. In these areas, the Loughlin 1 and 2

Figs 10-32a and b *Mesiofacial and distofacial line angle area of the defect being removed by the end and side cutting action of the Ochsenbein 1.*

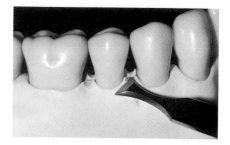
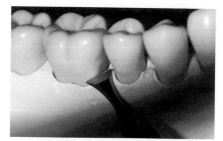

Fig 10-32c *(left) Distolingual line angle area of the defect being removed by the Loughlin 1 and 2. Note the significant reach of the blade interproximally and the angulation of the shaft to reach posteriorly.*

Fig 10-32d *(right) Distolingual line angle area of the defect being removed by the Rhodes 33 or 34.*

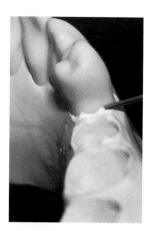
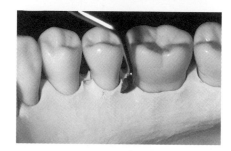

Figs 10-33a and b *Facial and proximal views following removal of the osseous defect in the line angle areas with the Ochsenbein chisel and Rhodes and Loughlin back action scalers. Some tooth aspect of the defect that is inaccessible with the above chisels remains.*

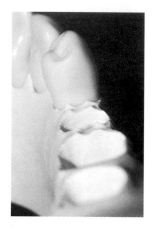

Figs 10-33c and d *Facial and proximal views using a narrow Wedelstadt chisel to remove the remaining inner aspects of the defect.*

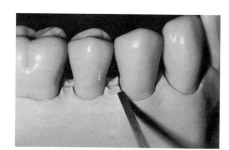

Figs 10-33e and f *Lingual view using Schluger bone file and Ochsenbein 3 chisel to remove the remaining inner aspects of the defect.*

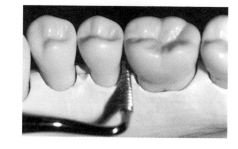
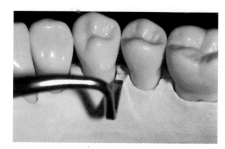

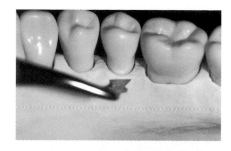

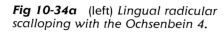
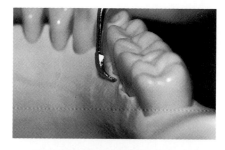

Fig 10-34a (left) *Lingual radicular scalloping with the Ochsenbein 4.*

Fig 10-34b (right) *Lingual radicular scalloping with the back action scalers (Loughlin or Rhodes as the anatomy permits).*

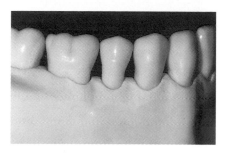
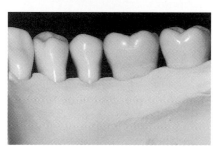

Figs 10-34c and d *Facial and lingual views upon completion of the initial scalloping. The osseous morphology requires careful evaluation to determine if it is the same as will be assumed by the gingiva based on its anatomic determining factors. Any additional modifications required are now made.*

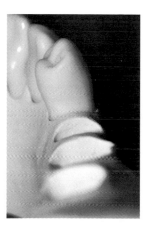

Fig 10-34e *Proximal view upon completion of the initial scalloping. Note the slightly peaked bony septa in the premolar area and the relatively flat bony septa in a faciolingual plane in the molar area.*

is most effective, especially in a mouth with a small opening. Once all the line angle areas are completed, the interdental areas are carefully inspected from the facial and lingual, following thorough aspiration and assisted with fiberoptics to note the osseous topography.

In hemiseptal defects and narrow faciolingual craters, there may still remain a significant amount of the tooth aspect of the defect (Figs 10-33b to d). These inner portions of the defects are best removed with narrow Wedelstadt chisels, curets, Fedi chisels, Ochsenbein 3 and bone files (Figs 10-33c to f). The Ochsenbein 3 and Fedi chisels and files may be used from a lingual approach as well. During this step it is very easy to gouge the root surface and this must be guarded against.

Following the elimination of the tooth aspect of the defect, a careful analysis of the determinants of gingival morphology for

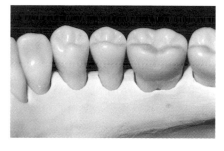
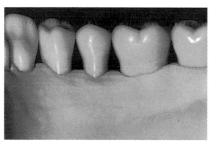

Figs 10-34f and g *Lingual view at less than 90 degrees (Fig 10-34f) to the long axis of the tooth following completion of the final osseous reshaping. Note how the scalloping appears very scalloped relative to Fig 10-34g, which is the same, but viewed at 90 degrees to the long axis of the teeth. In Fig 10-34f the therapist would be criticized for excessive ostectomy versus Fig 10-34g, yet they are the same viewed at different angles. The therapist must be knowledgeable of this "viewpoint distortion."*

this environment is again completed prior to the next step.

Shaping of Radicular Bone — Establish Physiologic Scallop: Ostectomy (Figs 10-34a to g)

This step is entirely ostectomy — removal of alveolar bone proper. Only the minimal amount of scalloping-ostectomy is done to establish a physiologic osseous / gingival architecture. A careful analysis of the determinants of gingival morphology for this environment is again completed. The minimal amount of scalloping is completed to establish a physiologic morphology and shallow probing depth. This is accomplished with a variety of instruments, providing access relative to the various anatomic limitations present.

Final Reshaping: Possibly Osteoplasty and Ostectomy

A detailed inspection of the osseous morphology is now completed using aspiration under direct, reflected, and fiberoptic light sources. The clinician must evaluate if this osseous morphology is that which the gingiva will assume relative to the anatomic factors that determine the gingival morphology. Any refinements that are indicated are now completed.

Viewpoint Distortion

The angle at which the osseous morphology and scalloping is viewed relative to the long axis of the teeth can significantly alter the visual appearance of the degree of scalloping. The marginal morphology should be viewed perpendicular to the long axis of the teeth, otherwise an altered form will be perceived. Note Figs 10-34e and f, which are of the same subject viewed perpendicular to the long axis (90 degrees) of the teeth (Fig 10-34f) and at less than

90 degrees to the long axis (Fig 10-34e). Note that even though they are the same, the one viewed at less than a 90-degree angle appears significantly more scalloped. This is the angle at which many lingual surgical photographs are taken. The uninformed evaluator then determines that too much ostectomy was performed. The clinician must place his / her mirror such that the marginal bone contour is viewed perpendicular to the long axis of the teeth. Photographic mirrors and patient detail mirrors are very helpful for this purpose.

Molar Areas

In the molar areas, additional considerations are involved that do not exist for single-rooted teeth. The level of the furcations and root trunk length relative to the interdental defect depth must be taken into consideration. In producing a scalloped margin, a therapeutic furcation is not to be created.

Determinants of marginal bone reduction in the molar area:

1. Extent of the interdental defect
2. Relationship of the facial and lingual (mandibular) furca to the marginal bone height
3. Width of the interdental space

The marginal radicular bone is removed in small stages, alternating between it and the facial and lingual lips of the interdental crater until the level of the furca is reached (Figs 10-35a and b). If some defect still remains and if the interdental septum is wide mesiodistally, some slight reverse contour may be established if it is believed the gingiva will assume this form. If the interdental septum is narrow mesiodistally, then some residual defect must remain.

Lingual Approach to the Posterior Mandible

A lingual approach to the posterior mandible is necessary due to the predominant lingual position of the interdental defects and the anatomic considerations in the area.

The mandible consists of (1) a horseshoe-shaped body joined at its posterior extent by two vertical ramii at an outward obtuse angle, and (2) the alveolar process joined to the upper portion of the body (Fig 10-36a). The curvature of the alveolar process differs from that of the body, curving inward in the posterior part more toward the midline (Fig 10-36b). This is reflected in the lingual inclination of the alveolus and teeth in the posterior region (Fig 10-36c). This inward curvature located distal to the second or third molar, in combination with the outward junction with the ramus in the same region, creates a marked outward curvature to the overall bony anatomy in this area, which is largely masked by the overlying soft tissue. This outward curvature must be considered when extending incisions distal to the second and third molars into the retromolar region (Figs 10-37a and b).

Only minimal facial marginal bone reduction is possible on the facial aspect of the molars, especially the second molars, due to the frequent shallow vestibule, prominent external oblique ridge and sometimes shelflike form, buccinator muscle attachment, and short root trunk. In conjunction with these anatomic limiting factors, the lingual location of the interdental defects, and the 20- to 25-degree lingual inclination of the molars, the interdental septum is ramped lingually (Figs 10-38 and 10-39a to j). The most coronal aspect of the septum in this case is not the base of the interdental

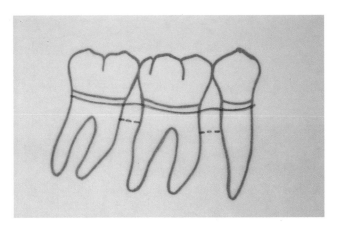

Fig 10-35a *Facial view of interdental craters, with their base represented by the dotted lines at the level of the furcations. Normal marginal bone levels are present.*

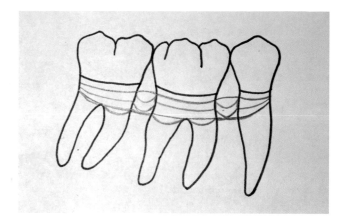

Fig 10-35b *Facial view (lingual would be similar), demonstrating the alternating stages in reduction of the marginal bone and the lip of the crater. Done in this judicious alternating manner, no therapeutic furcation or reversed architecture will be created.*

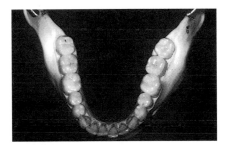

Fig 10-36a *Occlusal view of mandible demonstrating the horseshoe-shaped body of the mandible, the ramus joining the mandible at an outward angulation, and the alveolar process with a somewhat smaller arc of curvature than the body of the mandible.*

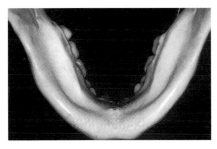

Fig 10-36b *Inferior or apical view of the mandible demonstrating the smaller curvature of the alveolar process and its position somewhat within the curvature of the mandible, particularly in the posterior areas.*

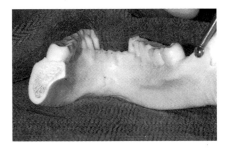

Fig 10-36c *Cross-sectional view in the molar area of the mandible demonstrating the alveolar process largely within the curvature of the mandibular body and the lingual inclination of the molars.*

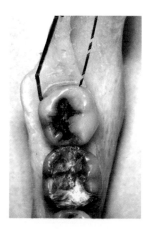 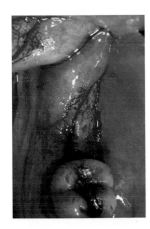

Fig 10-37a *(left) Occlusal view of the retromolar area. The dotted line represents the most frequently used incision line and the solid line the author's preferred incision line. This incision location makes it much easier to reflect the tissues lingually over the bulbous bony structure that frequently is present at the junction of the mandibular body and ramus in the area of the second or third molar. The lingual nerve is avoided by carefully palpating the bony anatomy and placing the incision to bone, and by carefully following the outward angulation of the ramus (not straight distally).*

Fig 10-37b *(right) Occlusal view of the lingual flap reflected using the author's preferred location for the incision. Note the surgical access and visibility of the lingual molar and retromolar area.*

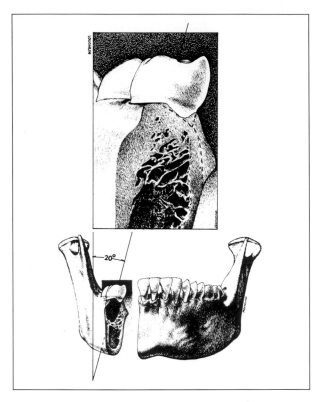

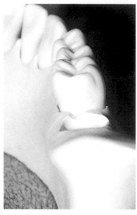

Fig 10-38 (left) *Cross-sectional drawing of the lingual inclination of the molars and a shallow interdental crater lingually positioned. The dotted line demonstrates the proposed osseous surgical reduction ramping the defect lingually. In this schematic, nearly all of the reduction is from the lingual. The most coronal aspect of the bony interdental system will be facially located rather than midfaciolingual.*

Fig 10-39a (below left) *Proximal view of an interdental crater somewhat lingually positioned. Two osseous craters only, one between the molars and one between the first molar and second premolar.*

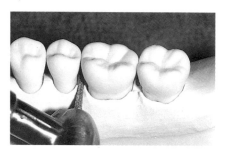

Fig 10-39b (below right) *Interdental reduction of the lingual lip of the crater from the lingual aspect using a narrow tapered diamond.*

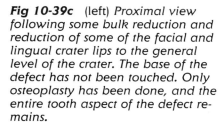

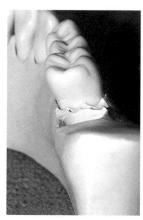

Fig 10-39c (left) *Proximal view following some bulk reduction and reduction of some of the facial and lingual crater lips to the general level of the crater. The base of the defect has not been touched. Only osteoplasty has been done, and the entire tooth aspect of the defect remains.*

Fig 10-39d (right) *Proximal view following the removal of the bone (ostectomy) in the line angle areas with the Ochsenbein 1 and 2 chisels and the Loughlin 1 and 2 back action scalers.*

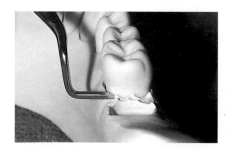

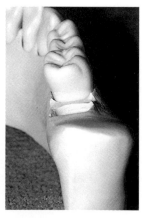

Fig 10-39e (left) *Proximal view demonstrating use of the Ochsenbein 3 chisel for removing the inaccessible aspect of the defect from the lingual. Files and curets may also be used for this step. In the premolar and incisor region, a small chisel may be used from the facial aspect.*

Fig 10-39f (right) *Proximal view following removal of the tooth aspect of the interdental crater. Note the general lingual inclination of the interdental bony septum.*

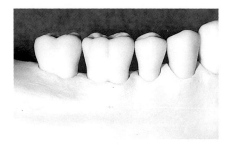

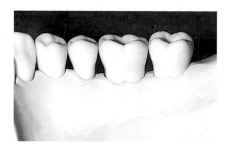

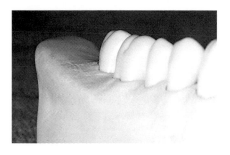

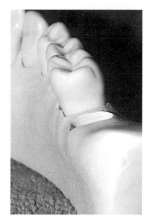

Fig 10-39g (left) *Lingual view following completion of the osseous surgery. Note the gradual scalloped pattern.*

Fig 10-39h (right) *Facial view following osseous surgery. Note the more scalloped morphology in the premolar area compared to the molar areas. Also note the gradual blending in of the osseous morphology into the area of the original defects between the molars and the first molar and second premolar.*

Figs 10-39i (left) *Facial view demonstrating minimal facial marginal bone reduction completed and in association with a prominent external oblique ridge and probable buccinator muscle attachment.*

Figs 10-39j (right) *Proximal view of the completed osseous resection. Note the lingual inclination of the interdental septum, the most coronal aspect of the septum facial to the midpoint, the facial marginal bone more coronal to the lingual marginal bone, and the general taper of the lingual bone compared to Fig 10-39a.*

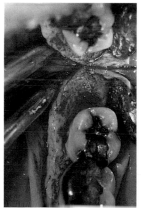

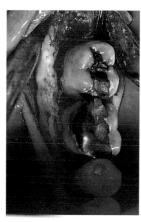

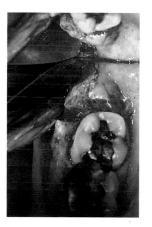

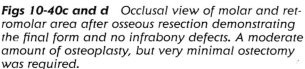

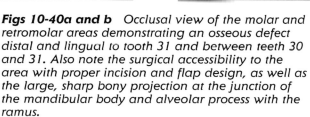

Figs 10-40a and b *Occlusal view of the molar and retromolar areas demonstrating an osseous defect distal and lingual to tooth 31 and between teeth 30 and 31. Also note the surgical accessibility to the area with proper incision and flap design, as well as the large, sharp bony projection at the junction of the mandibular body and alveolar process with the ramus.*

Figs 10-40c and d *Occlusal view of molar and retromolar area after osseous resection demonstrating the final form and no infrabony defects. A moderate amount of osteoplasty, but very minimal ostectomy was required.*

defect but rather an area facial to the defect. Greater lingual marginal reduction is also possible if required, due to the longer lingual root trunk.

By reducing the defect primarily to the lingual aspect rather than equally from the facial and lingual aspects, significantly less radicular bone proper is removed (Figs 10-40a to d). The chance of creating a therapeutic furcation is thus minimized. The apical gingival margin established on the lingual surface seems to be very stable, and facial esthetics is preserved.

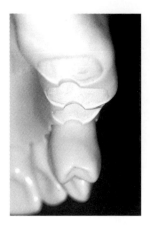
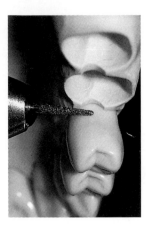

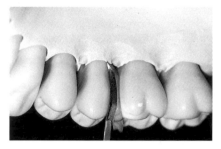
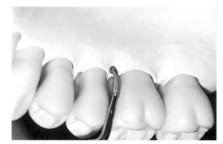

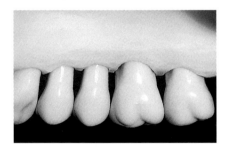
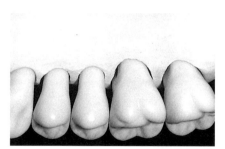

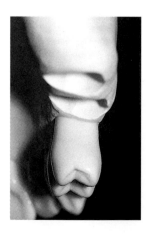
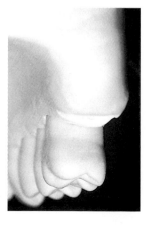

Fig 10-41a (left) *Proximal view of interdental craters somewhat palatally positioned between the first and second molars and the first molar and second premolar.*

Fig 10-41b (right) *Proximal view showing a tapered diamond about to initiate the reduction of the palatal lip of the crater. The diamond may be tipped to ramp the interproximal bony septum to the palate. The base of the defect must not be reduced. The most coronal position of the interdental bone will be facial to the faciolingual midpoint.*

Fig 10-41c (left) *Palatal view of the Ochsenbein 2 engaging alveolar bone proper at the distolingual line angle in a push-engage-twist action. This is very effective on distolingual line angles as far posterior as the patient can open for access.*

Fig 10-41d (right) *Palatal view of the back action scaler removing alveolar bone proper where the Ochsenbein 2 cannot gain favorable access. The Loughlin 1 and 2 are most effective for this.*

Fig 10-41e (left) *Palatal view following completion of osseous resection viewed at 90 degrees to the long axis of the teeth. Note the gradual rise and fall of the bony architecture blending into the originally noninvolved areas and the modest scalloping.*

Fig 10-41f (right) *Same view as Fig 10-41e but at less than 90 degrees to the long axis. This creates the appearance of excessive scalloping and excessive removal of alveolar bone proper. Understanding of viewpoint distortion is paramount for the clinician.*

Figs 10-41g and h *Proximal views following completion of osseous resection. Note the generalized slope of the interdental osseous crest to the palate. The most coronal aspect is located facially and the base of the original defect has not been altered.*

Figs 10-42a and b *Proximal and facial views of severe osseous defects, not fully correctable by osseous resection. Note the concavity in the faciolingual form of the interdental crest. There will be a minimal of 4 to 5 mm of probing depth at this point once the interdental soft tissues heal. The facial interdental lip of the crater has been reduced to the level of the adjacent furcations. There is no reversed architecture or therapeutic furcation invasion.*

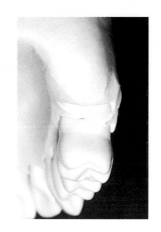
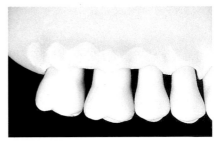

Lingual Approach to the Posterior Maxilla

A lingual approach to the posterior maxilla is also necessary due to the predominant lingual position of the interdental defects and the anatomic considerations in the area.

The interdental septum can be ramped primarily to the lingual aspect due to the lingual location of the interdental defect (Figs 10-41a to h). The coronal tip of the interdental septum then becomes located facially. Neither the base of the defect nor the midpoint faciolingually becomes the coronal tip of the interdental septum. Less facial marginal bone reduction is required, decreasing the chance of a therapeutic furcation involvement. The results are more esthetic and there is less total alveolar bone proper removal. Access to the mesial and distal furcations is impossible from the facial aspect because they are located lingually and behind the facial roots. The maxillary molars are essentially single-rooted teeth from the lingual aspect, and there is a widened mesiodistal embrasure that permits access to the mesial and distal furcations. There is less total alveolar bone proper removal, and the results are significantly

more esthetic. The apical position of the palatal masticatory mucosa seems to be very stable.

Severe Defect

A severe defect is not defined by depth of the defect and amount of attachment loss alone. The potential to correct the defect must also be considered relative to anatomic and esthetic considerations as well as the amount of attachment loss.

Residual defects must be accepted as a compromise in the presence of these anatomic factors and deep probing depths (Figs 10-42a and b). In these circumstances the following may be performed: no osseous surgery, osteoplasty only, or osteoplasty and limited ostectomy producing partial pocket depth reduction. It is up to the clinical judgment of the therapist to determine the most efficacious approach.

Root Surface Treatment in Osseous Resection

It is important that healthy root surfaces are not root planed as this would decrease the chance of reattachment of the flap connective tissue fibers. Root surfaces that are exposed to the periodon-

tal pocket and will be covered by the flap are thoroughly root planed. Root surfaces coronal to the flap margin are thoroughly scaled but not root planed, thus minimizing potential root hypersensitivity.

Suturing

Basic principles:

1. Use the least reactive material
2. Minimize the amount of suture material under the flap
3. Minimize potential entanglement of dressing with suture and suture knots
4. Remove in 5 to 10 days if nonresorbable
5. Intimate adaptation of tissues to the teeth and underlying bone
6. Avoid excessive tension that would compromise circulation and result in localized flap necrosis

Techniques The **interrupted suture** may be used when equal tension and coronal position of both the facial and lingual flap margins are desired. Examples would include the ENAP, open flap curettage, modified Widman flap, and regenerative procedures. There is the added safety in the event of the suture breaking or a knot becoming untied. There is the added risk of the dressing material becoming enmeshed in the surgical knots and presenting a problem at the time of dressing removal with nonresorbable suture material.

Sling sutures allow for localized positioning or adaptation of the flap around an individual tooth.

The **continuous sling** consists of two methods. A single facial-to-lingual suture and separate facial and lingual sutures. If equal tension and equal coronal positioning of the facial and lingual flap margins are desired, the single facial-to-lingual suturing method may be used (eg, mandibular anterior). However, if different marginal tension or coronal levels of the facial and lingual margins are desired, then separate facial and lingual sling sutures are used (eg, posterior maxilla). The sling suturing method is faster and there are fewer knots to become entangled with the dressing. However, if the suture breaks or the knot becomes untied, the whole flap may be dislodged.

Mattress sutures are used to help adapt the flap more intimately to the teeth and underlying bone and are useful with regenerative procedures to keep the suture above the tissue and not in the area of desired regeneration.

Anchor sutures are used for the suturing of a single papilla when it is not desired to suture it to the opposite flap.

QUICK REVIEW

I. Means of probing depth reduction
  • Increased resistance to sulcular probe penetration
    — decreased gingival inflammation and increased gingival tonus
  • Apical positioning of the free gingival margin
    — gingival shrinkage
    — gingival excision
    — gingival margin placement apically with and without osseous resection
  • Coronal positioning of the attachment
    — new attachment
    — orthodontics (relative coronal placement of the attachment level to the surrounding alveolar crest, not a net gain in attachment)

II. Probing depth reduction procedures
  • Plaque control
  • Scaling, root planing, and curettage
  • Gingivectomy
  • Repositioned flaps (unpredictable)
  • Apically positioned flap without osseous resection
  • Apically positioned flap with osseous resection
  • New attachment procedures
    — grafts (bone and alloplastic materials)
    — guided tissue regeneration (membranes, coronal flap positioning, and chemicals)
    — root biomodification
  • Orthodontics

III. Surgical procedures for moderate chronic adult periodontitis
  • Gingivectomy and gingivoplasty
    — internal beveled gingivectomy
    — external beveled gingivectomy
  • Flap procedures
    — repositioned flap (partial flap reflection — ENAP, modified ENAP, modified Widman / Ramfjord procedure. These procedures have also been referred to as a flap curettage by various authors)
    — apically positioned flap (with and without osseous resection)
    — regenerative procedures
  • Combined procedures

IV. Anatomic factors determining gingival morphology
  • The mesiodistal curvature of the facial and lingual root surface. A markedly curved root surface mesiodistally will have a pronounced scalloped margin. A relatively flat surface mesiodistally will have a more straight margin or flat scallop.

Quick Review continues on page 177.

- Mesiodistal width of the interdental space. The wider the interdental space, the more flat the architecture. The more narrow the interdental space, the more scalloped the architecture.
  - *proximal tooth morphology.* A flat proximal surface would have a narrow interdental space and a convex proximal surface would have a wider interdental space assuming normal alignment and contact relationship.
  - *tooth alignment.* Tipping of the teeth can make the space wider or narrower as the case may be.
  - *curve of Spee.* Tends to incline the roots of the maxillary molars together and diverge the mandibular molar roots.
  - *flaring of roots.* The distobuccal root of the maxillary first molar and the mesiobuccal root of the maxillary second molar flare and converge apically, producing a very narrow interdental space.
- Relationship of the tooth to bone or its position in the arch. A tooth in a prominent position in the arch facially or lingually would have a pronounced scalloped margin, and a tooth recessed in the arch would have a fairly flat margin.
- Width of the interdental space faciolingually. With a narrow width the papilla tends to be more pointed, and with it wide it tends to be more flat.

V. Changes in the gingival environment as a result of moving the gingival complex apically

- The interdental width mesiodistally usually becomes wider apically. This is due largely to the tapering shape of the roots. Less scalloping will be required, which means less marginal radicular bone on the facial and lingual surfaces will need to be removed.
- The interdental width mesiodistally may become more narrow apically. The narrower interdental space produces a greater gingival scalloping; therefore,

more marginal radicular bone on the facial and lingual will be need to be removed.
  - *tilting of the teeth*
  - *flaring of the molar roots.* A frequent occurrence between the distobuccal root of the maxillary first molar and the mesiobuccal root of the maxillary second molar. It may occur infrequently between the mandibular roots.
  - *curve of Spee.* Tends to narrow the interdental width between the maxillary molars and widen the interdental width mesiodistally between the mandibular roots.
- Apically the maxillary and mandibular arches in general become wider faciolingually. This means the interdental area will become wider faciolingually apically and the interdental papilla less pointed and more flat. There would therefore need to be less alveolar bone proper removal to achieve physiologic form.
- Tooth-to-bone relationships within the alveolus will change apically. The tooth may become more prominent or more recessed in the arch relative to the surrounding bony housing. The more prominent the root, the greater the scalloping. The more recessed the root, the less scalloping will be required. Be sure both the facial and lingual aspects are evaluated carefully. A tooth that is prominent facially may be recessed on the lingual and vice versa.
- Apically the roots become more curved mesiodistally. With greater mesiodistal curvature, more scalloping of the gingiva will occur and therefore increased scalloping must be placed in the marginal bone. Molars are a significant example, flat architecture at the CEJ area becoming quite curved apical to the furcation. There may be a progres-

Quick Review continues on page 178.

sion from a flat scallop to a prominent scallop with apical gingival placement in the molar areas.

VI. Considerations in the amount of attachment removal
Specific considerations prior to osseous resection therapy:
- Esthetics
- Root hypersensitivity
- Severity of defect
- Root length / attachment area
- Depth of interdental molar defects relative to furcation levels

VII. Dos and don'ts of osseous resection
- Must have adequate attachment remaining.
- Do not create roots so hypersensitive that the patient cannot perform adequate plaque control.
- Do not create an unesthetically acceptable result.
- Interdental defects generally cannot be reduced apical to adjacent furcation levels.
- Do not remove alveolar bone proper only to have a soft tissue defect or possibly soft tissue attachment remain in its place.

VIII. Severity of defect—anatomic considerations:
- Length and shape of root
- Apicocoronal level of furcations
- Root proximity
- External oblique ridge
- Ramus of the mandible
- Shallow hamular notch and short tuberosity
- Soft palate relationship to second molar
- Flat palatal vault
- Sinus approximation

IX. Marginal flap positioning
Marginal flap positioning depends on:
- Anatomic factors
  - adequate width and thickness of gingiva
  - adequate thickness of radicular bone

- Esthetics
- Attempting new attachment
- Desiring pocket depth reduction or elimination
- Accepting pocket depth postsurgically

Marginal flap location:
- CEJ
  - esthetics
  - attempting new attachment
  - adequate width of gingiva
- 1 to 2 mm coronal to the marginal alveolar crest
  - adequate width of gingiva
  - desire minimal probing depth
  - no esthetic concerns
- Even with the alveolar crest
  - minimal or no gingiva
  - desire minimal probing depth
  - no esthetic concerns
- Slightly apical to the alveolar crest (seldom done)
  - minimal / no gingiva
  - thick radicular bone
  - desire minimal probing depth
  - no esthetic concerns

X. Postoperative management
- Follow patient closely for 2 months
- Weekly postoperative visits for the first 4 to 6 weeks
- First week
  - remove dressing if placed
  - debridement of wound
  - suture removal if nonresorbable sutures placed
  - plaque control instructions
- Subsequent weeks
  - evaluate healing and tissue morphology
  - plaque control evaluation and instruction
  - desensitization as indicated
- Two-month interval
  - post surgical reevaluation, charting, and maintenance therapy
  - establish recall frequency and note special concerns

REFERENCES

1. Kepic TJ, O'Leary TJ, Kafrawy, AH: Total calculus removal: An attainable objective? *J Periodontol* 1990;61:16-20.

2. Robertson PB: The residual calculus paradox. *J Periodontol* 1990;61:65-66.

3. American Academy of Periodontology: *Current Procedural Terminology For Periodontics*. Chicago: American Academy of Periodontology, 1989.

4. Goodson JM, Haffajee AD, Socransky SS: The relationship between attachment level loss and alveolar bone loss. *J Clin Periodontol* 1984;11:348.

5. Prichard JF: *The Diagnosis and Treatment of Periodontal Disease*. Philadelphia: WB Saunders Co, 1979.

6. Barrington EP: An overview of periodontal surgical procedures. *J Periodontol* 1981;52:518.

7. Pihlstrom BL, McHugh RB, Oliphant TH, Ortiz-Campos C: Comparison of surgical and nonsurgical treatment of periodontal disease. A review of current studies and additional results after 6-1/2 years. *J Clin Periodontol* 1983;10:524.

8. Becker W, Becker B, Ochsenbein C, Keary GJ, Caffesse R: A longitudinal study comparing scaling and osseous surgery and modified Widman procedures — Results after 1 year. *J Periodontol* 1988;59:351.

9. Kaldahl WB, Kalkwarf KL, Patil KD, Dyer JK, Bates RE: Evaluation of four modalities of periodontal therapy. Mean probing depth, probing attachment level and recession changes. *J Periodontol* 1988;59:783.

10. Lindhe J, Nyman S, Karring T: Scaling and root planing in shallow pockets. *J Clin Periodontol* 1982;9:415.

11. Stambaugh RV, Dragoo M, Smith DM, Carasal L: The limits of subgingival scaling. *Int J Periodont Rest Dent* 1981;1(5):30.

12. Waerhaug J: Healing of the dento-epithelial junction following subgingival plaque control. II. As observed on extracted teeth. *J Periodontol* 1978; 49:119.

13. Kaldahl WB, Kalkwarf KL, Patil KD, Molvar M: Responses of four tooth and site groupings to periodontal therapy. *J Periodontol* 1990;61:173.

14. Badersten A, Nilvéus R, Egelberg J: Effect of nonsurgical periodontal therapy. I. Moderately advanced periodontitis. *J Clin Periodontol* 1981; 8:57.

15. O'Leary TS, Barrington EP, Gottsegen R: Periodontal therapy — A summary status report. *J Periodontol* 1988; 59:306.

16. Kakehashi S, Parakkal P: Proceedings from the state of the art workshop on surgical therapy for periodontitis. *J Periodontol* 1982;53:475.

17. Gottsegen R: A fresh look at the maintenance phase of periodontal therapy. *Alpha Omegan* 1983;76:85.

18. Ramfjord SP: Maintenance care for treated periodontitis patients. *J Clin Periodontol* 1987;14:433-437.

19. Ramfjord S: Surgical periodontal pocket elimination: Still a justifiable objective? *J Am Dent Assoc* 1987; 114:37.

20. Schluger S: Osseous resection — A basic principle in periodontal surgery. *Oral Surg Oral Med Oral Pathol* 1949;2:316.

21. Widman L: The operative treatment of pyorrhea alveolaris: A new surgical method. *Svensk Tandlakar* Tidskr 1918; December.

22. Ramfjord SP, Nissle RR: The Modified Widman flap. *J Periodontol* 1974; 45:601.

23. Ochsenbein C: A primer for osseous surgery. *Int J Perio Rest Dent* 1986;6(1):8.

24. Hancock EB: Regeneration procedures. In: *Proceedings of the World Workshop In Clinical Periodontics*. Chicago: American Academy of Periodontology, 1989.

25. Ramfjord SP, Caffesse RG, Morrison EC, et al: Four modalities of periodontal treatment compared over five years. *J Clin Periodont Res* 1987;22:222.

26. Kalkwarf K: Tissue attachment. In: *Proceedings of the World Workshop in Clinical Periodontics*. Chicago: American Academy of Periodontology, 1989.

27. Prichard J: Infrabony technique as a predictable procedure. *J Periodontol* 1957;28:202.

28. Becker W, Becker B, Beng I: Repair of intrabony defects as a result of open debridement procedures. Report of 36 treated cases. *Int J Periodont Rest Dent* 1986;6(2):8.

29. Isidor F, Attstrom R, Karring T: Regeneration of alveolar bone following surgical and non-surgical periodontal treatment. *J Clin Periodontol* 1985;12:687.

30. Patur B, Glickman I: Clinical and roentgenographic evaluation of the post-treatment healing of infrabony pockets. *J Periodontol* 1962;33:164.

31. Goldman HM, Cohen DW: Infrabony pocket classification and treatment. *J Periodontol* 1958;29:272.

32. Nabers CL: Repositioning the attached gingiva. *J Periodontol* 1954;25:38.

33. Friedman N: Mucogingival surgery: The apically repositioned flap. *J Periodontol* 1962;33:328.

34. Prichard J: Gingivoplasty, gingivectomy and osseous surgery. *J Periodontol* 1961;32:275.

35. Caffesse RG: Resective procedures. In: *Proceedings of the World Workshop in Clinical Periodontics*. Chicago: American Academy of Periodontology, 1989.

36. Axelsson P, Lindhe J: The significance of maintenance care in the treatment of periodontal disease. *J Clin Periodontol* 1981;8:281.

37. Lindhe J, Nyman S: Long-term maintenance of patients treated for advanced periodontal disease. *J Clin Periodontol* 1984;11:504.

38. McFall WT: Supportive treatment. In: *Proceedings of the World Workshop in Clinical Periodontics*. Chicago: American Academy of Periodontology, 1989.

39. Yukna R, Lawrence J: Gingival surgery for soft tissue new attachment. *Dent Clin North Am* 1980;24:705.

40. Ochsenbein C, Ross S: A reevaluation of osseous surgery. *Dent Clin North Am* 1969;13:87.

41. Selipsky H: Osseous surgery — How much need we compromise? *Dent Clin North Am* 1976;20:79.

42. Orban B: *Orban's Oral Histology and Embryology*. St Louis: CV Mosby Co, 1966.

43. Ritchey B, Orban B: Crests of the interdental alveolar septa. *J Periodontol* 1953;24:75.

Severe Chronic Adult Periodontitis

CURRENT CONCEPTS by James T. Mellonig

CLINICAL APPLICATION by James T. Mellonig

CURRENT CONCEPTS	CLINICAL APPLICATION
Introduction	Atlas of procedures
Bone grafts	
Bone substitutes (alloplasts)	QUICK REVIEW
Guided tissue regeneration	
	REFERENCES

C U R R E N T   C O N C E P T S

INTRODUCTION

The patient who presents with advanced chronic adult periodontitis will have clinical and radiographic evidence of severe periodontal destruction. The bone loss may be horizontal and / or vertical and localized or generalized in nature. Commonly the probing depths exceed 6 mm and clinical attachment loss is equal to or greater than the probing depth; this depends on whether or not there is gingival recession. In addition, grade II or III furcation invasion is a frequent finding. In order to correct these problems, a whole array of treatment modalities can be used. These usually include: extraction, scaling and root planing alone, osseous surgery, root amputation / hemisection, orthodontic repositioning, interdental denudation, coronally positioned flap, open flap debridement procedures with or without chemotherapeutic root conditioning, bone grafts, alloplastic grafts, and guided tissue regeneration with and without bone grafts. The clinician must weigh the advantages and disadvantages of each of these procedures and select the proper one based on the therapeutic objectives for a particular patient. If the desired goal is reconstruction of destroyed periodontal tissue, the selection is usually a bone graft, an alloplastic graft, or guided tissue regeneration; this section will focus on these therapeutic modalities since they are the most effective methods presently available.

BONE GRAFTS

Bone grafts can be used to reduce probing depth, gain clinical attachment, fill osseous defects, and reconstruct the attachment apparatus consisting of new bone, cementum, and periodontal ligament. Bone grafting is the only regenerative modality for which there is ample evidence of new attachment apparatus formation about a root surface previously exposed to the oral environment.[1,2]

Bone grafts may be either autogenous (patient's own bone) or allogeneic (bone from a nonrelated donor) and can be obtained either intraorally or extraorally. Intraoral grafts can be composed of cancellous bone and marrow, cancellous bone or cortical bone alone, or a combination of cortical and cancellous bone.

Intraoral cancellous bone and marrow autografts are usually taken from the maxillary tuberosity or a healing extraction socket. Cortical and / or cancellous bone is taken from a donor site within the surgical area. A graft of cortical and / or cancellous bone, when obtained with a bur and mixed with blood and saliva, is termed an osseous coagulum.[3] If removed with a trephine and triturated in an amalgam capsule to produce a small particle size, it is called a bone blend.[4] Clinical case reports have documented mean bone fill of 3 to 4 mm, with up to 12 mm in some osseous defects, and greater than 50% bone repair on a predictable basis following placement of intraoral autografts.[5-8]

Autogenous Bone Grafts

There is general agreement that autogenous iliac cancellous bone and marrow is a graft material of extremely high osteogenic potential. Furcation invasions, dehiscence-type defects, and osseous lesions of varying morphology have all been reconstructed with this type of graft.[8-12] In addition, mean bone apposition of 2.5 mm above the level of the previous alveolar crest has been obtained.[8] This type of graft can be used both fresh and frozen. Unfortunately, the fresh extraoral autograft has the unique postoperative problem of root resorption.[13-15] If diagnosed early, root resorption can be corrected by root planing and renewed efforts at plaque control.[15] Freezing the autograft prior to implantation apparently attenuates this problem.[14]

Allogeneic Bone Grafts (Allografts)

Frequently it occurs that insufficient quantities of intraoral autogenous bone are available to fill large or multiple osseous defects. Likewise, logistical and economic considerations in the procurement of iliac autografts and the root resorption associated with this type of material have dictated the need for an allogeneic source of bone. Bone allografts are commercially available from tissue banks. In order to preclude the possibility of disease transfer, the protocol for donor procurement of any tissue banks should include at a minimum the following exclusionary techniques: (1) omission of donors

from high-risk groups, (2) medical and social screening, (3) HIV antibody, (4) HIV antigen, (5) blood culture, (6) surrogate or proxy tests, ie, serology for hepatitis and syphilis, (7) special lymph node study, (8) histopathologic studies of donor tissue, and (9) followup study of grafts from the same donor.[16] The risk of disease transfer is calculated to be one in well over a million by average estimates when the above exclusionary techniques are applied.[16] The procedure of processing a bone allograft further reduces the risk to one in 8 million.[17]

Bone allografts are usually procured surgically under sterile conditions within 24 hours of the death of the donor. The cortical bone is defatted, cut into cortical strips or fragmented, cultured for bacterial contamination, washed in absolute ethanol, and deep frozen. Pending results of exclusionary assays, the bone may or may not be demineralized in 0.6 normal hydrochloric acid. It is repeatedly washed, pulverized to 250 to 750 μm, freeze-dried, and stored under a vacuum. Freeze-drying markedly reduces the antigenicity of a bone allograft.[18,19]

Two types of bone allografts are routinely available for clinical use: undemineralized freeze-dried bone allograft (FDBA) and demineralized freeze-dried bone allograft (DFDBA). In field trials, approximately 63% of the defects treated with FDBA showed complete or greater than 50% bone repair.[20] An even greater percentage of defects (80%) were successfully treated by combining FDBA with autogenous bone to form a composite graft.[20] Demineralization of a bone allograft (DFDBA) in 0.6 normal hydrochloric acid significantly enhances the osteogenic potential of the allograft by exposing bone morphogenetic protein (BMP).[21,22] BMP is

a hydrophobic glycoprotein that is located in the cortical bone matrix and induces new bone formation by the host.[22,23] The results from clinical studies in which DFDBA was inserted into bone defects showed an average gain of 2.4 to 2.6 mm of bone fill as measured from the bottom of the original defect.[24,25] Of special interest was that 78% of the sites demonstrated greater than 50% bone fill.[25]

Human controlled studies with autogenous or allogeneic bone grafts demonstrate that significantly better results of therapy are obtained in grafted compared to nongrafted sites for both types of graft materials.[7,9,25-32] Human histologic studies also show that regeneration of a new attachment apparatus composed of bone, cementum, and periodontal ligament is the normal outcome following implantation of a bone graft.[2,12,33-36]

BONE SUBSTITUTES (ALLOPLASTS)

Bone substitutes are implants of inert material composed of beta tricalcium phosphate, nonporous hydroxyapatite, or porous hydroxyapatite. Beta tricalcium phosphate is resorbable whereas the hydroxyapatite implants are not. Such bone substitutes are used to simply fill osseous defects, not for regeneration of periodontal tissues.

Healing after implantation of beta tricalcium phosphate and nonporous hydroxyapatite does not restore periodontal structures. Rather, the materials become encapsulated within connective tissue and act as merely inert space fillers.[37,38] Therefore, grafting with bone substitutes is reserved for those situations in which it is not possible to obtain a bone autograft and the patient objects to a bone allograft. A 5-year followup study suggests that sites treated with nonporous hydroxyapatite remain stable after surgery and result in a high frequency of clinical improvement. In contrast, areas treated by open flap debridement alone are not stable and regress at a rate three to five times that of the grafted sites.[39]

Porous hydroxyapatite is manufactured by a process in which the calcium carbonate skeleton of marine corals undergoes a chemical conversion to hydroxyapatite while the porous structure is preserved. This material appears to have more favorable outcomes than other alloplastic materials, as positive results have been reported in grade II furcation invasions.[1,40] Implantation of porous hydroxyapatite may result in the formation of osseous material in the pores and on the surface of the implant.[41,42] Adjacent to the root surface, however, healing is mainly by a long junctional epithelium, which extends apical to the coronal level of the implant.[41,42]

GUIDED TISSUE REGENERATION

The guided tissue regeneration procedure evolved from a biologically based concept relative to the healing of periodontal surgical wounds. This concept states that if healing proceeds from the epithelium, then a long junctional epithelium will result; if healing proceeds primarily from the gingival connective tissue, root resorption will occur. And finally, if healing proceeds from bone, ankylosis will be the result.[43-47] It is only when preference is given to cells migrating from the periodontal ligament that reconstruction of the periodontal tissues will be promoted.[48] This may be accomplished by placing a physical barrier (eg, a membrane composed of expanded polytetrafluoroethylene) between the root surface and the epithelium / gingival connective tissue.[49] This will occlude epithelium and connective tissue and will create a space between the root and the soft tissue into which cells from the periodontal ligament can migrate and

undergo amplifying cell division.[49]

The guided tissue regeneration procedure shows predictability for connective tissue attachment in intraosseous and grade II furcation invasions.[50,51] Clinically, the tissue filling the osseous defect is resistant to penetration by a periodontal probe and has a rubber-like consistency.[50] Bone fill has not been noted with any degree of frequency.[49-53] Therefore, the objective of the guided tissue regeneration procedure is closure of the periodontal lesion by new cementum with inserting connective tissue fibers.[49,53,54] Osseous fill may be more predictable if a bone graft is inserted into the lesion before the periodontal membrane is placed.[55] Problems associated with guided tissue regeneration are related to the technique-sensitivity of the procedure.[1] At times, the periodontal membrane becomes so well integrated with the host tissue that a gentle tug will not remove it; therefore, a secondary surgical procedure is need to remove the membrane.[1]

CLINICAL APPLICATION

Patient and site selection for periodontal regeneration
(Figs 11-1a and b)

The patient should be free of any major systemic complications, should have an acceptable level of plaque control and positive attitude toward therapy, and should be committed to life-long periodontal maintenance therapy. Sites selected should have deep probing depths, minimal soft tissue recession, a zone of keratinized gingiva of at least 2 mm, and radiographic evidence of vertical bone loss.

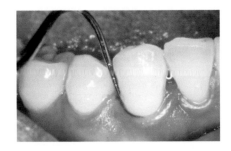
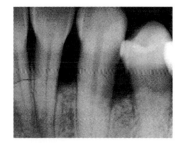

Anesthesia and incisions (Fig 11-2)

Block or infiltration anesthesia may be used. Good hemostasis is important for visualization of the bone defect and root surface prior to implantation. Inability to control bleeding at the defect site will impede root surface preparation and graft placement. Sulcular incisions to bone are made on both facial and lingual surfaces; they should be extended as far to the interproximal area as possible. Gingival thinning techniques should be avoided. The goal is maximum tissue conservation. The incisions are carried at least one tooth to the mesial and distal of the graft site to provide access for instrumentation and visualization of the wound site.

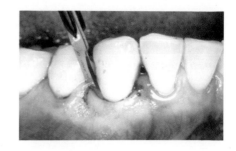

Flap reflection (Fig 11-3)

Once the incisions are made, the interproximal papillae are gently elevated to ensure they are freely movable. This will avoid any unintentional trauma and possible tearing of the papillae upon flap elevation. Full-thickness flaps are then reflected the minimum distance necessary to gain access to the underlying osseous defect; 2 or 3 mm beyond the alveolar crest is all that should be necessary.

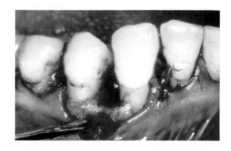

Adherent granulation tissue (Fig 11-4)

With the flaps reflected, excessive granulation tissue is removed from the inner surface of the flaps and papillae with a scissors. Excessive thinning of the flap and especially the papillae is to be avoided. A thin papilla will likely tear when suturing, and complete wound closure will be unobtainable.

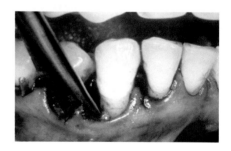

Soft tissue debridement (Fig 11-5)

All soft tissues, including the transseptal connective fibers located at the base of the osseous defect, are removed. This is accomplished initially with ultrasonic instrumentation followed by curets. Once all granulation tissue is removed, bleeding will rapidly subside.

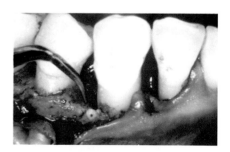

Root planing (Fig 11-6)

Meticulous removal of bacterial plaque debris, calcified deposits, and contaminated cementum is the essential prerequisite for success. Gross debris is removed via ultrasonic instrumentation. Hand instruments are used to plane the root surface. The goal is a root surface that is clean and smooth as determined with the aid of magnifying lenses, a fiberoptic light source, and a sharp explorer.

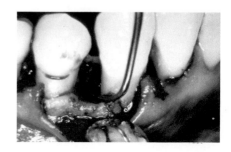

Visualization of defect site (Fig 11-7)

The surgical site is inspected to make sure that all soft tissue remnants have been removed from the osseous defect. Likewise, the root surface is carefully inspected to make sure that it is free of soft and hard accretions. Documentation should be done at this time for any future comparisons. A measurement is made from the cementoenamel junction to the alveolar crest; repeating this measurement at the time of reevaluation will determine how much alveolar crestal resorption has taken place. An additional measurement is taken from the cementoenamel junction to the base of the osseous defect, which will demonstrate the amount of bone fill that was achieved.

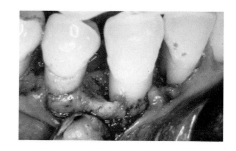

Intramarrow penetration (Fig 11-8)

To gain access to the underlying marrow spaces, a sharp instrument or small bur is used to penetrate the cortical bone lining the defect. Theoretically, this will allow for egress of the pluripotential cells of the marrow spaces to graft site. This may also aid in revascularization of the graft.

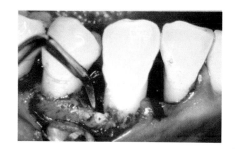

Bone graft material (Fig 11-9)

The bone graft material of choice is placed in a sterile dappen dish. If the material is autogenous, it is covered with moistened gauze to prevent dehydration. If a bone allograft is used, sterile saline or water is added to reconstitute the graft. Excess fluid is removed with gauze prior to graft insertion.

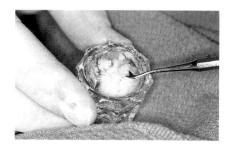

Graft placement (Fig 11-10)

The graft material is packed firmly into the defect in a step by step fashion until the entire defect is filled with bone. After each increment of graft material is placed, it is blotted with gauze moistened in saline to absorb excessive fluid; this will assist in condensing the graft. An overfill approach may be used if supracrestal apposition of bone is the desired outcome. However, overfilling the defect may impede complete wound closure.

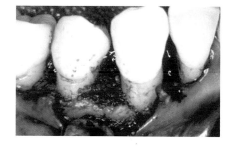

Flap closure (Fig 11-11)

Complete flap closure is important for a successful result. If after replacing the flaps the papillae do not abut (a), it may be necessary to scallop the facial gingival tissue to create a longer interdental papilla (b). If conditions permit, festooning of the interproximal bone may assist in flap closure (c). Care should be taken not to reduce the height of the bony walls lining the defect.

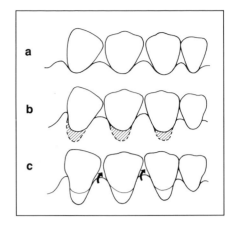

Suturing (Fig 11-12)

An interrupted or vertical matress suturing technique is used. The suture material of choice is a monofilament material.

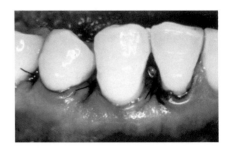

Flap adaptation (Fig 11-13)

Once sutured, firm finger pressure with gauze moistened in saline is applied to both facial and lingual flaps for 2 to 3 minutes. This will help to reduce the blood clot under the flap and aid the healing process.

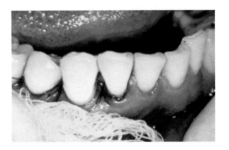

Immediate postsurgical management (Fig 11-14)

A periodontal dressing is placed to protect the wound. Written and verbal postoperative instructions are given, and a mild analgesic is prescribed. Systemic antibiotic coverage is prescribed at the discretion of the clinician. Antibiotic coverage may be important in controlling bacterial plaque and in collagen maturation. Systemic tetracycline is the drug of choice: 1.0 g per day for 10 days beginning the day before surgery.

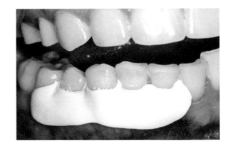

Postoperative management — First week (Fig 11-15)

The patient is seen 1 week postsurgery for suture removal. Superficial debris and bacterial plaque are gently removed. An irrigation solution such as hydrogen peroxide may be used as an adjuvant. The surgical site is dressed for an additional week.

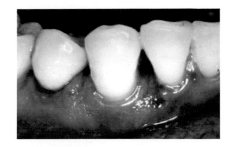

Postoperative management — Second week (Fig 11-16)

The periodontal dressing is removed and not replaced. The surgical site is inspected. Some soft tissue cratering may be evident at this time. This will resolve itself within 2 months if the patient maintains a high level of plaque control. A chlorhexidine rinse is prescribed for at least 1 month as an aid in the control of bacterial plaque.

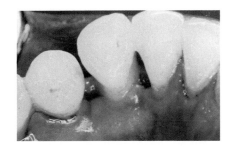

Supportive periodontal care (Fig 11-17)

The patient is placed in a periodontal program commensurate with his/ her needs for maintenance of probing depth reduction and gain in clinical attachment. The interval between supportive treatments may vary from a few weeks to several months. By 6 months the patient can usually return to the referring dentist for restorative and adjunctive care as needed.

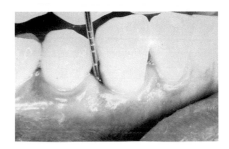

Reentry (Fig 11-18)

Reentry of the bone graft site is usually not necessary. However, surgical reentry of the graft site may be necessary for documentation purposes, to regraft (second stage procedure) a very deep lesion where complete repair was not expected, or to correct a shallow residual bone defect by osteoplasty. In the case depicted, a reentry was done for documentation purposes. There is no alveolar crestal resorption, and there is bone fill of at least 3 mm.

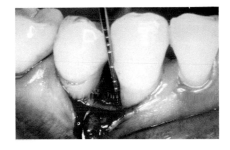

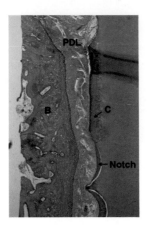

Histology after placement of a bone graft (Fig 11-19)

Regeneration of the attachment apparatus is the usual result following bone grafting. In the human histologic view shown, new bone (B), new cementum (C), and a new periodontal ligament (PDL) coronal to a notch is demonstrated 6 months after placement of a decalcified freeze-dried bone allograft. The notch was placed in calculus at the time of surgery. This indicates that the root surface coronal to the notch has lost its attachment apparatus and is contaminated by hard and soft bacterial debris. (Courtesy of Dr G.M. Bowers.)

Intraoral autogenous bone blend — Clinical results (Figs 11-20a to d)

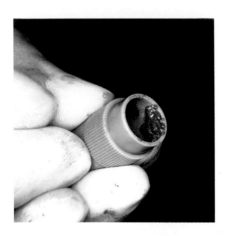

Fig 11-20a *Cortical and/or cancellous bone is collected from the surgical site, placed in a sterile amalgam capsule, and triturated for 10 seconds.*

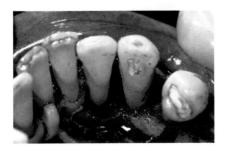
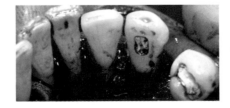
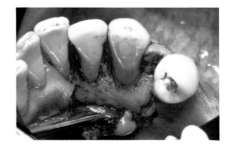

Fig 11-20b (left) *The osseous defect is debrided of all soft tissue and the root planed.*

Fig 11-20c (middle) *The bone is packed into the defect.*

Fig 11-20d (right) *Complete bone fill of the defect can be observed at a 6-month reentry. (Courtesy of Dr R.M. Zupnik.)*

Extraoral autograft — Clinical results (Figs 11-21a to c)

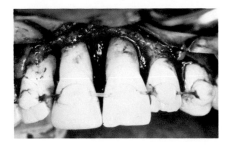 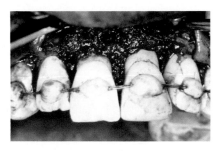 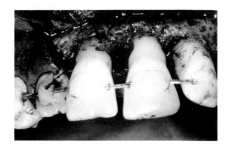

Fig 11-21a (left) *Horizontal bone loss of 7 mm as measured from the cementoenamel junction can be observed on the facial surface of the maxillary central incisors.*

Fig 11-21b (middle) *Extraoral cancellous bone and marrow autograft is placed in a supracrestal position.*

Fig 11-21c (right) *A 6-month reentry procedure demonstrates supracrestal new bone formation of greater than 4 mm. Root resorption can also be seen on the mesial and distal surfaces of these teeth. This problem may be managed by root planing and renewed efforts at plaque control. (Courtesy of Drs S. Martin and H.J. Towle.)*

Undemineralized freeze-dried bone allograft — Clinical results (Figs 11-22a to c)

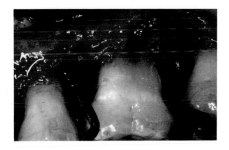 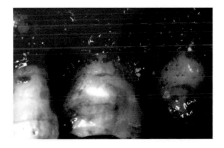 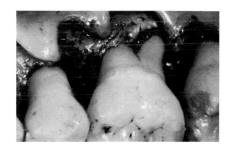

Fig 11-22a (left) *Advanced bone loss with grade II furcation involvement is evident about a maxillary first molar.*

Fig 11-22b (middle) *A composite graft of intraoral autogenous bone and freeze-dried bone allograft is inserted into the defect.*

Fig 11-22c (right) *Reconstruction of the defect as observed at a 1-year reentry. (Courtesy of Dr R.M. Zupnik.)*

Decalcified freeze-dried bone allograft compared with nongraft flap debridement surgery (Figs 11-23a to e)

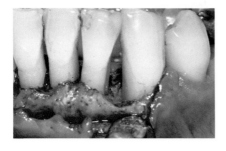 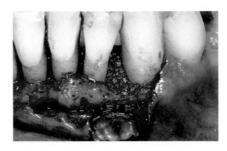 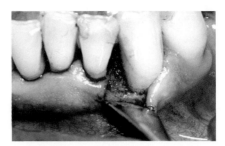

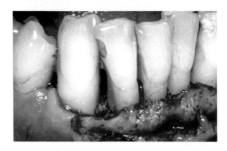

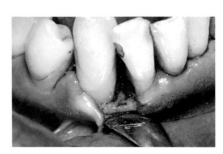

Fig 11-23a (above left) *Defect on the mesial surface of the left mandibular canine prior to graft placement.*

Fig 11-23b (above middle) *Decalcified freeze-dried bone allograft implanted into defect. An overfill approach has been used to gain crestal bone height.*

Fig 11-23c (above right) *Complete resolution of the defect and 2 mm of crestal apposition of new bone was recorded at a 6-month reentry.*

Fig 11-23d (right) *Osseous defect on the mesial surface of the right mandibular canine in the same patient.*

Fig 11-23e (bottom right) *Surgical reentry of the nongraft site at 6 months postsurgery. There is limited bone repair of the lesion.*

Synthetic graft — Clinical results (Figs 11-24a and b)

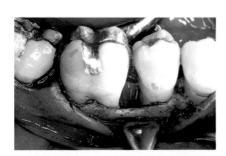

Fig 11-24a *A deep intraosseous defect with the lingual and buccal osseous walls remaining. The lesion was implanted with particulate porous hydroxyapatite and reentered at 6 months.*

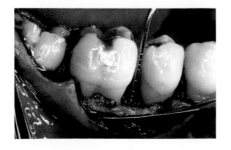

Fig 11-24b *The defect is completely filled. Particles of hydroxyapatite integrated into host bone can be noted on the surface. (Reprinted with permission from Bowen JA, Mellonig JT, Gray JL, Towle HT: Comparison of decalcified freeze-dried bone allograft and porous particulate hydroxyapatite in human periodontal osseous defects. J Periodontol 1989;60:647.)*

Histology after placement of a synthetic bone graft
(Fig 11-25)

The expected result of grafting with a synthetic bone graft material is full of the osseous defect, not regeneration. Healing is by a long junctional epithelium. The hydroxyapatite particles (HA) are well tolerated and surrounded by connective tissue (CT).

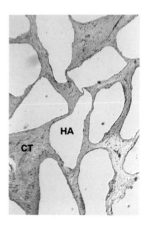

Guided tissue regeneration procedure (Figs 11-26a to e)

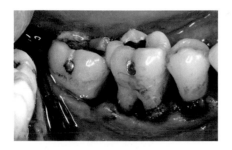
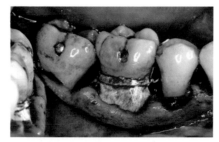
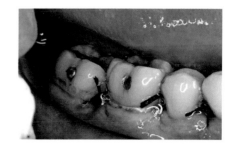
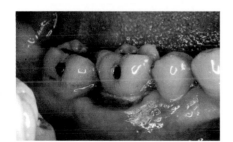
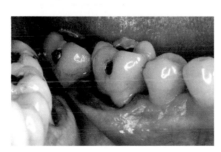

Fig 11-26a (top left) *The mandibular first molar has a grade II furcation involvement on the buccal surface. Granulation is removed from the lesion and the root surfaces are planed.*

Fig 11-26b (top middle) *An expanded polytetrafluroethylene membrane is sutured tightly to the tooth. The membrane is designed to exclude epithelium and gingival connective tissue from contacting the root surface and give preference to healing from the periodontal ligament space.*

Fig 11-26c (top right) *The flap is sutured to entirely cover the membrane.*

Fig 11-26d (bottom left) *The membrane is removed 4 to 6 weeks after it was placed.*

Fig 11-26e (bottom middle) *Dense connective tissue with a rubberlike consistency can be noted slightly above the gingival margin. This tissue is resistant to penetration by a periodontal probe.*

Guided tissue regeneration — Clinical results
(Figs 11-27a to c)

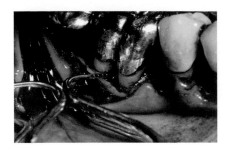
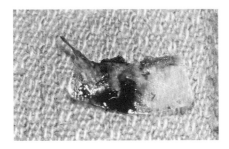
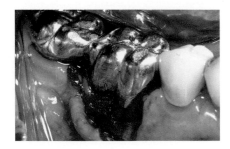

Fig 11-27a (left) *A deep grade II furcation invasion on the facial surface of the mandibular first molar can be observed.*

Fig 11-27b (middle) *The appearance of the periodontal membrane just after its removal 4 weeks postsurgery.*

Fig 11-27c (right) *Dense connective tissue firmly attached to the root surface now occupies the furcation.*

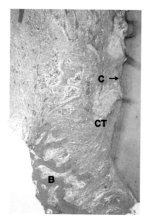

Histology of the guided tissue regeneration procedure
(Fig 11-28)
New cementum (C) with inserting connective tissue fibers (CT) is the expected result following the guided tissue regeneration procedure. Limited amounts of new bone formation (B) may or may not be present. (Courtesy of Dr William Becker.)

QUICK REVIEW   SEVERE CHRONIC ADULT PERIODONTITIS

I. Bone grafts
- Intraoral autografts have been shown to be effective in the treatment of intraosseous defects but are less successful in correction of crestal and furcation lesions.
- Extraoral autografts have been shown to be effective in management of intraosseous, supracrestal, and furcation defects.
- Freeze-dried bone allograft and freeze-dried plus autogenous bone have some indication as regenerative materials but have been supplanted by demineralized freeze-dried bone allograft due to its high osteogenic potential.
- There is clinical and histological evidence that implantation of demineralized freeze-dried bone allograft can result in regeneration in intraosseous defects.

II. Bone substitutes
- Bone substitutes or alloplasts are inert graft materials. Beta tricalcium phosphate and hydroxyapatite are the alloplasts used most often. Beta tricalcium phosphate is resorbable; placement of this material into a periodontal osseous defect results in clinical fill of the defect with fibrous encapsulation of the graft particles, but periodontal structures are not restored.
- Nonporous hydroxyapatite has a similar clinical and histological result as does beta tricalcium phosphate. There is evidence that the porous type of hydroxyapatite may result in periodontal regeneration that is localized at the base of the lesion. Formation of bone within the pores and on the surface of the material has been noted but healing is mainly by a long junctional epithelium.

III. Guided tissue regeneration
- Guided tissue regeneration is based on the biological concept which states that if preference is given to the cells from the periodontal ligament during healing, regeneration of periodontal tissue will be promoted. This is accomplished by placing a physical barrier between the root surface and the gingival flap. Healing from the epithelium and gingival connective tissue is effectively blocked and healing from the periodontal ligament enhanced.
- This procedure shows efficacy for connective tissue attachment in intraosseous defects and grade II furcation invasions. Regeneration of bone is unpredictable.

REFERENCES

1. American Academy of Periodontology: *Proceedings of the World Workshop in Clinical Periodontics*. Chicago: American Academy of Periodontology; 1989:VI-24.
2. Bowers GM, Schallhorn RG, Mellonig JT: Histologic evaluation of new attachment in human intrabony defects. A literature review. *J Periodontol* 1982; 53:509.
3. Robinson RE: Osseous coagulum for bone induction. *J Periodontol* 1969; 40:503.
4. Diem CR, Bowers GM, Moffitt WC: Bone blending: A technique for osseous implants. *J Periodontol* 1972; 43:295.
5. Hiatt W, Schallhorn R: Intraoral transplants of cancellous bone and marrow in periodontal lesions. *J Periodontol* 1973;44:194.
6. Rosenberg M: Free osseous tissue autografts as a predictable procedure. *J Periodontol* 1971;42:195.
7. Froum SJ, Oritz M, Witkins RT, Thaler R, Scopp IW, Stahl SS: Osseous autografts. III. Comparison of osseous coagulum-bone blend implants with open curettage. *J Periodontol* 1976;47:287.
8. Schallhorn R, Hiatt W, Boyce W: Iliac transplants in periodontal therapy. *J Periodontol* 1970;41:566.
9. Patur B: Osseous defects: Evaluation of diagnostic and treatment methods. *J Periodontol* 1974;45:523.
10. Schallhorn RG: The use of autogenous hip marrow biopsy implants for bony crater defects. *J Periodontol* 1968; 39:145.
11. Siebert JS: Reconstructive periodontal surgery: Case report. *J Periodontol* 1970;41:113.
12. Dragoo M, Sullivan H: A clinical and histologic evaluation of autogenous iliac bone grafts in humans. Part I. Wound healing 2 to 8 months. *J Periodontol* 1973;44:599.
13. Ross S, Cohen D: The fate of a free osseous tissue autograft. A clinical and histologic case report. *Periodontics* 1968;6:145.
14. Schallhorn RG: Postoperative problems associated with iliac transplants.

J Periodontol 1972;43:3.

15. Dragoo M, Sullivan H: A clinical and histologic evaluation of autogenous iliac bone grafts in humans. II. External root resorption. *J Periodontol* 1973; 44:614.

16. Buck B, Malinin T, Brown M: Bone transplantation and human immunodeficiency virus: An estimate of risk acquired immunodeficiency syndrome (AIDS). *Clin Orthop* 1989; 240:129.

17. Buck B, Resnick L, Shah S, Malinin T: Human immunodeficiency virus cultured from bone. Implications for transplantation. *Clin Orthop* 1990; 251:249.

18. Turner D, Mellonig J: Antigenicity of freeze-dried bone allograft in periodontal osseous defects. *J Periodont Res* 1981;16:89.

19. Quattlebaum J, Mellonig J, Hensel N: Antigenicity of freeze-dried cortical bone allograft in human periodontal osseous defects. *J Periodontol* 1988; 59:394.

20. Sanders J, Sepe W, Bowers G, Koch R, Williams J, Lekas J, Mellonig J, Pelleu G, Gambill V: Clinical evaluation of freeze-dried bone allograft in periodontal osseous defects. Part III. Composite freeze-dried bone allografts with and without autogenous bone grafts. *J Periodontol* 1983;54:1.

21. Urist MR: Bone formation by autoinduction. *Science* 1965;150:893.

22. Urist MR, Strates B: Bone morphogenetic protein. *J Dent Res* 1971; 50:1392.

23. Mellonig J, Bowers G, Baily R: Comparison of bone graft materials. Part I. New bone formation with autografts and allografts determined by strontium-85. *J Periodontol* 1981;52:291.

24. Quintero G, Mellonig J, Gambill V: A six month clinical evaluation of decalcified freeze-dried bone allografts in periodontal osseous defects. *J Periodontol* 1982;53:726.

25. Mellonig JT: Decalcified freeze-dried bone allograft as an implant material in human periodontal defects. *Int J Periodont Rest Dent* 1984;4(6):40.

26. Carraro J, Sznajder N, Alonso C: Intraoral cancellous bone autografts in the treatment of infrabony pockets. *J Clin Periodontol* 1976;3:104.

27. Movin S, Borring-Moller G: Regeneration of infrabony periodontal defects in humans after implantation of allogeneic demineralized dentin. *J Clin Periodontol* 1982;9:141.

28. Renvert S, Garrett S, Schallhorn R, Egelberg J: Healing after treatment of periodontal intraosseous defects. III. Effect of osseous grafting and citric acid conditioning. *J Clin Periodontol* 1985;12:441.

29. Hiatt W, Schallhorn R, Aaronian A: The induction of new bone and cementum formation. IV. Microscopic examination of the periodontium following human bone and marrow allograft, autograft, and nongraft periodontal regenerative procedures. *J Periodontol* 1978;49:495.

30. Listgarten M, Rosenberg M: Histological study of repair following new attachment procedures in human periodontal lesions. *J Periodontol* 1979;50:333.

31. Mabry T, Yukna R, Sepe W: Freeze-dried bone allografts combined with tetracycline in the treatment of juvenile periodontitis. *J Periodontol* 1985;56:74.

32. Pearson G, Rosen S, Deporter D: Preliminary observations on the usefulness of a decalcified, freeze-dried cancellous bone allograft material in periodontal surgery. *J Periodontol* 1981;52:55.

33. Bowers G, Chadroff B, Carnevale R, Mellonig J, Corio R, Emerson J, Stevens M, Romberg E: Histologic evaluation of new human attachment apparatus formation in humans, Part I. *J Periodontol* 1989;60:664.

34. Bowers G, Chadroff B, Carnevale R, Mellonig J, Corio R, Emerson J, Stevens M, Romberg E: Histologic evaluation of new human attachment apparatus in humans, Part II. *J Periodontol* 1989;60:675.

35. Bowers G, Chadroff B, Carnevale R, Mellonig J, Corio R, Emerson J, Stevens M, Romberg E: Histologic evaluation of human new attachment apparatus in humans, Part III. *J Periodontol* 1989;60:683.

36. Froum S, Kushner L, Stahl S: Healing responses of human intraosseous lesions following the use of debridement, grafting and citric acid root treatment. I. Clinical and histologic observations six months postsurgery. *J Periodontol* 1983;54:67.

37. Baldock W, Hutchens L, McFall W, Simpson D: An evaluation of tricalcium phosphate implants in human periodontal osseous defects of two patients. *J Periodontol* 1985;56:1.

38. Froum S, Kushner L, Scopp I, Stahl S: Human clinical and histologic responses to Durapatite implants in intraosseous lesions. Case reports. *J Periodontol* 1982;53:719.

39. Yukna R, Mayer E, Amos S: 5-Year evaluation of durapatite ceramic alloplastic implants in periodontal osseous defects. *J Periodontol* 1989;60:544.

40. Kenney E, Lekovic V, Elbaz J, Kovacvic K, Carranza F, Takei H: The use of a porous hydroxylapatite implant in periodontal defects. II. Treatment of Class II furcation lesions in lower molars. *J Periodontol* 1988;59:67.

41. Stahl SS, Froum S: Histologic and clinical responses to porous hydroxylapatite implants in human periodontal defects. Three to twelve months post-implantation. *J Periodontol* 1987; 58:689.

42. Carranza F, Kenney E, Lekovic V, Tal-amante E, Valencia J, Dimitrijevic B: Histologic study of healing of human periodontal defects after placement of porous hydroxylapatite implants. *J Periodontol* 1987;58:682.

43. Karring T, Nyman S, Lindhe J: Healing following implantation of periodontitis affected roots into bone tissue. *J Clin Periodontol* 1980;7:96.

44. Karring T, Nyman S, Lindhe J, Sirirat M: Potential for root resorption during periodontal wound healing. *J Clin Periodontol* 1984;11:41.

45. Nyman S, Karring T, Lindhe J, Planten S: Healing following implantation of periodontitis affected roots into gingival connective tissue. *J Clin Periodontol* 1980;7:394.

46. Gottlow J, Nyman S, Karring T, Lindhe J: New attachment formation as the result of controlled tissue regeneration. *J Clin Periodontol* 1984;11:494.

47. Magnusson I, Nyman S, Karring T, Egelberg J: Connective tissue attachment formation following exclusion of gingival connective tissue and epithelium during healing. *J Periodont Res* 1985;20:201.

48. Isidor F, Karring T, Nyman S, Lindhe J: The significance of coronal growth of periodontal ligament tissue for new attachment formation. *J Clin Periodontol* 1986;13:145.

49. Gottlow J, Nyman S, Lindhe J, Karring T, Wennstrom J: New attachment formation in the human periodontium by guided tissue regeneration. Case reports. *J Clin Periodontol* 1986;13:604.

50. Becker W, Becker B, Berg C, Prichard J, Caffesse R, Rosenberg E: New attachment after treatment with root isolation procedures: Report for treated Class III and Class II furcations and vertical osseous defects. *Int J Periodont Rest Dent* 1988;8(3):8.

51. Pontoriero R, Lindhe J, Nyman S, Karring T, Rosenberg E, Sanavi F: Guided tissue regeneration in degree II furcation involved mandibular molars. A clinical study. *J Clin Periodontol* 1988;15:247.

52. Lekovic V, Kenney E, Kovacevic K, Carranza F: Evaluation of guided tissue regeneration in Class II furcation defects. A clinical re-entry study. *J Periodontol* 1989;60:694.

53. Nyman S, Lindhe J, Karring T, Rylander H: New attachment following surgical treatment of human periodontal disease. *J Clin Periodontol* 1982; 9:290.

54. Nyman S, Gottlow J, Lindhe J, Karring T, Wennstrom J: New attachment formation by guided tissue regeneration. *J Periodont Res* 1987;22:252.

55. Schallhorn R, McClain P: Combined osseous composite grafting, root conditioning, and guided tissue regeneration. *Int J Periodont Rest Dent* 1988;8(4):8.

Supportive Periodontal Treatment for Patients With Inflammatory Periodontal Diseases

CURRENT CONCEPTS by Thomas G. Wilson, Jr

CLINICAL APPLICATION by Thomas G. Wilson, Jr

CURRENT CONCEPTS

What is supportive periodontal treatment (SPT)?

Is SPT effective?

Do most patients comply to suggested SPT intervals?

What happens if patients do not comply?

CLINICAL APPLICATION

Chart review

Operatory and instrument infection control

Health history update

Personal conversation with the patient

Clinical data collection

Radiographic examination

Microbiologic monitoring

Personal oral hygiene review

Removal of subgingival accretions

Removal of supragingival deposits

Behavior modification

Setting SPT intervals

Length of time for the average SPT visit

Who should be responsible for SPT?

QUICK REVIEW

REFERENCES

C U R R E N T   C O N C E P T S

WHAT IS SUPPORTIVE PERIODONTAL TREATMENT (SPT)?

The phase of treatment that follows active therapy has been variously named "recall" and "maintenance"; currently, "supportive periodontal treatment (SPT)" is the preferred term.

Supportive periodontal treatment is an integral part of periodontal care. These SPT visits serve to cement the positive relation between patient and therapist started in the early stages of therapy and help to ensure that patients have the opportunity to maintain their mouths in a healthy and comfortable state for the longest possible time. The monitoring done during this stage is essential since it indicates when additional active care is needed.

This stage of therapy is also important because the average patient, over time, will go back and forth between active therapy and SPT. This is a result of the constant examination and reappraisal performed at SPT visits and is needed to control the chronic nature of periodontal diseases.

IS SPT EFFECTIVE?

For Patients With Gingivitis

There is little question that periodic professional prophylaxis is effective in controlling gingivitis in children, especially when combined with routine reinforcement of personal oral hygiene.[1-4] However, there is little evidence that SPTs for children reduce the severity of periodontal problems they experience as adults. It must therefore be concluded, at present, that to be effective in the control of inflammatory periodontal lesions, SPT must be a lifelong process.

Studies in the 1960s and early 1970s showed that periodic professional prophylaxis combined with effective personal oral hygiene in adults resulted in improved periodontal health when compared to individuals not receiving this care.[5-7]

In one study,[8] when adult patients with gingivitis were treated with scaling and root planing but their personal oral hygiene was not reinforced, their gingival condition did not improve compared to individuals receiving prophylaxes at 6-month intervals. The test group's prophylaxes were regulated by the percentage of motile rods and spirochetes seen by darkfield microscopy. At the termination of this 18-month study, both groups experienced slightly increased pocket probing depths. This study demonstrated that either oral hygiene is an important facet in controlling gingivitis or that the relative number of organisms perceived to be causative were not relevant for setting SPT intervals, or both.

For Patients With Periodontitis

Over a 6-year study period, Axelsson and Lindhe[9] reinforced oral hygiene and scheduled SPTs from four to six times per year for a group of patients with periodontitis. A control group received only an initial prophylaxis. At the end of the study the test group had better oral hygiene, less gingivitis, and a significant reduction in pocket probing depths when compared to controls.

Badersten and co-workers[10] studied a group who had received nonsurgical debridement of nonmolar teeth with 5-mm pocket probing depths or greater. Baseline measurements were taken and oral hygiene was reinforced after completion of initial active therapy. The patients were then placed on SPT. Although this therapy controlled gingivitis and initially reduced pocket probing depths, individual sites lost attachment and oral hygiene scores worsened as the study progressed.

A series of studies on choosing the appropriate therapy(ies) for patients with inflammatory periodontal diseases was started at the University of Michigan in the 1960s and continued into the 1980s. Patients were placed on a 3-month SPT interval following active therapy.[11-17] It was concluded that the majority of the patients remained stable regardless of which therapy was used as long as the patients stayed on a regular SPT interval.[18]

As a result of these and other studies, it can be said that while SPT has limitations, regular intervals of SPT can maintain the dentition of patients with periodontitis when scheduled following active therapy. The question now arises, do most patients receive regular SPT?

DO MOST PATIENTS COMPLY TO SUGGESTED SPT INTERVALS?

Studies on compliance to SPT in clinical practice are limited. One study of approximately 1,000 patients seen over an 8-year period in a private practice found that 16% showed complete compliance to suggested SPT intervals; of the remainder, almost 35% never returned for maintenance care.[19] Another study in a private periodontal practice showed that although there was a high dropout rate before SPT was even begun, those patients who did start maintenance tended to comply to suggested intervals.[20] Dropout rates in university-based studies are also available and demonstrate a range of noncompliance from 11% to 45%.[21]

From the studies available, it can be concluded that many patients do not comply completely to suggested intervals for SPT and that compliance varies from setting to setting, between patients, and by the same patient over time.

WHAT HAPPENS IF PATIENTS DO NOT COMPLY?

Tooth Loss

Untreated Sri Lankan workers receiving no dental therapy lost 0.1 to 0.3 teeth per year per person between the ages of 15 and 40.[22] Another untreated group, this one in the United States, seen in a private periodontal practice and then an average of 4 years later, had a loss of 0.61 teeth per patient per year.[23] By contrast, Hirschfeld and Wasserman[24] found loss of 0.03 teeth per patient per year in a "well-maintained" group of treated patients who stayed in an SPT program for an average of 22 years. This result was later confirmed by McFall[25] in a study of 100 patients seen in his private practice.

In another study, Wilson[26] looked retrospectively at a group of 166 SPT patients whose compliance could be followed. Complete compliers to SPT lost no teeth, while erratic compliers lost 0.06 teeth per patient per year over the 5 years of the study. This can be contrasted to patients who underwent active therapy but not SPT and lost an average of 0.22 teeth per patient per year.[27]

In all of these studies, including the untreated Sri Lankans, most teeth lost were lost by a small percentage of the population in the study. This suggests that different patients may require different levels of supportive care. Currently, no method is totally predictable for determining the need for different levels of SPT. Therefore, until such studies are available, one should err by scheduling too frequent visits as opposed to too few.

Long-term studies comparing different periodontal therapies have evaluated therapeutic outcomes in "well-maintained" patients. There are currently no studies that provide insights relative to the best therapies for erratic or noncompliant patients. Studies that would provide information on appropriate therapy and SPT for noncompliant or erratically compliant patients would be helpful.

Periodontal Status

In contrast to "well-maintained" individuals, patients in one study receiving no SPT after surgical therapy showed continued periodontal breakdown regardless of the type of surgery performed.[28]

In another work, one third of a group of postsurgical patients returned to their general dentist for SPT. The remaining two thirds received SPT by a periodontist every 2 to 3 months. Infrequent maintenance care for the first group resulted in loss of attachment, whereas the status of the patients receiving SPT from the periodontist remained stable.[29]

Kerr[30] studied a group of 44 patients treated for periodontal problems. Five years after returning to their general dentists for SPT, this group was reexamined; the author reported a relapse in 45% of the patients.

Another private practice group[27] found increased periodontal problems (compared to baseline) in patients who received active therapy but who chose not to follow through with SPT.

It can be concluded that SPT can be effective in helping the average patient to retain his / her teeth and maintain periodontal tissue stability. To be effective, patients must present for care. Unfortunately, a large percentage of patients either never enter SPT or drop out after beginning this phase of treatment. In addition, large percentages of those who present for care do so erratically, often leading to less than optimal results.

CLINICAL APPLICATION

Supportive periodontal treatment (SPT) is an important but often overlooked phase of periodontal therapy. As detailed in the previous section of this chapter, without SPT, active therapy is often doomed to fail. This is true because most periodontal problems are chronic and are closely associated with the bacterial flora often found in the oral cavity. This scenario is complicated by the fact that many dental professionals have been selected and trained to deal with an active problem (car-ies) that can be removed and the damage readily repaired, then the professional moves on to the next acute problem. To successfully deal with periodontal lesions, one must realize that these problems are chronic. Periodontal lesions are dealt with and then must be monitored and retreated when appropriate. The concept of "cure" is a transient one, since the best treated case will usually break down without adequate SPT or personal oral hygiene. Although it may be possible to truly "cure" some patients, at present no technology is available to confirm the cessation of disease. This means that frequent visits to the professional for disease monitoring and appropriate therapy are needed.

The remainder of this chapter covers the specific procedures performed at a typical SPT visit for a patient with an inflammatory periodontal disease. Since offices and patients differ widely, these suggestions should be tailored (and improved upon) for each specific situation.

CHART REVIEW

The therapist will benefit from reviewing the patient's health history and record of the previous SPT visit before the patient arrives for treatment. Any medications needed before SPT (such as antibiotic prophylaxis to reduce the chance of subacute bacterial endocarditis in a patient with a heart murmur) or any special needs (such as local anesthesia) can be determined in this manner.

OPERATORY AND INSTRUMENT INFECTION CONTROL

Providing a safe, clean environment for patient care has always been important. However, the recent rise in highly infectious viral diseases has heightened the need for these procedures. On the positive side, when infection control procedures are used, less cross contamination occurs. On the negative side, a great deal of time and material must be expended toward infection control, which has an impact on the economics of the delivery of care.

HEALTH HISTORY UPDATE

Patients can undergo significant medical and dental health changes in the few weeks between SPT visits. The questions that follow often uncover important new information for the health history. Any changes should be recorded in the patient's chart.

1. Has there been any change in your health or medications, or have you been hospitalized since your last visit?
2. Is there anything about your mouth or jaws that is of concern to you?
3. Have you had any dental work since your last visit?
4. What do you routinely do to clean your teeth?

PERSONAL CONVERSATION WITH THE PATIENT

The recent trend has been to deliver dental care rapidly to more and more patients. Professionals sometimes then fall into the trap of seeing patients as "mouths to be repaired," not people who have dental problems. Taking a few moments during each visit to get to know one another will have long-term benefits for both the therapist and the patient. Such interchanges can lead to better care and compliance for the patient and more satisfaction for the professional.

CLINICAL DATA COLLECTION

Dental and Periodontal

1. **Probing pocket depth.** This parameter has been defined as the distance from the gingival margin to the apical depth of periodontal probe tip penetration.[31] These measurements should be taken and recorded at six points around each tooth. The readings are best obtained by moving a periodontal probe through the sulcus (pocket), with the long axis of the probe parallel to the long axis of the tooth. Records are made of the midfacial and midlingual depths as well as the mesiolingual and distolingual and me-

siobuccal and distobuccal (facial) aspects of the tooth. Interproximal readings are best made not at the line angles of the tooth, but by placing the probe tip in the deepest part of the pocket (usually under the contact area) while keeping it as parallel as possible to the tooth's long axis. This parameter should be checked at each SPT visit and any changes from baseline recorded. As discussed earlier in this book (see chapter 1), the accuracy and reproducibility of this measurement depend on the diameter of the probe, on how forcefully the probe tip is introduced into the pocket, on the relative health of the tissue, and on the skill and experience of the operator. Recent advances in the Florida Probe make this machine very desirable when it becomes more cost effective for the dentist and more comfortable for the patient.[32]

2. **Gingival recession.** As long as the clinician measures pocket probing depth and not attachment levels, gingival recession must be included in routine measurements at SPT visits. This is important not only to document any continued recession, but also to provide a perspective for probing pocket depth measurements. A 3-mm probing pocket depth associated with 7 mm of recession is of more concern than the same depth where no recession is found.

3. **Disease activity.** In the foreseeable future a number of more accurate tests for disease activity should be available. At present it is helpful to assess bleeding upon probing and suppuration. These parameters are found by dragging a probe through the sulcus. A force of 25 g has been suggested as optimal to measure bleeding.[33] These data are important because they may provide information about disease activity

(see chapter 4) and therefore should be measured and recorded at each SPT visit. Suppuration can also be detected by applying coronal pressure on the gingival tissues using a football-shaped burnisher.

4. Fremitus. Movement of the teeth during function (fremitus) is simple to measure (see page 31) and has been associated with advancing disease.[34] Therefore, it should be checked, noted, and eliminated (when possible) if it is found on a tooth that has clinical signs of active periodontal breakdown.

5. Assessment of prostheses. Any prostheses, fixed or removable, should be examined at each SPT visit and repairs or replacements made when indicated.

6. Caries examination. Each tooth should be checked clinically for caries at each SPT visit. Radiographs, if available, should be reviewed.

7. Soft tissue examination. The intraoral and extraoral soft tissues should be examined for any abnormalities and the findings recorded.

In many practices an integrated record keeping system can be helpful in recording and evaluating much of the data mentioned in this section (Fig 12-1).

SPT for Implants and Peri-implant Tissues
(see chapter 21)

Fig 12-1 Entries made into a readily readable form such as this allow comparison of data from one SPT interval to the next. (Form courtesy of Perio Access, 450 Sutter, San Francisco, Calif.)

RADIOGRAPHIC EXAMINATION

Conventional parallel or right-angle radiographs, while limited to showing only gross amounts of bone loss, still provide important information, especially when several sets exposed over a number of years are available for comparison. The number of radiographs should be limited for safety reasons, but in cases of apparently active disease, a full-mouth series every 2 years with seven vertical bite-wing radiographs in intervening years is helpful in making an accurate assessment of bone stability.

MICROBIOLOGIC MONITORING

For those patients who appear to have a form of aggressive periodontitis (see chapter 6), microbiologic monitoring and antibiotic sensitivity testing can be useful. When used in these cases and combined with traditional approaches to therapy, including subgingival scaling and root planing, the appropriate antibiotic and antimicrobial therapy often yields results superior to scaling and root planing alone. When possible causal organisms remain after this therapy, periodic microbial monitoring is suggested.

PERSONAL ORAL HYGIENE REVIEW

Patients who clean their teeth well tend to keep their teeth longer than those who do not clean optimally. Therefore, personal oral hygiene is of great importance. Unfortunately, a large percentage of our patients do not brush well, much less clean between their teeth.[21] Newer electric toothbrushes offer improved results when compared with manual brushes and have been well accepted by patients. Both a multiple rotating bristle brush[35] and a single rotating tuft brush[36] have been helpful additions for those patients who do not clean well using traditional manual methods.

Most disease starts between the teeth, however, and when no interproximal gingival recession exists, patients must use dental floss. The problem remains that the average patient does not floss at all or does it incorrectly.

Most of us are looking for a single problem-free method to rid our patients of dental plaque, but this method does not exist. However, in some patients who will not comply otherwise, chlorhexidine rinses have been shown to be useful on a short-term basis.

REMOVAL OF SUBGINGIVAL ACCRETIONS

After monitoring and reinforcing personal oral hygiene, removal of subgingival accretions is the next most important step. This is technically one of the most difficult procedures performed by the dental professional. Inadequate removal of deposits by subgingival scaling and root planing will often produce a positive gingival response that may lead the inexperienced clinician to believe that the disease process has been arrested, when in fact only gingival health has been improved and bone loss continues.

Several studies[37,38] have shown that with long and diligent effort, the clinician can successfully remove subgingival tooth-borne plaque and calculus from teeth that have 3-mm probing depths using closed subgingival scaling and root planing. These same studies show that as pocket probing depths move past 5 mm, the probability of removing all subgingival accretions diminishes; this in spite of up to three quarters of an hour per tooth spent cleaning. In these deeper probing depths, surgery is often needed to provide easier access to the dental accretions and to reduce the pocket probing depths so as to facilitate access by the patient and the professional.[39]

If time for this segment of the SPT visit is short, then areas that have been deemed to have active disease should be the first to receive closed subgingival scaling and root planing. The patient should then be reappointed for removal of the remaining accretions.

REMOVAL OF SUPRAGINGIVAL DEPOSITS

It is unfortunate but true that a great deal of time that could be best spent on removing subgingival deposits is used for mechanical removal of supragingival accretions. For this reason the dental professional providing the care at the SPT visit should complete needed subgingival scaling and root planing before beginning to remove materials that have accumulated supragingivally. This may require additional visits by the patient.

BEHAVIOR MODIFICATION

Patient compliance to professional suggestions is critical to long-term success when treating inflammatory periodontal diseases. However, the average patient does not completely comply to recommendations concerning personal health. On a personal level, most people understand that compliance to suggestions made by health care providers can lengthen and enrich their lives. Still, most people find it difficult to adhere to the myriad rules needed for positive change. Why then do clinicians become agitated when patients fail to comply? Is it not more important for patients to take the time to improve their cardiovascular fitness than to floss? It is suggested that since all of us have limited time and energy to devote to personal health, the professional be realistic when placing demands on patients.

We can also assume that the average patient will not make sweeping behavioral changes, especially in the long term. This is not to say that we will never be able to turn a noncomplier into a complete complier, only that these victories will be few and far between. Since we deal with chronic diseases for the most part, we must take these facts into consideration during all phases of dental therapy. Expecting a patient with a past history of noncompliance to suggested oral hygiene and SPT to respond well to procedures that require compliance is illogical. Therapy should be based on facilitating compliance, not making it more difficult.

It is possible to improve patient compliance to some degree in almost every case using accepted practices for behavior modification. This discussion, while very important, is beyond the scope of this text; appropriate techniques are described elsewhere.[40,41]

SETTING SPT INTERVALS

Traditionally, 6 months was the interval most often suggested between SPT visits. A few periodontal patients do well with this interval, but most seem to require more frequent care. At present, the average suggested time between SPTs for patients with inflammatory periodontal problems is every 3 months[42]; however, this interval must often be varied. The correct time between visits should be based on disease activity, not on the calendar.

LENGTH OF TIME FOR THE AVERAGE SPT VISIT

The average SPT visit for a patient with inflammatory periodontal disease requires about an hour.[43] This is only the average; many patients may require a longer time for completion of required SPT.

WHO SHOULD BE RESPONSIBLE FOR SPT?

The 1989 World Workshop in Clinical Periodontics[44] advised that gingivitis and early (Class I and II) forms of periodontitis be treated in the general practitioner's office, but the more advanced the disease, the more the case should be the periodontist's responsibility. Using the diagnoses established earlier in chapter 5, the author suggests the following modifications to the ideas of the World Workshop:

1. Patients with a form of chronic gingivitis or chronic periodontitis (Classes I and II) should be the primary responsibility of the general dentist.
2. Other forms of gingivitis should be treated and maintained by the periodontist.
3. Those patients with moderate chronic periodontitis (Class III) usually do well by alternating between the general dentist's and periodontist's office.
4. Severe chronic periodontitis patients should have their SPT at the periodontist's office.
5. While patients with aggressive forms of periodontitis should be seen by the periodontist for SPT, it is important for these patients to have periodic restorative checks by their general dentist.

<table>
<tr><td>

QUICK REVIEW

I. Current concepts
- "Supportive periodontal treatment (SPT)" has replaced "maintenance" and "recall" as the preferred term for the phase of treatment that follows active periodontal therapy.
- Patients who adhere to suggested SPT intervals have healthier dentitions and less progression of periodontal destruction than those who do not comply.
- A large percentage of patients do not comply or comply erratically to suggested SPT.
- The fate of the average noncomplier or the erratic complier is greater tooth loss and more periodontal destruction than found in patients who do comply to suggested SPT.

II. Clinical application
- Supportive periodontal treatment is an integral part of periodontal therapy.
- The following is an outline of a typical SPT visit:
  1. Review the chart before the patient arrives
  2. Provide a clean environment for therapy
  3. Update the health history
  4. Talk with the patient
  5. Collect the following clinical data at each SPT visit

</td><td>

SUPPORTIVE PERIODONTAL TREATMENT

- probing pocket depth
- gingival recession
- information on disease activity
- fremitus
- prosthesis and caries assessment
- soft tissue examination

6. A full-mouth series of radiographs should be taken at least every 2 years for patients with active periodontal problems.
- Periodic microbiologic monitoring is often needed for patients with aggressive periodontal problems.
- Where appropriate, personal oral hygiene should be reviewed and modified.
- Removal of subgingival accretions is more critical than removal of supragingival accretions.
- Supragingival deposits should be removed as time allows.
- Noncompliers or erratic compliers to suggested oral hygiene or SPT often can benefit from behavior modification.
- SPT intervals should be set by disease activity, not the calendar.
- The average SPT visit takes about 1 hour.
- The more advanced or aggressive the disease, the more SPT should be the responsibility of the periodontist.

</td></tr>
</table>

REFERENCES

1. Badenstern A, Egelberg J, Koch G: Effects of monthly prophylaxis on caries and gingivitis in school children. *Community Dent Oral Epidemiol* 1975;3:1.
2. Poulsen S, Agerbaek N, Melsen B, Konts D, Glavind L, Roolla G: The effect of professional tooth cleansing on gingivitis and dental caries in children after 1 year. *Community Dent Oral Epidemiol* 1976;4:195.
3. Axelsson P, Lindhe J: Effect of oral hygiene instruction and professional toothcleaning on caries and gingivitis in schoolchildren. *Community Dent Oral Epidemiol* 1981;9:251.
4. Bellini H, Campi R, Denardi J: Four years of monthly professional tooth cleaning and topical fluoride application in Brazilian school children.1. Effects on gingivitis. *J Clin Periodontol* 1981;8:231.
5. Lövdal A, Arno A, Schei O, Waerhaug J: Combined effect of subgingival scaling and controlled oral hygiene on the incidence of gingivitis. *Acta Odontol Scand* 1961;19:537-555.
6. Suomi JD, Greene JC, Vermillion JR, Chang JJ, Leatherwood EC: The effect of controlled oral hygiene procedures on the progression of periodontal disease in adults. Results after two years. *J Periodontol* 1969;40:416.
7. Suomi JD, Greene JC, Vermillion JR, Doyle J, Chang JJ, Leatherwood EC: The effect of controlled oral hygiene procedures on the progression of periodontal disease in adults: Results after third and final year. *J Periodontol* 1971;42:152-160.
8. Listgarten MA, Schifter C: Differential darkfield microscopy of subgingival bacteria as an aid in selecting recall intervals: Results after 18 months. *J Clin Periodontol* 1982;9:305.
9. Axelsson P, Lindhe J: Effect of controlled oral hygiene procedures on caries and periodontal disease in

adults. Results after 6 years. *J Clin Periodontol* 1981;8:239-248.

10. Badersten A, Nilvéus R, Egelberg EJ: Effect of nonsurgical periodontal therapy. I. Moderately advanced periodontitis. *J Clin Periodontol* 1981;8:57-72.

11. Ramfjord SP, Nissle RR, Shick RA, et al: Subgingival curettage versus surgical elimination of periodontal pockets. *J Periodontol* 1968;39:167.

12. Ramfjord SP, Knowles JW, Nissle RR, Shick RA, Burgett FG: Longitudinal study of periodontal therapy. *J Periodontol* 1973;44:66-77.

13. Ramfjord SP, Knowles JW, Nissle RR, Burgett FG, Shick RA: Results following three modalities of periodontal therapy. *J Periodontol* 1975;46:522.

14. Knowles JW, Burgett FG, Nissle RR, Shick RA, Morrison EC, Ramfjord SP: Results of periodontal treatment related to pocket depth and attachment level. Eight years. *J Periodontol* 1979;50:225-233.

15. Knowles JW, Burgett FG, Morrison EC, Nissle RR, Ramfjord SP: Comparison of results following three modalities of periodontal therapy related to tooth type and initial pocket depth. *J Clin Periodontol* 1980;7:32.

16. Ramfjord SP, Morrison EC, Burgett FG, Nissle RR, Schick RA, Zann GJ, Knowles JW: Oral hygiene and maintenance of periodontal support. *J Periodontol* 1982;53:26-30.

17. Morrison EC, Ramfjord SP, Burgett FG, Nissle RR, Shick RA: The significance of gingivitis during the maintenance phase of periodontal treatment. *J Periodontol* 1982;53:31.

18. Shick RA: Maintenance phase of periodontal therapy. *J Periodontol* 1981;52:576.

19. Wilson TG, Glover ME, Schoen J, Baus C, Jacobs T: Compliance with maintenance therapy in a private periodontal practice. *J Periodontol* 1984;55:468.

20. Schmidt JK: *Patient compliance with suggested maintenance recall in a private periodontal practice.* Master's Thesis, University of Michigan, 1990.

21. Wilson TG: Compliance. A review of the literature with possible applications to periodontics. *J Periodontol* 1987;58:706.

22. Löe H, Anerud A, Boysen H, Smith M: The natural history of periodontal disease in man. Tooth mortality rates before 40 years of age. *J Periodont Res* 1978;13:563.

23. Becker W, Berg L, Becker BE: Untreated periodontal disease: A longitudinal study. *J Periodontol* 1979;50:234.

24. Hirschfeld L, Wasserman B: A long-term survey of tooth loss in 600 treated periodontal patients. *J Periodontol* 1978;49:225.

25. McFall WT Jr: Tooth loss in 100 treated patients with periodontal disease. A long-term study. *J Periodontol* 1982;53:539.

26. Wilson TG, Glover ME, Malik AK, Schoen JA, Dorsett D: Tooth loss in maintenance patients in a private periodontal practice. *J Periodontol* 1987;58:231.

27. Becker W, Becker BE, Berg LE: Periodontal treatment without maintenance. A retrospective study in 44 patients. *J Periodontol* 1984;55:505.

28. Nyman S, Lindhe J, Rosling B: Periodontal surgery in plaque-infected dentitions. *J Clin Periodontol* 1977;4:240-249.

29. Axelsson P, Lindhe J: The significance of maintenance care in the treatment of periodontal disease. *J Clin Periodontol* 1981;8:281-294.

30. Kerr NW: Treatment of chronic periodontitis. 45% failure rate after 5 years. *Br Dent J* 1981;150:222.

31. Caton J: Periodontal diagnosis and diagnostic aids. In: *Proceedings of the World Workshop in Clinical Periodontics.* Chicago: American Academy of Periodontology; 1989:I-1 to I-6.

32. Gibbs CH, Hirschfeld JW, Lee JG, Low SB, Magnusson I, Thousand RR, Yernen P, Clark HB: Description and clinical evaluation of a new computerized periodontal probe — The Florida Probe. *J Clin Periodontol* 1988;15:137-144.

33. Proye M, Caton J, Polson A: Initial healing of periodontal pockets after a single episode of root planing monitored by controlled probing forces. *J Periodontol* 1982;53:296.

34. Pihlström BL, Anderson KA, Aeppoli D, Schaffer EM: Association between signs of trauma from occlusion and periodontitis. *J Periodontol* 1986;57:1.

35. Schifter CC, Emiling RC, Seibert JS, Yankell SL: A comparison of plaque removal effectiveness of an electric versus a manual toothbrush. *Clin Prev Dent* 1983;5:15.

36. Killoy WJ, Love JW, Love J, Fedi PF, Tira DE: The effectiveness of a counter-rotary action powered toothbrush and conventional toothbrush on plaque removal and gingival bleeding. A short term study. *J Periodontol* 1989;60:473.

37. Waerhaug J: Healing of the dento-epithelial junction following subgingival plaque control. II. As observed on extracted teeth. *J Periodontol* 1978;49:119-134.

38. Stambaugh RV, Dragoo M, Smith DM, Carasal L: The limits of subgingival scaling. *Int J Periodont Rest Dent* 1981;1(5):30-41.

39. Caffesse RG, Sweeney PL, Smith BA: Scaling and root planing with and without periodontal flap surgery. *J Clin Periodontol* 1986;13:205.

40. Merchenbaum D, Turk DC: *Facilitating Treatment Adherence.* New York: Plenum Press, 1987.

41. Haynes RB, Sackett DC: *Compliance with Therapeutic Regimens.* Baltimore: Johns Hopkins University Press, 1976.

42. American Academy of Periodontology: Consensus Report, Supportive Treatment. *Proceedings of the World Workshop in Clinical Periodontics.* Chicago: American Academy of Periodontology; 1989:II-1 to IX-25.

43. Schallhorn RG, Snider LE: Periodontal maintenance therapy. *J Am Dent Assoc* 1981;103:227.

44. American Academy of Periodontology: *Proceedings of the World Workshop in Clinical Periodontics.* Chicago: American Academy of Periodontology; 1989:II-1 to II-20.

PART III

Adjunctive Therapy, Esthetics, and Considerations for Medically Compromised Patients

Occlusal Trauma

CURRENT CONCEPTS by Raul G. Caffesse

CLINICAL APPLICATION by Thomas J. Fleszar

C U R R E N T   C O N C E P T S

DEFINITION

It is universally accepted today that inflammatory periodontal diseases are the response to the effects of bacterial plaque components.[1] However, certain factors influence the host / bacteria balance, thus accentuating the injurious effects of this bacterial load. These modifying factors may be local or systemic. Among the local factors, tooth malposition, overhanging margins of restorations, caries, and mouth breathing are examples.

Occlusal trauma may also fall in this category. It is defined as an injury to the attachment apparatus as a result of occlusal forces.[2] It may affect the supporting tissues of the teeth (periodontal ligament, bone, and cementum), and will manifest itself with increasing mobility and / or migration of the teeth and pain to percussion or upon biting. Additionally, radiographic signs may include discontinuity of the lamina dura surrounding the tooth roots, and the presence of a widened periodontal space.[3]

THE ROLE OF OCCLUSAL INTERFERENCES AND BRUXISM IN THE ETIOLOGY OF OCCLUSAL TRAUMA

Tooth malposition or occlusal discrepancies are almost universally present, unless the occlusion has to be treated. However, they do not necessarily produce signs or symptoms of occlusal trauma since adaptation is the rule.[4] Adaptation to interferences is dependent upon the level of psychic tension or stress to which the individual is subjected. Consequently, the functional impact of an occlusal discrepancy cannot be predicted and could change over time. An overloaded tooth may adapt to the excessive force by having increased, but not increasing, mobility or by moving away from the excessive force (migration). Under stress, however, the effect of an occlusal discrepancy may become significant enough to overcome adaptation, and thus become a traumatic interference.

The interplay between stress

and occlusal interferences may trigger the production of *bruxism*. Bruxism can be defined as any nonfunctional tooth contact, either continuous or intermittent. It is the first manifestation of lack of adaptation to occlusal relationships, but, once again, its true detrimental role depends on the degree of adaptation of the particular individual. If well adapted, teeth may depict wear facets, minimal increased mobility, and, radiographically, a well-defined periodontal support. This represents hyperfunction. If adaptation is overridden, this parafunctional habit may trigger symptomatology, and an occlusal dysfunction develops. Injury may affect any of the components of the masticatory system (ie, muscles, temporomandibular joints, or supporting structures of the teeth). When the latter happens, the lesion of occlusal trauma is present.

In summary, it can be stated that occlusal trauma will develop as a consequence of a lack of adaptation to the forces acting upon the teeth. It will be generally mediated by the production of bruxism because of the presence of occlusal interference and tension.

CLASSIFICATION OF OCCLUSAL TRAUMA

Occlusal trauma can be classified as primary and secondary.[2] **Primary occlusal trauma** is defined as an injury resulting from excessive occlusal forces acting upon a tooth or teeth with an adequate support.

Secondary occlusal trauma may result from the effect of normal occlusal forces causing an injury to the attachment apparatus of a tooth or teeth with reduced periodontal support. Consequently, the greater the amount

of periodontal support lost due to periodontitis, the more important the occlusion becomes.

THE LESION OF OCCLUSAL TRAUMA

Occlusal trauma affects the supporting mechanism of the tooth. The lesion involves the periodontal ligament, bone, and cementum. Basically, the connective tissue of the periodontal ligament depicts an inflammatory response with vascular dilation, increased vascular permeability, infiltration of the connective tissue, hyaline degeneration of the collagen fibers, and necrosis. Bone resorption (frontal, but also undermining), as well as cementum resorption, is associated with the aseptic inflammatory response seen in the periodontal ligament. The result is a widened, funnel-shaped periodontal space in which the fibers have lost their normal functional orientation.[4-7]

The lesion of occlusal trauma is reversible once adaptation is reached or the forces subside. The only sequela may be self-limited mobility.[8]

OCCLUSAL TRAUMA AND PERIODONTAL BREAKDOWN

Several studies have tried to elucidate the role of occlusal trauma in the initiation and progression of periodontal breakdown, as well as its effect upon the therapeutic response.

Initiation of Disease

It has been shown conclusively that occlusal trauma is not capable of initiating marginal inflammation or pocket formation in the ab-

sence of bacterial plaque, nor will it aggravate gingivitis.[5]

Progression of Disease

Although occlusal trauma will not affect the progression of gingivitis into periodontitis, excessive forces associated with preexisting periodontitis may increase the rate of spread of inflammation into deeper structures. It is conceivable that the presence of the inflammatory infiltrate curtails the possibilities for adaptation to the excessive forces. Several animal studies where jiggling forces were established support this concept.[9-11] It has also been found that more severe bone loss may take place, although it may not be accompanied by increased connective tissue attachment loss.[12,13] Rarely do intrabony pockets develop. Clinically, and only in cases where jiggling forces do not allow for adaptation or migration of the tooth, an increased rate of destruction and the possibilities of intrabony defects occur.

It needs to be stressed that not every intrabony pocket is the result of trauma superimposed on inflammation. Other factors, such as the anatomy of the area, the pattern of vascularization, or the presence of food impaction, may also contribute to the development of intrabony pockets.[3]

Therapeutic Response

In dogs in which both occlusal trauma and periodontitis were present, it was found that removal of the excessive forces had no effect in the periodontal healing achieved, or in the maintenance of the attachment levels. Only an increased mobility persisted on those teeth still subjected to the jiggling forces. The elimination of the inflammatory response made it possible for adaptation to be achieved.[14,15] In studies performed using the squirrel monkey as a model, it was found that after cessation of occlusal trauma, bone regeneration will occur in the absence of marginal periodontitis but not when periodontitis is present. Furthermore, if both factors are treated, bone regeneration without gain in connective tissue attachment will result.[13,16]

Considering that mobility is the main clinical sign of occlusal trauma (with the limitations discussed above), several studies have tried to evaluate the effect of mobility on periodontal healing. Earlier studies reported no effect of mobility upon periodontal healing,[17-20] a concept that was also supported by histologic evidence.[21] Recently, however, reports have suggested the beneficial effects of reduced tooth mobility on posttreatment clinical gains of attachment. Fleszar et al[22] published long-term results of several modalities of periodontal therapy related to the degree of tooth mobility prior to therapy. The results indicated that the initial gain in clinical attachment levels was inversely related to the degree of mobility. The less the mobility, the more favorable the posttreatment gain in clinical attachment. These results were seen for all original probing depths and all therapeutic modalities.

More recently, another report[23] evaluated the effects of occlusal adjustment in a population of 50 periodontitis patients with the diagnosis of occlusal trauma, treated with modified Widman flap and scaling and root planing. Two year results of this randomized trial demonstrated significantly greater gain in clinical periodontal attachment in patients who received occlusal adjustment. Conversely, compared to those patients in whom occlusal adjustment was not performed, no effect

fects on probing depth reductions were seen.

These results seem to indicate that periodontal healing may be more advantageous in nonmobile than in mobile teeth.[24] Thus, it seems reasonable to support the role of occlusal therapy in the treatment of certain patients suffering with periodontal diseases where occlusal trauma could be diagnosed. The information available is still controversial, however. Different models and experimental designs may explain the different results reported. The role that occlusal trauma plays in the pathogenesis of periodontal diseases may vary among animal species, and also between animals and humans.[25]

OCCLUSAL FACTORS

Several occlusal factors may be related to periodontal breakdown and its therapy, although not directly associated with the lesion of occlusal trauma.

Malocclusion

The role malocclusion plays in periodontics has represented a controversial issue for many years. Although some epidemiological reports[26-28] indicate a certain degree of relationship between various types of malocclusions and gingivitis, other studies[29-38] failed to find any relationship between malocclusion and periodontal health.

If, however, a malocclusion is diagnosed as being responsible for the lesion of occlusal trauma, its correction is indicated. Only those malocclusions conducive to the establishment of jiggling forces that are not adapted to have a great potential to cause occlusal trauma.

Tooth Malposition

Tooth malposition may play the role of a secondary factor in periodontics by modifying the local environment. Malposed teeth may make plaque control a more difficult procedure. However, this may be overcome by properly educating the patient in oral hygiene procedures. Crowding of teeth is a good example of such a situation. Similarly, malposed teeth and crowding in particular may create sites of close root proximity that are highly susceptible to the effects of marginal inflammation and are poor candidates for regeneration therapy unless the proximity of the roots is corrected.

Uneven marginal ridges and open contacts have also been associated with increased marginal inflammation, although these factors seem to be less significant than once considered, according to more recent reports.[39]

Teeth in severe buccal or lingual version may be associated with very thin or nonexistent alveolar bone, with the development of fenestrations or dehiscences. This would set the stage for localized gingival recessions to develop.

Mesially tilted molars are usually associated with deep mesial periodontal pockets as a result of combined hyperplastic tissue growth and actual loss of attachment due to the modified local environment.

Habits

Certain habits produce excessive forces upon a particular tooth or group of teeth for variable periods of time.[4] These habits may involve the use of a foreign object in a particular tooth location, creating a localized defect. They may include, but are not limited to, biting objects such as pens and pencils, using the teeth to open hairpins, and nail biting. Soft tissue habits, such as tongue thrusting or cheek and lip biting may also be responsible for such lesions (Figs 13-1a and b). Although these localized defects may be associated with the occlusion, occlusal therapy will have very limited benefit unless the habit is corrected.

Soft Tissue Trauma

Impinging overbite is the typical example of gingival trauma of occlusal origin. It may produce significant destruction of the marginal gingiva by direct contact of the opposing dentition with loss of attachment by stripping off the gingiva. The deleterious effects of an impinging overbite will be seen particularly when in association with a collapsed posterior dentition.

Food impaction, usually associated with the presence of plunger cusps, could also be responsible for the development of a localized area of periodontal breakdown.[40]

INDICATIONS FOR OCCLUSAL THERAPY

The need for occlusal therapy as part of periodontal treatment is still a matter of controversy. Undoubtedly, the main objective of periodontal therapy must be to control the bacterial infection and maintain the existing support, and secondly, if possible, to restore lost attachment. The need to include occlusal therapy as part of the treatment varies according to different clinicians. Its inclusion is mainly based on clinical beliefs more than scientific evidence. Clinical research results have indicated that the only treatment required was the control of the in-

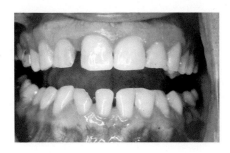

Fig 13-1a *A 23-year-old woman complained about migration of teeth and diastemata between right central and lateral incisors in both arches that developed during a 1-year period and were increasing over time.*

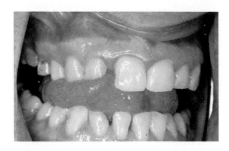

Fig 13-1b *The patient had a tongue habit, which placed significant forces on the teeth and produced the migration and diastemata.*

flammatory marginal periodontitis by means of conventional therapy.[13,14] However, clinical reports from two Michigan longitudinal studies point to the beneficial effects of treating the occlusion when indicated.[22,23] In essence, in a comprehensive periodontal treatment plan, all aspects of the diagnosis must be addressed. Consequently, if the diagnosis of occlusal trauma has been established, its therapy is indicated. This means that a functional evaluation of the occlusion is required in order to make the proper diagnosis. It has been stated that one of the reasons for the present controversy is the inability to develop criteria to identify the lesion of occlusal trauma.[25]

The objective of therapy should be to obtain occlusal stability and optimal function and reduce tooth mobility, which should not interfere with normal function.[41]

Occlusal therapy also can be indicated when factors such as food impaction, tooth crowding that interferes with plaque control, or root approximation precluding proper response to therapy are

encountered. In these instances, the objective of the occlusal therapy will be to facilitate proper periodontal treatment and maintenance.

In instances where teeth have migrated as a consequence of periodontal disease or previous extractions, occlusal therapy may also be applied to improve tooth positioning, achieve stability, and facilitate reconstruction.

Contrary to what was once proposed,[42] it is agreed today that no prophylactic treatment of the occlusion should be instituted.[2,25] It is advisable to introduce reversible treatment approaches whenever possible or when in doubt. The control of bruxism fits this category.

THERAPEUTIC APPROACHES

Depending on the situation, one or more techniques can be applied to the treatment of the occlusal needs of a patient. The goal of therapy should be optimal function and stability.

Occlusal Adjustment/ Selective Grinding

Occlusal adjustment is defined as "reshaping the occlusal surfaces of teeth by grinding to create harmonious contact relationships between the upper and lower teeth."[43] The World Workshop in Clinical Periodontics found agreement in the following indications[2]: *(1)* to reduce traumatic forces to teeth exhibiting increasing mobility or discomfort during function; *(2)* to achieve functional relationships and efficiency associated with restorative treatment, orthodontics, orthognathic surgery, or jaw trauma when indicated; *(3)* as adjunctive therapy that may reduce the damage from habits; *(4)* to reshape teeth that produce soft tissue trauma; and *(5)* to adjust marginal ridge relationships and cusps that contribute to food impaction.

Generally, occlusal adjustment should be performed, when indicated, after marginal inflammation has been controlled by scaling and root planing. However, this sequence may be changed if circumstances indicate the initial need for occlusal adjustment.

Occlusal Bite Plane Splints

Stabilization occlusal splints covering the occlusal and incisal surfaces of one arch (usually the maxillary) are used to control occlusal trauma during periodontal therapy. They provide stabilization of teeth, ideal occlusal relationships, and axial distribution of forces. This type of splint represents a noninvasive reversible approach that can be easily adjusted (Fig 13-2).[4]

Occlusal splints may represent the only treatment needed to control bruxism in periodontal patients, with the added advantage

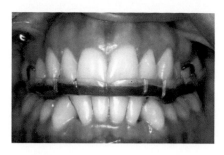

Fig 13-2 *Maxillary occlusal bite splint used as a noninvasive reversible method to control excessive forces acting on the teeth. A completely flat occlusal surface provides even contacts in centric throughout the arches, while the incorporation of a canine guidance design allows for smooth working and protrusive movements with minimal contacts and elimination of balancing interferences.*

that the occlusal surface of the teeth will be protected from excessive wear.

Patients treated for advanced periodontitis may be provided with an occlusal splint at the completion of active therapy, to control the effects occlusal factors may have upon a reduced periodontium.

Orthodontics

Adult orthodontics has become an integral part of the treatment of many patients with periodontitis (Figs 13-3a to e). Fixed or removable appliances can be used to produce minor tooth movements or comprehensive treatment in adults with the objective of improving stability, function, and also esthetics.[44]

The World Workshop in Clinical Periodontics[2] recognized the following indications for orthodontic treatment in periodontics: *(1)* to facilitate occlusal and restorative treatment; *(2)* to aid in the treatment of gingival and osseous defects; *(3)* for forced tooth exception for crown lengthening; *(4)* to improve plaque control by the correction of crowded or malposed teeth; *(5)* to correct root proximity problems; *(6)* to correct food impaction by closing open contacts that fail to close following reduction of inflammation and/or occlusal adjustment; *(7)* to treat gingival impingement caused by severe overbite; *(8)* to help to create a lip seal in patients with gingivitis aggravated by mouth breathing; *(9)* to correct flared and/or mobile teeth associated with a tongue thrusting habit (improper swallowing pattern); and *(10)* for forced eruption of unerupted teeth.

Orthodontic movement should be performed only after tissue inflammation has been controlled by scaling and root planing. However, since gingival and bony morphologies may be modified by orthodontic therapy, periodontal surgery should be delayed until after completion of orthodontics.[45] There is general agreement that orthodontic treatment, when properly performed with close monitoring and light forces applied, causes no detrimental effects to the periodontium.[46-49]

Several studies have also documented the beneficial effects of specific orthodontic procedures on the periodontal tissues, such as molar uprighting, extrusion, and forced eruption.[50-53]

Restorative Dentistry

Restorative dentistry becomes a key factor in periodontal treatment planning when teeth need to be replaced or treated teeth need permanent splinting for stabilization. Any restoration should provide a stable occlusion, promote periodontal health, and permit adequate professional and pa-

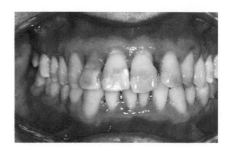

Fig 13-3a *A 38-year-old man had generalized moderate to advanced periodontitis. His concern was the labial rotation of the maxillary left central incisor. Significant amount of plaque and calculus has accumulated throughout the mouth, and the gingival tissues exhibit the expected inflammatory response. Probing depths ranged from 4 to 8 mm, with clinical loss of attachment of 4 to 10 mm.*

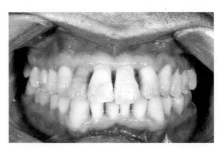

Fig 13-3b *Response of the tissues after the hygiene phase of therapy was completed. It included patient education, oral hygiene instruction, and scaling and root planing. At reevaluation, inflammation was controlled with no bleeding present.*

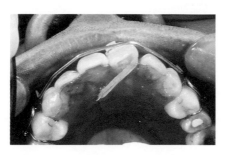

Fig 13-3c *A modified Hawley appliance was fabricated with a special hook placed on the palate. A plastic bracket was acid etched to the labial surface of the rotated incisor. Observe the orthodontic rubber band anchored to the bracket and the palatal hook.*

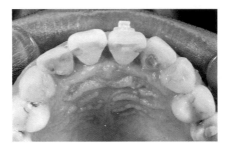

Fig 13-3d *Four months later the rotation of the maxillary left central incisor has been completed. Notice the alignment achieved. The clinical health of the periodontal tissues has been maintained.*

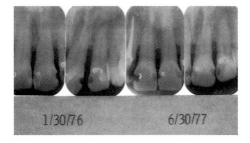

Fig 13-3e *Radiographs of the maxillary anterior sextant, showing improvement of the periodontal support after periodontal therapy and minor tooth movement. Followup radiographs taken 18 months after initiation of treatment.*

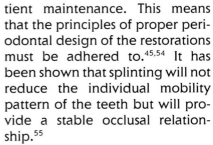

tient maintenance. This means that the principles of proper periodontal design of the restorations must be adhered to.[45,54] It has been shown that splinting will not reduce the individual mobility pattern of the teeth but will provide a stable occlusal relationship.[55]

Although it is not routinely used, temporary splinting may be required to achieve stabilization of a tooth or teeth during treatment. Different types of temporary splints may be used depending on the circumstances (eg, amalgam splints, A-splints, acid-etched composite resin splints, etc). Whenever possible, extracoronal splints should be used because they do not commit the case to a permanent restoration.

In certain patients with occlusal trauma, splinting may represent the only approach to treatment that will allow achievement of functional stability and comfort. The World Workshop in Clinical Periodontics[2] has accepted the following indications for this therapy: *(1)* to stabilize teeth with in-creasing mobility that have not responded to occlusal adjustment and periodontal treatment; *(2)* to stabilize teeth with advanced mobility that have not responded to occlusal adjustment and periodontal therapy when there is interference with normal function and patient comfort; *(3)* to facilitate treatment of extremely mobile teeth by splinting them prior to periodontal instrumentation and occlusal adjustment procedures; *(4)* to prevent tipping or drifting of teeth and the extrusion of unopposed teeth; *(5)* to stabilize teeth, when indicated, following orthodontic movement; *(6)* to create adequate occlusal stability when replacing missing teeth; *(7)* to splint teeth so that a root can be removed and the crown retained in its place; and *(8)* to stabilize teeth following acute trauma.

GOAL OF OCCLUSAL THERAPY

Irrespective of the treatment approach followed, when occlusal trauma needs to be corrected, the overall goal of therapy must be the achievement of an optimal functional occlusion with stable tooth relationships, where comfort, function, and esthetics are restored, protected, and maintained.

CLINICAL APPLICATION

INTRODUCTION

For years, researchers and practitioners have struggled with occlusal trauma and cofactor destruction[56,57] in periodontal patients. Because both are dynamic and potentially harmful, experimental design for verification and quantification has been difficult. However, as in most fields, progress has been made.

The reaction of periodontal tissues to traumatic forces initiated by the occlusion is understood. When unilateral forces are exerted on teeth, tension and pressure zones develop within the periodontium corresponding directly to areas of bone apposition and destruction. This is the biologic phenomenon that allows the orthodontic movement of teeth. With the exception of orthodontics, however, such unilateral trauma is rare in humans. More common are occlusal forces that act alternately in one then the opposite direction. Such forces have been termed "jiggling" forces.[7] In this type of trauma no clear cut tension and pressure zones can be identified, rather, areas that exhibit a combination of the two exist on both sides of the affected tooth. Microscopically, these combination areas appear remarkably similar to the pressure zone seen in conjunction with orthodontically moved teeth. Tissue destruction is evident. Ultimately, the destruction ceases as the traumatic forces are compensated for. The tooth is left with increased clinical mobility and a radiographically widened periodontal membrane space. Adaptation occurs without any attachment loss.[58]

The scenario changes when periodontitis is introduced to the "jiggling" model. In a series of experiments during the 1970s and early 1980s, Swedish scientists succeeded in demonstrating cofactor destruction.[5,8,9,11,14,15,59-63] The coexistence of occlusal trauma and periodontitis was shown to accelerate attachment loss during periods of increased tooth mobility.[9,62,63]

The adaptive capacity of the periodontium and the episodic nature of periodontitis ensure that most periods of active interaction are likely transient. Only when mobility steadily increases should the effect be sustained. This has been viewed as justification for focusing treatment on the plaque-induced lesion rather than on occlusal trauma.[58] The presumption is reasonable. Resolution of periodontal inflammation will halt attachment loss.[19,64] However, clinicians have long suspected that the presence of occlusal trauma impairs or inhibits this healing.[65-67] Recent studies seem to be confirming these suspicions.[22,23] Occlusal adjustments improved the therapeutic results when occlusal trauma was diagnosed.[23] Gains in attachment were inversely related to pretreatment mobility levels[22]; firm teeth appeared to heal better than loose teeth.[22]

Occlusal trauma, therefore, is significant not only in the progression of periodontitis, but also in its resolution. Optimum therapeutic results depend upon occlusal therapy when occlusal trauma is diagnosed. Herein lies the problem. Definitive clinical criteria for the diagnosis of occlusal trauma are still lacking. Increasing tooth mobility is extremely difficult to detect chairside. As a consequence, some clinical judgment is required for diagnosis.

To facilitate sound judgement, clinicians must integrate their understanding of the dynamic, interactive, and adaptive nature of the entire masticatory system with a detailed and comprehensive patient evaluation.

PATIENT HISTORY

Information gathering begins with the review of the patient's health questionnaire. If the following questions are included, affirmative answers will help identify existing or potential occlusal / dysfunctional problems and the impact they may have on treatment planning.

1. Do you think your teeth are drifting or changing position?

Most people are very aware of their teeth and will be able to point out immediately a tooth or group of teeth that has changed position. Often they will point to a "new" diastema or a widened preexistent one. Maxillary anterior teeth and teeth adjacent to extraction sites are those most affected. Drifting is often an indication that the periodontium is reacting to the influence of occlusal forces (Fig 13-4).

2. Are you dissatisfied with the appearance of your teeth? This provides patients with another opportunity to point out drifted teeth or "new" diastemata. An affirmative answer may also alert the clinician to the fact that the patient intends to seek corrective therapy after periodontal treatment. If occlusal trauma is diagnosed in such a patient, the approach to occlusal therapy may be altered to complement the comprehensive treatment plan.

3. Do you have any difficulty chewing? Inadequate, uncomfortable, and unstable occlusal schemes are identified with this question. It is also an opportunity to note the presence of some temporomandibular disorders.

4. Have you noticed any loose teeth? Besides identifying areas of potentially advanced periodontal destruction, a positive answer may indicate the presence of traumatic occlusal forces and / or parafunctional habits. The question also allows one to assess the patient's comfort with their occlusion. If they deny noticing any looseness and the clinical exam reveals some, then the increased mobility may be within the adaptive capacity of their periodontium.

5. Do your teeth ever feel sore when you bite on them? Similar to the question above, an affirmative answer may indicate the presence of occlusal trauma or parafunctional activity. It may in-

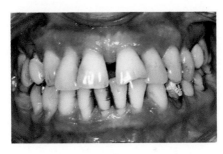

Fig 13-4 *The patient sought treatment to correct these recently widened spaces, a phenomenon that is often an indication the periodontium is reacting to occlusal forces.*

dicate a tooth fracture. Most likely, however, it will merely indicate the presence of caries or pulpal problems.

6. Do you ever have pain in the region in front of your ears? This is often an indication of a temporomandibular disorder. If confirmed and coexistent with occlusal trauma, the therapeutic approach to controlling the trauma may be altered.

7. Do your jaws click or pop when you chew? Like the preceding question, this may signal a temporomandibular disorder. It should also alert the clinician to the presence of occlusal schemes that have a high potential for generating nonaxial forces (eg, severe malocclusions or heavy balancing interferences).

8. Do you clench, grit, or grind your teeth in the daytime or while sleeping? Positive answers here definitely indicate the presence of parafunctional tooth contact and a high potential for occlusal trauma.[68-70]

9. Do you have any habits such as biting your nails, chewing a pencil or pen, etc? Similar parafunctional habits can lead to tooth movement and to traumatic injury.[71]

10. Does food wedge between any of your teeth? Specific areas of food impaction may

identify recently opened contacts or caries, or fractured or faulty restorations. Each abnormality is capable of altering occlusal harmony and function.[40]

11. Are your teeth sensitive to cold, heat, sweets, or touch? While most positive answers will relate to root exposure, some may be an indication of parafunctional activity. Increased bruxism (centric or eccentric) can cause hypersensitive teeth.

12. Have you ever had orthodontic treatment? Knowledge of this can be helpful when performing an occlusal analysis. Many postorthodontic patients have heavy balancing interferences associated with their second molars. Also, some adults may have sought orthodontic care originally to correct a developing maxillary anterior diastema.

13. Have you been under increased nervous tension lately? This alerts the clinician to increased psychic stress and to a possible initiation or exacerbation of parafunctional activities.

14. Do you have frequent headaches? Again, this is a possible sign of parafunctional activity.

15. Do you have arthritis? Arthritis may account for some temporomandibular symptomatology and may predispose to occlusal trauma due to altered occlusal function.

CLINICAL EXAMINATION

A clinical examination will enable detection of the signs and symptoms of occlusal trauma. Figure 13-5 displays a chart that may be used to record the examination findings. Locations for recording missing teeth, tooth mobility, and open contacts are not evident; this information is usually placed on a

OCCLUSAL ANALYSIS

Angles I II III ☐ Cross Bite _____

☐ Crowding/Impinging _____

☐ Slide in Centric ☐ Vert. ___ ☐ Hor. ___ ☐ R ___ ☐ L ___

☐ Cr-Co Prematurity _____

☐ Working   R _____ L _____

☐ Balancing   R _____ L _____

☐ Protrusive   R _____ L _____

☐ Fremitus   _____

☐ Bruxism   _____

☐ Adj.   ☐ Non. Adj.

Pres. Function: ☐ Adeq.   ☐ Inadeq. _____

TMJ and MUSCLES

☐ Normal

☐ Crepitation   R _____ L _____

☐ Clicking   R _____ L _____

☐ Subluxation   R _____ L _____

☐ Deviation   R _____ L _____

☐ Hypertonicity _____

☐ Hypertrophy _____

☐ Pain _____

_____

_____

TEETH

Percussion _____

Abrasion: ☐ None   ☐ Slight   ☐ Moderate   ☐ Severe

Attrition: ☐ None   ☐ Slight   ☐ Moderate   ☐ Severe

Vitality: ☐ Ice _____ ☐ Pulp tester _____

Caries _____

Other _____

PROSTHESES

Type _____   Yr. made _____

Type _____   Yr. made _____

Type _____   Yr. made _____

RADIOGRAPHIC

Lamina Dura: Discont.   ☐ Crestal _____ ☐ Lateral _____ ☐ Apical _____

Bone Resorption: ☐ Incipient ☐ Moderate ☐ Severe ☐ Furcations _____ ☐ Traumatic Defects _____

Defective Restorations: _____

Caries: _____

Periapical Radiolucency: ☐ None   ☐ _____

Effective Crown/Root Ratio: ☐ Good   ☐ Moderate   ☐ Poor

Endodontic Treatment: ☐ _____

Other _____

Fig 13-5 *This sample chart will facilitate recording the clinical signs and symptoms of occlusal trauma. Tooth mobility and the presence of diastemata can be recorded elsewhere.*

chart used for pocket depths and attachment levels.

Occlusal Analysis

In most instances a detailed occlusal analysis can be performed chairside. However, for those practitioners just developing their skills, or for particularly complex cases, use of casts mounted on a fully adjustable articulator is encouraged.

Angle's Classification/Occlusal Scheme

Most studies have failed to find a relationship between periodontal health and malocclusion,[29-38,72-77] but this does not mean that analysis is without merit. Clinically relevant information regarding occlusal trauma and its treatment can be obtained. The most obvious example is that of direct gingival trauma. Usually evidenced in impinging overbites, this condition requires corrective occlusal therapy.[4,54]

For the most part, severe malocclusions (skeletal and acquired) have the greatest potential to affect periodontal health. Discrepancies in jaw size and tooth alignment can alter masticatory function, often changing the direction of occlusal forces and increasing the occlusal load on individual teeth.

Patients with **skeletal bimaxillary protrusion** often exhibit buccal movement and drifting of the maxillary anterior teeth when suffering from moderate to advanced periodontitis. Their occlusal scheme contributes to the development of trauma, "unlimited" mobility (see page 215), and tooth migration. If drifting has occurred, these patients will require orthodontic repositioning of their teeth and some type of retainer, possibly an occlusal bite plane.

Similar findings are often observed in **dentitions missing posterior teeth.** Therapeutic stability will require reconstruction to reestablish posterior support and redirect the occlusal forces.

The **anterior open bite,** particularly if occlusal contact is limited to the molars, is another malocclusion with tremendous potential for occlusal trauma. Functional load demands usually precipitate jiggling mobility. If a tongue thrust coexists, there is also potential for maxillary and/or mandibular anterior tooth migration. An orthodontic consultation should be sought. If orthodontic therapy is declined, then an occlusal bite plane should be considered along with an occlusal adjustment to ensure the even distribution of the biting forces.

There is a rare but particularly disturbing **variation of the anterior open bite.** The anomaly is characterized by an anterior open bite that seems to progressively develop and worsen during middle age. Arthritic changes within the temporomandibular joint have been linked to this condition. However, a number of patients with this malocclusion are asymptomatic and seemingly free of joint pathology. Managing treatment for these patients is difficult. The potential for occlusal trauma is high and the changing occlusal scheme requires constant vigilance. A clinician can identify these cases by noting the presence of functional or parafunctional attrition on the incisal edges of the anterior teeth where no demonstrated tooth contact can occur. Questioning the patient about recent changes in their ability to open bags with their teeth or to eat lettuce from sandwiches will often elicit a surprised look and confirmation of their newly discovered inability to do so. In the absence of joint pathology, these patients are treated as discussed above.

Tooth migration is a red flag signaling the presence of occlusal trauma and periodontitis. The most common example is that of the migrated maxillary central incisor (Fig 13-6). It is important to identify how it developed. Was it due to an occlusal habit such as pen chewing, or was it due to the occlusion? Movement may have been due to a high occlusal contact on a new restoration or from the original occlusal scheme. Both may have been "tolerated" for a time, and for a time the tooth may have been able to adapt to these excessive forces. As the periodontitis progressed, however, adaptation was no longer possible and the tooth attempted to "escape" by moving buccally. When similar overloads occur in the posterior region and sound mesiodistal tooth contacts are present, such an escape will not be possible, and increased mobility will result.

If minimal drifting has occurred, then an occlusal adjust-

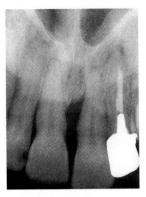

Fig 13-6 This radiograph reveals a maxillary left central incisor that has migrated. A new diastema has opened and the tooth has "dropped" incisally. This is often an indication of the presence of periodontitis and occlusal trauma.

ment may be all that is required. Removing or reducing the violating contact will allow lip pressure to return the tooth to its prior position. It may be necessary to repeat the process several times. If displacement has been more significant, minor orthodontic therapy might be needed. In either case, if protrusive bruxism was involved, an occlusal bite plane will serve to control these forces and act as a retainer.

Another approach to correcting the problem would be to consider using the bite plane as an orthodontic appliance by incorporating a Hawley wire and additional finger springs as needed. By relieving the acrylic resin on the palatal surface, the migrated tooth will have the space needed to be repositioned. Once in place, the splint can be relined, and from that point on it will serve as both a retainer and guard for bruxism.

Missing teeth are an indication of an altered occlusal scheme because the remaining teeth will have had to assume all functional demands.[69,71] If the result is functional instability, increased mobility, occlusal trauma and tooth migration are likely sequelae. All are commonly evidenced in lone standing posterior teeth. While prosthetic appliances may have been placed to prevent or correct this, they have to have been properly designed and constructed. Each should be evaluated for its compatibility with the overall occlusal scheme. If care was not taken in their placement, they can be the initiators of occlusal trauma. Abutment teeth for removable partial dentures are the all-too-frequent recipients of nonaxially directed forces.[78]

Occlusal Contact Relationships

The presence of occlusal discrepancies such as centric relation prematurities or balancing, protrusive, and working interferences does not automatically predispose occlusal trauma. The torquing or nonaxial forces generated by these tooth contacts are usually well tolerated. They become significant only when the adaptive capacity of the periodontium is exceeded, as in cofactor destruction.

Carefully analyzing these occlusal contacts will greatly aid the clinician in deciding on the best approach to occlusal therapy when trauma is diagnosed. To illustrate: occlusal trauma is most often treated by an occlusal adjustment. Since contact points from interferences or a slide in centric are capable of generating damaging forces, they ideally should be eliminated. If the clinician blindly proceeds, mutilation of the dentition might occur. In certain malocclusions, notably Class II's and particularly those with "double bites," an occlusal adjustment cannot provide stability without destroying significant amounts of tooth structure. Obviously, this is not advised. There are prudent alternatives.

Analysis also helps detect new, poorly adjusted restorations. Their presence can precipitate episodes of parafunctional activity such as bruxism that place periodontally compromised dentitions "at risk."

Tooth Mobility

When evaluating the periodontal patient, tooth mobility is arguably the most important clinical test for occlusal trauma. Like the masticatory system, tooth mobility is dynamic. The stability of a tooth is dependent upon the resistance of its supporting structures and the character of the forces directed against it.[79] When either changes, so does mobility.[56,69,71,79-83] Mobility can be classified as either physiologic[84-86] or as pathologic,[9,63,71,80,87-91] self-limited, or progressive. Each carries its own significance.

Physiologic mobility represents the range of mobility levels considered normal.

Self-limited mobility is a greater than normal, but constant, tooth mobility based on a balance between the occlusal forces and the adaptive capacity of the periodontium. "Self-limited" implies that the progression of tooth movement has been stopped without splinting or other mechanical stabilization of the teeth. The best example of this involves the mandibular incisors. The mobility of these teeth is often limited buccally and lingually by the lingual surfaces of the maxillary incisors and the tongue, respectively. This provides stability not evidenced in the maxillary incisors and enhances the prognosis even when only minimal periodontal support remains.[54]

The maxillary incisors often migrate when severely involved periodontally. As discussed earlier, certain occlusal schemes promote this drifting. Without a barrier on the buccal surfaces, these teeth experience unlimited or steadily increasing mobility.

Until recently, mobility was considered pathologic only when it was increasing.[9] New research seems to indicate that all levels of mobility have some pathologic significance in the response of periodontal patients to treatment.[22]

Within patients, the greater the mobility of a tooth, the less favorable will be the therapeutic response in terms of attachment loss or gain in pockets around it. This statistically significant relationship is irrespective of initial pocket depth.[22] While not to be interpreted as meaning mobile teeth have a poor prognosis, this information does indicate that optimum healing can only be expected around clinically firm teeth.[22]

Underscored is the need to evaluate tooth mobility and its causes. When pathologic or unlimited, mobility must be reduced or controlled. This is also true whenever tooth mobility causes discomfort or functional impairment.

The method most commonly used to detect tooth mobility is luxation. With this technique teeth are evaluated according to the ease and the extent of their movement. They are held firmly between two instruments, two fingers, or one of each and are moved back and forth. The use of two instruments appears to be ideal, since it avoids the drawback of a possible depression of a finger pad; this depression might be mistaken for tooth movement or might mask slight variations in existing mobility.[92,93]

There are many systems for rating tooth mobility.[36,92,94] Clinicians should pick one they are comfortable with and strive to remain consistent in its use. This will provide some capability to detect changes in looseness. Below is the simple yet reproducible system[94] used to score patients in the Michigan Longitudinal Study,[95,96] the study from which the healing data originated.

Tooth mobility:

M-0 = physiologic mobility; firm tooth

M-1 = slightly increased mobility

M-2 = definite but considerable increase in mobility, but no impairment of function

M-3 = extreme mobility; a "loose" tooth that cannot be used for normal function

Fremitus

Fremitus refers to the visible or palpable displacement of a tooth from its resting position during occlusal function or parafunction.[89,93] Some prefer the term "functional" mobility.[97,98] It is checked by having the patient tap their teeth in centric and then glide into all excursions (Fig 13-7). Tooth movements are then noted visually or are palpated by fingertips that have been placed lightly on the buccal surfaces. While this assessment technique is limited to only the maxillary teeth, a very small degree of tooth mobility can be detected.[99] Assessing fremitus enables the practitioner to identify those teeth that will be most effectively treated by an occlusal adjustment. It also helps in obtaining an even distribution of working and protrusive forces.

Most importantly, the presence of functional mobility or fremitus is useful in detecting occlusal trauma. When this type of mobility is present and accompanied by

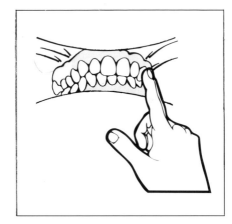

Fig 13-7 *A technique for detecting fremitus or functional mobility. The buccal tooth surfaces are lightly palpated. Tooth movements can be detected when the patient taps the teeth in centric and slides into excursions.*

a radiographically widened periodontal ligament space, loss of clinical attachment is greater than around teeth without similar findings.[97]

Percussion

Percussion has been claimed to be useful in detecting tooth mobility[89] or occlusal trauma.[100] Its value for the former is doubtful, but it can provide information on discomfort. A tooth that causes discomfort may be a sign of trauma. However, the possibility of periapical or sinus problems cannot be discounted.

Attrition

The presence of attrition is an excellent sign of occlusal abnormalities and possible parafunction.[4] The importance of identifying parafunctional forces in the periodontal patient cannot be overstated. The forces generated during bruxism (both centric and eccentric) frequently exceed the

adaptive capacity of the periodontium, initiating occlusal trauma and cofactor destruction.

By having a patient move into excursions, it is possible to determine the pattern of the parafunctional activity. Incisal edges will match up like a jigsaw puzzle. Occasionally, patients will deny current bruxism even with the presence of the aforementioned patterns of attrition. Questioning family members may confirm their contentions. Clinically, there are also some aids. By lightly running the tip of one's finger over the edge of the attrition, much can be learned. If the slide is impeded by a "catching," as it would be on a very sharp knife, then there is a high probability that the patient still bruxes. Conversely, if the finger slides easily, the edge is rounded and excursive bruxism may not be the factor it once was. Incisal edges should also be evaluated for thinning or chipping. Both are good indicators of a current problem.

Detecting isolated areas of attrition is also helpful. Such areas may indicate the presence of occlusal habits such as pen or pencil chewing. These habits and similar ones can lead to isolated trauma.

The absence of attrition does not necessarily mean there is no parafunctional activity. Some patients acknowledge gritting or clenching of their teeth. Under proper conditions, this centric bruxism can also lead to occlusal trauma. It is most often treated by means of a comprehensive occlusal adjustment eliminating nonaxially directed forces in and around centric occlusion. Final decisions regarding the therapeutic approach should be delayed until the initial root preparation has been completed. In many patients, parafunctional activities, particularly clenching, seem to be closely related to the level of gingival inflammation. As the inflammation subsides, often the clenching does as well.

The most difficult case to manage is one that combines eccentric bruxism with clenching in an eccentric position. Individuals with these problems often have accompanying temporomandibular disorders. Often splints must be constructed to prevent the individual from reaching the eccentric position.

Caries, Broken/Missing Restorations, and Open Contacts

The presence of these problems may lead to altered chewing patterns due to food impaction or an unstable occlusal relationship. In doing so, occlusal trauma may be precipitated by overburdening those teeth required to bear the load. Repair of the defects may be all that is required to reestablish occlusal harmony.

Open contacts may depict recent tooth movement. Broken restorations may be a result of heavy or misdirected occlusal forces. Both may be a clue to aid in identifying ongoing trauma or hyperfunction.

Temporomandibular Joint and Masticatory Muscle Analysis

This portion of the examination is essential, but a comprehensive review is beyond the scope of this chapter. These structures are an integral part of the occlusal system. Identification of joint pathology or of temporomandibular disorders may necessitate an altered therapeutic approach to the management of occlusal trauma.

Radiographic Analysis

After mobility, radiographs prove to be the best means of detecting signs of occlusal trauma and/or signs of adaptation to heavy occlusal forces. Traditionally, a discontinuous lamina dura, particularly around the apical one third of the root, has been considered evidence of occlusal trauma (Fig 13-8). Failure to detect this lesion does not preclude the existence

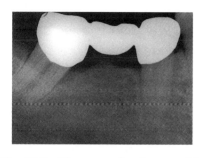

Fig 13-8 *The premolar has a widened periodontal ligament space and no discernable lamina dura. Traditionally this has been considered evidence of occlusal trauma.*

of trauma, however. Many variables can influence the diagnostic quality of radiographs, perhaps the most significant of which are those encountered when attempting to view an irregular, three-dimensional object in two dimensions. Changes in the width of the periodontal membrane space are significant. The presence of a widened space suggests increased occlusal loading and represents radiographic evidence of the supporting mechanism's attempt to adapt to these forces (Figs 13-9a and b).

The "classical" defects associated with occlusal trauma and cofactor destruction can also be detected radiographically. They appear as areas of vertical or "cupped-out" bony destruction (Figs 13-10a and b). While their direct association with trauma has been disputed, their presence is often accompanied by increased clinical tooth mobility. To aid in the identification of these often overlooked radiographic signs, an experiment can be performed as shown in Fig 13-11.

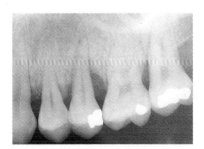
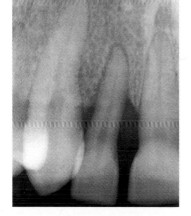

Figs 13-9a and b *The maxillary premolar* (left) *and incisor* (right) *have distinctly widened periodontal ligament spaces. This is consistent with heavy occlusal loading.*

Functionally, this experiment represents a tooth being driven forward by an opposing tooth during mastication. When the teeth disocclude, the involved tooth returns to its former position. Repetition leads to a widening of the periodontal membrane space and, if periodontitis happens to coexist, a more rapid loss of attachment. This is often depicted in radiographs of free-standing second molars (Fig 13-12).

The experiment shown in Fig 13-11 can be taken one step further, as described in Figs 13-13 and 13-14. And one can continue

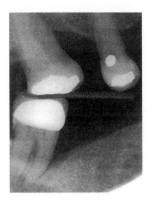

Fig 13-12 *This radiograph clearly depicts the vertical defects created by the cofactors of periodontitis and occlusal trauma. Both free-standing second molars exhibited a high degree of mobility.*

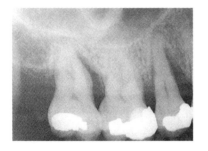 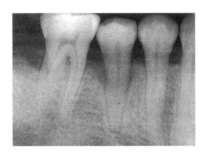

Figs 13-10a and b *These radiographs represent examples of the "classical" osseous defects associated with occlusal trauma. The vertical and/or "cupped-out" lesions are usually accompanied by increased tooth mobility.*

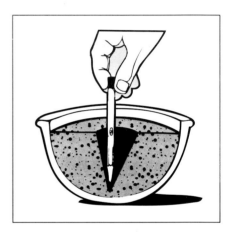

Fig 13-13 *This illustration aids in understanding the type of osseous lesion that would be expected to develop if occlusal forces from many directions were impacting the tooth. Using the same model described in Fig 13-11, move the pencil in all directions. Again, sagittally section the bowl and view it from the side. The soil should have a concave or cupped-out appearance. This will be seen often when examining a radiograph of a premolar that is an abutment for a removable partial denture (see Figs 13-14a and b).*

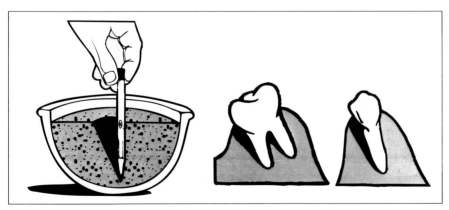

Fig 13-11 *The following experiment shows how an osseous lesion will develop when occlusal forces repeatedly drive a tooth in one direction. Take a glass bowl filled with moistened potting soil and push a pencil into it vertically. The periodontium has just been re-created. Gently, but repeatedly, apply force in one direction. Next, imagine a sagittal section made along the same plane as the force application, splitting the pencil and bowl in half. View the model from the side. The soil should appear compressed on one side of the pencil (call it the mesial) and there should be a widened space adjacent to the pencil.*

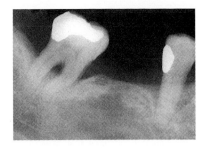 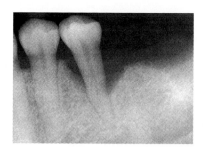

Figs13-14a and b *These radiographs are clear examples of the lesion shown in Fig 13-13. In Fig 13-14a (left), the mandibular premolar served as an abutment for a malfitting removable partial denture. The traumatic lesions seen in Fig 13-14b (right) developed in a patient who was a heavy bruxer.*

to "play" with the model, creating different situations. For example, the pencil can be moved "buccally, lingually, or both." The location of the sagittal section can be changed to represent different thicknesses of bone. The ability to interpret radiographs and to detect classical, traumatic defects will be enhanced using this model.

Finally, radiographs are helpful in detecting periapical and other pathology, the amount of remaining osseous support, and irregular root forms. Each can influence clinical tooth mobility.

DIAGNOSIS

As previously stated, a diagnosis of occlusal trauma is difficult to make. The adaptive capacity of the periodontium rapidly eliminates many of the signs and symptoms. Even so, there should be a definable injury.[54] This means one or more of the following should be detectable: increasing tooth mobility, fremitus, radiographic evidence of active bone resorption, and pulpal or tooth discomfort. Given radiographic limitations and the unlikelihood of detecting increasing mobility chairside, many diagnoses will

continue to be based on the judgment and experience of the clinician.

That judgment and experience will tell the clinician that occlusal trauma is most likely to exist in patients who have moderate to advanced periodontitis and increased tooth mobility or fremitus. Confirmation is assured if the radiographic changes reviewed above are also present. Most closely scrutinized will be those patients deemed to be "at risk," that is, those with parafunctional habits, compromised dentitions, or malocclusions.

TREATMENT TECHNIQUES

The elimination or control of occlusal trauma in periodontal therapy can be accomplished in many ways. Each case is different but the goal is the same: a healthy, stable, functionally adequate, and esthetically pleasing occlusion.[3]

The task of achieving that goal is simplified, regardless of the therapy chosen, when the following principles of occlusion are kept in mind: *(1)* stability in centric relation, centric occlusion, and in

the area from centric relation to centric occlusion; *(2)* axial distribution of occlusal forces; *(3)* freedom of movement of the mandible in all lateral and protrusive excursions; *(4)* absence of balancing contacts; and *(5)* maintenance of a correct vertical dimension and of a functional interocclusal space.[3,4]

Occlusal Adjustment

Occlusal adjustment is the primary technique for occlusal therapy.[3] It may be comprehensive or limited, and it is frequently used in concert with other therapeutic modalities. Detailed discussions of the basic techniques can be found elsewhere[4] and should be reviewed. Compliance with their recommendations and those highlighted below will benefit the clinician as well as patients with occlusal trauma. Properly performed occlusal adjustments have the demonstrated ability to reduce tooth mobility.[71,82,89,101-103]

To achieve axially directed forces, occlusal prematurities in centric relation, centric occlusion, and the region between the two must be removed. This will establish a "freedom in centric" and the elimination of any vertical and lateral component of the slide in centric. By preserving centric stops, stability will be achieved without altering vertical dimension or the patient's "normal" occlusion.

Balancing interferences should be eliminated. These contacts often prohibit free mandibular movement[4] and are capable of delivering damaging lateral forces to the periodontium.

Some form of working and protrusive guidance is needed. For some patients that means a canine-protected occlusion; for others that means group function. When occlusal trauma affects one or more of the teeth providing the guidance, the functional burden should be shifted to those teeth most capable of handling it. For example, if occlusal trauma is noted affecting the molars but not the canine and the occlusal scheme allows for canine guidance, adjust to it. The posterior teeth then would disengage in all movements except within the CR-CO range. If the canine is suffering from trauma, then shift to group guidance. If the canine and the posterior teeth are all afflicted, then use group guidance, carefully establishing an even distribution of the forces / contacts.

Testing for fremitus is extremely helpful in obtaining this even distribution of forces. It is also useful in finalizing the centric adjustment.

Detection of the last deflective contacts can be best accomplished by using 28-gauge green wax.

Occlusal Bite Planes

Bite planes are extremely useful and versatile appliances for the treatment of occlusal trauma in the patient with advanced periodontitis. The bite plane should provide complete occlusal coverage of one arch and be made of a heat-cured acrylic resin. The bite plane should be adjusted so that all teeth of the opposing arch contact evenly on a smooth, relatively flat surface. "Freedom in centric" and canine guidance of excursive movements should be established. This arrangement allows for excellent stability, free lateral movements without balancing contacts, and an axial distribution of occlusal forces.

The bite plane is important for the patient who also has parafunctional habits such as bruxism. The damaging occlusal forces are dissipated by the appliance. These individuals should wear the bite plane at times when the para-

functional activities are active. For most, this means during sleep, when the subconscious assumes control. For them and most others, the bite plane should be placed in the maxillary arch where it is most stable and easiest to adjust. Some patients require protection during the waking hours; a mandibular bite plane is usually the best choice because it makes clear speech easier.

Bite planes are also used for their ability to splint teeth. They allow retention of teeth when an occlusal adjustment alone would be ineffective. An excellent example is controlling the unlimited mobility observed in anterior teeth of periodontal cases with lost vertical dimension (no posterior occlusion) or bimaxillary protrusion. Another would be the retention of teeth in postorthodontic patients who also have parafunctional habits.

In complex periodontal reconstruction cases, bite planes can temporarily splint teeth during healing to allow for a better assessment of abutment stability.

Similarly, a bite plane can stabilize the occlusion while a molar is being orthodontically uprighted.

One of the greatest benefits of a bite plane of this design is its ability to treat concomitantly occlusal trauma and some temporomandibular disorders. Bite plane therapy relaxes the masticatory musculature.

There is one final advantage. Bite plane usage allows occlusal therapy to be effected without causing permanent change. Occlusal surfaces are not altered.

Orthodontics

As with the nonperiodontal patient, orthodontics can be used to achieve the optimum occlusal relationships described at the be-

ginning of this section. Through the movement of teeth, traumatic occlusal forces and their sequelae can be eliminated. Some malocclusions can be corrected, diastemata closed, impingements eliminated, and teeth uprighted.

Even a patient with advanced periodontitis is a candidate for orthodontic therapy. However, since their support is already compromised, the use of light forces and slow tooth movement is advocated. Contrary to what has been advocated in the past,[2,66] it is also recommended that periodontal therapy be completed prior to beginning orthodontic therapy on these patients. Root planing alone often is insufficient treatment to resolve the deepest defects in moderate to advanced periodontitis. This means residual inflammation. Coupled with the fact that orthodontic movement produces transient occlusal trauma, the risk of unintentionally inducing cofactor destruction is great. Thus, in the process of correcting one problem, another might be created. Proper maintenance can minimize the risk, but patient compliance often is lacking. This is less of a factor for minor tooth movement. Minor tooth movement can and probably should be performed immediately after the initial root preparation. Doing so allows more flexibility in determining the method for retention.

Permanent and Temporary Splinting

Permanent splinting is used widely to replace missing teeth, to restore occlusal function, and to stabilize teeth. When constructed, these splints should possess an occlusal scheme compatible with the principles detailed under the occlusal adjustment section. Too often, these restorations create interferences or disturb occlusal function and harmony.

The splinting of teeth can positively increase the effective ligament area of each tooth, but it will not provide immunity to traumatic forces.[104] The act of splinting also will not reduce individual tooth mobility, but properly constructed, it can stabilize the mobility.[55,71,82,105-108]

Posttherapeutic tooth mobility is not justification for splinting unless the mobility is unlimited or uncomfortable to the patient.[109,110] Whether pretreatment, permanent, or temporary splinting will help promote a more favorable gain in attachment levels has not yet been determined.

Temporary splinting will definitely aid a tooth or teeth that have suffered acute trauma. It will provide stability and allow function during healing.

Temporary splinting can also be useful in evaluating the response of some potential abutment teeth and in maintaining tooth position during delays in treatment. Usually, the involved teeth would be unstable if left unsecured. Composite bridges reinforced with Kevlar fibers have proven effective in this regard. They are both durable and cost effective.

TREATMENT PLANNING

When occlusal trauma is diagnosed in a patient with periodontitis, therapy should be performed to eliminate or control those factors causing the trauma. If there is an acute injury, pain, or discomfort, corrective steps should be taken immediately. The tooth that has received a direct blow should be temporarily splinted. The new restoration with the faulty occlusion should be adjusted. The tooth with unlimited or uncomfortable mobility should be temporarily splinted.

In the absence of acute symptomatology, it is prudent to defer occlusal therapy until after the initial root planing and oral hygiene instruction have been completed. The resultant reduction in inflammation will lead to reduced tooth mobility. This will ease the task of obtaining a stable occlusion. When the tissues are ready, occlusal adjustments and bite plane construction are the techniques of choice in attaining the stability.

From this point, however, treatment plans can be as different as individuals. Each case will have its own variables. These variables are not just dental. Patient desires, compliance, and economic restrictions will greatly influence what procedures are performed and when.

Thus, if fixed bridgework is planned for a patient who will be unable financially to complete treatment for an indeterminate period of time and the patient has moderate to advanced periodontitis with mobile teeth, it may be prudent to consider temporary splinting. This will aid in preserving occlusal stability and function. Healing may benefit as well by limiting the temporary increase in mobility[82,111-113] that accompanies periodontal surgical procedures.

As discussed earlier, comprehensive orthodontic therapy should be postponed until after periodontal therapy has been completed. Minor tooth movement can be performed at any time following the initial root preparation.

Regardless of the therapeutic approach to treating occlusal trauma, the occlusal relationships should always be monitored after treatment for change and stability. Corrections, refinements, and adjustments should be performed as needed.

I. Current concepts
- Occlusal trauma:
  - represents an injury to the attachment apparatus
  - is the result of lack of adaptation to occlusal forces
  - will affect periodontal ligament, bone, and cementum
  - will show increasing mobility or migration of teeth, pain to percussion or biting, and discontinuity of the lamina dura surrounding the roots and a widened periodontal space on radiographs
- Occlusal interferences coupled with stress can trigger bruxism and develop into occlusal trauma.
- There are two types of occlusal trauma: primary and secondary.
- The role of occlusal trauma in periodontics is still controversial.
- Trauma will not initiate marginal inflammation, nor will it aggravate gingivitis.
- Excessive forces associated with periodontitis may speed up the process of periodontal breakdown if no adaptation is possible.
- If periodontitis and trauma are present, treating the marginal inflammation may allow for adaptation to the excessive forces.
- Reduced mobility may promote more favorable gains in clinical attachment levels.
- When the diagnosis of occlusal trauma is made, treatment of the occlusion is justified.
- Therapy may include occlusal adjustment, bite splints, orthodontics, restorative dentistry, and splinting.
- Occlusal therapy must achieve an optimal functional occlusion with stable tooth relationships.

II. Clinical application
- Occlusal trauma and periodontitis interact as follows:
  - increasing tooth mobility will accelerate attachment loss when periodontitis is also present
  - occlusal trauma impairs or inhibits periodontal healing
- Diagnosis of occlusal trauma requires an understanding of the entire masticatory system. A comprehensive patient history and examination is also needed. This includes:
  - review of a detailed health questionnaire
  - an occlusal analysis evaluating the occlusal scheme, tooth contact relationships, tooth mobility, fremitus, percussion, attrition, and the integrity of the arches and restorations
  - a radiographic analysis focusing on the integrity of the lamina dura and the width of the periodontal ligament space
  - an analysis of the TMJ and masticatory masticulation
- Diagnosis of occlusal trauma requires a definable injury. One or more of the following should be detectable:
  - increasing tooth mobility
  - fremitus
  - radiographic evidence of active bone resorption: discontinuous lamina dura, widened periodontal ligament spaces, or "cupped" out defects
  - pulpal or tooth discomfort
- Those patients "at risk" have:
  - moderate to advanced periodontitis
  - increased mobility or fremitus
  - parafunctional habits
  - compromised dentitions
  - severe malocclusions
- Optimum therapeutic results depend upon eliminating or controlling occlusal trauma when it is diagnosed in periodontal patients.
- The method(s) of occlusal therapy and the attendant treatment plans can be as varied as the patients themselves. While each case must be judged on its own variables, the goal is always the same: a healthy, stable, functionally adequate, and esthetically pleasing occlusion.
- The following are the treatment techniques most often used to achieve that goal:
  - occlusal adjustment
  - occlusal bite planes
  - orthodontics
  - permanent and temporary splinting

REFERENCES

1. Williams RC: Periodontal disease. *N Engl J Med* 1990;322:373-382.
2. American Academy of Periodontology: *Proceedings of the World Workshop in Clinical Periodontics.* Chicago: American Academy of Periodontology; 1989:III-15 to III-22.
3. Caffesse RG: Management of periodontal disease in patients with occlusal abnormalities. *Dent Clin North Am* 1980;24:215.
4. Ramfjord S, Ash M: *Occlusion.* 3rd ed. Philadelphia: WB Saunders Co, 1983.
5. Svanberg G: Influence of trauma from occlusion on the periodontium of dogs with normal or inflamed gingivae. *Odontol Rev* 1974;25:165.
6. Reitan K: Initial tissue reaction incident to orthodontic tooth movement as related to the influence of function. An experimental histological study on animal and human material. *Acta Odontol Scand* 1951;(Suppl 6):9.
7. Wentz F, Jaraback J, Orban B: Experimental occlusal trauma imitating cuspal interferences. *J Periodontol* 1958;29:117.
8. Svanberg G, Lindhe J: Experimental tooth hypermobility in the dog. A methodological study. *Odontol Rev* 1973;24:269.
9. Lindhe J, Svanberg G: Influence of trauma from occlusion on progression of experimental periodontitis in the beagle dog. *J Clin Periodontol* 1974;1:3.
10. Nyman S, Lindhe J, Ericsson I: The effect of progressive tooth mobility on destructive periodontitis in the dog. *J Clin Periodontol* 1978;5:213.
11. Ericsson I, Lindhe J: The effect of long standing jiggling on experimental marginal periodontitis in the beagle dog. *J Clin Periodontol* 1982;9:497.
12. Meitner S: Co-destructive factors of marginal periodontitis and repetitive mechanical injury. *J Dent Res* 1975; Spec no. C:78.
13. Polson A, Meitner S, Zander H: Trauma and progression of marginal periodontitis in squirrel monkeys. IV: Reversibility of bone loss due to trauma alone and trauma superimposed upon periodontitis. *J Periodont Res* 1976;11:290.
14. Lindhe J, Ericsson I: The influence of trauma from occlusion on reduced but healthy periodontal tissues in dogs. *J Clin Periodontol* 1976; 13:110.
15. Lindhe J, Ericsson I: Effect of elimination of jiggling forces on periodontally exposed teeth in the dog. *J Periodontol* 1982;53:562.
16. Kantor M, Polson A, Zander H: Alveolar bone regeneration after removal of inflammatory and traumatic factors. *J Periodontol* 1976;47:687.
17. Glickman I, Smulow J, Voger B, Passamonti G: The effect of occlusal forces on healing following mucogingival surgery. *J Periodontol* 1966;37:319.
18. Nyman S, Rosling B, Lindhe J: Effect of professional tooth cleaning on healing after periodontal surgery. *J Clin Periodontol* 1975;2:80.
19. Rosling B, Nyman S, Lindhe J: The effect of systematic plaque control on bone regeneration in infrabony pockets. *J Clin Periodontol* 1976; 3:38.
20. Polson A, Heijl L: Osseous repair in infrabony periodontal defects. *J Clin Periodontol* 1978;5:13.
21. Kohler C, Ramfjord S: Healing of gingival mucoperiosteal flaps. *Oral Surg Oral Med Oral Path* 1960;13:89.
22. Fleszar TJ, Knowles JW, Morrison EC, Burgett FG, Nissle RR, Ramfjord SP: Tooth mobility and periodontal therapy. *J Clin Periodontol* 1980;7:495.
23. Burgett F, Charbeneau T, Nissle R, Morrison E, Ramfjord S, Caffesse R: A randomized occlusal adjustment in periodontitis patients. *J Dent Res* 1988;67:124 (Abstr no. 93).
24. Ericsson I, Lindhe J: Lack of significance of increased tooth mobility in experimental periodontitis. *J Periodontol* 1984;55:447.
25. Hoag P: Occlusal treatment. In: *Proceedings of the World Workshop in Clinical Periodontics.* Chicago: American Academy of Periodontology; 1989;39:III-1 to III-14.
26. Poulton D, Aaronson S: The relationship between occlusion and periodontal status. *Am J Orthod* 1961; 47:691.
27. Sutcliffe P: Chronic anterior gingivitis—An epidemiological study in school children. *Br Dent J* 1968; 125:47.
28. Alexander A, Tipins A: The effect of irregularity of teeth and the degree of overbite and overjet on the gingival health. *Br Dent J* 1970; 128:539.
29. Geiger AM: Occlusal studies in 188 consecutive cases of periodontal disease. *Am J Orthod* 1962;48:330.
30. Geiger AM, Wasserman BH, Thompson RH, et al: Relationship of occlusion and periodontal disease. Part I. A system for evaluating periodontal status. *J Periodontol* 1971;42:364.
31. Wasserman BH, Thompson RH Jr, Geiger AM, et al: Relationship of occlusion and periodontal disease. II. Periodontal status of the study population. *J Periodontol* 1971;42:371.
32. Thompson RH, Geiger AM, Wasserman BH, Turgeon LR: Relationship of occlusion and periodontal disease. 3. Relation of periodontal status to general background characteristics. *J Periodontol* 1972;43:540.
33. Wasserman BH, Geiger AM, Thompson RH, Turgeon LR: Relationship of occlusion and periodontal disease. IV. Relationship of inflammation to general background characteristics and periodontal destruction. *J Periodontol* 1972;43:547.
34. Geiger AM, Wasserman BH, Thompson RH, Turgeon LR: Relationship of occlusion and periodontal disease. Part V. Relation of classification of occlusion to periodontal status and gingival inflammation. *J Periodontol* 1972;43:554.
35. Geiger AM, Wasserman BH, Turgeon LR: Relationship of occlusion and periodontal disease. Part VI. Relation of anterior overjet and overbite to periodontal destruction and gingival inflammation. *J Periodontol* 1973; 44:150.
36. Wasserman BH, Geiger AM, Turgeon LR: Relationship of occlusion and periodontal disease. VII. Mobility. *J Periodontol* 1973;44:572.
37. Geiger AM, Wasserman BH, Turgeon LR: Relationship of occlusion and periodontal disease. Part VIII. Relationship of crowding and spacing to periodontal destruction and gingival inflammation. *J Periodontol* 1974; 45:43.
38. Geiger AM, Wasserman BH: Relationship of occlusion and periodontal disease. Part X. Incisor inclination and periodontal status. *J Periodontol* 1977;48:785.
39. Kepic T, O'Leary T: Role of marginal ridge relationships as an etiologic factor in periodontal disease. *J Periodontol* 1978;49:570.
40. Hirschfeld I: Food impaction. *J Am Dent Assoc* 1930;17:1504.
41. Beyron H: Optimal occlusion. *Dent Clin North Am* 1969;13:537.
42. Winslow M: Preventive role of occlusal balancing of the natural dentition. *J Am Dent Assoc* 1954;48:293.
43. American Academy of Periodontology: Glossary of Periodontic Terms. *J Periodontol* 1986;57(Suppl).
44. Marks M, Corn H: *Atlas of Adult Orthodontics.* Philadelphia; Lea & Febiger, 1989.
45. Genco R, Goldman H, Cohen D: *Contemporary Periodontics.* St Louis: CV Mosby Co, 1990.
46. Polson A, Reed B: Long term effect of orthodontic treatment on crestal alveolar bone levels. *J Periodontol* 1984;55:28.
47. Reitan K: Some factors determining the evaluation of forces in orthodontics. *Am J Orthod* 1957;43:32.

48. Zachrisson B, Alnaes L: Periodontal condition in orthodontically treated and untreated individuals. I. Loss of attachment, gingival pocket depth and clinical crown height. *Angle Orthod* 1973;43:402.

49. Zachrisson B, Alnaes L: Periodontal condition in orthodontically treated and untreated individuals. II. Alveolar bone loss: Radiographic findings. *Angle Orthod* 1974;44:48.

50. Brown IS: The effect of orthodontic therapy on certain types of periodontal defects. I. Clinical findings. *J Periodontol* 1973;44:742.

51. Kraal J, Digiancinto J, Dail R, Lemmerman K, Peden J: Periodontal conditions in patients after molar uprighting. *J Prosthet Dent* 1980; 43:156.

52. Marks M, Corn H: Adult tooth movement: Alteration of the occlusal vertical dimension preparatory to tooth movement. *Alpha Omegan* 1977; 70:54.

53. Everett F, Baer P: A preliminary report on the treatment of the osseous defect in periodontosis. *J Periodontol* 1964;35:429.

54. Ramfjord S, Ash M: *Periodontology and Periodontics.* Philadelphia: WB Saunders Co, 1979.

55. Renggli H: Splinting of teeth — An objective assessment. *Helv Odont Acta* 1971;15:129.

56. Cohen DW, Friedman L, Shapiro J, Kyle GC: A longitudinal investigation of the periodontal changes during pregnancy. *J Periodontol* 1969; 40:563.

57. Glickman I: Inflammation and trauma from occlusion, co-destructive factors in chronic periodontal disease. *J Periodontol* 1963;34:5.

58. Lindhe J: *Textbook of Clinical Periodontology.* 2nd ed. Copenhagen: Munksgaard, 1989.

59. Ericsson I, Lindhe J: Lack of effect of trauma from occlusion on the recurrence of experimental periodontitis. *J Clin Periodontol* 1977;4:115.

60. Ericsson I, Thilander B, Lindhe J, Okamato H: The effect of orthodontic tilting movements on the periodontal tissues of the infected and non-infected dentitions in dogs. *J Clin Periodontol* 1977;4:278.

61. Ericsson I, Thilander B: Orthodontic forces and recurrence of periodontal disease. An experimental study in the dog. *Am J Orthod* 1978;74:41.

62. Nyman S, Lindhe J, Ericsson I: The effect of progressive tooth mobility on destructive periodontitis in the dog. *J Clin Periodontol* 1978;5:213.

63. Svanberg G, Lindhe J: Vascular reactions in the periodontal ligament incident to trauma from occlusion. *J Clin Periodontol* 1974;1:58.

64. Nyman S, Rosling B, Lindhe J: Effect of professional tooth cleaning on healing after periodontal surgery. *J Clin Periodontol* 1975;2:80.

65. Glickman I: *Clinical Periodontology; Prevention, Diagnosis and Treatment of Periodontal Disease in the Practice of General Dentistry.* 4th ed. Philadelphia: WB Saunders Co, 1972.

66. Goldman HM, Cohen DW: *Periodontal Therapy.* 5th ed. St Louis: CV Mosby Co, 1973.

67. Lemmerman K: Rationale for stabilization. *J Periodontol* 1976;47:405.

68. Hirt A, Muhlemann HR: Diagnosis of bruxism by means of tooth mobility measurements. *Parodontologie* 1955;9:47.

69. Schei O, Waerhaug J, Lövdal A, Arno A: Tooth mobility and alveolar bone resorption as a function of occlusal stress and oral hygiene. *Acta Odontol Scand* 1959;17:61.

70. O'Leary TJ, Rudd KD, Nabers CL, Stumpf AJ: The effect of a "tube type" diet and stress-inducing conditions on tooth mobility. *J Periodontol* 1967;38:222.

71. O'Leary TJ: Tooth mobility. *Dent Clin North Am* 1969;13:567.

72. Ainamo J: Relationship between malignment of teeth and periodontal disease. *Scand J Dent Res* 1972;80:104.

73. Beagrie GS, James GA: The association of posterior tooth irregularity and periodontal disease. *Br Dent J* 1962;113:239.

74. Gould MSE, Picton DCA: The relation between irregularities of the teeth and periodontal disease. *Br Dent J* 1966;121:21.

75. Grewe JM, Chadha JM, Hagan D, Zermeno JA: Oral hygiene and occlusal disharmony in Mexican-American children. *J Periodont Res* 1969;4:189.

76. Steiner GG, Pearson JK, Ainamo J: Changes of the marginal periodontium as a result of labial tooth movement in monkeys. *J Periodontol* 1981;52:314.

77. Reitan K: To what extent can orthodontics be a contributory factor in the treatment of periodontal cases? *Am J Orthod* 1962;48:934 (Abstr).

78. Carlsson G, Hedegard B, Koivumaa K: Studies in partial denture prosthesis. IV. Final results of a 4-year longitudinal investigation of dentogingivally supported partial dentures. *Acta Odontol Scand* 1965;23:443.

79. Morris ML: The diagnosis, prognosis and treatment of the loose tooth. *Oral Surg* 1953;6:957, 1037.

80. Muhlemann HR: Tooth mobility: A review of clinical aspects and research findings. *J Periodontol* 1967;38:686.

81. Nyman S, Lindhe J: Persistent tooth hypermobility following completion of periodontal treatment. *J Clin Periodontol* 1976;3:81.

82. Rateitschak KH: Therapeutic effect of local treatment on periodontal disease assessed upon evaluation of different diagnostic criteria. I. Changes in tooth mobility. *J Periodontol* 1963;34:540.

83. Rateitschak KH: Tooth mobility changes in pregnancy. *J Periodont Res* 1967;2:199.

84. Amsterdam M: Periodontal prosthesis. Twenty-five years in retrospect. *Alpha Omegan* 1974;67:8.

85. Amsterdam M, Fox L: Provisional splinting — Principles and techniques. *Dent Clin North Am* 1959;3:73.

86. Lindhe J, Nyman S: The role of occlusion in periodontal disease and the biologic rationale for splinting in treatment of periodontitis. *Oral Sci Rev* 1977;10:11.

87. Muhlemann H: Clinical implications of tooth mobility measurements. In: *The Mechanisms of Tooth Support; A Symposium* (Oxford, 1965). London: J. Wright and Sons, Ltd; 1967:144.

88. Laster L, Laudenbach KW, Stoller NH: An evaluation of clinical tooth mobility measurements. *J Periodontol* 1975;46:603.

89. Reichborn-Kjennerud I: Development, etiology and diagnosis of increased tooth mobility and of traumatic occlusion. *J Periodontol* 1973;44:326.

90. Rudd KD, O'Leary TJ, Stumpf AJ Jr: Horizontal tooth mobility in carefully screened subjects. *Periodontics* 1964;2:65.

91. Stahl SS: The role of occlusion in the etiology and therapy of periodontal disease. *Angle Orthod* 1970;40:347.

92. Miller SC: *Textbook of Periodontia.* 1st ed. Philadelphia: Blakiston, 1938.

93. Weatherford TW 3d: Tooth mobility: Mechanisms and treatment. *Ala J Med Sci* 1977;14:32.

94. Ramfjord SP: Indices for prevalence and incidence of periodontal disease. *J Periodontol* 1959;30:51-59.

95. Ramfjord SP, Knowles JW, Nissle RR, Burgett FG, Shick RA: Results following three modalities of periodontal therapy. *J Periodontol* 1975;46:522.

96. Ramfjord SP, et al: Longitudinal study of periodontal therapy. *J Periodontol* 1973;44:66.

97. Pihlstrom BL, Anderson KA, Aeppoli D, Schaffer EM: Association between signs of trauma from occlusion and periodontitis. *J Periodontol* 1986; 57:1.

98. Vogel RI, Deasy MJ: Tooth mobility: Etiology and rationale of therapy. *N Y State Dent J* 1977;43:159.

99. Posselt U, Maunsbach O: Clinical and roentgenographic studies of trauma from occlusion. *J Periodontol* 1957;28:192.

100. Prichard JF: *Advanced Periodontal*

Disease; Surgical and Prosthetic Management. 2nd ed. Philadelphia: WB Saunders Co, 1972.

101. Goldberg H: Changes in tooth mobility during periodontal therapy. *I A D R* 1962;40:69.

102. Muhlemann HR, Herzog H, Rateitschak K: Quantitative evaluation of the therapeutic effect of selective grinding. *J Periodontol* 1957;28:11.

103. Vollmer WH, Rateitschak K: Influence of occlusal adjustment by grinding on gingivitis and mobility of traumatized teeth. *J Clin Periodontol* 1975;2:113.

104. Glickman I, Stein R, Smulow J: The effect of increased functional forces upon the periodontium of splinted and non-splinted teeth. *J Periodontol* 1961;32:290.

105. Heringlake CB, Goodwin RJ: The effect of a cantilever posterior fixed partial denture on abutment mobility. A clinical study. *N W Dent* 1973;52:111.

106. Plotnick IJ, Beresin VE, Simkins AB: The effects of variations in the opposing dentition on the changes in the partially edentulous mandible. Part III. Tooth mobility and chewing efficiency with various maxillary dentitions. *J Prosthet Dent* 1975; 33:529.

107. Renggli HH, Schweizer H: Splinting of teeth with removable bridges — Biological effects. *J Clin Periodontol* 1974;1:43.

108. Rudd KD, O'Leary TJ: Stabilizing periodontally weakened teeth by using guide plane removable partial dentures: A preliminary report. *J Prosthet Dent* 1966;16:721.

109. Lindhe J, Hamp SE, Löe H: Experimental periodontitis in the beagle dog. *Int Dent J* 1973;23:432.

110. Nyman S, Lindhe J, Lundgren D: The role of occlusion for the stability of fixed bridges in patients with reduced periodontal tissue support. *J Clin Periodontol* 1975;2:53.

111. Burch JG, Conry CW, Ferris RT: Tooth mobility following gingivectomy. *Periodontics* 1968;6:90.

112. Forsberg A, Hagglund B: Mobility of the teeth as a check of periodontal therapy. *Acta Odontol Scand* 1958;15:305.

113. Selipsky H: Osseous surgery — How much need we compromise? *Dent Clin North Am* 1976;20:79.

Restorative Dentistry

C U R R E N T   C O N C E P T S by Richard D. Wilson

C L I N I C A L   A P P L I C A T I O N by Richard D. Wilson

CURRENT CONCEPTS
Morphology
Margin quality
Margin location
Periodontal diagnosis in planning
    restorative therapy

CLINICAL APPLICATION
A proper restorative environment
Interim restorations

Full-coverage restorations
Composite resin restorations
Porcelain laminate veneers
Amalgam restorations
Restoration of endodontically
    treated teeth

QUICK REVIEW

REFERENCES

C U R R E N T   C O N C E P T S

The tooth and its surrounding structures are continually challenged by microbial flora, and restorative dentistry may exacerbate this challenge (Fig 14-1).[1] The dentogingival unit has been described by Schroeder and Listgarten[2] as a heterogenous and interconnected "sandwich," with its most vulnerable component being the gingival crevice. Frequently entered, but rarely understood, the crevice remains an enigma to many restorative dentists (Fig 14-2).

Periodontal attachment loss begins when the epithelial integrity of the dentogingival unit is breached. Injury may be produced by microbial flora, by trauma, or by both.[3] The progression of this injury appears to be related to host resistance, the competence of the surrounding tissue, and the bacterial pathogens.[4] In turn, each of these elements may be influenced by the three aspects of a dental restoration: morphology, margin quality, and margin location.

MORPHOLOGY

The morphology (ie, form and surface characteristics) of a restoration affects bacterial plaque retention.[5] Improperly contoured and rough restorations not only hinder oral hygiene,[5] they also "change a nondestructive subgingival flora to a destructive one."[6]

When the contours of a dental restoration exceed the original profile of the tooth, the gingival crevice is distended and the papilla is displaced.[7] Studies have demonstrated that most crowned teeth are overcontoured[8] and conclude that a protective, dou-

ble-deflective cervical bulge created to defend the gingiva actually brings about increased plaque accumulation and resulting inflammation. The "transitional line angle," as described by Amsterdam and Abrams,[9] is fundamental to physiologically shaped restorations and encourages restorations that have a relatively flat profile, thus diminishing bacterial retention and soft tissue distention (Fig 14-3).

An area that is sensitive to excessive restorative contours is the interdental embrasure.[10,11] As the restoration emerges from the crevice, it should be flat or even concave.[12] The occlusal housing of the embrasure should not impinge on the papilla. Solder joints should be rounded and smooth as they approach the tissue (Figs 14-4a to e). The interproximal surfaces should have a contact area,

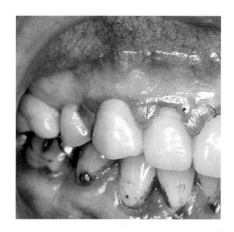

Fig 14-1 *Periodontal tissues severely violated by full-coverage restorations.*

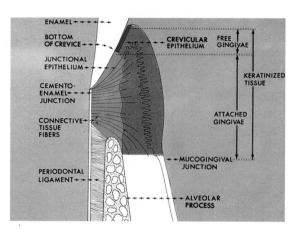

Fig 14-2 *A diagrammatic cross section of the three physiologic dimensions that make up the dentogingival unit:* (1) **superficial physiologic dimension:** *includes both the free gingivae and the attached gingivae (keratinized tissue);* (2) **crevicular physiologic dimension:** *extends from the free gingival margin to the junctional epithelium;* (3) **subcrevicular physiologic dimension:** *includes the junctional epithelium and the supra-alveolar connective tissue fibers. Restorations and the procedures that create them should defend, not violate, these arenas.*

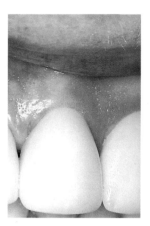

Fig 14-3 *Single porcelain/metal crown illustrating relatively flat emergence profile, which lessens bacterial intention and soft tissue distention.*

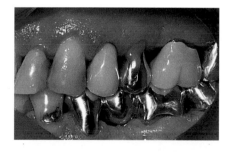

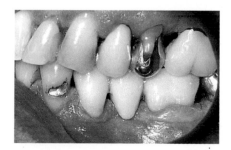

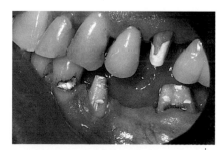

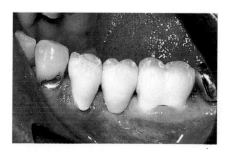

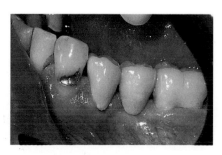

Figs 14-4a to e *Cosmetic demands of patient required remaking a mandibular three-unit gold bridge and a maxillary single gold crown. Restorations had been in place for 19 years. Such demands compel very serious consideration on the part of the practitioner and candid review of the risks with the patient. The alveolar mucosa tissue margin on the mandibular premolar required a supragingival restorative margin. Note the health of the tissue upon removal of the provisional bridge. The unglazed porcelain allows the dentist control of tooth shape and color and permits careful contouring of the interproximal areas.*

not a contact point.[13] A contact point may deceptively "snap" floss but often opens under occlusal loading, allowing vertical food impaction. For the patient who has longer clinical crowns, the annoyance of lateral food impaction may be avoided by creating restorations that have a long (in an inferior-superior dimension) and broad contact area, while taking care not to violate the soft tissues.[14]

From a patient perspective, the contours of some pontics are especially bothersome. The "bullet"-shaped pontic will often collect debris, usually on the lingual surface.[15] A fully shaped pontic that allows complete access for floss is more desirable,[16] especially if the edentulous area is keratinized[17] and free of plaque-accumulating irregularities.

MARGIN QUALITY

No restoration meets the tooth with a perfect margin,[18] and in the cemented restoration, the luting agent is like an Achilles' heel.[19] At the microscopic level, dental cements are rough and inconsistent and accelerate the accumulation of plaque.[20] These sites could be especially insidious and damaging when placed in the gingival crevice.[21] This situation is aggravated by margins that are open or of poor quality, and inflammation invariably ensues.[22] Even heroic plaque control on the part of the patient often cannot compensate for an inferior restoration margin placed within the gingival crevice. In those restorations that are directly inserted, such as silver alloy or composite resin, the quality of the margin is equally significant.[23] These restorations are of great benefit to the patient when used following accepted precepts. However, disparities are often found in these margins. Studies[24-30] indicate that the prevalence of inferior and overhanging restoration margins is very high — at least 33% in adult patients.

Although it was originally postulated that poor margins mechanically irritated the periodontium, Waerhaug's[31] findings, followed by the studies of Highfield and Powell[32] and Jeffcoat and Howell[33] indicated that rough margins increase plaque mass and also increase the number of specific periodontal pathogens in the plaque.[6] Lang et al[34] conclude that poor margins "resulted in a change in the composition of the subgingival microflora at that site to one that may be associated with periodontitis, rather than by harboring increased plaque masses."

In commercial dental laboratories, the most commonly prescribed porcelain-fused-to-metal (PFM) margin is that which joins metal and porcelain just at the edge of the restoration. This margin has many shortcomings. The metal is very thin and flexible whereas the porcelain is not. This leads to small fractures of the margin porcelain when the crown is seated. In addition, this margin requires that metal, opaque, porcelain, and usually an overglaze terminate within microns of each other. This creates an overcontoured and rough margin. Plaque readily accumulates and inflammation results. No conscientious dentist would accept this type of margin on the buccal surface of an onlay, and yet it is inserted into gingival crevices on a daily basis and with apparent universal approval.[35]

Restoration margins are significantly influenced by biomaterials.[36] The large number of new restorative materials has left many questions. Phillips[37] states: "Every year clinical studies are published that present 1-, 3-, and even 4-year results on materials no longer available or so significantly altered as to render much of the data of questionable value." The problem is compounded by disparities in research methodologies. As a consequence, broad differences in supposedly similar clinical studies are published. In addition, commercial companies accept no responsibility for failures of the materials that they have only recently marketed so aggressively. Thus, the dentist in daily practice may be left confused and dependent on his/her own experiences and on lectures based on empirical knowledge.

There appear to be differences in the plaque retainability of some of the dental materials. Possibly through a surface tension phenomenon, castable ceramic appears to be the least plaque retentive,[38] while resins used as cementing agents seem to retain a greater amount of plaque.[39] Data suggest that in thin sections, resin (such as a luting agent) demonstrates notable roughness.[40] Others have shown that the cohesive bond strength of ionomer luting agents is reduced by 25% to 30% when joining rigid surfaces in vitro.[41] Resulting microcracks and faults in these luting agents collect plaque that is inaccessible to cleansing.[42] The persistent complaints of dentists about pulpal symptoms after crowns are cemented with ionomer is also troubling.[43] Nevertheless, ionomers and resins are evolving materials that show unique potential as luting agents.[44]

When resins are used as luting agents for crowns, for porcelain laminate veneers, and for porcelain and composite resin inlays and onlays, the efficacy of the bond depends, at least in part, on dentin bonding.[45] Because dentin bonding lacks the quality of enamel bonding,[46] the microscopic gaps and voids that develop at the margin may well be responsible for seemingly inexplicable inflammation around restorations that appear to fit well clinically.

Poor restorative margins initiate inflammation. Initially, portions of the gingival fiber unit are lysed. The lysis is superficial and may demonstrate no attachment loss. This inflammatory response may persist for years, but the level of attachment may never change (gingivitis). However, once lysis extends, the epithelium migrates apically and a periodontal pocket occurs (periodontitis).[3] At present it is not possible to predict which inadequate restoration will lead to gingivitis only and which will lead to periodontitis.

MARGIN LOCATION

The space between the most apical part of the gingival crevice and the alveolar crest houses the junctional epithelium and the connective tissue attachment. This tissue connection has been termed the "biologic width."[47] Although it has been suggested that measurements of the biologic width were somewhat consistent,[48] clinical experience supports the concept that this subcrevicular dimension varies from patient to patient and from tooth surface to tooth surface in the same patient.[49] This biologic width is three dimensional and may be invaded laterally as well as apically. Healthy unaltered crevices are quite shallow, especially in the anterior region,[50] which often leads the restorative dentist to encroach into this subcrevicular dimension.[51] Injuries may occur during tooth preparation, gingival retraction methods (Fig 14-5), during impression making, by the extrusion of luting materials as restorations are cemented, and by overextended restorations that are "sunk" into the gingiva to hide the margin.[52] The effects of these injuries may be reversible, but only if tissue is permitted to heal against smooth and acceptable tooth surfaces[53] and not against a restorative material.

Carnevale et al[54] reported in a retrospective study of 1,020 teeth, 510 of which were crowned, "precise crown margins located in a slightly subgingival position are not prejudicial to the health of the periodontium." It therefore appears that in order to avoid a negative tissue response, dental restorations that must be taken subgingivally should be intracrevicular (Figs 14-6a and b).[55] Intracrevicular restorations are those confined to the limits of the gingival crevice. The term *intracrevicular* is more accurate and descriptive than *subgingival*, which implies the restoration is apical to the gingival margin and does not specify where the restoration terminates. Intracrevicular restorative dentistry protects the periodontal structures and should be used where supragingival restorations are not to be used.[56] Supragingival restorations are relatively harmless to the adjacent tissues and are easier to impress,

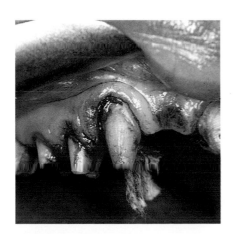

Fig 14-5 An example of an abusive restorative endeavor that extended well beyond limits to the gingival crevice but is still considered "subgingival."

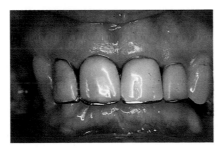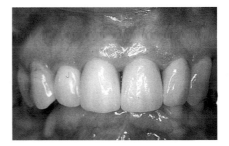

Figs 4-6a and b Four porcelain/metal crowns replacing gold-acrylic resin crowns. The margins are intracrevicular and the surrounding tissue is healthy.

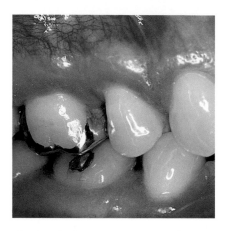

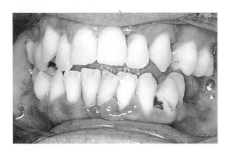

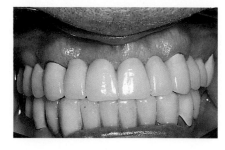

Figs 14-8a and b *Severely involved dentition demonstrating advanced periodontal disease. Unilateral function, occlusal trauma, and inadequate plaque control exacerbated the problem. Multiple extractions, periodontal surgery, and extensive restorations became necessary. In these instances, the patient must be informed that the activity state of periodontal disease may be unknown and consequently could affect the long-term prognosis.*

Fig 14-7 *Even restorations that are considered supragingival, such as the illustrated onlay, usually have margins that, at some surfaces, enter the gingival crevice.*

finish, and cleanse. However, many restorations have margins that enter the gingival crevice, if only at one or two tooth surfaces (Fig 14-7). There are legitimate reasons for such margins, including the removal of caries and existing restorations and the esthetic requirements of the patient. It is illusory at present to advocate that all restoration margins be supragingival.

PERIODONTAL DIAGNOSIS IN PLANNING RESTORATIVE THERAPY

The dilemma of determining the activity of the patient's periodontal disease is even more formidable if extensive restorative therapy is anticipated (Figs 14-8a and b). To date, a simple, economical, and accurate means of risk factoring remains elusive. In its absence, the evaluation of collected data coupled with good judgment must suffice in periodontal diagnosis.[57]

Circumferential probing is imperative to diagnosis, as are recordings of dimensions between the cementoenamel junctions and the apical depths of pockets.[58] Evaluation of plaque indices, furca involvements, and the ability of marginal tissue to withstand intracrevicular restorative care are especially significant to the restorative dentist. Sites of bleeding must be noted and compared with those observed after root planing and scaling. Root sensitivity also influences restorative treatment planning, as this may guide margin placement. Tooth mobility and whether it is increasing must also be scrupulously monitored.

Mounted casts are important in planning complex interdisciplinary treatment. Recent, good quality right-angle periapical radiographs are also necessary. Somewhat less helpful, but occasionally useful, are panographic radiographs.[59] Root shape and size, caries, bone-to-tooth and tooth-to-tooth interfaces, unexpected pathoses, and proximity of anatomical structures (maxillary sinus, mental foramen, mandibular canal, etc) should be carefully noted on radiographs before treatment is begun. An intellectual summary of conclusions drawn from these and other diagnostic tools must be integrated with the patient's health history, esthetic preferences, and perceived commitment prior to treatment.

CLINICAL APPLICATION

The clinical application of restorative dental treatment must be compatible with periodontal health. Sometimes, well-intentioned efforts to obtain an accurate impression, to hide a crown margin, or to reach and remove decay could permanently harm periodontal tissues. The clinical evidence of this damage may become apparent quickly or not for some years. Therefore, guidelines should be established that allow quality restorative care and at the same time would also protect the periodontium.

Before implementing final restorative dentistry, the total environment that is to surround the restoration must be evaluated. This evaluation should be ongoing, should be punctuated with appropriate reevaluation, and, with complex restorative care, should seldom take place at the first visit. Much can be learned from both tissue and patient reaction as early treatment evolves.

Whereas a simple supragingival restoration may require only periodontal health and sustained plaque control as restorative prerequisites, complex or multi-tooth restorations demand far more. Tooth proximity, the amount of attached gingiva, the depth of existing restorations, and many other factors affect restorative success.[60] The therapist must project how the anticipated restorations will influence, or will be influenced by, the restorative environment.

A PROPER RESTORATIVE ENVIRONMENT

A proper restorative environment is defined as the sum of those factors that enables a restoration to coexist in sustained health, comfort, and function with teeth and adjacent tissue. Components of a proper restorative environment include:

1. Adequate plaque control
2. Arrested dental caries
3. Proper nutrition
4. Periodontal health
5. Competence of marginal tissue
6. Tooth position / posture
7. Craniomandibular harmony
8. Adequate clinical crown
9. Nonpathogenic occlusion

Adequate Plaque Control

The level of patient plaque control must be carefully considered before any restorative treatment is begun. Judgment of plaque control should not only be made on the amount of plaque retained, but perhaps more importantly on where it is retained. A millimeter or less of recalcitrant retained plaque at the cervical area in an otherwise plaque-free mouth is both deceptive and damaging. The patient (or even the practitioner) may believe that plaque control is quite good; in reality that site is exquisitely susceptible to root caries and usually contributes to the potential of gingival and periodontal disease.[61-63]

Many patients may not fulfill a dentist's home care expectations in a few weeks or even in a few months. Large numbers of patients who remain in one's practice eventually respond very favorably to persuasive, persevering, and positive education. The dental hygienist is invaluable in this regard, especially if his / her primary mission is not viewed as root planing and scaling; more correctly, the role of the hygienist is to modify patient behavior. It may be stated, therefore, that although restorative care ideally should take place in a plaque-free mouth, evidence of substantial and ongoing improvement is often sufficient to initiate treatment.

Chlorhexidine mouthrinsing continues to be of singular benefit in controlling plaque.[64-66] In implementing complex restorative care, the patient receives a final session of root planing, scaling, and polishing, is placed on chlorhexidine rinses for 7 days, and is then scheduled for tooth preparation. If the patient has been reasonably compliant, the tissue surrounding the teeth to be prepared is far less hemorrhagic, friable, and inflamed. Continuation of chlorhexidine rinsing is also imperative at least during the succeeding 6 weeks after tooth preparation. The patient is informed of the associated staining, which is compensated for via polishing of the provisional restoration. As plaque is controlled, inflammation and tenderness are greatly diminished, as is the patient halitosis that is sometimes noticed with multiple acrylic resin interim restorations.

The use of tetracycline mixed in with a temporary cement was first suggested by P. K. Thomas during the 1960s.[67] Strictly from an empirical perspective, this technique seems to lessen plaque accumulation, tissue inflammation, and halitosis. The mechanism of this is speculative but may relate to the

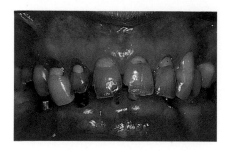
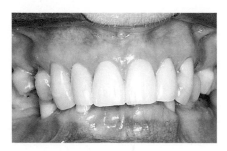
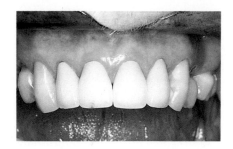

Figs 14-9a to c *This patient underwent placement of four individual porcelain/metal crowns. The provisional restorations are splinted together to withstand dislodgement. The final crowns have porcelain shoulders and have been designed to allow access for home hygiene care.*

benefits of gradual subgingival tetracycline release through a collagen-carrying agent.[68,69] Fluoride appears to have little value in reducing gingivitis.[70] Nonetheless, appropriate fluoride rinses are recommended during and after restorative treatment to diminish caries potential. To be effective, plaque control must take place before, during, and after restorative treatment. Interim and final restorations must be designed to allow access for home hygiene care (Figs 14-9a to c).[71,72]

Arrested Dental Caries

Because dental caries can lead to pulpal disease, pain, additional treatment and patient expense, and possibly tooth loss, intercepting these lesions should take priority in treatment planning. Arrest should be accomplished with materials that do not harm the periodontium; this rules out zinc oxide and eugenol provisional restorative materials, overcontoured aluminum shell crowns (Fig 14-10), and hastily fabricated acrylic resin provisional restorations.

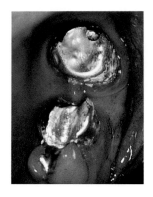

Fig 14-10 *Poorly contoured and hastily inserted aluminum shell provisional crowns. Soft tissue damage is inevitable.*

Proper Nutrition

In a review article, Walker and Cleaton-Jones[73] raise a question about the role of refined sugar in dental caries but conclude that "the overriding culpability of sugar continues to be asserted." The cariogenicity of refined sugar appears to be especially important in those patients who have diminished salivary flow. Long-term use of tobacco, a history of significant alcohol ingestion, Sjögrens syndrome, and the aging process all contribute to reduced salivation.[74] The most frequent culprit in dry mouth, however, is medication. Over 400 medications influence the flow or the

quality of saliva.[75] In patients who have exposed roots, a high intake of sugar, or a dry mouth, root caries becomes an ongoing problem. Therefore, nutrition counseling is necessary for the restorative patient, especially the patient taking certain medications. Great prudence should be taken with the patient who enters treatment with numerous restorations recently placed in the cervical area.

Periodontal Health

A healthy periodontium means different things to different people. To the purist, such an ideal may not exist. To the restorative dentist, it means one that has adequate alveolar support and pocket probing depths within normal limits and that lacks clinical signs of inflammation.

Periodontal health must precede final restorative treatment.[76] Debate continues as to whether pocket elimination is a reasonable goal before extensive restorative care. Although the judgment is empirically based, most restorative dentists would concur that pocket reduction is important.

Porphyromonas gingivalis (*Bacteroides gingivalis*), *Prevotella intermedia* (*Bacteroides intermedius*) and *Actinobacillus actinomycetemcomitans* have been implicated as pathogens in periodontal disease.[77-82] Various studies[83-88] have found that improved patient oral hygiene coupled with root planing and scaling have yielded reduced bleeding and improved levels of clinical probing depths at treated sites. This same therapy was found by VanWinkelhoff et al[89] and Loos et al[90] to reduce the counts of black-pigmented *Bacteroides* in periodontal pockets. Renvert et al[91] compared root planing and flap surgery and concluded that the procedures produced similar results in diminishing *A. actinomycetemcomitans*. Therefore, from the micropathologic perspective, reclamation of periodontal health by root planing or by flap surgery might seem to be equally acceptable for the restorative dentist.

Quite to the contrary, flap surgery appears imperative as a prerestorative prerequisite in mouths with periodontal disease. Various researchers[92-95] offer valid evidence that closed instrumentation in periodontal pockets does not remove all radicular calculus. Because all restorative margins that extend into the crevice accumu-

late plaque submarginally, it would appear that retained calculus on a tooth that is to receive a restoration should be avoided as it could accelerate the deposition of microbial flora. In addition, retained calculus exacerbates bleeding, which in turn interferes with impression accuracy and often produces inferior restorative margins. The periodontal implications of this are obvious.

Many patients with periodontitis who are to receive new restorations already have existing restorations that are faulty. These restorations may impede effective scaling and root planing and often present an additional indication for surgical flap procedures, often with some osseous reshaping. Moreover, the lengthened clinical crown that is attendant to pocket elimination procedures *(1)* allows restorative access for removal of caries and inadequate restorations, *(2)* offers opportunities for well-defined margins and therapeutically shaped restorations, and *(3)* provides additional retention. Consequently, most restorative dentists prefer some type of

surgical flap procedure as a prerestorative step in the periodontally involved dentition.

Competence of Marginal Tissue

When recession is arrested and no soft tissue pathosis is found, the amount of attached gingiva may be of little significance if no intracrevicular restorative treatment is planned. If such care is anticipated, the competence of the marginal tissue must be evaluated.[96]

When the external or superficial covering of the crevice is composed of alveolar mucosa, intracrevicular restorative margins may cause tissue recession.[97] (Because the soft tissue curbing of a tooth may either be alveolar mucosa or gingiva, the term *marginal tissue recession* is more appropriate than *gingival recession*.[98]) Intracrevicular restorative dentistry is traumatic to the crevicular epithelium in the best of circumstances.[99] The extent of that trauma is influenced by the competence of the marginal tissue (Figs 14-11a to c).[100]

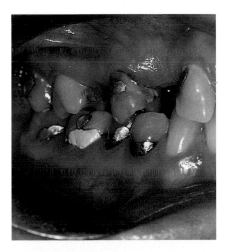
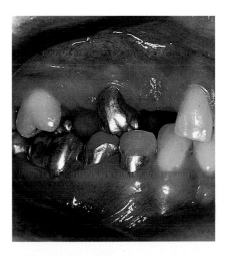
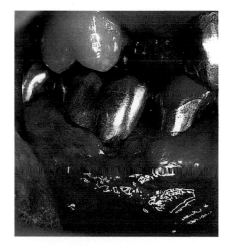

Fig 14-11a *Preoperatively, patient's mandibular first molar shows caries extending to the mucogingival junction.*

Figs 14-11b and c *A 3-year postoperative view shows marginal tissue recession coupled with root caries. Incompetent marginal tissue should have received a graft prior to restorative dentistry.*

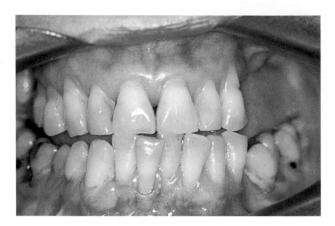

Fig 14-12a *Prerestorative view illustrates inadequate dimension of attached gingiva on facial surfaces of canines. Autogenous gingival grafts were done before restorative care was begun.*

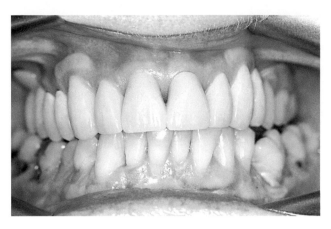

Fig 14-12b *Four-year postrestorative view.*

Crevices surrounded by an adequate dimension of attached keratinized tissue resist marginal tissue recession when subjected to insult; there also appears to be resistance to attachment loss.[101] Clinical judgment dictates that 2 or 3 mm of attached gingiva constitute an "adequate dimension." If that adequate dimension is lacking, the marginal tissue should be augmented, usually by an autogenous soft tissue graft (Figs 14-12a and b) but only if intracrevicular restorative dentistry is anticipated.

The establishment of competent marginal tissue should precede intracrevicular restorative dentistry by about 2 months. If a restoration is already present and ongoing marginal tissue recession is noted, an autogenous gingival graft should be done. Although obtaining a satisfactory esthetic result is not always predictable, incisal "creep" of the graft may occur, occasionally covering the restorative margin.

Tooth Position / Posture

The position of the tooth in the arch may prevent acceptable restorative dentistry. Teeth that are tilted, extruded, or are too close together make restorative care extremely difficult, impede patient plaque control, and usually diminish a good prognosis.[102] To overcome these problems, tilted teeth can be uprighted[103] and extruded teeth shortened, which occasionally requires endodontic therapy. Root proximity often requires tooth movement (eg, between maxillary first and second molars) or a combination of root resection and endodontic treatment, followed by full-coverage restorations.[104,105] Teeth with poor posture / position may not require intervention unless they play a role in restorative dentistry.

If the position of a tooth is not relatively stable, judgments must be made as to whether the mobility is increasing, whether the tooth is migrating, or whether the mobility is leading to food impaction or patient discomfort. Reduction of tooth mobility often follows scaling and root planing and elevation of plaque control, especially when combined with occlusal adjustment therapy. If mobility increases in spite of these efforts, joining the teeth together with restorations is usually indicated.

Craniomandibular Harmony

In the past, severe malocclusions were often addressed with compromised treatment. In 1927, Wassmund introduced a surgical procedure for moving the entire maxilla. The operation, since called a LeFort I osteotomy, was based on the work of Rene LeFort in 1901.[106] Since that time, surgical intervention linked with orthodontic treatment has created opportunities for greatly improved restorative and prosthetic results.[107] Patient desires for better esthetics, mastication, and self-image all have compelled continuing clinical research and new surgical techniques. As a consequence, profiles of patients can be improved and occlusal function and comfort can be significantly enhanced. However, time in therapy and expense continue to be impediments to patient acceptance.

In achieving craniomandibular

harmony, the sequencing of treatment is critical. Caries arrest, plaque control, and eliminating local factors contributing to periodontitis are implemented before either orthodontic or oral surgery care is started. Tooth movement in the presence of regularly scheduled supportive periodontal treatment is then initiated until intervention by the oral surgeon is deemed appropriate.[108] After 6 to 8 weeks, a stabilizing phase is followed by final tooth movement. Frequent monitoring and consultation with the restorative dentist for input regarding tooth posture and pontic spaces is important. The orthodontic appliance should be removed by the restorative dentist, and fixed or removable retention should be placed immediately; this minimizes the possibility of relapse. A stable occlusion in these cases is absolutely imperative. As with all complex cases, diagnosis and treatment planning must be thorough and well conceived. Haste leads to failure.

Adequate Clinical Crown

A tooth must have enough volume of clinical crown to support a restoration. In some cases this is achieved with a post / core or simply a core (Figs 14-13a to d).[109] In other instances, orthodontic ex-

trusion or surgical crown lengthening or a combination of these is indicated. These techniques increase the height of the clinical crown.

Caries, an existing faulty restoration, or a fractured tooth may not only affect the amount of coronal support but may also extend apically into connective tissue. In these instances, surgical extension of the clinical crown is imperative if apical overextension of the subsequent restoration is to be avoided.[110,111]

Unless abundant gingiva is present and accompanied by significant circumferential clinical, probeable depth (a rare occurrence indeed), surgical crown extension cannot be accomplished by removing soft tissue alone. Gingivectomy is virtually useless in crown extension procedures. The tissue merely rebounds to its approximate original height. If a restoration has been placed in the meantime, reattachment is impeded, plaque is retained, and inflammatory periodontal disease results. Surgical crown extension requires osseous resection (Figs 14-14a to c).[27,112,113]

Nonpathogenic Occlusion

There are several occlusal concepts, and most are successful. Care must be taken, however, not

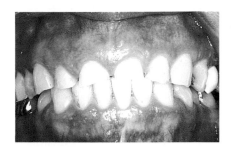

Fig 14-14a *Restorative therapy of a bulimic patient. Note the classic loss of tooth structure.*

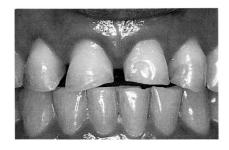

Fig 14-14b *In these instances, surgical crown extension is mandatory.*

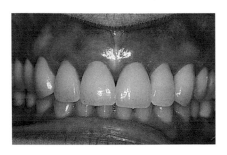

Fig 14-14c *Final restorations.*

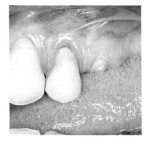 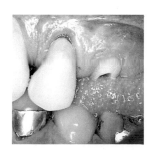 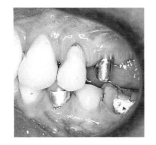 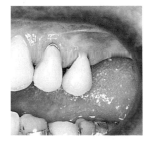

Figs 14-13a to d *Commonly encountered situation of a fractured tooth, requiring a post / core. Where little clinical crown volume is available, a cast post / core with a circumferential ferrule is mandatory to minimize the risk of root fracture that is so frequently observed with prefabricated posts.*

to impose one's own occlusal convictions on a comfortable and healthy dentition.

Prior to final restorative treatment, occlusal discrepancies that produce severe tooth mobility, fremitus, discomfort, gross deviations from the sagittal pathway, or balancing interferences should be eliminated. To accomplish these objectives, the recontouring of articulating surfaces of teeth, tooth movement, or even extraction may be necessary (see chapter 13). The recontouring of articulating surfaces, in turn, may be developed during the creation of a new restoration (Fig 14-15).

Frequently, a removable occlusal appliance is necessary prior to restorative treatment to allow the patient to return to a more relaxed mandibular position. With some completed restorative cases, patients should still wear a device nocturnally. The best of occlusions can be abused by the inveterate clencher — fractured porcelain,

broken solder joints, and even fractured teeth under full crowns are not infrequent in one who is a confirmed parafunctionist.

INTERIM RESTORATIONS

The quality of an interim restoration influences the longevity of the permanent restoration.[114] The fact that a restoration is temporary does not preclude that it may cause permanent damage. Gingival inflammation and also attachment loss can result from hastily shaped acrylic resin provisional crowns, aluminum shells with rough overextended margins, and temporary cement extruded into subcrevicular areas, even though these may be in place only a few weeks.

The interim restoration should protect both the dentogingival unit and the tooth. It should prevent the tooth from drifting or extruding. It should allow flossing without being dislodged and should not interfere with occlusal function (Figs 14-16a to c). In the anterior region, interim restorations should allow normal phonetics and should duplicate or improve upon prior esthetics.[115] The tongue and lip act as guides in the shaping of anterior restorations.

When interim restorations are removed, the surrounding tissue should be reasonably normal in appearance. Improperly constructed interim restorations can obviate the benefits of recently performed periodontal therapy. If multiple teeth are being restored with full-coverage restorations, some or all of these interim restorations should be luted together to enhance retention. However, care must be taken to avoid violating embrasure tissue and to allow access for personal oral hygiene.[116]

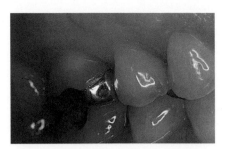

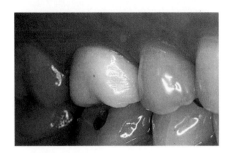

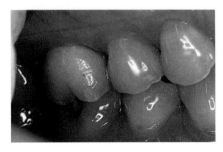

Figs 14-16a to c *Even single crowns require carefully shaped interim restorations, which maintain tooth position, prevent between-visit saliva leakage and discomfort, and enhance esthetics. The final crown has a porcelain shoulder.*

With maxillary full-coverage restorations, tooth preparation is followed by the interim restoration. The patient is reappointed at least 14 days later for impression making. This allows the marginal tissue to heal. If slight recession does occur, the clinician has the option to re-dress a facial margin. If the interim restoration reveals inadequate tooth reduction by temporary cement "showing

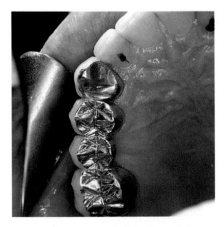

Fig 14-15 *Occlusal surfaces of restored teeth. Especially in the periodontally involved patient, occlusal contours have singular importance. Inappropriate occlusion can precipitate unacceptable trauma, patient discomfort, or damaging parafunction.*

through," these sites may be re-prepared as well, prior to final impressions.

Contours may also be examined and adjusted at the impression visit. The lower lip should govern the facial-incisal prominence of interim and final restorations. Excessive labial projections should also be adjusted if necessary. Once corrected, the lower lip will feel comfortable during function. The now properly shaped interim restoration may be photographed and impressed with irreversible hydrocolloid. Casts and photographs are sent to the laboratory technician as a guide. Otherwise, the dentist is totally dependent upon a technician to shape the patient's crowns, possibly resulting in final restorations that interfere with phonetics, esthetics, occlusion, or periodontal health.[117]

Impressions

Prepared teeth may be accurately impressed with a variety of materials and techniques. A clinician should be familiar with multiple impression methods. Impressions should not permanently damage the dentogingival unit. To ensure that the margin of the prepared tooth will be captured, some tooth structure slightly beyond the margin should be observed in the impression. This also gives the technician guidance relative to the emergence profile. Impression accuracy must not be hindered by bleeding in the crevice. Guesswork concerning the margin on the die then becomes inevitable.

A poorly contoured, rough interim restoration or poor patient plaque control may elicit bleeding. Reshaping and polishing of the interim restoration coupled with postponement of the impression may be necessary. Uncon-

trollable bleeding may also be caused by apical or lateral over-extension of rotary instruments into the subcrevicular connective tissue during the preparation visit. Bleeding from minor laceration of the crevicular epithelium is routinely arrested with retraction cords. Retraction with epinephrine-impregnated cords is no longer acceptable or necessary, due to the potential of cardiovascular stress.

Imprudently placed retraction cords can cause severe damage to the dentogingival unit. In some cases, retraction cords have been forced 5 and 6 mm under connective tissue.[118] Gentle seating of the cord is imperative. A judiciously placed thin cord exposes the preparation margin and may be left in place during the impression, as it eliminates bleeding and ensures accuracy while being kind to soft tissue.[119]

FULL-COVERAGE RESTORATIONS

It is an intimidating and imposing challenge to completely restore the clinical crown of a tooth with porcelain, metal, or some combination of these. Few dentists appear to be daunted, however. The number of full crowns being done today per general dentist represents a tenfold increase in the number done 25 years ago.[120] Frequently observed inflammatory gingival and periodontal disease may be traceable to this impressive expansion in crown-and-bridge therapy.[121]

Although some crowns are responsible for soft tissue pathosis, many exist in harmony with their environment. Selecting the desirable qualities that are common denominators to successful crowns and emulating them as new ones

are created is fundamental to quality restorative care.

A successful full crown begins with a properly prepared tooth surrounded by competent and healthy tissue. Crown margins that enter the gingival crevice must be confined to the crevice. A crevice depth of 1 mm imposes far more restriction than does one of 3 mm. Ignorance of the crevice depth invites subcrevicular tooth preparation and margin placement. Classic "purple-itis" of the marginal tissue results, often resulting in eventual attachment loss (Figs 14-17a to e).

If the tooth is to be restored with a material that is 1.5 mm thick, that tooth must be reduced at least 1.5 mm. The tooth must be "retracted" from the surrounding tissue and from adjacent and articulating teeth to allow for this thickness. The final crown must replicate or improve upon original tooth form. In most maxillary anterior porcelain/metal crowns, the facial-cervical margins should have porcelain shoulders.[122] This margin has no metal at the facial/tissue interface (Fig 14-18), is esthetically pleasing, and offers a high-quality fit,[123] especially if the shoulder is hand-planed.[124] It also allows a lingual surface of metal to function against an opposing tooth, thereby obviating frequently observed wear of opposing teeth. Because this restoration has no facial metal collar to "hide," it is not necessary to place the margin deep into the crevice. An extension of 0.5 mm beyond the entrance to the crevice is usually all that is required (Figs 14-19a and b). This same margin is also used in the all-ceramic crown,[125] which is the most esthetically acceptable crown but has a few material shortcomings, indicating that further research is needed.[126]

When operator preference dictates a porcelain/metal crown

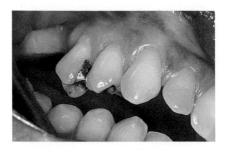

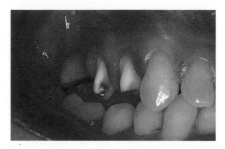

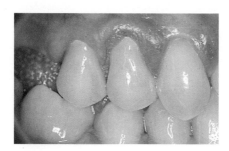

Figs 14-17a and b   *Result of apical overextension of a restoration. The preoperative view shows the fractured first premolar and the defective restoration on the second. The preparation view shows deep overextension.*

Fig 14-17c   *Two-year posttreatment view.*

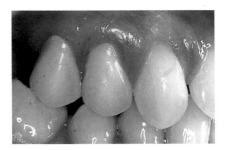

Fig 14-17d (left)   *Seven-year posttreatment view.*

Fig 14-17e (right)   *A 6-mm attachment loss is shown — the only periodontal pathosis in the entire mouth.*

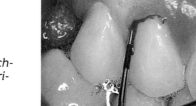

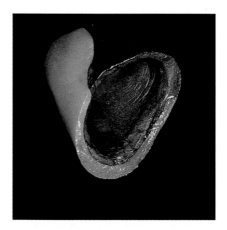

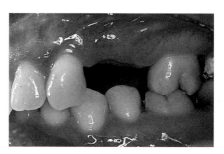

Figs 14-19a and b   *Four-unit bridge with canine retainer showing porcelain shoulder. The shallow crevice militated against a metal collar "sunk" into subcrevicular connective tissue.*

Fig 14-18   *Internal view of a porcelain/metal crown with a porcelain shoulder. The metal lingual surface minimizes wear of opposing teeth. The width of the porcelain shoulder should be approximately 1 to 1.5 mm.*

with a metal collar, care must be taken that the junction of the porcelain and the metal not display a "hump." Otherwise, plaque will accumulate there as well as at the terminus of the collar, where the unavoidable minute amount of plaque that is submarginal in all restorations exists.[127] Often, this duality of plaque growth is the cause of restoration-induced gingivitis, even in well-fitting crowns.

All crown margins should be supragingival or intracrevicular. The concept that a tooth preparation should be finished just to the attachment is conceivable, but only intellectually. It is unrealistic to expect that the tip of a diamond or bur rotating at speeds in excess of 400,000 rpm within a crevice and in the presence of a water spray be placed exactly at the attachment level. Some advocate that intracrevicular tooth preparation be preceded by the placement of one, thin retraction cord or suture in the crevice.[128] If this technique is used, prudence is required relative to the vigor of the cord placement.

Periodontal therapy may result in "long teeth." The length of these clinical crowns and the exposure of root concavities and furcations usually alter classic tooth preparation concepts. Provided appearance is not an issue, shoulder or shoulder-with-bevel preparations may not be necessary and may even be contraindicated due to the potential of pulpal exposure. Metal collars of a millimeter or more may be used to allow a gradual sloping of the restoration from the gingiva to the incisal edge and to provide room for the cosmetic material where it would be noticeable.

Teeth that have been sectioned require an untraditional preparation,[129-132] and access for cleansing is paramount. Few endeavors in dentistry challenge the clinician as do the requirements of full-coverage preparation. Only the neophyte and the unconcerned believe it to be simple.

COMPOSITE RESIN RESTORATIONS

Composite resin restorations are esthetically pleasing, functional, and widely used in our profession. However, leakage, contraction, and margin gaps continue to be troublesome.[133] Contraction perpendicular to the walls of the preparation, which may reach a value almost three times that of linear shrinkage,[134] may cause tooth discomfort. As cusps are pulled toward each other, stress occurs in both enamel and dentin, which precipitates low-grade pain.[135] This is increased with occlusal loading.

Margin leakage of Class II composite resin restorations seems about the same with bulk placement as with incremental placement.[136] Leakage at the cervical area may be more noticeable because the enamel is thin, and these areas often exhibit plaque retention.

In one study of 60 Class II composite resin restorations in children, clinical evaluation showed success, whereas radiographs revealed gingival margin defects in 40% of the restorations. The conclusions were that tooth preparation, contamination of the field, and difficulty of condensation at the gingival seat were primarily the causes of failure. Clinical examination may not detect early failure in these restorations, especially in the embrasure area.[137]

Composite resin inlays/onlays that are cured extraorally mitigate a number of the current shortcomings inherent in the intraoral cured composite resins.[138] The former allow proper contact areas and smoothly polished surfaces and decrease the contraction problem. However, these restorations have a higher cost and, if a laboratory is involved, an extra visit for the patient.

Regrettably, a great many Class II and Class V composite resin restorations that are cured intraorally demonstrate inadequate margins and plaque retention.[139-140] Marginal and interproximal tissue inflammation is often observed.

PORCELAIN LAMINATE VENEERS

As the profession has evolved, it has become apparent that new materials must still be applied within the existing guidelines of biologic health. Porcelain laminate veneers restore esthetics quite well and usually extend into the gingival crevice only slightly (Figs 14-20a and b). However, if the margins are open, bulky, or overextended, they will create the same circumadjacent inflammation noted with other inadequate restorations. Also, the porcelain laminate veneer restoration is very technique-sensitive. Patient selection is critical. Diastemata may be closed somewhat with these restorations, but prognoses are diminished due to the lateral extension of unsupported porcelain.[141] Clinical experience will reveal much about these innovative but still untested-by-time restorations.

AMALGAM RESTORATIONS

Still the profession's most commonly used restorative material, silver amalgam alloy is economical, is not technically demanding, and is relatively long-lasting. Even when used for large restorations, the material can be shaped to duplicate tooth form (Figs 14-21a and b). Efforts to avoid interproximal overhangs require firm and careful wedging. Unfortunately, the more conscientious the wedging, the more likely the trauma to interproximal tissue. Frequently, this results in irreparable damage to the COL and loss of the papilla with ensuing lateral food impactions. Small, difficult to detect overhangs are often left in interproximal concavities of posterior

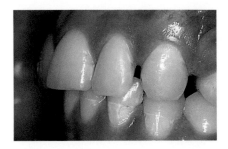

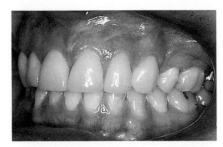

Figs 14-20a and b Appropriately implemented porcelain laminate veneers.

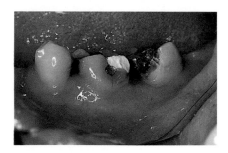

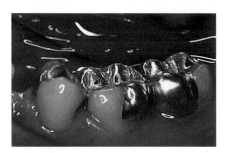

Figs 14-21a and b Properly contoured and finished amalgam restorations.

teeth, especially on the mesial and distal surfaces of maxillary molars. Floss is not adequate in these instances to remove such overhangs. Thin curets or scalers are most effective but must be used before the material is finally set.

RESTORATION OF ENDODONTICALLY TREATED TEETH

The increasing use of endodontic treatment leaves the dentist with a difficult legacy. Endodontically treated teeth often have a minimal amount of tooth structure coronal to the alveolar bone, making them susceptible to fracture. These fractures may be supragingival, may extend into connective tissue, or may even split the tooth

to the apex. Restorations for these teeth should strive for adequate retention; more importantly, they should be designed to protect the tooth from fracture. Therefore, amalgam, resin, or ionomer cores retained by pins, posts that extend into canals, or a combination should only be used if the circumferential clinical crown has 3 mm or more of height. If the clinical crown is shorter, a cast post/core with a ferrule encompassing the circumference of the tooth is mandatory.

Extending posts deep into molar roots, especially those with significant mesial and distal concavities, should be avoided. These posts often create root fracture or perforations and consequent tooth loss. In mandibular molars, there is usually enough of the coronal portion remaining to sup-

port an amalgam core extending less than 2 mm into each canal. These molar cores are usually successful and offer conservative solutions for the root perforation or root fracture problem.

In teeth that have been previously restored with full crowns, access through a porcelain occlusal surface remains a problem. Fracturing, chipping, and crazing are seen frequently, especially in the all-ceramic crown.[142] It is strongly suggested that endodontically treated existing crowns receive a metal post/core as soon as possible after the endodontic treatment is completed. The use of a cast glass ceramic post/core has been proposed to supply missing tooth structure under porcelain crowns subsequent to endodontic therapy.[143] Its ability to resist fracture has yet to be evaluated.

QUICK REVIEW

Microbial flora and the character of host response constitute the most important factor in the cause and progress of inflammatory periodontal disease. Restorative dentistry may be the second most important factor.

Rough, hasty, and ill-conceived procedures coupled with open and apically overextended margins and poor restorative contours all contribute to gingival and periodontal disease. The symbiotic support of a restoration and its surrounding tissues must lead to mutual and long-term health, function, and comfort. The chapter suggests guidelines for restorative dental care that defend and sustain the integrity of the dentogingival unit.

I. Current concepts
- **Morphology.** Restorations should defend the integrity of the dentogingival unit by duplicating physiologic tooth profiles and by allowing for proper home oral hygiene.
- **Margin quality.** The margins of restorations should be smooth and not catch dental floss, should demonstrate no voids, openings or overhangs and should not diminish in quality with time.
- **Margin location.** Those restoration margins that enter the gingival crevice should be confined to that crevice, as apical overextension frequently causes or contributes to inflammatory periodontal disease.

- **Periodontal diagnosis in planning restorative therapy.** For those patients requiring both periodontal and restorative care, the evaluation of the periodontium and of the teeth should precede final restorative treatment and should use all diagnostic tools currently available.

II. Clinical application
- **A proper restorative environment.** Complex or multitooth restorations require far more than periodontal health and plaque control as treatment prerequisites.
- **Interim restorations.** The objectives of an interim restoration are more demanding than merely covering and protecting tooth structure.
- **Full-coverage restorations.** Only the neophyte or the unconcerned believe that high-quality full-coverage restorations are quickly and easily achieved.
- **Composite resin restorations.** Esthetically pleasing, functional and widely used, these restorations nevertheless continue to raise clinical concerns.
- **Porcelain laminate veneers.** Technically demanding and esthetically excellent, porcelain laminate veneers are still maturing as a restoration
- **Restoration of endodontically treated teeth.** When restoring the endodontically treated tooth, the potential of root perforation, tooth fracture, and inadequate retention leave the restorative dentist with multiple dilemmas.

REFERENCES

1. Leon AR: The periodontium and restorative procedures: A critical review. *J Oral Rehabil* 1977;4:105-117.
2. Schroeder HE, Listgarten MA: Fine structure of the developing epithelial attachment of human teeth. *Monogr Dev Biol* 1971;2:1-134.
3. Stahl SS: Speculations on periodontal attachment loss. *J Clin Periodontol* 1986;13:1-5.
4. Abbas F, van der Velden U, Moorer WR, Everts V, Vroom TM, Scholte G: Experimental gingivitis in relation to susceptibility to periodontal disease. II. Phase-contrast microbiological features and some host-response observations. *J Clin Periodontol* 1986;13:551-557.
5. Campbell SD: Evaluation of surface roughness and polishing technique for new ceramic materials. *J Prosthet Dent* 1989;61:563-568.
6. Brunsvold MA, Lane JJ: The prevalence of overhanging dental restorations and their relationship to periodontal disease. *J Clin Periodontol*

1990;17:67-72.

7. Wilson RD, Maynard JG: The relationship of restorative dentistry and periodontics. In: Clark JW, et al, eds. *Clinical Dentistry*. New York: Harper and Row, 1983.

8. Parkinson CF: Excessive crown contours facilitate endemic plaque niches. *J Prosthet Dent* 1976;35:424.

9. Amsterdam M, Abrams L: Provisional splinting — principles and techniques. *Dent Clin North Am* 1964;3:73-99.

10. Boner C, Boner N: Restoration of the interdental space. *Int J Periodont Rest Dent* 1983;3(2):30.

11. Nevins M: Interproximal periodontal disease — The embrasure as an etiologic factor. *Int J Periodont Rest Dent* 1982;2 (6):8.

12. Stein RS, Kuwata M: A dentist and a dental technologist analyze current ceramo-metal procedures. *Dent Clin North Am* 1977;21:729.

13. Trott JR, Sherkat A: Effect of Class II amalgam restorations on health of the gingiva: A clinical survey. *J Can Dent Assoc* 1964;30:766-770.

14. Kay HB: Esthetic considerations in the definitive periodontal prosthetic management of the maxillary anterior segment. *Int J Periodont Rest Dent* 1982;2(3):44.

15. Kay HB: Criteria for restorative contours in the altered periodontal environment. *Int J Periodont Rest Dent* 1985;5(3):42-63.

16. Weisgold A: *Coronal Forms of the Full Crown Restoration — Their Clinical Applications*. Chicago: Quintessence Publ Co, 1981.

17. Maynard JG, Wilson RD: Attached gingiva and its clinical significance. In: Prichard JF, ed. *The Diagnosis and Treatment of Periodontal Disease in General Dental Practice*. Philadelphia: WB Saunders, 1979.

18. Löe H: Reactions of marginal periodontal tissues to restorative procedures. *Int Dent J* 1968;18:759-778.

19. Abbate MF, Tjan AH, Fox W: Comparison of the marginal fit of various ceramic crown systems. *J Prosthet Dent* 1989;61:527-531.

20. Tullberg A: An experimental study of the adhesion of bacterial layers to some restorative dental materials. *Scand J Dent Res* 1986;94:164-173.

21. Sorensen JA: A rationale for comparison of plaque-retaining properties of crown systems. *J Prosthet Dent* 1989;62:264-269.

22. Tarnow D, Stahl SS, et al: Human gingival attachment responses to subgingival crown placement. Marginal remodelling. *J Clin Periodontol* 1986;13:563-569.

23. Keszethelyi G, Szabo I: Influence of Class II amalgam fillings on attachment loss. *J Clin Periodontol* 1984;11:81-86.

24. Gilmore N, Sheiham A: Overhanging dental restorations and periodontal disease. *J Periodontol* 1971;42:8-12.

25. Burch JG, Garrity T, Schnecker D: Periodontal pocket depths related to adjacent proximal tooth surface conditions and restorations. *J Kentucky Dent Assoc* 1976;28:13-18.

26. Hakkarainen H, Ainamo J: Influence of overhanging posterior tooth restorations on alveolar bone height in adults. *J Clin Periodontol* 1980; 7:114-120.

27. Than A, Duguid R, McKendrick A: Relationship between restorations and the level of the periodontal attachment. *J Clin Periodontol* 1982;9:193-202.

28. Lervick T, Riordan P, Haugejorden O: Periodontal disease and approximal overhangs on amalgam restorations in Norwegian 21 year olds. *Community Dent Oral Epidemiol* 1984;12:264-268.

29. Coxhead LJ: Amalgam overhangs: A major cause of periodontal disease. *New Zealand Dent J* 1987;82:99-101.

30. Claman L, Koidis P, Burch J: Proximal tooth surface quality and periodontal probing depth. *J Am Dent Assoc* 1986;113:890-893.

31. Waerhaug J: Effect of rough surfaces upon gingival tissue. *J Dent Res* 1956;35:323-325.

32. Highfield JE, Powell RN: Effects of removal of posterior overhanging metallic margins of restorations upon the periodontal tissues. *J Clin Periodontol* 1978;5:169-181.

33. Jeffcoat MK, Howell TH: Alveolar bone destruction due to overhanging amalgam in periodontal disease. *J Periodontol* 1980;51:599-602.

34. Lang NP, Kiel RA, Anderhalden K: Clinical and microbiological effects of subgingival restorations with overhanging and clinically perfect margins. *J Clin Periodontol* 1983; 10:563-578.

35. Wilson RD: Fundamental restorative dentistry. *Tennessee Dent J* 1988; 68(2):35-38.

36. McLean JW: Long-term esthetic dentistry. *Quintessence Int* 1989;20:701-708.

37. Phillips RW, Jendresen MD, Klooster J, McNeil C, Preston JD, Schallhorn RG: Report of the committee on scientific investigation of the American Academy of Restorative Dentistry. *J Prosthet Dent* 1990;64:74-110.

38. Sheth JJ, Jensen ME, Sheth PJ, Versteeg J: Effect of etching glass-ionomer cements on bond strength to composite resin. *J Dent Res* 1989;68:1082.

39. Thomas M, Wickens J: Microleakage of resin-retained porcelain veneers (abstract). *J Dent Res* 1989;68:590.

40. Staninec M, Giles WS, Saiku JM, Hattori M: Caries penetration and cement thickness of three luting agents. *Int J Prosthodont* 1988; 1:259-263.

41. Van Zeghbroeck LM, Feilzer AJ, Davidson CL, et al: Spontaneous failure of glass ionomer cements (abstract). *J Dent Res* 1989;68:613.

42. Van Zeghbroeck LM, Davidson CL, DeClercq M: Cohesive failure due to contraction stress in glass ionomer luting cements (abstract). *J Dent Res* 1989;68:1014.

43. Charbeneau GT, Klausner LH, Brandau HE: Glass ionomer cements in dental practice: A national survey (abstract). *J Dent Res* 1988;67:283.

44. Wilson AD: Developments in glass-ionomer cements. *Int J Prosthodont* 1989;2:438-446.

45. Hansen EK, Asmussen E: Efficacy of dentin-bonding agents in relation to application technique. *Acta Odontol Scand* 1989;47:117.

46. Hansen EK, Asmussen E: Marginal adaptation of posterior resins: Effect of dentin-bonding agent and hygroscopic expansion. *Dent Mater* 1989;5:122.

47. Ingber JS, Rose LF, Coslet TG: The "biologic width" — a concept in periodontics and restorative dentistry. *Alpha Omegan* 1977; 70(3):62-65.

48. Garguilo AW, Wentz FM, Orban B: Dimensions and relations of the dentogingival junction in humans. *J Periodontol* 1961;32:261.

49. Maynard JG, Wilson RD: Physiologic dimensions of the periodontium significant to the restorative dentist. *J Periodontol* 1979;50:170-174.

50. Dragoo MR, Williams GB: Periodontal tissue reactions to restorative procedures. *Int J Periodont Rest Dent* 1981;1(1):8-23.

51. Wilson RD: Restorative dentistry and total oral health, advances in tissue management. ADA "Emphasis" Series. *J Am Dent Assoc* 1985; 111(4):550-564.

52. Wilson RD, Maynard JG: The relationship of restorative dentistry to periodontics. In: Prichard JF, ed. *The Diagnosis and Treatment of Periodontal Disease in General Dental Practice*. Philadelphia: WB Saunders Co, 1979.

53. Newcomb GM: The relationship between the location of subgingival crown margins and gingival inflammation. *J Periodontol* 1974;45:151-154.

54. Carnevale G, de Febo G, Fuzzi MA: A retrospective analysis of the perio-prosthetic aspect of teeth re-prepared during periodontal surgery. *J Clin Periodontol* 1990;17:313-316.

55. Nevins M, Skurow HM: The intracrevicular restorative margin, the biologic width, and the maintenance of the gingival margin. *Int J Periodont Rest Dent* 1984;4(3):30-49.

56. Wilson RD, Maynard G: Intracrevicular restorative dentistry. *Int J Peri-*

odont Rest Dent 1981;1(4):34-49.

57. Lytle JD, Skurow H: An interdisciplinary classification of restorative dentistry. *Int J Periodont Rest Dent* 1987;7(3):8-41.

58. Rosenberg MM, Kay HB, Keough BE, Holt RL: *Periodontal and Prosthetic Management for Advanced Cases.* Chicago: Quintessence Publ Co, 1988.

59. Prichard JF: *Advanced Periodontal Disease; Surgical and Prosthetic Management.* 2nd ed. Philadelphia: WB Saunders Co, 1972:142-196.

60. Amsterdam M: Periodontal prosthesis. Twenty-five years in retrospect. *Alpha Omegan* 67(3):8-52.

61. Sanz M, Newman MG: Dental plaque and calculus. In: Newman MG, Nisengard R, eds. *Basic and Applied Oral Microbiology and Immunology.* Philadelphia: WB Saunders Co, 1988.

62. Page RC, Schroeder HE: *Periodontitis in Man and Other Animals. A Comparative Review.* Basel, Switzerland: S. Karger, 1982.

63. Beck JD, Hunt RJ, Hand JS, Field HM: Prevalence of root coronal caries in a noninstitutionalized older population. *J Am Dent Assoc* 1985;111:964-967.

64. De Paola LG, Overholser CD, Meiller TF, Minah GE, Niehaus C: Chemotherapeutic inhibition of supragingival dental plaque and gingivitis development. *J Clin Periodontol* 1989;16:311-315.

65. Gjermo P: Chlorhexidine and related compounds. *J Dent Res* 1989; 68:1602-1608.

66. Southard SR, Drisko CL, Killoy WJ, Cobb CM, Tira DE: The effect of 2% chlorhexidine digluconate irrigation on clinical parameters and the level of *Bacteroides gingivalis* in periodontal pockets. *J Periodontol* 1989;60:302-309.

67. Thomas PK: Lecture Series, Medical College of Virginia, 1963.

68. Minabe M, Takeuchi K, Tomomatsu E, Hori T, Umemoto T: Clinical effects of local application of collagen film — immobilized tetracycline. *J Clin Periodontol* 1989;16:291-294.

69. Minabe M, Takeuchi K, Tamura T, Hori T, Umemoto T: Subgingival administration of tetracycline on a collagen film. *J Periodontol* 1989; 60:552-556.

70. Wolff LF, Pihlstrom BL, Bakdash MB, Aeppi DM, Brand CL: Effect of toothbrushing with 0.4% stannous fluoride and 0.22% sodium fluoride gel on gingivitis for 18 months. *J Am Dent Assoc* 1989;119:283-289.

71. Amsterdam M, Fox L: Provisional splinting — Principles and techniques. *Dent Clin North Am* 1959;3:73-79.

72. Reider CE: Use of provisional restorations to develop and achieve esthetic expectations. *Int J Periodont Rest Dent* 1989;9:123-139.

73. Walker AR, Cleaton-Jones PE: Sugar intake and dental caries: Where do we stand? *J Dent Child* 1989;56:30-35.

74. Tseng CC, Wolff LF, Rhodus N, Aeppli DM: The periodontal status of patients with Sjögrens syndrome. *J Clin Periodontol* 1990;17:329-330.

75. Atkinson JC, Fox PC: Clinical pathology conference: Xerostomia. *Gerodont* 1986;2:193-197.

76. Waerhaug J, Philos D: Periodontology and partial prosthesis. *Int Dent J* 1968;18:101-107.

77. Zambon JJ, Christersson LA, Slots J: *Actinobacillus actinomycetemcomitans* in human periodontal disease: Prevalence in patient groups and distribution of biotypes and serotypes within families. *J Periodontol* 1983;54:707-711.

78. Tanner AC, Goodson JM: Sampling of microorganisms associated with periodontal disease. *Oral Microbiol Immunol* 1986;1:15-20.

79. Dzink JL, Tanner AC, Haffajee AD, Socransky SS: Gram-negative species associated with active destructive periodontal lesions. *J Clin Periodontol* 1985;12:648-659.

80. Slots J: Bacterial specificity in adult periodontitis. A summary of recent work. *J Clin Periodontol* 1986; 13:912-917.

81. Slots J, Bragd L, Wikstrom M, Dahlen G: The occurrence of *Actinobacillus actinomycetemcomitans*, *Bacteroides gingivalis* and *Bacteroides intermedius* in destructive periodontal disease in adults. *J Clin Periodontol* 1986;13:570-577.

82. Haffajee AD, Dzink JL, Socransky SS: Effect of modified Widman flap surgery and systemic tetracycline on the subgingival microbiota of periodontal lesions. *J Clin Periodontol* 1988;15:255-262.

83. Badersten A, Nilvéus R, Egelberg J: Effect of nonsurgical periodontal therapy. II. Severely advanced periodontitis. *J Clin Periodontol* 1984;11:63-76.

84. Lindhe J, Westfelt E, Nyman S, Socransky SS, Haffajee AD: Long-term effects of surgical/non-surgical treatment of periodontal disease. *J Clin Periodontol* 1984;11:448-458.

85. Loos B, Kiger R, Egelberg J: An evaluation of basic periodontal therapy using sonic and ultrasonic scalers. *J Clin Periodontol* 1987;14:29-33.

86. Nordland P, Garrett S, Kiger R, Vanooteghem R, Hutchens LH, Egelberg J: The effect of plaque control and root debridement in molar teeth. *J Clin Periodontol* 1987;14:231-236.

87. Ramfjord SP, Caffesse RG, Morrison EC, et al: Four modalities of periodontal treatment compared over five years. *J Periodont Res* 1987; 22:222-223.

88. Claffey N, Loos B, Gantes B, Martin M, Heins F, Egelberg J: The relative effect of therapy in periodontal disease on loss of probing attachment after root debridement. *J Clin Periodontol* 1988;15:163-169.

89. van Winkehoff AJ, Van der Velden U, De Graff J: Microbial succession in recolonizing deep periodontal pockets after a single course of supra and subgingival debridement. *J Clin Periodontol* 1988;15:116-122.

90. Loos B, Claffey N, Egelberg J: Clinical and microbiological effects of root debridement in periodontal furcation pockets. *J Clin Periodontol* 1988;15:453-463.

91. Renvert S, Wikstrom M, Dahlen G, Slots J, Egelberg J: On the inability of root debridement and periodontal surgery to eliminate *Actinobacillus actinomycetemcomitans* from periodontal pockets. *J Clin Periodontol* 1990;17:351-355.

92. Jones WA, O'Leary TJ: The effectiveness of in vivo root planing in removing bacterial endotoxin from the roots of periodontally involved teeth. *J Periodontol* 1978;49:337-342.

93. Waerhaug J: Healing of the dentoepithelial junction following subgingival plaque control. II. As observed on extracted teeth. *J Periodontol* 1978;49:119-134.

94. Rabbani GM, Ash MM, Caffesse RG: The effectiveness of subgingival scaling and root planing in calculus removal. *J Periodontol* 1981;52:119-123.

95. Stambaugh RV, Dragoo M, Smith DM, Carasa L: The limits of subgingival scaling. *Int J Periodont Rest Dent* 1981;1(5):30-41.

96. Nevins M: Attached gingiva — mucogingival therapy and restorative dentistry. *Int J Periodont Rest Den* 1986;6(4):9-27.

97. Kramer GM. *Periodontal Therapy.* St Louis: CV Mosby Co, 1980.

98. Wilson RD: Marginal tissue recession in general dental practice: A preliminary study. *Int J Periodont Rest Den* 1983;3(1):40.

99. Hall WB: *Pure Mucogingival Problems.* Chicago: Quintessence Pub Co, 1984.

100. Hangorsky J, Bissada NF: Clinical assessment of free gingival graft effectiveness on the maintenance of periodontal health. *J Periodontol* 1980;51:274.

101. Ericsson I, Lindhe J: Recession in sites with inadequate width of the keratinized gingiva. An experimental study in the dog. *J Clin Periodontol* 1984;11:95-103.

102. Miller TE: Orthodontic therapy for the restorative patient. Part II: The esthetic aspects. *J Prosthet Den* 1989;61:402-411.

103. Wagenberg BD, Eskow RN, Langer B: Orthodontics: A solution for the advanced periodontal or restorative problem. *Int J Periodont Rest Dent* 1986;6(6):36-45.

104. Eastman JR, Backmeyer J: A review of the periodontal, endodontic and prosthetic considerations in odontogenous resection procedures. *Int J Periodont Rest Dent* 1986;6(2):34-51.

105. Kastenbaum F: The restoration of the sectioned molar. *Int J Periodont Rest Dent* 1986;6(6):8-23.

106. Bell WH, Profitt WR, White RP: *Surgical Correction of Dento-facial Deformities.* Philadelphia: WB Saunders Co, 1980.

107. Vanarsdall R: American Academy of Crown & Bridge Prosthodontics, Chicago, 1990.

108. Marks MH: Tooth movement in periodontal therapy. In: Goldman HM, Cohen DW, eds. *Periodontal Therapy.* St Louis: CV Mosby Co, 1973.

109. Tjan AH, Chiu J: Microleakage of core materials for complete cast gold crowns. *J Prosthet Dent* 1989;61:659-664.

110. Parma-Benfenati S, Fugazzotto PA, Ruben MP: The effect of restorative margins on the postsurgical development and nature of the periodontium. Part I. *Int J Periodont Rest Dent* 1985;5(6):30-51.

111. Flores-de-Jacoby L, Zafiropoulous GG, Ciancio S: The effect of crown margin location on plaque and periodontal health. *Int J Periodont Rest Dent* 1989;9:197-205.

112. Carnevale G, et al: Soft and hard tissue wound healing following tooth preparation to the alveolar crest. *Int J Periodont Rest Dent* 1983;3(6):36.

113. Parma-Benfenati S, Fugazzotto PA, Ferreia PM, Ruben MP, Kramer GM: The effect of restorative margins on the postsurgical development and nature of the periodontium. Part II. Anatomical considerations. *Int J Periodont Rest Dent* 1986;6(1):65-75.

114. Shavell HM: Mastering the art of tissue management during provisionalization and biologic final impressions. *Int J Periodont Rest Dent* 1988;8(3):24-43.

115. Lowe RA: Esthetic restoration of the maxillary anterior region: A case report. *Int J Periodont Rest Dent* 1989;9:354-363.

116. Skurow HM, Nevins M: The rationale of the preperiodontal provisional biologic trial restoration. *Int J Periodont Rest Dent* 1988;8(1):8-29.

117. Lowe RA: The art and science of provisionalization. *Int J Periodont Rest Dent* 1987;7(3):64-73.

118. Bartlett JA: Impression techniques utilizing the mercaptan rubbers. In: Baum L, ed. *Advanced Restorative Dentistry: Modern Materials and Techniques.* Philadelphia: WB Saunders Co, 1973.

119. Schmitt SM, Brown FH: A rationale for management of the dentogingival junction. *J Prosthet Dent* 1989;62:381-385.

120. Gilliam R: Personal communication.

121. Douglas CW: Estimating periodontal treatment needs from epidemiological data. *J Periodontol* 1989;60:417-419.

122. Sozio R: Precision ceramometal restoration with facial butted margin. *J Prosthet Dent* 1977;37:517-521.

123. Ishii M, Satoh N: Fabrication of collarless porcelain fused to metal restorations without using a platinum matrix. *Int J Periodont Rest Dent* 1986;6(3):64-73.

124. Zena RB, Kahn Z, von Fraunhofer JA: Shoulder preparations for collarless metal ceramic crowns: Hand-planing as opposed to rotary instrumentation. *J Prosthet Dent* 1989;62:273-277.

125. Donovan T, Daftary F: Alternatives to metal ceramics. *J Can Dent Assoc* 1988;16:10-17.

126. McLean JW: Lectures to the American Academy of Crown and Bridge Prosthodontics. Chicago: American Academy of Crown and Bridge Prosthodontics, 1990.

127. Waerhaug J: Tissue reactions around artificial crowns. *J Periodontol* 1983;24:172-185.

128. Toffenetti F: La Conservativa — Manuale Atlante. 2nd ed. Milan: Instituto per la Communicazione Audio Visiva I.C.A., 1985.

129. Marin C, Carnevale G, De Febo G, Fuzzi M: Restoration of endodontically treated teeth with interradicular lesions before root removal and/or root separation. *Int J Periodont Rest Dent* 1989;9:143-157.

130. Baima RF: Considerations for furcation treatment. Part I: Diagnosis and treatment planning. *J Prosthet Dent* 1986;56:138-142.

131. Schmitt SM, Brown FH: The hemisected mandibular molar: A strategic abutment. *J Prosthet Dent* 1987;58:140-145.

132. Baima RF: Considerations for furcation treatment. Part III: Restorative therapy. *J Prosthet Dent* 1987;58:145-147.

133. Torstenson B, Oden A: Effects of bonding agent types and incremental techniques on minimizing contraction gaps around resin composites. *Dent Mater* 1989;5:218.

134. Feilzer AJ, De Gee AJ, Davidson CL: Increased wall-to-wall curing contraction in thin bonded resin layers. *J Dent Res* 1989;68:48.

135. Leinfelder K: Lectures to the American Academy of Crown and Bridge Prosthodontics. Chicago: American Academy of Crown and Bridge Prosthodontics, 1990.

136. Koenigsberg S, Fuks A, Grajower R: The effect of three filling techniques on marginal leakage around Class II composite resin restorations in vitro. *Quintessence Int* 1989;20:117.

137. Eidelman E, Fuks A, Chosack A: A clinical, radiographic and SEM evaluation of class 2 composite restorations in primary teeth. *Oper Dent* 1989;14:58.

138. Biederman JD: Direct composite resin inlay. *J Prosthet Dent* 1989;62:249-253.

139. McLean JW: Limitations of posterior composite resins and extending their use with glass ionomer cements. *Quintessence Int* 1987;18:517-529.

140. McLean JW, Powis DR, Prosser HJ, et al: The use of glass-ionomer cements in bonding composite resins to dentine. *Br Dent J* 1985;158:410-414.

141. Dickinson AJG, Moore BK, Harris RK, et al: A comparative study of the strength of aluminous porcelain and all-ceramic crowns. *J Prosthet Dent* 1989;61:297-304.

142. Sutherland JK, Teplitsky PE, Moulding MB: Endodontic access of all-ceramic crowns. *J Prosthet Dent* 1989;61:146-149.

143. Kwiatkowski S, Geller W: A preliminary consideration of the glass-ceramic dowel post and core. *Int J Prosthodont* 1989;2:51-55.

Mucogingival Surgery: Esthetic Treatment of Gingival Recession

C U R R E N T   C O N C E P T S by Henry H. Takei

C L I N I C A L   A P P L I C A T I O N by Laureen Langer / Burton Langer

---

CURRENT CONCEPTS
Historical review
A clinical opinion

CLINICAL APPLICATION
Pedicle graft
Autogenous free gingival graft
Subepithelial connective tissue
 graft for root coverage
Removal of restorations prior to
 grafting

Damaged root surfaces
Multiple wide recessions
Coverage of existing crown mar-
 gins
Ten most common mistakes in soft
 tissue grafting

QUICK REVIEW

REFERENCES

C U R R E N T   C O N C E P T S

HISTORICAL REVIEW

The predictable coverage of denuded roots with keratinized gingiva has been one of the goals in periodontal surgery for as long as surgery has been performed on the gingiva. In the early history of mucogingival surgery, the maintenance or gaining of attached, keratinized gingival tissue and concurrent problems of a shallow vestibular depth were managed by numerous surgical procedures. The problems of crestal bone resorption with bone denudation procedures[1,2] to gain keratinized gingiva were followed by other techniques such as the apically repositioned flap.[3]

The double flap technique[4] as advocated by Ochsenbein attempted to manage the twofold problems of gaining keratinized gingiva and deepening the vestibule. A three-part study by Bohannan[5-7] demonstrated that vestibular deepening (ie, denudation, periosteum retention, vestibular incision) using several techniques all presented results that were poor when evaluated months after the final healing. Corn[8] reported in 1962 that the periosteal separation technique presented a better result in maintaining vestibular depth. However, the large, open granulating wound and exposure of the crestal bone were negative aspects to this technique. Friedman and Levine[9]

in 1964 summarized the current status of mucogingival surgery by stating that the apically repositioned flap, frenotomy, the laterally repositioned flap, and the double flap were the most accepted forms of surgical procedures to either gain or maintain keratinized tissue and to deepen the vestibule. From these studies and reports it was evident that a predictable gain in keratinized, attached gingiva and the concurrent increase in vestibular depth could only be achieved by the use of a gingival graft.

Early Grafting Procedures

The early attempts to gain keratinized gingiva by grafting

procedures[10] involved either the root coverage attained by the lateral pedicle flap, as reported by Grupe and Warren[11] in 1956, or the addition of keratinized gingiva apical to the area of gingival recession. As early as 1966, Nabors[12,13] reported cases in which he used free gingival grafts for vestibular extension procedures and subsequently used a graft to gain attached gingiva and to cover denuded root surfaces. A series of reports by Sullivan et al[14-16] in the late 1960s gave the initial impetus to our current understanding of gingival grafting and eventually to the predictable covering of denuded root surfaces with gingiva. Their initial classification of the recipient site and description of the histology enabled us to better understand the clinical and histological aspects of the principles of gingival grafting. Increasing the zone of attached gingiva and the depth of the vestibular fornix along with the coverage of denuded root surfaces by the use of the free, autogenous, gingival graft is described in a summary report by Sullivan and Atkins.[17]

Sullivan and Atkins,[16] in their final report of a three-part study on free autogenous gingival grafting principles, stated that 1 to 2 mm of new tissue will survive over the apical avascular area of recession when a free gingival graft is used. This partial "take" is possible due to the collateral circulation from the three vascular areas adjacent to the apical area of recession. From these early studies several clinicians had reported[18] that root coverage was possible with free gingival grafts if there was adequate tissue lateral to the area of recession to provide collateral circulation for the graft.

As stated earlier, root coverage by means of pedicle grafts had been reported by Grupe and War-

ren as early as 1956.[11] The oblique rotated flap,[19] double papillae repositioned flap,[20] and coronally repositioned periodontal flap[21] are all modifications of the pedicle flap. They have the advantage of offering vital blood supply to the graft, which is placed over the avascular root surface. All of the pedicle grafts obviously have the shortcoming of the need for donor tissue, which may not always be available adjacent to the recipient site. It is at this juncture in the history of mucogingival surgery that connective tissue began to be considered as graft donor tissue.

Connective Tissue as Graft Material

The use of connective tissue beneath the keratinized epithelium as a graft material has been studied and attempted clinically by numerous investigators. Sullivan and Atkins[16] had stated that the use of a thick gingival graft resulted in the loss of the surface epithelial cells by desquamation and degeneration, but this is not important in the final outcome since the cells from the deeper portion will re-epithelialize the surface. Studies by other investigators[22-24] confirmed the initial findings of Sullivan and Atkins. These studies, as well as several others, state that the cells which dictate the type of epithelium that eventually re-epithelializes the surface are found in the underlying connective tissue or the basal epithelial cells at the epithelium-connective tissue junction. Edel[25] clinically evaluated the use of free connective tissue grafts in humans to increase the zone of attached gingiva. From this study, he also found that the information that dictates the type of epithelium which will eventually cover the recipient site is found in the connective tissue.

Since these early studies, Becker and Becker[26] have published a study on the use of connective tissue autografts to treat mucogingival problems successfully.

It was not until the early 1980s that several clinical findings were published[27-29] on predictable coverage of denuded root surfaces using free gingival grafts. Miller[27,29] emphasized the use of citric acid as a means to obtaining connective tissue attachment to the root surface. Recent studies by Bertrand and Dunlap[30] report good root coverage both with and without the use of citric acid application. Miller[31] also published a classification of marginal tissue recession. This classic classification provided the clinician with a guide to better predict the type of recession that can be covered, and it also placed root coverage on a sounder clinical basis for treatment (Fig 15-1). The classification emphasized the need for intact papilla and bone adjacent to the graft site to provide adequate collateral circulation to the graft. Even though the coverage of denuded roots using free gingival grafts became a predictable procedure, the gingival color and the open wound created on the palate in obtaining the donor tissue were drawbacks.

In 1985, Langer and Langer[32] published an important paper reporting a technique of using a free connective tissue graft placed between a split-thickness flap adjacent to and apical to the area of gingival recession. The blood supply to this double-sided donor tissue placed between the periosteum and the flap increases the collateral circulation. The possibility for the survival of the connective tissue over the avascular root surface is increased by this technique, which also provides a closed wound over the donor site. The gingival color match of the

Fig 15-1 *Miller's classification of gingival recession.*
I. *Recession not reaching the mucogingival junction. Complete root coverage is expected.*
II. *Recession past the mucogingival junction with no interproximal tissue loss. One hundred percent root coverage can be anticipated.*
III. *Recession with interproximal tissue loss, thus negating the chances for complete coverage.*
IV. *Severe recession and soft and hard tissue loss to the extent that root coverage should not be expected. (From Miller.[31] Reprinted with permission.)*

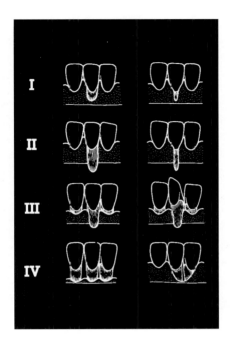

connective tissue to the adjacent gingiva is esthetically superior to that of a gingival graft. It is this technique that is most commonly used today in the treatment of root coverage. A modification of this technique published by Nelson in 1987[33] using a pedicle to cover the exposed connective tissue over the avascular root surface enhances the blood supply to this portion of the connective tissue. This bilaminar flap design incorporates the use of a double-sided blood supply donor tissue sandwiched between the split-thickness pedicle flap to cover and add another source of collateral circulation to that portion of the donor tissue covering the avascular root surface.

The present knowledge of root coverage techniques encompasses the contribution of numerous researchers and clinicians. The pioneers in this field have used past knowledge and experiences to continuously improve the techniques to allow us to predictably achieve a result that at one time was considered unpredictable.

A CLINICAL OPINION

The historical review of literature for mucogingival surgery as it pertains to increasing keratinized, attached gingiva, and the eventual evolution to covering denuded root surfaces is an interesting study of biological knowledge and technical skills coming together to produce predictable procedures that can enhance periodontal function and esthetics. The need for adequate blood supply to the donor tissue is the principle on which grafting procedure is based. Therefore, the early attempts at root coverage were based on pedicles such as lateral, coronal, or double papillae pedicle grafts. The blood supply at the base of the flap is the obvious source. It was not until the classic classification of Miller, published in the mid 1980s and indicating the clinical conditions necessary for successful grafting, that free gingival grafts were used for root coverage on a predictable basis.

There have been many refine-

ments to the initial use of free gingiva as the donor tissue. The use of free, subepithelial, connective tissue taken from beneath keratinized gingiva and the many changes in surgical design at the recipient site have allowed for increased blood supply to the donor tissue, therefore leading to a predictable result. The importance of suturing to accurately adapt and hold the donor tissue to the recipient area has been noted by numerous clinicians. The elimination of the "dead space" between the donor tissue and the recipient site by accurate and precise suturing and the selection of the proper type of donor tissue (free gingival or subepithelial connective tissue) has been emphasized to increase the chances for good root coverage. Recipient surfaces that may have concavities or convexities are better suited for "soft" donor tissue, such as the subepithelial connective tissue, since it better conforms to the irregular recipient site. The knowledge and application of these factors have been invaluable in the predictability of root coverage and the management of mucogingival problems.

On a day-to-day clinical use of root coverage procedures, the clinician must address many aspects of clinical problems. Color matching of the gingiva, donor site wound, vestibular depth, and anatomic contour of the recipient site are some of the factors to consider. For most of the situations encountered in practice, it has been the experience of this clinician that the use of the subepithelial, connective donor tissue used between a split-flap recipient area (as first published by Langer and Langer[32]) has been the most versatile and useful procedure of all grafting techniques. Obviously, where possible, the pedicle donor tissue should be used since this tissue best suits the adjacent tissue in color and offers the best blood supply and other factors necessary for successful grafting.

The Langer technique obviously is kinder to the donor area than a free graft since the tissue is removed from beneath the palatal flap and the donor area is closed with primary intention. The subepithelial, connective tissue is better esthetically in gingival color matching. The white, "tire patch-like" appearance, as sometimes seen with the free gingival graft, is not apparent with the subepithelial tissue. The lateral and apical portion of the subepithelial connective tissue has a "double-sided" connective tissue surface. This surface is sandwiched between the split-thickness recipient flap; thus the blood supply to the

donor tissue is increased twofold. Only that area of the donor tissue covering the denuded root surface is devoid of blood supply other than from the lateral and apical borders beneath the flap. From a histologic aspect, it may be possible that any attachment of the connective tissue of the donor tissue to the root surface is enhanced by using donor tissue, which is devoid of epithelium. This may eliminate or lengthen the time for epithelium to migrate between the root surface and the connective tissue, therefore reducing the chances of a long junctional epithelial attachment. It has been the experience of this clinician and several others in personal communication that the application of citric acid on the root sur-

face during the root coverage procedures has not made any appreciable difference on the result. There has been a difference of opinion amongst numerous clinicians regarding this interesting subject. Further research and long-term careful evaluation of clinical cases regarding the use or nonuse of citric acid is needed.

The progress made in clinical periodontal surgery as it applies to mucogingival problems has certainly advanced both in biologic knowledge and technical procedures. This progress may now be referred to as "periodontal plastic and reconstructive soft tissue surgery." The future is exciting and promising.

CLINICAL APPLICATION

Historically, indications for treatment of gingival recession consisted of halting progressive recession, enhancing plaque control, preserving a band of keratinized gingiva, decreasing frenum pull,[13,14,34] and preventing post-orthodontic[35,36] and post-prosthetic[37] marginal recession. Occasionally attempts were made to cover denuded roots for cosmetic purposes and to decrease root sensitivity.[11,20] However, total coverage of denuded roots remains a problem for most clinicians because the avascular nature of the root surface hampers the ability of most grafts to survive. Consequently, the wider the area of root exposure, the more difficult a problem for the clinician. The objective of any health professional is not only to arrest and cure a disease process but, if possible, to regenerate any lost tis-

sue. Such is the goal of root coverage procedures.

In daily clinical practice, decisions must be made to determine which procedures will best resolve the particular type of recession defect presented by the patient. In general, the anatomy of the area involved dictates the treatment. Following are several graft techniques.

PEDICLE GRAFT
(Figs 15-2a to d)

The first major breakthrough in root coverage procedures was the lateral sliding flap "pedicle graft." Narrow isolated mandibular recessions (Fig 15-2a) with adequate interproximal bone height and adequate keratinized adjacent donor tissue can be suc-

cessfully treated with a lateral sliding flap as described by Grupe and Warren.[11] This is a one-stage surgical procedure whereby a pedicle flap (Fig 15-2b) is elevated by split-thickness dissection from an adjacent area of keratinized tissue. The blood supply that nourishes the flap over the avascular root surface is supplied by the wide base of the flap and the underlying periosteum surrounding the denuded roots. The pedicle is secured in position over the denuded root with interrupted silk sutures (Fig 15-2c). The color blend and root coverage of an isolated defect in the mandibular anterior region is excellent (Fig 15-2d). However, in cases of wide isolated recessions or multiple recessions, the horizontal sliding flap has had limited success.

Fig 15-2a Preoperative condition. There is a labial dehiscence and cleft formation on the mandibular left central incisor and an accompanying mucogingival problem and a frenum pull. The adjacent tissue is healthy and an adequate band of attached keratinized gingiva is present. The vestibular fold is of adequate length to allow the lateral movement of tissue used in a horizontal sliding flap or pedicle graft.

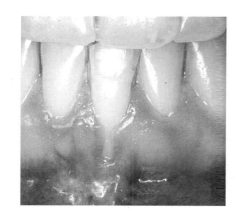

Fig 15-2b Initial incision — bed preparation. An incision is made one and a half teeth away from the defect. This is a rectangular partial-thickness flap whose base is angulated toward the mandibular left central incisor. This cutback allows easier mobilization of the pedicle graft toward the recipient site. Another incision is made around the perimeter of the defect on the mandibular left central incisor. This exposes the connective tissue and periodontal ligament space around the recipient site. The recipient root is planed to reduce some of its convexity in preparation for the pedicle.

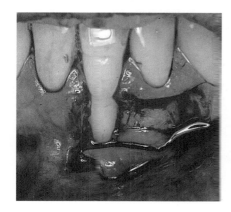

Fig 15-2c Suturing. The pedicle is positioned over the recipient labial defect and sutured into position with interrupted silk sutures. The pedicle should have minimal muscle pull after it has been secured in place.

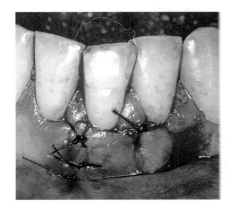

Fig 15-2d Six-year postoperative result. This shows a clinically healthy condition in which the defect over the mandibular left central incisor has been eliminated. There is an adequate band of attached keratinized gingiva and the frenum pull has been eliminated. The color blend is good and the root coverage is stable.

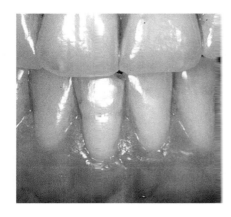

AUTOGENOUS FREE GINGIVAL GRAFT
(Figs 15-3a to c)

The autogenous free gingival graft introduced by Nabers in 1966[13] is designed to increase the width of keratinized gingiva. Unlike the pedicle graft, this procedure takes keratinized palatal connective tissue and epithelium away from its original site, the palate, and relocates it to a remote site. The tissue is placed over a freshly cut bed of connective tissue and sutured in place. Within approximately 4 days, the underlying connective tissue nourishes the graft until it rebuilds its own blood supply and thus survives and functions as keratinized gingiva.

Because this graft retains none of its own blood supply and is totally dependent upon the bed of recipient blood vessels, it was originally intended to change alveolar mucosa into keratinized gingiva, not specifically to cover denuded roots.[16] However, several excellent modifications have improved this procedure's root coverage capabilities. Maynard[38] developed two procedures: the initial placement of a free gingival graft to create a band of keratinized gingiva, followed by a second procedure in which the graft is pulled coronally. Holbrook and Ochsenbein[28] used thick, stretched, free gingival grafts with intricate suturing to improve the graft's adaptation to the recipient bed and limit the amount of dead space, which could hinder vascularization. Miller[27,29] emphasized root planing and thick butt-jointed free gingival grafts placed over denuded roots that had been treated with saturated citric acid burnished into the root for 5 minutes.

All of these modifications have improved the capability of free gingival grafts to survive over avascular root surfaces. But although coverage of wide-deep, wide-shallow, and multiple recessions has been improved greatly, the greatest success of the free gingival graft for root coverage remains on the mandible (Figs 15-3a to c) or on isolated maxillary teeth.

SUBEPITHELIAL CONNECTIVE TISSUE GRAFT FOR ROOT COVERAGE (Figs 15-4a to o)

The ridge augmentation procedure as described by Langer and Calagna[39,40] combined the positive features of the pedicle and free gingival graft to build out edentulous ridges. Its use was expanded by Langer and Langer[32] to

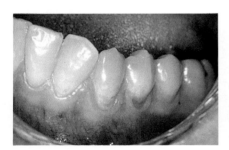

Fig 15-3a **Multiple shallow-wide recessions.** *Note minimal keratinized gingiva apical to the mandibular left canine and premolar with shallow-wide root denudations, which exhibited hypersensitivity.*

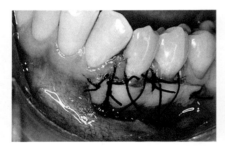

Fig 15-3b **Placement of thick free gingival graft.** *A thick butt-jointed autogenous free graft is placed on the prepared recipient bed and secured with three interrupted sutures coronally, which pass through the graft. The two circumferential sutures and the one vertical interdental suture do not pass through the graft. This suturing technique aids in adapting the graft to the undulating convexities and concavities of the area and promotes rapid revascularization.*

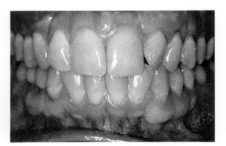

Fig 15-3c **Two-year postoperative result.** *The mandibular left canine and premolar were treated with a thick free gingival graft. The maxillary left lateral incisor, canine, and first premolar were treated with a subepithelial connective tissue graft on the same day. Note thickness and lighter color on the mandible.*

Figs 15-4a to o A 21-year-old woman presented with a chief complaint of extreme sensitivity to cold liquids, air, and toothbrush use bilaterally in the maxilla. The marginal gingiva of the maxillary right first and second premolars is erythematous due to her inability to cleanse the area adequately as well as to the subsequent plaque accumulation. On the maxillary left lateral incisor, canine, and first premolar, the prominent root position contributed to the pronounced recession.

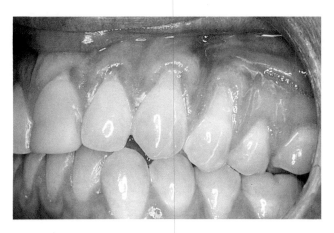

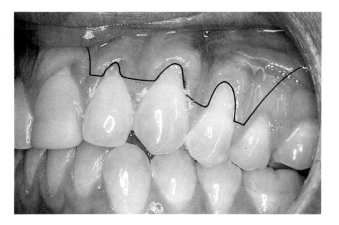

Fig 15-4a   Preoperative condition — maxillary left quadrant. *The wide-deep recessions as seen on the maxillary left canine and first premolar are best treated with the subepithelial connective tissue graft. The visible clinical recession is: lateral incisor = 2 mm x 2 mm, canine = 3 mm x 4 mm, first premolar = 5 mm x 4 mm.*

Fig 15-4b   Flap design — recipient site. *A horizontal incision is made at or incisal to the cementoenamel junctions of the involved teeth with a no. 15 scalpel, taking care not to lift the papillae. The horizontal incisions are connected by sulcular split-thickness incisions. The mesial and distal vertical incisions extend well beyond the mucogingival junction to create a wide base for the flap.*

Fig 15-4c   Flap elevation. *A split-thickness flap is elevated by sharp dissection using the 1 x 2 tissue forceps to lift a corner of the flap to create tension. Care must be taken not to perforate the flap as this will adversely affect the blood supply, which is the main source of nourishment to the future connective tissue graft. The recipient flap is freed apically so that there will be very little tension when pulled coronally. The actual or hidden recession is: lateral incisor = 5 mm x 3 mm, canine = 5 mm x 5 mm, first premolar = 7 mm x 4 mm. The size of the graft needed is determined by measuring the length of the recipient bed and the height. The graft must be large enough to cover the recession and the connective tissue bed in all directions, as this is the second source of blood supply to the overlying graft.*

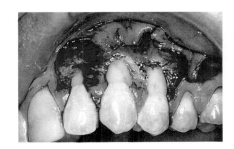

Fig 15-4d   Flap design — donor site. *Palatally, two horizontal beveled incisions are made with a no. 15 scalpel parallel and 3 mm apical to the free gingival margin of the posterior teeth from the canine to the first molar area. Since the graft is taken internally, the rugae are of no concern and the connective tissue is thicker and well vascularized in this area. A split-thickness flap is raised with or without vertical releasing incisions. A wedge of connective tissue 1.5 mm thick with its border of epithelium is dissected free, leaving the epithelialized flap to be replaced for primary intention wound closure. (CTG) connective tissue graft; (EPI) epithelium.*

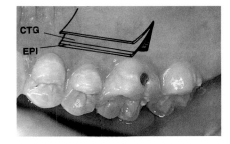

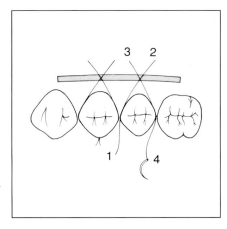

Fig 15-4e   Donor site suturing (diagram). *It is advisable to suture the palatal flap back into position immediately after taking the donor tissue; this will reduce the size of the blood clot, which might cause tissue necrosis. Hemostasis is best accomplished with horizontal mattress sutures which begin by (1) passing through a mesial interproximal space on the buccal surface, (2) penetrating the palatal mucosa apical and distal to the base of the graft site, (3) exiting the palate mesially, and (4) crossing to the distal interproximal space to be tied on the buccal surface.*

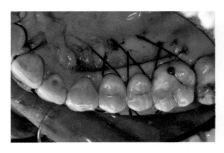

Fig 15-4f   Donor site suturing (clinical). *This method of suturing provides compression of the palatal flap, approximation of the wound edges, and hemostasis. Since there is no denuded palatal area, the patient reports less discomfort than with a free gingival graft and less bleeding problems. Dressing on the palate is optional.*

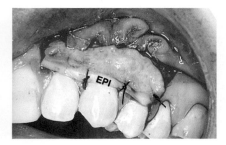

Fig 15-4g   Graft stabilization. *The subepithelial connective tissue graft measuring 7 mm x 20 mm x 1.5 mm is positioned over the denuded roots and stretched slightly to extend mesially and distally to cover the prepared bed. Next, 4-0 silk and a CE-2 atraumatic needle or chromic gut interrupted sutures can be used to secure the graft through the papillae interproximally. The thin border of epithelium left on the graft helps with the color blend and suturing and should be placed incisal to the cementoenamel junction. (EPI) epithelium.*

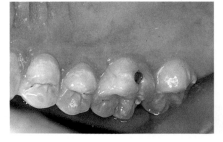

Fig 15-4i   Palatal healing. *The 10-day palatal healing demonstrates early wound closure.*

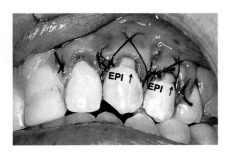

Fig 15-4h   Recipient overlying flap. *The recipient flap is repositioned coronally to cover as much of the subepithelial connective tissue graft as possible using 4-0 silk sutures interproximally. On prominent roots a better flap adaptation and avoidance of a dead space may be obtained with the use of a circumferential suture through the periosteum apical to the denuded root. This is then passed through the distal interproximal, carried around the cervical region of the canine palatally, passed back through the mesial interproximal, and tied with slight tension. The epithelial border of the connective tissue graft may be visible incisal to the cementoenamel junction. The area may be covered with Barricaid (LD Caulk) dressing or Coe-Pak (Coe Laboratories).*

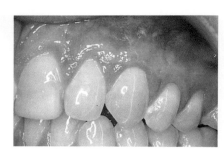

Fig 15-4j   Recipient site healing. *Three-year postoperative healing. The area exhibits good color blend of the grafted area to the adjacent site and continued total root coverage with minimal probing depth less than 2 mm. Compare to Fig 15-4a.*

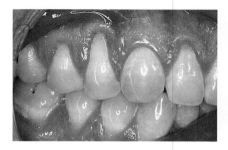

Fig 15-4k *Preoperative condition — maxillary right quadrant.*

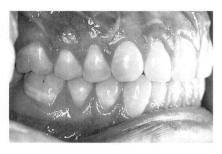

Fig 15-4l *Two weeks postoperative. The right side of this same patient 2 weeks after placement of an epithelial connective tissue graft. Note small scarring mesial to the first premolar and distal to the second premolar, which could be corrected by gingivoplasty.*

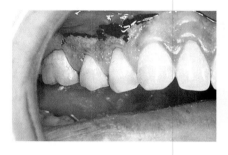

Fig 15-4m *Plasty. Gingivoplasty may be accomplished by sharp dissection with a no. 15 scalpel, electrosurgical needle, or a diamond stone under local anesthesia. At 3 weeks, the connective tissue is firmly attached and resilient. A Barricaid dressing may be placed if desired.*

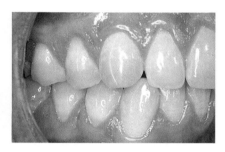

Fig 15-4n *Healing. One week postplasty, the epithelium has covered the area and produced a smooth, pink surface.*

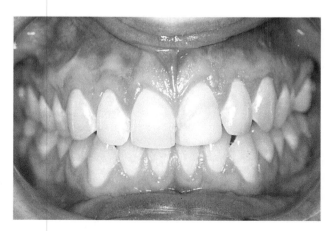

Fig 15-4o *One year postoperative. The result shows obliteration of the recessions in both treated areas.*

gain total root coverage in cases of severe recession on isolated and multiple teeth, especially in the maxilla where root coverage is most difficult to obtain.

In actuality, the subepithelial connective tissue graft for root coverage is a combination of a pedicle graft and an autogenous free connective tissue graft performed simultaneously.

First, the recipient bed is prepared by carefully elevating a split-thickness flap with a wide base dissected well beyond the mucogingival junction. This is the pedicle aspect of the procedure. Because the flap contributes the overlying blood supply that will nourish the graft to be taken from the palate, it must not be perforated. A perforation is a major contributing factor to obtaining a poor result.

Second, a connective tissue graft is dissected from the palate and placed on the recipient bed, which consists of a thin layer of periosteum and connective tissue overlying the bone surrounding the tooth or teeth involved with the recession. This is the autogenous free gingival graft part of the procedure. The recipient bed contributes the second underlying blood supply to the graft and enhances its survival.

Bed Preparation — Root Preparation

The recipient bed is composed of a thin layer of periosteum and connective tissue overlying the bone. The roots are planed with sharp, Gracey curets to remove debris, composite resin restorations (if present), and endotoxins. It may be necessary in some cases to shave overly convex root surfaces to bring them within the bony housing of the maxilla; this can be accomplished using curets or a diamond stone *with caution.*

Root Conditioning (Optional)

The roots may be additionally treated with citric acid as described by Miller[41] or a tetracycline hydrochloride solution applied with a cotton pellet for 3 minutes then rinsed with water for 1 minute. Research has shown that citric acid widens the lumens of the dentinal tubules, creates tufts of collagen,[42] and removes endotoxin[43] and the smear layer created by scaling.[44] Tetracycline hydrochloride accomplishes these goals and additionally offers the benefits of substantivity, plaque inhibition, and epithelial cell migration inhibition.[45]

Chemical root conditioning research on animals has been encouraging,[46,47] and although the results in the few human studies have been conflicting,[48,49] it has been shown that chemical root conditioning does not adversely affect the result.[50,51]

REMOVAL OF RESTORATIONS PRIOR TO GRAFTING (Figs 15-5a to h)

Deep recessions (Fig 15-5a) of maxillary canines often present as challenging problems, which can be complicated by previous placement of composite resin restorations. Although the procedure of the subepithelial connective tissue graft is the same as outlined in Figs 15-4a to j, additional consideration must be given to the complete removal of the composite resin material and aggressive root planing by means of curets (usually Gracey 7/8) to ensure that no foreign material will be left beneath the graft.

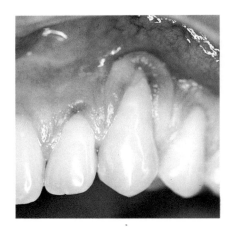

Fig 15-5a   Wide deep recession. A 26-year-old man presented with severe hypersensitivity on the maxillary left canine. The tooth had previously been treated by a composite resin restoration that continually chipped away at the most apical margin. The patient was most unhappy with his appearance and felt that his best efforts to keep this area plaque-free were in vain.

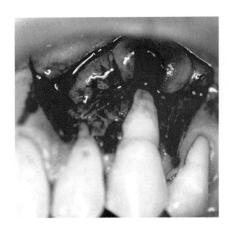

Fig 15-5b   Composite resin removal and flap elevation. The composite resin restoration was removed with an acrylic bur before the initial incision was made. The root surface was planed with Gracey curets 5/6 and 7/8 until an air stream directed at the root revealed no composite resin remnants. A horizontal incision was then made at the level of the CEJ with a vertical releasing incision mesially and distally. A split-thickness flap was elevated beyond the mucogingival junction to expose a thin layer of connective tissue and periosteum.

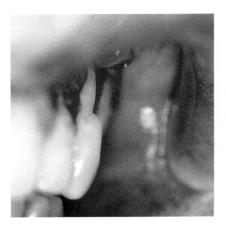

Fig 15-5c   Root shaving. A side view reveals the extent to which the tooth had been prepared for the original restoration and that it is within the bony housing of the adjacent alveolus. This is helpful in that the decreased convexity of the labial surface diminishes the area of avascular surface that the connective tissue graft must cover.

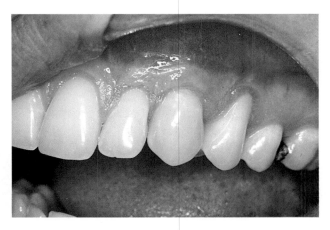

Fig 15-5d   One-year postoperative healing. *Maxillary left canine shows no loss of original coverage of the denuded root.*

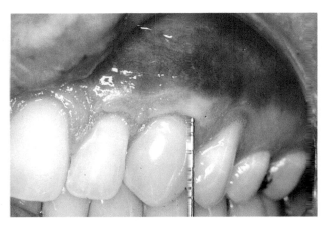

Fig 15-5e   Three-year postoperative result. *Probing with pressure reveals minimal sulcus depth and continued root coverage to the cementoenamel junction.*

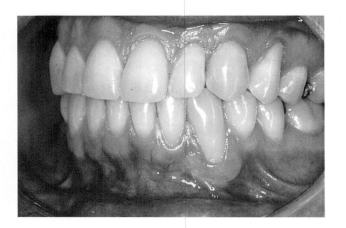

Fig 15-5f   Free gingival graft vs subepithelial connective tissue graft recipient site. *On the same day that a subepithelial connective tissue graft (SCTG) was performed on the maxillary left canine, an autogenous free gingival graft was performed on the mandibular left canine to increase the zone of keratinized gingiva. A slight difference in the color match is evident. The gingiva on the mandibular canine appears somewhat thicker and lighter than the SCTG on the maxillary canine.*

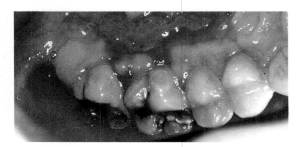

Fig 15-5g   Palatal healing — free gingival graft donor site. *One week healing of the right side of the palate after a thick free gingival graft was harvested from the same patient on the same day. The poor healing was attributed to the thick nature of the graft needed for root coverage. Thinner free gingival grafts used to widen the band of attached gingiva usually show better palatal healing.*

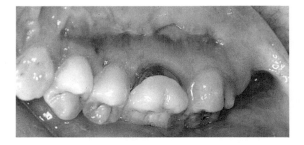

Fig 15-5h   Palatal healing — subepithelial connective tissue graft donor site. *One week healing of the left side of the palate after the SCTG was harvested. A smoother course of healing and less postoperative pain is the result of primary intention healing with this palatal approach (see Fig 15-4e).*

DAMAGED ROOT SURFACES (Figs 15-6a and b)

Previously damaged root surfaces present a particular challenge to the clinician. In many cases previous failures can be reversed by employing a subepithelial connective tissue graft.

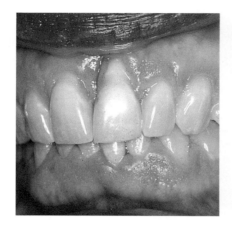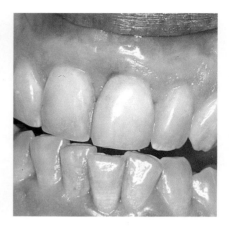

Fig 15-6a (left) ***Preoperative view.*** *A 29-year-old woman presented with severe recession on the maxillary left central incisor and incipient recession on the maxillary right central incisor, which had been treated previously by a coronally repositioned graft and two pedicle grafts on different occasions. Each procedure increased the recession on the left central incisor and eventually involved the right central incisor. Both teeth were extremely sensitive and increasingly unsightly. Additionally, there was a marked area of hypermineralization from the midlabial to the distal line angle on the left central incisor. Following flap elevation, the root was shaved with a diamond stone and treated with citric acid rubbed on the root with a cotton pellet for 5 minutes. A subepithelial connective tissue graft was taken from the palate, as outlined in Fig 15-4e.*

Fig 15-6b (right) ***Postoperative view.*** *One year postoperative healing shows 90% root coverage on the right central incisor and 100% root coverage on the left central incisor.*

MULTIPLE WIDE RECESSIONS
(Figs 15-7a and b)

In order to cover the multiple recessions in this 32-year-old woman in one session, both sides of the palate were used from the canine to the distal surface of the first molar. Since the connective tissue graft is taken internally, the rugae in the canine–first premolar areas is not a problem. The overlying flap is composed of the existing labial gingivae, which nourishes the graft and provides a good color blend. Using a free gingival graft in this instance would have denuded an extensive area of the palate.

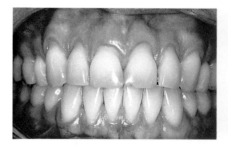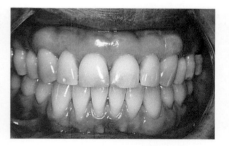

Fig 15-7a ***Multiple wide maxillary recession.*** *The roots of teeth 7, 8, 9, 10, and 11 are prominent apically. The patient had been using a horizontal scrub method of toothbrushing that accomplished excellent plaque control but contributed to the increasing recession.*

Fig 15-7b ***Five-year postoperative result.*** *Continued total root coverage of the labial surfaces after 5 years.*

COVERAGE OF EXISTING CROWN MARGINS (Figs 15-8a to e)

One of the more exasperating situations in restorative dentistry occurs when a gingival margin pulls away from a recently placed crown margin. The patient's attention becomes focused on this one area of the entire reconstruction.

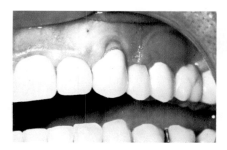

Fig 15-8a Recession adjacent to an existing crown margin. *Maxillary right canine showing buccal recession apical to the margin of an existing crown within a maxillary reconstruction.*

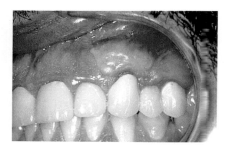

Fig 15-8b First subepithelial connective tissue graft placed. *A portion of the recession has been eliminated after placement of a subepithelial connective tissue graft. Residual recession was still present and the decision was made to attempt a second procedure.*

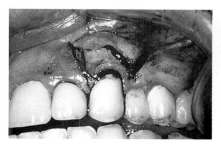

Fig 15-8c Internal incision. *The new thickness of the buccal tissue obviates the need of a second surgical site. A split-thickness flap is elevated to expose the underlying connective tissue. The trapezoid-shaped tissue is incised along its lateral and apical borders and then moved coronally.*

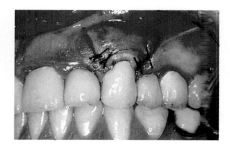

Fig 15-8d Suturing. *The underlying connective tissue is sutured over the residual area of recession and over the crown margin. The overlying flap is then sutured on top of the connective tissue graft using interrupted sutures.*

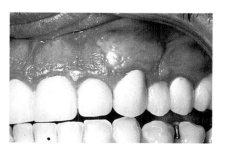

Fig 15-8e Postoperative view. *Thick coverage of the denuded root surface. Some of the gold margin is now obscured by the graft. A gingivoplasty could be performed if desired.*

TEN MOST COMMON MISTAKES IN SOFT TISSUE GRAFTING

Gingival grafting for root coverage is technique-sensitive. Most failures in obtaining total coverage of a denuded root are due to operator error, such as lack of judgment of the biologic or anatomic situations that do not lend themselves to graft survival, or errors in performing the technique itself. The most common errors are:

1. Not enough interproximal bone and soft tissue height for the procedure
2. Initial horizontal incision made apical to the CEJ (Fig 15-9a)
3. Lifting the interproximal papilla entirely
4. Perforations of the overlying flap
5. Roots not planed well enough

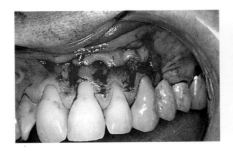

Fig 15-9a Common mistakes: initial incision. *Initial horizontal incision made apical to CEJs (arrows) of denuded roots, which makes it impossible to achieve total root coverage as graft placement will also be apical to the CEJ.*

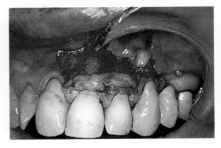

Fig 15-9b Common mistakes: graft size and placement. *The connective tissue graft is too small in the vertical dimension. It is not receiving the benefit of the collateral blood supply from the nondenuded area of the roots and the adjacent connective tissue and periosteum.*

6. Recipient bed not wide enough to provide collateral blood supply
7. Connective tissue graft too small (Fig 15-9b)
8. Connective tissue graft too thick
9. Connective tissue graft not positioned coronally enough to cover entire denuded area
10. Overlying flap not positioned coronally enough to cover the graft

I. Current concepts
- Early attempts at root coverage failed because of inadequate understanding of wound healing.
- Techniques for more predictable root coverage were developed in the 1980s.
- The subepithelial connective tissue graft used beneath a split-thickness flap at the graft site has proved most useful for root coverage.

II. Pedicle graft
Indications:
- Isolated narrow-deep or shallow recessions on mandibular teeth
- Adequate band of keratinized gingiva on neighboring teeth
- Adequate vestibular depth
- Isolated wide-shallow recession on maxillary or mandibular teeth

Advantages:
- Good color blend
- One-stage procedure
- Blood supply from base of flap and underlying periosteum adjacent to denuded root
- No necessity for second surgical site
- Minimal postoperative sequela

Disadvantages:
- Limited to narrow or shallow isolated recessions
- Not for multiple recessions
- Limited success with wide maxillary recession, especially on canines
- Must have adequate donor source on adjacent teeth

III. Free gingival graft for root coverage (thick stretched)
Indications:
- Isolated narrow or wide recession, usually on mandibular teeth
- To increase width of attached gingiva
- To increase vestibular depth

Advantages:
- One-stage procedure

- Increases amount of keratinized gingiva
- Eliminates frenum attachments
- Covers multiple shallow-wide defects

Disadvantages:
- Usually poor color blend with adjacent tissue: the thicker keratinization of the palate appears whiter than the buccal gingiva
- Large denuded area of he palate, which may be painful during healing
- Precise suturing technique
- Technique-sensitive
- May be two-stage procedure if free gingival graft is placed first then coronally repositioned at a later date
- Limited success with multiple wide-deep recessions of the maxilla due to inadequate blood supply

IV. Subepithelial connective tissue graft for root coverage
Indications:
- Inadequate donor site for pedicle graft
- Isolated wide recessions not usually amenable to free gingival grafting, especially on the maxilla
- Multiple root exposures
- Multiple root exposures in combination with minimal attached gingiva
- Recession adjacent to an edentulous area that also required ridge augmentation

Advantages:
- Double blood supply to the graft
- Minimal palatal denudation, primary intention healing
- One-step procedure
- Excellent color blend
- Coverage of existing unsightly crown margins

Disadvantages:
- Technique-sensitive
- Complicated suturing

REFERENCES

1. Wilderman M, Wentz FM, Orban BJ: Histogenesis of repair after mucogingival surgery. *J Periodontol* 1960;31:283.

2. Carranza F, Carraro JJ: Effect of removal of periosteum on postoperative result of mucogingival surgery. *J Periodontol* 1963;34:223.

3. Friedman N: Mucogingival surgery: The apically repositioned flap. *J Periodontol* 1962;33:328.

4. Ochsenbein C: Newer concepts of mucogingival surgery. *J Periodontol* 1960;31:175.

5. Bohannan H: Studies in the alteration of vestibular depth: I. Complete denudation. *J Periodontol* 1962;33:120.

6. Bohannan H: Studies in the alteration of vestibular depth: II. Periosteal retention. *J Periodontol* 1962;33:354.

7. Bohannan H: Studies in the alteration of vestibular depth: III. Vestibular incision. *J Periodontol* 1963;34:209.

8. Corn H: Periosteal separation — Its clinical significance. *J Periodontol* 1962;33:140.

9. Friedman N, Levine L: Current approaches to periodontal therapy, mucogingival surgery: Current status. *J Periodontol* 1964;35:5.

10. Bjorn H: Free transplantation of gingiva propia. *Sverige Tandlakarforb Tidn* 1963;22:684.

11. Grupe HE, Warren RF: Repair of gingival defects by a sliding flap operation. *J Periodontol* 1956;27:92.

12. Nabors J: Extension of the vestibular fornix utilizing a gingival graft — Case history. *Periodontics* 1966;4:77.

13. Nabors J: Free gingival grafts. *Periodontics* 1966;4:243.

14. Sullivan HC, Atkins JH: Free autogenous gingival grafts, I. Principals of successful grafting. *Periodontics* 1968;6:121.

15. Gordon HP, Sullivan HC, Atkins JH: Free autogenous gingival grafts. II. Supplemental findings — Histology of the graft site. *Periodontics* 1968;6:130.

16. Sullivan HC, Atkins JH: Free autogenous gingival grafts, 3. Utilization of grafts in the treatment of gingival recession. *Periodontics* 1968;6:152.

17. Sullivan HC, Atkins JH: The role of free gingival grafts in periodontal therapy. *Dent Clin North Am* 1969;13:133.

18. Douglass GL: Mucogingival repairs in periodontal surgery. *Dent Clin North Am* 1976;20:107.

19. Pennel B et al: Oblique rotated flap. *J Periodontol* 1965;36:305.

20. Cohen DW, Ross S: The double papillae repositioned flap in periodontal therapy. *J Periodontol* 1968;39:65.

21. Bernimoulin J: Coronally repositioned periodontal flap. *J Clin Periodontol* 1975;2:1.

22. Oliver R, Löe H, Karring T: Microscopic evaluation of the healing and revascularisation of free gingival grafts. *J Periodont Res* 1968;3:84-95.

23. Lange DE, Bernimoulin JP: Exfoliative cytological studies in evaluation of free gingival graft healing. *J Clin Periodontol* 1974;1:89-96.

24. Karring T, Ostergaard E, Löe H: Conservation of tissue specificity after heterotophic transplantation of gingiva and alveolar mucosa. *J Periodont Res* 1971;6:282-293.

25. Edel A: Clinical evaluation of free connective tissue grafts used to increase the width of keratinized gingiva. *J Clin Periodontol* 1974;1:185-196.

26. Becker B, Becker W: Use of connective tissue autografts for treatment of mucogingival problems. *Int J Periodont Rest Dent* 1986;6(1):88.

27. Miller PD: Root coverage using a free soft tissue autograft following citric acid application. Part I. *Int J Periodont Rest Dent* 1982;2(1):65.

28. Holbrook T, Ochsenbein C: Complete coverage of denuded root surface with a one stage gingival graft. *Int J Periodont Rest Dent* 1983;3(3):8.

29. Miller PD Jr: Root coverage using the free soft tissue autograft following citric acid application. Part III. A successful and predictable procedure in areas of deep-wide recession. *Int J Periodont Rest Dent* 1985;5(2):14.

30. Bertrand PM, Dunlap RM: Coverage of deep, wide gingival clefts with free gingival autografts: Root planing with and without citric acid demineralization. *Int J Periodont Rest Dent* 1988;8(1):64.

31. Miller PD Jr: A classification of marginal tissue recession. *Int J Periodont Rest Dent* 1985;5(2):8.

32. Langer B, Langer L: Subepithelial connective tissue graft technique for root coverage. *J Periodontol* 1985;56:715.

33. Nelson S: The subpedicle connective tissue graft. A bilaminar reconstructive procedure for the coverage of denuded root surfaces. *J Periodontol* 1987;58:95.

34. Lang NP, Löe H: The relationship between the width of keratinized gingiva and gingival health. *J Periodontol* 1972;43:623.

35. Alstad S, Zachrisson BV: Longitudinal study of periodontal condition associated with orthodontic treatment in adolescents. *Am J Orthod* 1979;76:277.

36. Dorfman HS: Mucogingival changes resulting from mandibular incisor tooth movement. *Am J Orthod* 1978;74:286.

37. Silness J: Periodontal conditions in patients treated with dental bridges. 3. The relationship between the location of the crown margin and the periodontal condition. *J Periodont Res* 1970;5:225.

38. Maynard JG: Coronal positioning of a previously placed autogenous gingival graft. *J Periodontol* 1977;48:151.

39. Langer B, Calagna L: The subepithelial connective tissue graft. *J Prosthet Dent* 1980;44:363.

40. Langer B, Calagna L: The subepithelial connective tissue graft. A new approach to the enhancement of anterior cosmetics. *Int J Periodont Rest Dent* 1982;2(2):22.

41. Miller PD Jr: Root coverage using a free soft tissue autograft following citric acid application. II. Treatment of the carious root. *Int J Periodont Rest Dent* 1983;3(5):38.

42. Sterret JD, Murphy HJ: Citric acid burnishing of dentinal root surfaces. A scanning electron microscopy report. *J Clin Periodontol* 1989;16:98.

43. Aleo J: The presence and biologic activity of cementum bound endotoxin. *J Periodontol* 1974;45:672.

44. Polson A, Frederick G, Ladenheim S, Hanes P: The production of a root surface smear layer by instrumentation and its removal by citric acid. *J Periodontol* 1984;55:443.

45. Wikesjo UME, Baker PJ, Christersson LA, et al: A biochemical approach to periodontal regeneration: Tetracycline treatment conditions dentin surfaces. *J Periodont Res* 1986;21:322.

46. Register A, Burdick F: Accelerated reattachment with cementogenesis to dentin, demineralized in situ. I. Optimum range. *J Periodontol* 1975;46:676.

47. Nilvéus R, Bogle G, Crigger M, Egelberg J, Selvig K: The effect of topical citric acid application on the healing of experimental furcation defects in dogs. II. Healing after repeated surgery. *J Periodont Res* 1980;15:544.

48. Common J, McFall WT: The effects of citric acid on attachment of laterally positioned flaps. *J Periodontol* 1983;54:9.

49. Moore JA, Ashley FP, Waterman CA: The effect on healing of the application of citric acid during replaced flap surgery. *J Clin Periodontol* 1987;14:130.

50. Ririe C, Crigger M, Selvig K: Healing of periodontal connective tissue following surgical wounding and application of citric acid in dogs. *J Periodont Res* 1980;15:314.

51. Crigger M, Renvert S, Bogle G: The effect of topical citric acid application on surgically exposed periodontal attachment. *J Periodont Res* 1983;18:303.

Esthetic Reconstruction of Alveolar Ridge Defects

by Oded Bahat / Mark Handelsman

INTRODUCTION

Repair of lost oral structures and prevention of unacceptable esthetic deformities are the goals of several current periodontal reconstructive procedures. Many of these reconstructive efforts are limited in their efficacy due to inadequate flap coverage and vascular perfusion.[1-7] To address these limiting factors, one must have a basic understanding of the oral mucosa and gingiva as they relate to surgical design. In addition, efforts to increase vascular perfusion can only enhance our ability to correct larger defects.

The interface between soft and hard tissues and a fixed partial denture is critical to achieving the desired esthetic result. Where esthetics is a concern, the primary objective is to prevent ridge collapse after tooth extraction. Procedures to prevent the collapse of the alveolar ridge[8] and to augment the edentulous ridges are

technique-sensitive and require different surgical designs depending on the size of the defect. Traumatic extractions and tooth avulsions often leave large deformities and traditionally have required either removable restorations (to replace the tremendous amount of soft tissue loss) or modification of the pontic design. Both solutions leave a compromised esthetic result. Various procedures[9-11] and materials presently available allow augmentation of these large defects in combination with fixed restorations.

It is important to plan the restorative treatment of the entire dentition prior to any tooth extraction. When the edentulous ridge is considered a future site for dental implants, the donor material should be carefully selected. Recent studies[12-14] on guided tissue regeneration indicate that using a membrane isolation procedure might be the most predictable procedure in these cases

because it allows for autogenous bone cells to repopulate the defect (see chapter 21 for additional information)

PERIODONTAL RECONSTRUCTIVE FLAPS — CLASSIFICATION

Periodontal reconstructive flaps have been previously classified according to flap types[15] or their intended direction.[16] Such a classification is confusing[17] and, in the opinion of the authors, unclear, because it is based on mismatched elements of the flap design, direction of transfer, geometry, number, and varied angles of rotation. To classify the uniqueness of flap design and to allow the placement of all flaps into a specific category, it is suggested that information from the general surgery and plastic surgery literature be adapted to periodontics.

Rationale for Classification

All periodontal reconstructive flaps share two similar characteristics:

1. They are all random pattern flaps (cutaneous flaps).[18,19] They receive their name due to their mode of blood supply, which arises from segmental and axial arteries. These vessels perforate the base of the flap via musculocutaneous arterioles.
2. All are local flaps since they are adjacent to the defect. This gives them improved ability to match the texture, color, and thickness of the surrounding tissues.

Mechanism of Classification

Periodontal reconstructive flaps can be separated by the direction of transfer and geometry (Table 16-1).

Mode of Transfer

1. **Rotational.** All rotational flaps share the common characteristic of movement around a pivot point. The radius of the arc of rotation is the line of greatest tension. The greater the rotation, the greater the actual shortening of the flap.
2. **Advancement.** Advanced flaps reach their final site without rotation or any lateral movement. They can consist of one or more pedicles. The advanced flap consists of two straight line vertical incisions with or without 100-degree to 110-degree back cuts. These incisions bring the wound edges together into their newly assumed position and coordinate their motion.

Both the advanced flap and the rotation flap can be further clas-

TABLE 16-1 *Classification of periodontal reconstructive flaps*

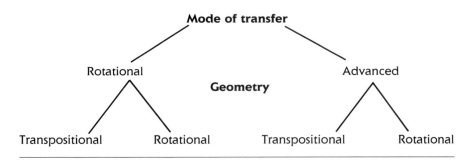

sified according to the geometry of the flap.

Geometry

1. **Transpositional.** A rectangular segment of gingiva and mucosa is used.
2. **Rotational.** A semi-circular segment of gingiva or mucosa is used.

This classification, which is based on accepted general surgical principles and is further modified to accurately describe the reconstructive periodontal flap, can assist the surgeon in visualizing presurgical designs, which will subsequently ensure optimal reconstructive efforts. No other subdivisions are needed. The simplicity of this classification precludes further esoteric division.

CLINICAL EXAMINATION

The following factors should be documented when examining the patient in preparation for periodontal reconstructive flap surgery:

1. The smile line.[20] At what level does the upper lip rest in the natural position and while smiling?
   Low = upper lip coronal to CEJ

Average = at level of CEJ
   High = at level above (apical) to the CEJ (a "gummy" smile)
2. Type and extent of deformity expected after tooth extraction or that is already present. This can be evaluated with radiographs to determine the height of the interproximal bone and clinical evaluation of the papilla.

Seibert classification[5,6]:
   Class I = buccolingual loss of tissue with normal apicocoronal ridge height
   Class II = apicocoronal loss with normal buccal lingual ridge width
   Class III = combination of buccolingual and apicocoronal loss.

3. General arch form, tooth form (shape, length, width), position of teeth, or future dental implant sites.
4. Future relationship of the pontic to the abutment teeth and gingiva.
5. Type of restoration supported by teeth, dental implants, or a combination of teeth with implants.
6. Type of periodontium. A thick periodontium is easier to manage the soft tissue and prevent loss of the papilla.[21] Thin tissue requires more

gentle manipulation and greater augmentation to scaffold the papilla.
7. Presence or absence of bone and its shape.
8. The interrelationship of maxillary and mandibular alveolar ridges.
9. The interrelationship of the alveolar ridges to the surrounding orofacial structures (eg, lips, soft tissue profile)
10. The position of the mucobuccal fold and mucogingival junction.

RIDGE PRESERVATION / AUGMENTATION TECHNIQUES

Ridge Preservation[8]
(Figs 16-1a to c)

Preserving the ridge at the time of extraction helps reduce future damage but usually requires further surgical augmentation procedures prior to final prosthetic construction.

Advantages

- Reduces subsequent ridge collapse.
- Reduces the number of subsequent reconstructive procedures.

Disadvantages

- Presurgical restorative planning must be done before the surgical procedure.

- Requires tooth preparation prior to the surgical procedure.
- Provisional restorations must be placed immediately after tooth extraction and ridge preservation.
- Thorough surgical debridement must be done in areas of periapical pathosis.

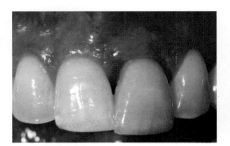

Fig 16-1a *Preoperative clinical view of left central incisor.*

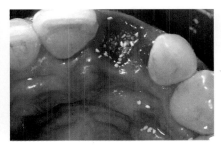

Fig 16-1b *Palatal view of hydroxyapatite placed at the most coronal aspect of the gingival margin. The graft is covered and secured with freeze-dried skin. This skin is removed 10 days postoperatively.*

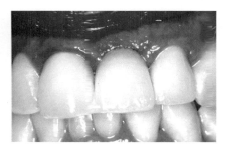

Fig 16-1c *Final reconstruction 8 months postoperatively. (Courtesy of Dr Jack Preston.)*

Immediate Ridge Augmentation[9]
(Figs 16-2a to e)

This technique can be performed at the time of tooth extraction. It enables the operator to reduce the number of surgeries and to achieve optimal ridge architecture.

Advantages

- It eliminates the need for multiple surgical interventions to augment volume loss.
- Overcontouring of the edentulous area allows for later gingival plasty to optimize pontic-to-soft tissue relationship.

Disadvantages

- Flap management and survival over large augmentation areas.
- All above-mentioned disadvantages of preservation procedures.

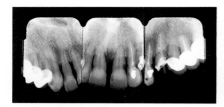

Fig 16-2a Preoperative radiograph shows advanced bone loss on the incisors.

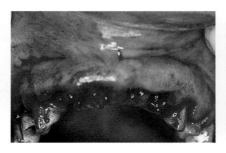

Fig 16-2b Teeth extracted. Sockets are extensively debrided to remove granulation tissue.

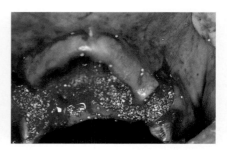

Fig 16-2c Graft material is placed into sockets and sutured.

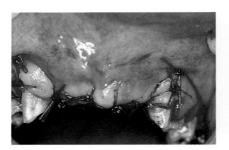

Fig 16-2d Anterior advanced flap is extended to cover graft site with primary coverage.

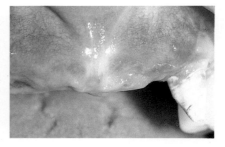

Fig 16-2e Postoperative healing of preserved ridge.

TECHNIQUES DEPENDING ON VASCULAR PERFUSION

These techniques are best suited to smaller defects but can also be used in large defects. The major drawback is the amount of donor material that the operator is able to harvest from the palate without leaving a large residual defect for secondary intention healing. Further limitations include the reliance on tissue perfusion for survivability of the graft.

Onlay Graft[5,6] (Figs 16-3a to f)

Indication

- The onlay graft is of value and is predictable in smaller areas.

Advantage

- Increases the dimension of gingiva.

Disadvantages

- Limited amount of donor material.
- Two surgical sites are necessary.
- Limited survivability due to reliance on vascular perfusion at the recipient bed.

- The need for multiple surgical interventions to augment larger defects.
- Color matching is unfavorable because of the degree of keratinization of the donor graft.
- Unpredictable postoperative soft tissue shrinkage.

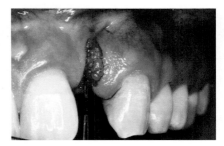

Fig 16-3a Preoperative frontal view shows congenital ridge defect (cleft palate).

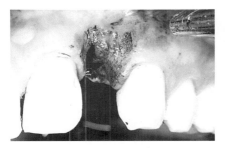

Figs 16-3b and c Frontal and occlusal views show recipient site preparation. Area is completely de-epithelialized.

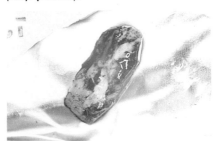

Fig 16-3d Graft from palate. Elliptical shape is desired.

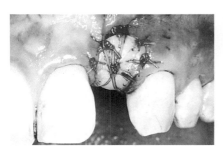

Fig 16-3e Frontal view showing graft tightly adapted to site with gut sutures. Stabilization of the graft is critical.

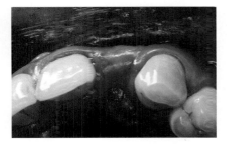

Fig 16-3f Postoperative healing at 6 months.

Inlay Graft[1-3]

Indication

- The inlay graft is of value and is predictable in small areas.

Advantages

- Good color matching.
- Improved (over onlay grafts) vascularity through flap coverage over the donor graft.
- Able to stabilize the donor graft at the desired site.

Disadvantages

- Two surgical sites are necessary.
- Limited amount of donor material.
- Unpredictable donor tissue shrinkage.
- Flap design, management, and transformation, especially in the interproximal papillary area.

Inlay-Onlay Graft[22]
(Figs 16-4a to g, 16-5a to c)

This is a combination of the above-described techniques. It has all the advantages and disadvantages of each individual technique.

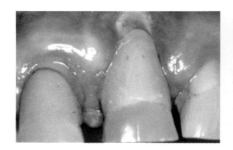

Fig 16-4a *Preoperative clinical view shows advanced attachment loss on buccal aspect of the left central incisor.*

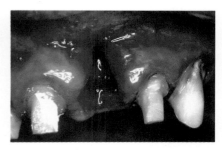

Fig 16-4b *Frontal view at time of extraction of left central incisor.*

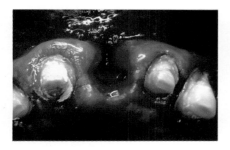

Fig 16-4c *Occlusal view after extraction.*

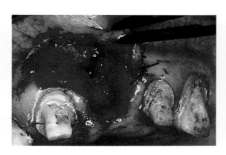

Fig 16-4d *Pedicle partial-thickness flap elevated from buccal surface of right central incisor and sutured to mesial aspect of left lateral incisor to create a buccal wall.*

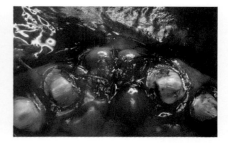

Fig 16-4e *Occlusal view of donor material secured in defect with reconstruction of buccal ridge contour.*

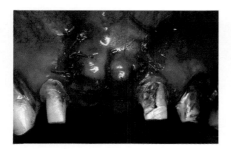

Fig 16-4f *Frontal view of final suturing.*

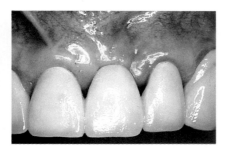

Fig 16-4g *Final reconstruction.*

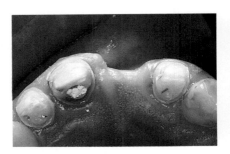

Fig 16-5a *Preoperative view. Note buccal ridge defect (Seibert Class I).*

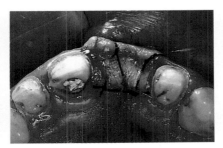

Fig 16-5b *Soft tissue graft from the palate is secured with silk sutures.*

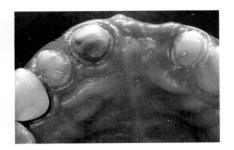

Fig 16-5c *The view 6 months postoperative. Note reconstruction of buccal ridge contour.*

TECHNIQUES BASED ON LOCAL FLAPS

Subperiosteal Tunnel (Pouch)[7]

Indication

- Usually for Class I type defects but also may be used for slight vertical (apicocoronal) augmentation.

Advantages

- Only one surgical site is needed.
- There is abundant donor material (eg, synthetic, alloplastic, autogenous).

Disadvantages

- Risk of loss of donor material through sequestration.

- Flap perforation over thin tissue bound to sharp alveolar ridge deformities.
- Similar to the inlay graft procedure, but donor material can be either soft tissue or synthetic (eg, hydroxyapatite, etc). The problem is the limited amount of augmentation because of limited flap extension and no versatility to manipulate the flap to desired dimensions. It is contraindicated in areas where the tissue is very thin because perforation during flap elevation will compromise the final result.

Roll Technique[4]

Abrams described this technique in 1980. Class II and III type defects can be augmented but in such small amounts that it does not make it a practical procedure. This procedure might be useful for papilla augmentation secondary to other reconstructive efforts.

Advantage

- Blood supply is maintained to the donor graft tissue.

Disadvantage

- It is limited to the relative thickness of the palatal tissue adjacent to the edentulous area.

Coronally Positioned Flap[7] (With Autogenous or Alloplastic Graft)

Indication

- Refer to advanced flap.

TECHNIQUES BASED ON LOCAL AND DISTANT FLAPS

Anterior Advanced Flap[9]
(Figs 16-6a to l)

The anteriorly advanced flap can be modified so that desired predictable results can be achieved. It can be used successfully in multiple clinical conditions. In the past, it was referred to as the coronally positioned flap. Its range was reduced by the minimal degree of mobilization and dissection. When periodontal reconstruction was attempted, it was used exclusively to achieve root coverage[23] alone, or subsequent to gingival augmentation, or in order to correct ridge defects of small to moderate dimension.

The therapeutic scope of the advancement flap can be expanded into areas of immediate ridge preservation and augmentation, papilla augmentation, and large ridge deformities.

In order to achieve such goals, various modifications in the surgical design of the "coronally positioned flap"[23] should be considered. These specific changes are compatible with the surgical and anatomical landmarks of gingiva, mucosa, submucosa, adipose tissue, and submucosa.

Advantages

- Provides flap coverage over large defect augmentation.
- Maintains excellent vascularity with extended distance transfer.
- Reduces the number of surgical interventions.
- Useful in combination with implant placement.
- Surgical access and visibility.

Disadvantages

- Extremely technique-sensitive.
- Secondary procedure because of the new location of the mucogingival junction (the further the transfer, the more coronal the junction).

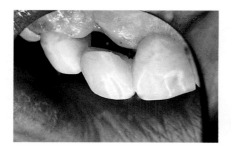

Fig 16-6a Note extent of ridge defect, both horizontal and vertical dimensions.

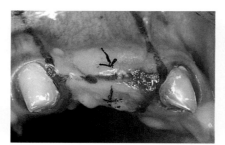

Fig 16-6b Edentulous ridge with surgical marking pen used to outline the "advanced flap" design.

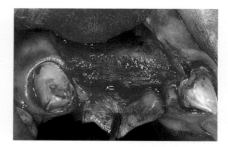

Fig 16-6c Ridge defect. Note palatal "edge flap" reflected.

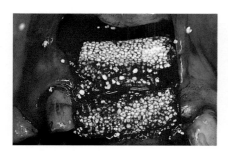

Fig 16-6d Donor material is easily shaped and positioned into defect.

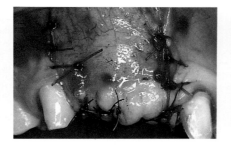

Fig 16-6e Advanced flap is sutured. Note that no tension is created on flap. Prolene sutures are used on the edge flap margin. Chromic gut is used to secure the buccal margins.

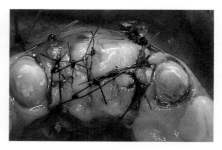

Fig 16-6f Occlusal view showing flap closure and amount of augmentation achieved in buccal dimension.

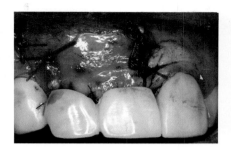

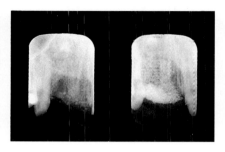

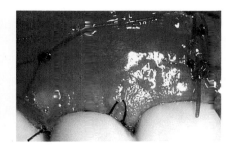

Fig 16-6g *Provisional restoration is adapted to allow for swelling during initial healing.*

Fig 16-6h *Preoperative and postoperative radiographs.*

Fig 16-6i *Healing at 1 week.*

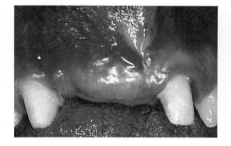

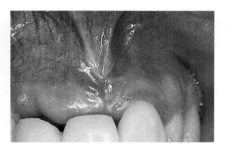

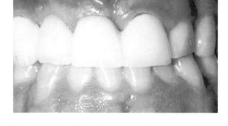

Figs 16-6j and k *Healing at 4 weeks. Provisional restoration can now be adapted to ideal ridge form.*

Fig 16-6l *Final restorative result. (Courtesy of Dr Bruce Coye.)*

Surgical Design An important principle for the advanced flap is that two vertical incisions are made on either side of the recipient site, which allows a rectangular flap to be advanced anteriorly. This advancement is achieved due to the elasticity of the surrounding tissue[10] and to existing excess tissue on the lateral aspect of the base, and it permits an even advancement between the flap sides and the wound edges.[24] Further modification can be achieved by two back-cut incisions at approximately 100 degrees on each side of the base. Each of these cuts will open up into a V shape upon advancement, thus increasing the effective range of the flap.[10,25] Further modification in the extension of the two vertical incisions allows for an increase of the desired range. This increase in turn provides for optimal coverage over augmentations of much larger deformities.

In order to obtain a successful result, further increase in sharp dissection beyond the mucobuccal fold is required. The shorter the vestibular depth, the larger the incision into the lip substance. These extensions reduce undue tension on the perforating vessels, increase tissue thickness over the defect, and improve vascularity due to musculocutaneous arterioles traversing through the lip submucosa. Special care should be directed towards the edge flap. The edge flap should not have vertical incisions at interproximal papilla; this avoids irreversible esthetic damage. It should be elevated sufficiently to provide a minimum of 3 mm (thickness) of effective length. The periosteum should be severed to allow reflection with minimal tension.

The formation of the edge flap (when ridge augmentation is considered) is essential in order to accurately determine the desired range of the advanced flap. The surgeon should keep in mind that upon raising the advanced flap, its effective length appears shorter due to the elasticity of the soft tissue. However, the original dimension can be evaluated by stretching the flap to its original dimension with pickup forceps, and the use of suture material as a measuring tape. Provided these modifications are executed, the versatility of this flap is enhanced beyond its original therapeutic scope. The suturing sequence of the flap is essential. Usually the flap's mesiocoronal and distocoronal edges are secured. This allows the operator to evaluate the optimal mesiodistal dimensions. The remaining interface between the advanced flap and the edge flap can be approximated with continuous sutures or multiple interrupted sutures. Prolene 4-0 suture material is commonly used at this interface. The lateral edges

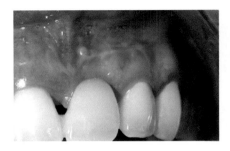

Fig 16-7a *Preoperative frontal view with provisional restoration showing lack of papilla (soft tissue) between the central incisors.*

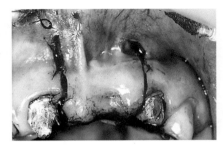

Fig 16-7b *Initial incisions illustrating design of advanced flap extending into the mucobuccal fold with back-cut incisions.*

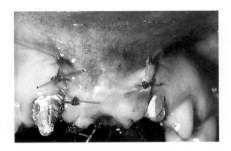

Fig 16-7c *Flap secured over graft material.*

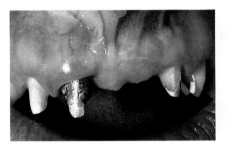

Fig 16-7d *Postoperative view shows excess tissue in pontic area.*

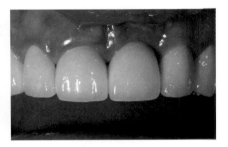

Fig 16-7e *Final restorations. (Courtesy of Dr Lane Ochi.)*

are approximated in a similar fashion using chromic gut 4-0 suture material.

Papilla Augmentation
(Figs 16-7a to e)

The loss of the interproximal papilla can inflict an esthetic and phonetic insult to patients. Reconstruction of this area is often a surgical nightmare with catastrophic results. An essential ingredient for successful reconstruction is the operator's ability to maintain adequate soft tissue coverage and intact vascularity at the surgical site. The advanced flap can be useful in reaching these therapeutic goals. Specific consideration should be given to the mode of anesthesia, amount of vasoconstrictor agents, length-to-base ratio, sequence of suturing, and the location of the perforating needle relative to the wound edge.

Local Anesthesia and Vasoconstrictors The interproximal papilla, due to its dimension and its specific blood supply pattern, acts like an end artery organ. Thus, even minimal amounts of a vasoconstricting agent may cause irreversible necrosis. When a narrow interproximal papilla is to be augmented, the operator should therefore avoid both the use of a vasoconstrictor agent at the site and excessive infiltration of any local anesthetic agent. Instead, in order to achieve hemostasis, improved surgical techniques to achieve clean, sharp dissection and use of other agents to achieve surface coagulation should be used.[10]

Length-to-Base Ratio When one papilla is to be augmented via an advanced flap the length-to-base ratio becomes unfavorable. Although it has been shown[26-30]

that the length of a viable flap can survive independent to its width, this flap may be extremely thin since care should be taken not to extend the vertical incision over the adjacent teeth. In order to increase the width, further consideration should be given to minor orthodontic tooth movement (root separation) prior to augmentation, in order to achieve a transient increase in width of the edge flap and subsequent similar increase in the width of the advanced flap.

Suturing Sequence and Location Due to the increased need for precision in readapting the flap, special consideration should be given to suturing technique. Trial closure without tension prior to flap apposition is the essential ingredient for success. The needle should perforate the flap 1 to 2 mm from its cut edge in order to ensure edge control. One should avoid perforating into the deep aspect of the papilla (especially when it is thin) in order to avoid vascular embarrassment. The needle should perforate the flap at an angle exceeding 90 degrees, thus everting the edge and gaining additional essential height. Sutures should be removed after 48 to 72 hours since initial approximation has been achieved.

Clearly, this procedure tests the outer limits of surgical precision and soft tissue manipulation, without which failure is assured.

Pantographic Lip Expansion for Ridge Augmentation[10]
(Figs 16-8a to j)

This technique allows for flap coverage over extensive defects, usually inflicted by traumatic avulsion of anterior teeth and severe alveolar ridge loss.

Advantages

- All the advantages of the advanced flap.
- Additional flap availability in areas of very shallow vestibular depth.

Disadvantages

- All the disadvantages of the advanced flap.
- Extremely technique-sensitive because of the surgical demands required to manipulate two dissimilar surfaces (lip mucosa and gingiva) and achieve an even junction.
- Eliminates or shallows the vestibular depth.

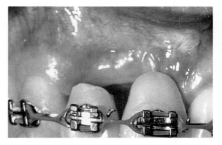

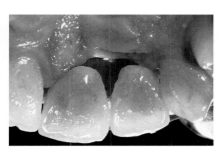

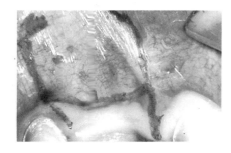

Figs 16-8a and b *Preoperative buccal and palatal views.*

Fig 16-8c *Outline of the edge and advanced flap is marked with a surgical pen prior to dissection.*

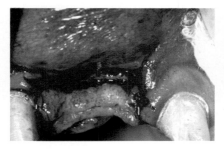

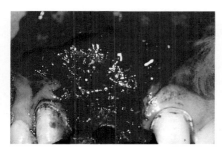

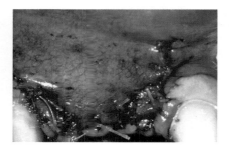

Fig 16-8d *Flap design showing future edge flap.*

Fig 16-8e *Flaps elevated. Note extent of ridge deformity.*

Fig 16-8f *Gut sutures used to accurately approximate the flap margins.*

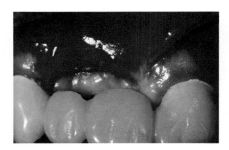

Fig 16-8g *One month postoperatively. Note loss of vestibule.*

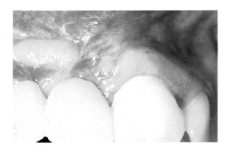

Fig 16-8h *Buccal and palatal views subsequent to the second procedure, which used a free gingival graft on the buccal surface to reestablish the depth of the vestibule.*

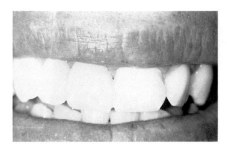

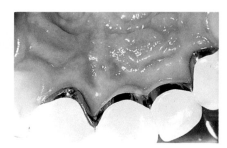

Figs 16-8i and j *Final restorative result. (Courtesy of Dr Albert Solnit.)*

CONTROLLED TISSUE EXPANSION[11] (Figs 16-9a to d and 16-10a to l)

Controlled tissue expansion is a new modality that may assist in achieving excess tissue, which is so desirable during reconstructive procedures.

Advantages

- Generates sufficient tissue at the defect site.
- Good color matching.
- Avoids the need for multiple phases of flap transfer or a residual defect with subsequent secondary intention healing.
- Expanded flaps have increased vascularity, hence their transfer may be safer.[31]

Disadvantages

- Requires an altered clinical judgment in evaluation of the site (tissue thickness of the gingiva and mucosa, bone irregularities, vestibular depth).
- Multiple office visits for gradual expansion of the expander.
- Possible infections.
- Tissue necrosis is possible because of overexpansion.
- Possible perforation of the reservoir bag during suturing or because of sharp bone aberrations.
- The tubing may interfere with the movement of oral tissue (lip, cheek, tongue).

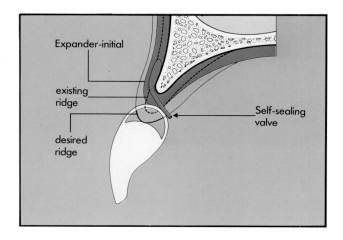

Fig 16-9a *Cross-sectional view of alveolar ridge with expander (blue) placed subperiosteally. Note the extent of ridge resorption and future pontic–soft tissue relationship.*

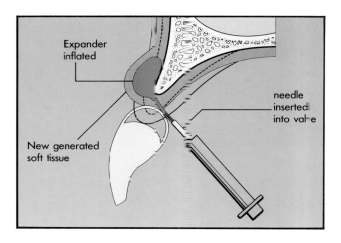

Fig 16-9b *Expander inflated with saline solution. Note amount of new tissue generated by expansion technique. A syringe with a 25-gauge needle is inserted into self-sealing valve for inflation.*

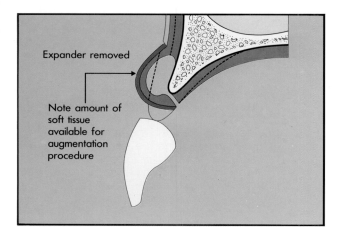

Fig 16-9c *At the second surgical procedure the expander is removed with the flap elevated from the palatal aspect. Note the extra soft tissue that is available for augmentation purposes.*

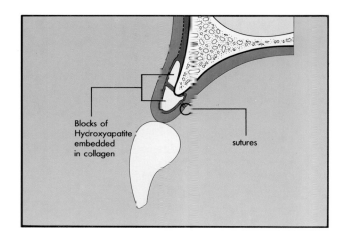

Fig 16-9d *Augmentation to desired ridge form is achieved with blocks (hydroxyapatite crystals embedded in collagen) placed subperiosteally. Passive flap closure is achieved with the newly generated soft tissue.*

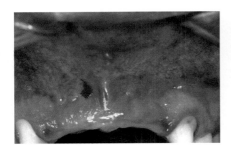

Fig 16-10a *Frontal view of alveolar ridge deformity. Structural loss includes vertical and horizontal loss. Observe the adequate tissue thickness and favorable location of the mucogingival junction.*

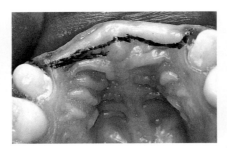

Fig 16-10b *Occlusal view of the edentulous area, illustrating the junction of the advanced flap (buccal) and the edge flap.*

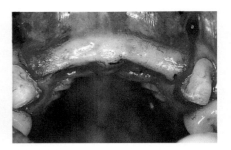

Fig 16-10c *Initial incisions completed.*

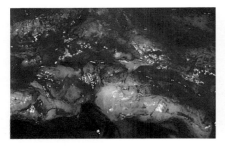

Fig 16-10d *Palatal view of the edge flap; 4 to 5 mm of edge is required for approximation and accurate suturing of the advanced and edge flaps.*

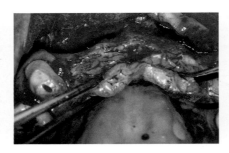

Fig 16-10e *Occlusal view shows the extent of the bony ridge deformity.*

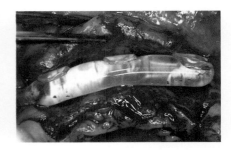

Fig 16-10f *The expander is placed into the surgical area that requires tissue expansion. The exit of the inflation tubing through the tissue should be predetermined in order to avoid mechanical trauma to mobile tissue and to allow for optimal patient comfort and easy access to the valve for inflation.*

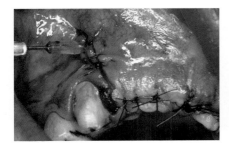

Fig 16-10g *Self-sealing valve extends out through the tissue and lies in the vestibule. Note that a 23-gauge needle is inserted and inflated with saline until tissue blanching occurs.*

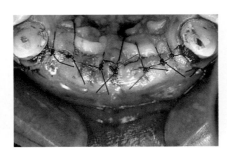

Fig 16-10h *Occlusal view of the suturing pattern at the junction of the advanced and edge flaps.*

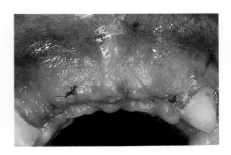

Fig 16-10i *Frontal view of the surgical site 2 weeks after the initial surgical procedure. Note the overcontoured tissue on the buccal aspect prior to removal of the expander.*

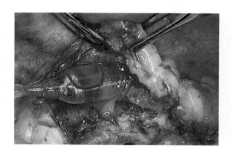

Fig 16-10j *Flap elevation to remove expander. Design is same as initial surgery.*

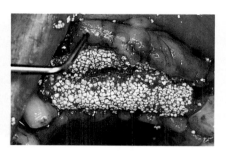

Fig 16-10k *Blocks of hydroxyapatite crystals embedded in collagen are placed to reconstruct the edentulous ridge.*

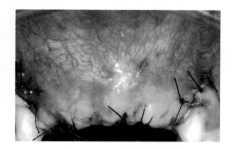

Fig 16-10l *Frontal view showing complete coverage over hydroxyapatite graft using expanded newly generated soft tissue with no tension on the flap.*

Expander

The Subperiosteal Tissue Expander (CUI, Santa Barbara, Calif) consists of two parts: *(1)* a silicon body (the bag) with *(2)* a tubing that contains a self-sealing valve to allow inflation of the bag with saline. The expander (bag) can be custom made both in dimension and curvature in order to fit specific requirements at the defect site. Custom-made tags can extend from the reservoir bag. These assist in securing it with resorbable sutures to the appropriate location on the ridge deformity. A 23-gauge needle or even finer needle can be used for internal (surgical) inflation.

Surgical Procedure

Prior to the surgery it is essential for the surgeon to evaluate the ex-act dimension, location, bony boundaries, and relationship to the oral (dynamic) structures (ie, lip, cheek).

With the patient under local anesthesia, an incision wide enough to accept the expander is placed on either side of the defect or bilaterally. This incision should allow adequate reflection and undermining with minimal tension.

The tissue is undermined so that continuous contact with bone is maintained.[32] The expander and its attached tubing is safely secured in place, so that it will not hinder the oral tissues. Extra care for suture placement and suturing technique is needed in order to avoid the perforation of the reservoir bag during the procedure. The expander is inflated with sterile saline until tissue blanching occurs. Overinflation may cause sequestration of the bag through the oral tissue or a break in suture line. Repeated addition of saline can be practiced with minimal patient discomfort in order to generate sufficient tissue.

When sufficient tissue has been generated, it can thereafter be used for tissue coverage over large donor material.

Complications

The most common complication is necrosis of the oral tissue overlying the expander bag. This complication can be avoided if adequate dissection has been achieved, and if judicious expansion is practiced.

The intraoral protocol follows guidelines similar to those used for skin expansion.[33-35] Prophylactic broad-spectrum antibiotics are given to the patient during the initial phase of expansion.

QUICK REVIEW

- Recent advances in periodontal plastic surgery allow the clinician to reconstruct deficit alveolar ridges in more predictable ways than previously possible.
- Gingival flaps used for ridge augmentation may be classified by mode of transfer (rotational or advanced) or by geometry (transportational or rotational).
- Clinical examination before ridge augmentation procedures should include:
  — smile line
  — type of ridge deformity
  — arch form and interarch relations
  — restorative / ridge relationship
  — type, character, and position of soft tissues and bone
  — relation of ridges to surrounding orofacial structures

- Ridges may be augmented in several ways:
  — technique depending on vascular perfusion
    (1) autogenous onlay soft tissue grafts
    (2) autogenous inlay soft tissue grafts
    (3) combination of *(1)* and *(2)*
  — local flap approaches
    (1) subperiosteal tunnel
    (2) roll technique
    (3) coronally positioned flap
  — local and distant flaps
    (1) anterior advanced flap
    (2) controlled tissue expansion
- These various methods allow the clinician a number of approaches to esthetically enhance deficit ridges.

REFERENCES

1. Langer B, Calanga L: The subepithelial connective tissue graft. *J Prosthet Dent* 1980;44:363.
2. Langer B, Calanga L: The subepithelial connective tissue graft. A new approach to the enhancement of anterior cosmetics. *Int J Periodont Rest Dent* 1982;2:22.
3. Garber DA, Rosenberg ES: The edentulous ridge in fixed prosthodontics. *Compend Contin Educ Dent* 1981;2:212.
4. Abrams L: Augmentation of the deformed residual edentulous ridge for fixed prosthesis. *Compend Contin Educ Dent* 1980;1:205.
5. Seibert J: Reconstruction of deformed, partially edentulous ridges, using full thickness onlay grafts. Part I. Technique and wound healing. *Compend Contin Educ Dent* 1983;4:437.
6. Seibert J: Reconstruction of deformed, partially edentulous ridges, using full thickness onlay grafts. Part II. Prosthethic / periodontal interrelationships. *Compend Contin Educ Dent* 1983;4:549.
7. Allen EP, Gainza GS, Farthing GG, et al: Improved technique for localized ridge augmentation. A report of 21 cases. *J Periodontol* 1985;56:195.
8. Bahat O, et al: Preservation of ridges utilizing hydroxyapatite. *Int J Periodont Rest Dent* 1987;7(6):35.
9. Bahat O, Handelsman M: Periodontal reconstructive flaps — Classification and surgical considerations. *Int J Periodont Rest Dent* 1991;11:481-487.
10. Bahat O, Koplin M: Pantographic lip expansion and bone grafting for ridge augmentation. *Int J Periodont Rest Dent* 1989;9:345.
11. Bahat O, Handelsman M: Controlled tissue expansion in reconstructive periodontal surgery. *Int J Periodont Rest Dent* 1991;11:25-30.
12. Becker W, et al: Bone formation at dehisced dental implant sites treated with implant augmentation material: A pilot study in dogs. *Int J Periodont Rest Dent* 1990;10:93-101.
13. Nyman S, Lang NP, Buser D, Brägger U: Bone regeneration adjacent to titanium dental implants using guided tissue regeneration: A report of two cases. *Int J Oral Maxillofac Implants* 1990;5:9-14.
14. Seibert J, Nyman S: Localized ridge augmentation in dogs: A pilot study using membranes and hydroxyapatite. *J Periodontol* 1990;61:157-165.
15. Friedman N: Mucogingival surgery. *Tex Dent J* 1957;75:358.
16. Hall WB: *Pure Mucogingival Problems.* Chicago: Quintessence Publ Co, 1984.
17. Hall WB: Gingival augmentation / mucogingival surgery: Review of the literature for the World Workshop in Periodontics. In: *Proceedings of the World Workshop in Periodontics.* Chicago: American Academy of Periodontology, 1989.
18. McGregor IA, Morgan G: Axial and random pattern flaps. *Br J Plast Surg* 1973;26:202.
19. McGregor IA: The Z plasty. *Br J Plast Surg* 1966;19:82.
20. Abrams L: Clinical Examination Chart. Personal Communication, 1987.
21. Schluger S, Youdelis RA, Page RC: *Periodontal Disease.* Philadelphia: Lea & Febiger, 1977.
22. Seibert JS, Cohen DW: Periodontal considerations in preparation for fixed and removable prosthodontics. *Dent Clin North Am* 1987;31:529-555.
23. Bernimoulin J: Coronally repositioned periodontal flap. *J Clin Periodontol* 1975;2:1.
24. Converse JM: *Reconstructive Plastic Surgery.* Philadelphia: WB Saunders Co, 1964.
25. Stark RB: The pantographic expansion principle as applied to advancement flap. *Plas Reconstr Surg* 1955;9:222.

26. Milton SH: Pedicled skin flaps: The fallacy of the length: width ratio. *Brit J Surg* 1970;57:502.

27. Milton SH: Experimental studies on island flaps: 1. The surviving length. *Plast Reconstr Surg* 1971;48:574.

28. Daniel RK, Williams HB: The free transfer of skin flaps by microvascular anastomoses. *Plast Reconstr Surg* 1973; 52:16.

29. Myers MB, Cherry G: Causes of necrosis in pedicle flaps. *Plast Reconstr Surg* 1968;42:43.

30. Patterson TJS: Survival of skin flaps in pigs. *Br J Plastic Surg* 1968;21:113.

31. Cherry GW, Austad ED, et al: Increased survival and vascularity of random pattern skin flaps elevated in controlled expanded skin. *Plast Reconstr Surg* 1983;72:680.

32. Bonomo D: Subperiosteal tissue expands for ridge augmentation. *CDS Review* 1986;79:34-39.

33. Hallock CG: Tissue expansion techniques in burn reconstruction. *Ann Plast Surg* 1987;18:274-282.

34. Heggers JP, Robson MC: Infection control in burn patients. *Clin Plast Surg* 1986;13:39-47.

35. Cullen KW, Clarke JA, McLean DR: The complications of tissue expansion in the burned scalp. *Burns* 1986;12:273-276.

The Diabetic Patient

CURRENT CONCEPTS by Terry D. Rees

CLINICAL APPLICATION by Joan Otomo-Corgel

C U R R E N T   C O N C E P T S

Diabetes mellitus is a complex multifactorial genetic disorder of unknown etiology. It is characterized by a relative or absolute decrease in insulin secretion or effect, which ultimately results in disturbed glucose metabolism and hyperglycemia. The disorder also features a specific type of vascular defect or microangiopathy that involves a thickening of the basement membrane of many blood capillaries throughout the body.[1,2] Symptoms suggestive of diabetes have been described since antiquity, and by the middle of the 19th century the condition was associated with elevated blood sugar levels. Treatment primarily consisted of controlling dietary intake of calories, carbohydrates, fats, and protein, until the discovery of insulin in the 1920s.[3]

Primary diabetes mellitus manifests with two major forms, both of which may result in hyperglycemia. The more severe form, **insulin-dependent diabetes mellitus (IDDM), or Type I,** was formerly referred to as *juvenile onset diabetes* because it frequently manifested in childhood. In the absence of insulin supplementation, Type I diabetes usually results in systemic ketosis or acidosis. Approximately 15% of all diabetics are insulin dependent.

Noninsulin-dependent diabetes (NIDDM), or Type II, was formerly referred to as *maturity onset diabetes* since the condition often occurs in midlife or later. In Type II diabetes, the pancreas is still capable of producing some insulin, at least in early stages of the disease, but the amount is insuf-

ficient to regulate blood glucose levels. This may be the result of increased resistance to the effects of insulin on body tissue cells.[4] NIDDM patients are often obese; onset of symptoms is generally gradual; and there is less tendency to develop ketoacidosis than in IDDM. These patients use insulin poorly, although circulating blood levels may be normal. Type II diabetics, however, often require insulin supplementation in more advanced stages of their disease, so some overlap exists between the two basic categories.[5]

EPIDEMIOLOGY

The true incidence of diabetes mellitus in the United States and

Western countries is unknown. Variations in standards used in diagnosis have resulted in large differences in reported disease rates. It appears, however, that approximately 2.4% of the US population are known diabetics, while a slightly higher percentage of the population may have glucose imbalance, which may ultimately lead to development of diabetes.[2] It has been estimated that at least as many diabetics are currently undiagnosed. Some racial differences have been reported with incidence higher in blacks, native Hawaiians, and some tribes of American Indians than in whites.[6,7]

Overall, approximately 10 million Americans are affected with the disease, and its incidence increases at a rate of 6% per annum.[8] It is reasonable, therefore, to assume that virtually every practicing dentist in the United States will encounter undiagnosed or known diabetic patients in his or her practice.[9] Consequently, a detailed knowledge of the disease and its management is necessary in order to safely and effectively manage dental patients.

SIGNS AND SYMPTOMS

The signs and symptoms of diabetes mellitus are related to pathophysiologic alterations associated with the disease process and may be generally reversible if proper treatment is started before permanent damage has occurred. Basically, the metabolic imbalance produced by impaired insulin function results in the breakdown of fat to yield free fatty acids or ketone bodies. Meanwhile, all body tissues perform as if in a fasting state leading to excess production of glucose and keto acids by the liver. In se-

vere circumstances, this may lead to polyuria, dehydration, ketoacidosis, hypovolemia, and diabetic coma.[2] It is interesting to observe that anorexia nervosa is sometimes associated with hypoglycemic coma identical to diabetic coma.[10] The altered metabolic state results in increased hunger (polyphagia), increased thirst (polydipsia), and frequent urination (polyuria). This may be accompanied by restlessness, irritability, and apathy. Weakness and fatigue are also common, and weight loss may occur. Nausea and vomiting are common due to increasing ketoacidosis. These symptoms usually occur relatively suddenly in IDDM, although there is some evidence that the destruction of beta cells occurs rather insidiously in Type I diabetes.[11,12]

NIDDM features similar signs and symptoms, but ketoacidosis is generally less severe and onset of classic symptoms is more gradual. Patients may experience blurring of vision; irritation and itching of skin, rectum, or vagina; chronic skin infections; delayed healing of cuts or wounds; numbness of extremities; and oral symptoms such as xerostomia, parotid enlargement, multiple or recurrent periodontal abscesses, and gingival hyperplasia.

ORAL MANIFESTATIONS

Seiffert in 1862 is reported to be the first to describe oral features of diabetic patients.[13] He described xerostomia and burning mouth or tongue as common complaints that have subsequently been substantiated by other investigators. Diminished salivary flow and enlargement of the parotid glands have been reported to occur in undiagnosed or poorly controlled diabetics.[14] This may be

the result of abnormalities of parotid gland ductal basement membrane[5] or other histopathologic changes. In some instances, parotid enlargement is at least partially reversible when the diabetic status is brought under control. Recently, slightly decreased salivary flow and increased salivary glucose content were reported in controlled diabetics of both long and short duration.[15]

Xerostomia is often associated with increased oral disease. Dry mucosa is more easily irritated and susceptible to infection. Increased infection with Candida albicans has often been described. General alteration in salivary microorganisms in diabetic patients, possibly as a result of the xerostomia, has also been suggested.[16-18] Increased plaque accumulation may also occur. It is important to remember that many diabetic patients may be receiving drug therapy for associated complications of their disease. Drug-induced xerostomia, therefore, may play a role in oral manifestations of diabetes mellitus.

Increased salivary glucose found in diabetics may relate to glandular secretory changes, but it is also probable that some salivary glucose increase may be derived from crevicular fluid, which also demonstrates increased glucose content in diabetics. Gingival fluid glucose increases might alter the plaque environment, leading to overgrowth of specific microorganisms. Conversely, gingival fluid has been found to increase with increasing periodontal inflammation, suggesting that in some instances, periodontal disease severity may influence salivary and gingival fluid glucose levels.[14]

Microangiopathy has been reported in periodontal tissues,[8,1] but to date, the phenomenon has not been demonstrated to directly correlate with the presence of increased periodontitis.[19] In theory, thickening of the basement membrane of the periodontal microvasculature could alter cellular oxygenation, nutrition, and waste exchange, thus modifying host resistance to advancing plaque-related periodontitis. Not all diabetics develop microangiopathies, and a genetically derived susceptibility may be required to do so. This may explain, in part, why some diabetic patients do not display an increased frequency or severity of periodontal disease.

Oral changes associated with diabetes appear to be consistent with those changes that occur in other body tissues.[20-22] There is general agreement that the uncontrolled or poorly controlled disease state is associated with increased oral/facial infection,[20,22,23] periodontitis,[24-28] and gingival hyperplasia.[26,29,30] In addition, wound healing may be delayed and caries incidence increased. Conversely, the presence of infection may disrupt control of the disease by increasing insulin resistance.[31,32] Although all studies do not agree,[33] candidiasis and other fungal infections tend to increase in incidence and severity even in controlled diabetes mellitus,[34-37] especially under dentures.[37]

Many studies have examined the relationship between diabetes mellitus and periodontal disease with conflicting results. Obviously, patients diagnosed with diabetes cannot remain untreated. Consequently, the effects of the uncontrolled condition on the periodontium have been determined by case reports that describe increased gingival hyperplasia, multiple or recurrent periodontal abscesses, and rapid alveolar bone loss in the presence of plaque-induced periodontal disease. Larger studies evaluating

diabetes-associated periodontitis yield variable results due, in part, to differences in the patient populations studied. Early papers tended to report findings from all diabetic patients identified, regardless of the type. Later, however, attempts were made to separate and study patients by disease type, age, duration of disease, degree of control, and presence or absence of complications.[38-41] The methods of testing and monitoring blood glucose levels currently in use can more accurately assess the interrelationship between periodontitis and diabetes.

The incidence and severity of marginal gingivitis appears to increase[39,42-44] in young patients with IDDM, especially in children with more severe systemic complications[44] or poor metabolic control.[45,46] Diabetic children with good metabolic control may exhibit no differences[17,47,48] or only slight differences[49] when compared to nondiabetic children.

Onset of puberty influences the incidence of gingivitis in IDDM children, but this occurs independently of the degree of diabetic control.[47] In one report, gingivitis was more severe in diabetic versus nondiabetic children, even when plaque scores were similar.[43] In other instances, however, increased plaque levels have been found in diabetic patient groups.[16-18]

Periodontitis does not appear to increase in diabetic children even when the diabetes is relatively poorly controlled.[17,49] Cianciola et al[43] studied young IDDM patients longitudinally. They found a very low incidence of periodontitis in children under 12 years of age; however, a marked increase occurred as the children progressed to young adulthood. This increased prevalence was more strongly related

to the age of the patient than to the duration of the diabetes.

Several studies have described an increased incidence of gingivitis or periodontitis among adults with diabetes mellitus,[13,39,50-54] whereas others have not found such a relationship.[55-58] Bacic et al[57] found deep periodontal pockets to be more common in diabetics with advanced retinopathy. As mentioned earlier, some studies have reported increased levels of plaque and calculus in diabetics, but others have found no increase or even lower plaque indices in diabetic patients.[40,52] Despite this disparity, the incidence of gingivitis and periodontitis is higher in diabetic groups.[52]

The establishment of metabolic control in previously undiagnosed diabetic patients may be associated with dramatic improvement in associated gingival hyperplasia and other manifestations of periodontitis even without extensive periodontal therapy.[26,59] In general, however, efforts to compare the degree of periodontitis with the degree of metabolic control have yielded conflicting results.[51,58,60] For example, a carefully studied group of diabetic Pima Indians was found to have increased incidence of periodontal disease even when their diabetes was relatively well controlled.[61] In other studies in which the blood glucose levels of diabetic patients were closely monitored, however, the differences in periodontal status were minimal. Information such as this suggests that diabetic patients must be carefully evaluated on an individual basis. Many or even most controlled diabetics can be anticipated to respond favorably to periodontal therapy.[41,62] A small group, however, may manifest a persistent life-long tendency to increased incidence and severity of periodontal destruction.

As mentioned earlier, microangiopathy in the periodontium may predispose diabetics to periodontal disease. Other predisposing factors suggested by studies among diabetic patients and experimentally induced diabetic animals include decreased collagen synthesis and increased collagenase activity, theoretically making the patient or the animal susceptible to periodontal connective tissue breakdown.[5,63-65] Meanwhile, increased nephropathy in diabetic rats may be associated with secondary hyperparathyroidism and accelerated alveolar bone destruction.[66] Bone mineral content is reduced in IDDM,[67] which may lead to accelerated alveolar bone destruction in the presence of periodontitis. El Deeb et al[68] recently reported a lack of connective tissue encapsulation of hydroxyapatite granules in diabetic rats treated with alveolar ridge augmentation. They indicated that this result occurs due to poor collagen formation in the diabetic animals.

Several reports have suggested that the oral flora is altered in diabetic patients, perhaps contributing to increased severity of periodontal disease. Mashimo et al[69] identified an increase of *Capnocytophaga* and anaerobic vibrio in IDDM patients, while Gusberti et al[47] found *Capnocytophaga* and *Actinomyces naeslundii* to increase at puberty. More recent studies, however, have failed to identify these organisms in greater quantities among diabetics.[70] Instead, periodontitis in diabetic patients has been correlated with increases in the microflora commonly associated with periodontal inflammation in healthy patients.[70-74]

Diabetes mellitus, especially IDDM, has long been associated with altered host resistance to infectious agents. Impaired polymorphonuclear leukocyte (PMN) chemotaxis or phagocytosis has been reported among diabetic patients.[75] McMullen et al[76] described depressed PMN chemotaxis in healthy individuals with a family history of diabetes mellitus when compared to healthy individuals without such a family history. Animal research and case studies in humans indicate that altered PMN chemotaxis may contribute to periodontal disease severity,[77-79] but diabetes mellitus does not always precipitate PMN dysfunction. Accelerated periodontal destruction is more likely to occur, however, in diabetics who also display altered PMN activity.[80,81] Periodontal disease itself may decrease PMN chemotaxis and phagocytosis regardless of diabetic status.[78] One study has indicated that diabetic rats with periodontitis and impaired PMN function experienced improved PMN chemotaxis when treated for their diabetes, but not to the level found in healthy controls. Therefore, if this information can be applied to humans, some controlled diabetics may continue to be susceptible to accelerated periodontal breakdown in the presence of local etiologic factors.

The incidence of dental caries in diabetics also remains controversial.[13] Uncontrolled or poorly controlled diabetes is associated with high caries prevalence in experimental animals and in humans.[53,82,83] The well-controlled diabetic, however, may exhibit no differences from nondiabetics or even a reduced caries rate.[13,16,17,48,49,82] These findings may relate to the control of carbohydrate intake in diabetic patients and to the degree of metabolic control of the diabetes[16-18,75,84] or to patient compliance with dental care and oral hygiene procedures.[85]

ORAL INFECTIONS

Severe infections have often been demonstrated to interfere with control of diabetes and, on occasion, to be life-threatening.[9,20,23] The primary effect appears to be an increase in insulin resistance caused by release of substances associated with the infectious process such as catecholamines, growth hormone, glucagon, and cortisol.[31,34-86]

Therefore, meticulous control of periodontal disease is an essential feature of establishing metabolic control in diabetics.[31,32] It is interesting to observe that both periodontitis and diabetes are considered to be diseases that are controlled rather than cured, and both rely to a marked extent on patient compliance to maintenance protocols. Patient motivation and compliance, or lack of it, can affect the two diseases simultaneously. That is, patients who carefully monitor and control their metabolic state also tend to maintain meticulous oral hygiene. Conversely, those who are careless regarding their metabolic control also tend to be less conscientious regarding oral hygiene procedures. Therefore, the patient's psychologic attitude may, in part, account for the association between poor metabolic control and increased incidence and severity of periodontal disease.[85]

OTHER MUCOSAL DISEASES

An association between lichen planus and diabetes mellitus has been suggested. Lichen planus is a mucocutaneous disorder of unknown but possible immunologic etiology. The rationale for a relationship with diabetes is unclear, but IDDM has been demonstrated to be occasionally associated with immunologic changes in general. Several early studies suggested the presence of impaired glucose tolerance in lichen planus patients,[87,88] but not all investigators agreed.[89] Plemons et al[90] studied 248 lichen planus patients and reported an increased incidence of diabetes mellitus in those patients (8.06%) versus age- and sex-matched controls (4.44%), but differences were not statistically significant. It should be noted that sulfonylurea drugs used in treatment of NIDDM may occasionally produce lichenoid reactions.[91]

Altered taste sensations are occasionally reported as an early manifestation of diabetes,[92] especially a decreased taste sensation for sucrose. This may result from disordered glucose receptors. Impaired taste, however, may relate to a mild, clinically unappreciated, diabetic neuropathy or to a genetically derived mechanism in susceptible NIDDM patients, but the precise relationship remains unclear.

SCREENING TESTS

There are some circumstances in which the dentist may wish to perform screening tests for altered blood glucose levels. The presence of certain oral signs and symptoms may suggest the possibility that the patient is an undiagnosed or poorly controlled diabetic. In other instances, screening tests may be indicated before performing definitive periodontal therapy. Several tests are available. Ideally, the dentist should chose one that is reasonably simple yet accurate. The glucose tolerance test (GTT) is a long and laborious procedure that must be accomplished under carefully controlled circumstances. It is pri-

marily useful as a medical diagnostic test and is of little practical value in dentistry. Urine glucose testing is a relatively simple procedure, but it is also somewhat insensitive. The renal threshold for glucose in the adult usually begins at 160 to 180 mg/dL, so lower blood glucose levels may not be detected. The renal threshold of glucose often varies among different individuals and also in the same person over time.[93] Additionally, the urine test may not accurately reflect present glucose concentrations since urine may collect in the bladder for many hours before voiding.

Patient screening is often performed using one or more fasting blood sugar (FBS) tests or a combination of FBS with a 2-hour test after glucose loading. These are accurate methods, but they require the use of a medical laboratory, a controlled diet several days prior to the testing, 12 hours of prediet fasting, and multiple venipuncture. Consequently, these tests are usually best performed by the physician, although they have been used for many years by periodontists and others for patient screening.[94]

Dry reagent strips have long been advocated for dental office screening. With this system, a blood sample is obtained by finger puncture or from gingival bleeding. This is used with a reflectance meter or color chart to assess blood glucose levels.[95] The system is probably adequate for monitoring known diabetics before performing periodontal procedures, but it should not be considered a diagnostic mechanism.

In recent years, glycated hemoglobin testing has been advocated for measuring blood glucose levels. This test is of value because glucose binds to blood hemoglobin molecules and remains for the life of the erythro-

cyte, which is approximately 120 days. Measurements of glycated hemoglobin reflect sustained blood sugar levels over a period of 1 to 2 months, with more recent glucose concentrations having proportionally more impact. This test was developed for monitoring blood glucose levels in known diabetics, but recently it has come into use as a diagnostic mechanism. The glycosylated hemoglobin test (HbA_{1c}) has several advantages: it reflects blood glucose levels over an extended period of time; it is accurate under less than ideal conditions; it requires only one laboratory visit; it is relatively inexpensive; and it does not have to be obtained in a fasting state.

The dentist should never tell a patient that he/she has diabetes based on screening tests. Many variables are involved in elevated blood glucose levels and only a physician should attempt to evaluate diagnostic findings. For example, glycosylated hemoglobin concentrations are modified by any condition that shortens red blood cell survival. High levels of fetal hemoglobin, sickle hemoglobin, or other conditions may interfere with test accuracy. Deficiency states of iron, vitamin B_{12}, or zinc may also influence test results.[93,96]

The National Diabetes Data Group has recommended the following diagnostic standards for diabetic diagnosis in nonpregnant adults:

1. Fasting plasma glucose equal to or greater than 140 mg/dL (7.77 mmol/L)
2. Glucose tolerance test showing two plasma glucose values of at least 200 mg/dL (11.1 mmol/L) including the 2-hour plasma glucose and an earlier value

Normal range for glycosylated

hemoglobin is considered to be 4.8% to 7.8% by Corning electrophoresis,[94] but different assays of glycosylated hemoglobin are used, so the practitioner must determine the normal values established for the laboratory that is performing the testing.[93]

THERAPY

An increasing body of evidence indicates that both NIDDM and IDDM patients experience reduced symptoms and fewer complications if effective metabolic control is achieved and blood glucose is stabilized at near-normal levels.[95] This is best achieved by techniques designed to simulate normal insulin secretion, for example, multiple daily insulin injections accompanied by frequent home self-monitoring. Injections of short-duration insulin may be administered before each meal plus a daily injection of long-lasting or intermediate-duration insulin to achieve basal concentrations. This approach is only successful in extremely well motivated and cooperative individuals.[97]

External or implanted insulin pumps are capable of simulating normal insulin output, but such techniques are not without problems.[98,99] Hypoglycemic episodes may occur with insulin pumps, and severe hyperglycemia and even death have been reported due to pump failure. Patients using insulin pumps may lose their awareness of the effects of insulin excess or deficiency.

Insulin has been administered experimentally in an encapsulated liposome or as an intraoral or intranasal spray,[99] but it is not known if this will prevent microangiopathy. Research is being directed toward development of an implantable insulin pump that will release insulin in proportion to blood glucose levels.

Eighty percent of NIDDM patients are overweight. In many instances, diet control leading to sufficient weight loss will establish a satisfactory level of blood glucose and enhance insulin sensitivity.[100,101]

Oral hypoglycemic agents (sulfonylureas) will stimulate insulin release from the beta cells and reduce blood glucose levels. Often, however, insulin is required in management of NIDDM as well as IDDM. In some instances, supplementation with hydroxychloroquine is helpful in controlling blood sugar levels, perhaps by inhibiting insulin degradation in the liver.[102] It is important to remember that diabetic patients are often treated vigorously if early signs of hypertension or renal dysfunction are present. Angiotensin-converting enzyme inhibitors and calcium channel blocking agents have been demonstrated to reduce hypertension in diabetics and to improve renal function.[103] Calcium channel blockers will occasionally cause gingival hyperplasia. Therefore, the dentist must not only consider the severity of diabetic complications present, but also the potential effects of drugs used in their treatment.

Pancreatic transplants or transplantation of pancreatic beta cells offer promise for the future and have been performed with some success in animals and humans. The ultimate goal of diabetic management, however, is prevention. Recent progress in detecting factors involved in the autoimmune process leading to IDDM may enable physicians to identify susceptible individuals.[12,104] These individuals might be protected from beta cell deterioration by use of immunosuppressive agents such as cyclosporin, corticosteroids, or azathioprine. There are potential problems with use of immunosuppressive drugs, however, and a more sophisticated method might be the development of agents that will selectively impair that part of the immune system involved in autoimmune attack on the beta cells.[12] All of these developments will impact on periodontal management of the diabetic patient.

C L I N I C A L   A P P L I C A T I O N

SCREENING FOR DIABETES IN THE DENTAL PRACTICE

Patient Evaluation

There is a likelihood that recognition of signs and symptoms of diabetes mellitus in the dental office may lead to the initial diagnosis of this disease. It is imperative that the clinician be aware that periodontal disease (advanced or progressive for the patient's age), multiple or recurrent periodontal abscesses, oral ulcerations with delayed healing, moniliasis, xerostomia, intraoral numbness or burning, and/or mucormycosis may require further questioning and medical evaluation. Also, key symptoms of polyphagia, polydipsia, recent weight loss and loss of strength, and polyuria require a physician's consultation.

If there is reason to believe a patient may be diabetic or if the patient is a diagnosed diabetic, further investigation via history taking and laboratory studies should be performed. In the confirmed diabetic, the clinician should know the patient's classification: Type I, which is insulin-dependent or IDDM; Type II, which is noninsulin dependent or NIDDM; Type III, which includes drug-associated, hormonal, or pancreatic disease; IGT (impaired glucose tolerance); gestational diabetes mellitus; pre-AGT (previous abnormalities of glucose tolerance); or pot-AGT (potential abnormalities of glucose tolerance).[105,106] Treatment may be altered depending on the individual's diagnosis. It is imperative

to know and record the patient's current medications, dosage, route, and time(s) of administration, the date of the initial diabetic diagnosis, most recent laboratory results, history of diabetic control (ie, previous laboratory results, incidence of insulin reactions, frequency of testing, and patient compliance), normal laboratory results for that patient, current level of control, and treating physician[107] (Table 17-1).

TABLE 17-1 Interviewing the diagnosed diabetic patient

- Approximate date of initial diagnosis of diabetes
- Current medications
  - dosage(s)
  - route of administration
  - time(s) of administration
- Name of treating physician
  - address
  - phone numbers
  - date of last visit
- History of diabetic control
  - most recent laboratory results
  - medical treatment and frequency rendered by physician
  - insulin reaction: date of last reaction; how often?
  - patient at-home testing: frequency; normal (usual) level for the patient

If there is a suspicion that the patient is an undiagnosed diabetic, review the signs and symptoms with the patient. Inform the patient of the possible other medical complications of diabetes mellitus (discussed further in this section). Be concerned if individuals are at risk for the disease based on hereditary predisposition, obesity, age (over 40 years), women with high birthweight babies (9 to

10 lbs), or a history of multiple spontaneous abortions or stillbirths.[108] These individuals should be screened or referred for further laboratory evaluation (Table 17-2).

TABLE 17-2 Interviewing the possible undiagnosed diabetic

- Review signs and symptoms of diabetes mellitus with the patient
- Review complications of diabetes mellitus with the patient
- Consider high-risk individuals:
  - heredity
  - obesity
  - age (over 40 years)
  - women who have had high birthweight babies (>9–10 lb)
  - women with a history of multiple spontaneous abortions or stillbirths
- Patient's last laboratory test for blood glucose (confirm results)
- Laboratory testing in office or referral to medical laboratory or physician

In-Office Laboratory Testing for Diabetes Mellitus

There are two laboratory screening tests that can be performed easily in the dental office: (1) fasting blood glucose or (2) 2-hour postprandial blood glucose. More recently, glycated hemoglobin (HbA_{1c}) has been indicated as a valuable screening laboratory test for periodontal therapy because it may reflect elevated glucose levels over time.[59] This test is referred to a medical laboratory, and results will vary with the methodology used (Figs 17-1 to 17-4). The oral glucose tolerance

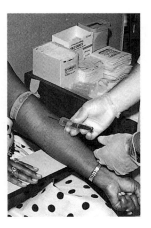

Fig 17-1 Laboratory venipuncture.

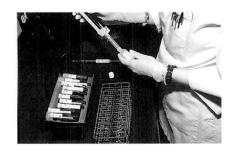

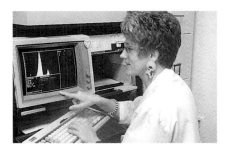

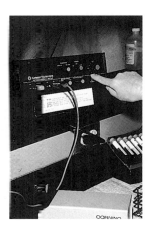

Figs 17-2 to 17-4 (top left, above, bottom left) Analysis of sample will depend on laboratory methodology utilized. Must be performed by a laboratory, but patients do not need to fast.

test is not a standard test for diabetes mellitus but is for screening patients with impaired glucose tolerance and gestational diabetes.

Fasting Blood Glucose Test In order to perform the fasting venous blood glucose test, the following are required: (1) overnight fast, (2) blood draw in the early morning (8 am to 9 am, preferably), (3) diet with a minimum of 250 g of carbohydrates on each of the 3 days prior to testing, and (4) avoidance of excessive physical activity (lowers blood glucose). The method of laboratory collection and analysis is indicated in Figs 17-5 to 17-8. The sample is best drawn on the lateral surface of the fourth digit due to thinner epithelium; also, it is a finger of lesser use. A fasting blood glucose of 140 mg/100 mL or greater over multiple draws requires further medical evaluation. Multiple

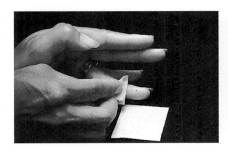

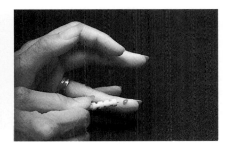

Fig 17-5 (left) Use an alcohol wipe on the area to be sampled for the fasting blood sugar test.

Fig 17-6 (right) The lateral surface of the fourth digit is the preferred site because it has thin epithelium and is an area of minimal use.

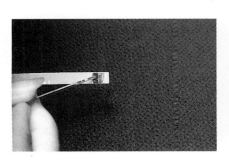

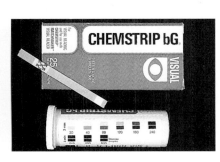

Fig 17-7 (left) Place a drop of blood on the test strip.

Fig 17-8 (right) The sample can be read in the office within 3 minutes.

draws of these levels are diagnostic for diabetes mellitus[109] (Table 17-3).

Two-Hour Postprandial Blood Glucose Test When performing the 2-hour postprandial blood glucose test, one must follow the same requirements as the fasting blood glucose with the exception that at the 8 am to 9 am blood draw, 75 g of glucose is ingested by the patient (glucose load). The blood sample is taken 2 hours later. With levels of 200 mg / 100 mL or greater, the patient should be referred for medical evaluation.

Glycated Hemoglobin Test The glycated hemoglobin test reflects the patient's glucose levels over the previous 6 to 8 weeks. It does not require fasting and is valuable in evaluating recent diabetic history and progress of the patient. The American Diabetic Association recommends the HbA_{1c} be used for followup laboratory tests for known diabetics and for patients with unstable conditions. There are different methods that provide different laboratory values, so it is imperative that the clinician be aware of the particular technique used (ie, electrophoresis versus columnar methods).

Urinary Glucose / Acetone Testing Urinary glucose and acetone testing are not "diagnostic" for diabetes. Individuals may have high blood glucose yet not spill glucose or acetone in the urine. Blood chemistry is the recommended method of laboratory testing.

When to Refer to the Physician

If the dental practitioner recognizes signs or symptoms of disease in an undiagnosed or diagnosed

TABLE 17-3 *Laboratory testing for diabetes*

TEST	VALUES	
Fasting blood glucose	50–100 mg / 100 mL	= Normal
	>100 mg / 100 mL	= Suggestive
	>140 mg / 100 mL	= Diagnostic (over multiple draws)
Two-hour postprandial	>170–200 mg / 100 mL over 2–3 draws	= Diagnostic
Glycated hemoglobin* (electrophoresis)	% total hemoglobin	
	4–8	= Normal adult
	<7.5	= Good control
	7.6–8.9	= Fair control
	9–20	= Poor control

*Laboratory results for glycated hemoglobin will vary with the laboratory and methodology used.

diabetic patient, a referral is recommended. Many clinicians are uncomfortable with in-office laboratory screening and may prefer to refer to the medical laboratory or directly to the physician. Periodontal therapy in the uncontrolled diabetic patient is not advised unless treatment is provided with the aid of medical advice and care. If the periodontal procedure is extremely stress provoking, long term, surgical, or involves orofacial infection, a physician's consultation is advised. Also, if the patient is an insulin-dependent diabetic, it is wise to contact the patient's physician for advice and treatment recommendations. It is the dentist's responsibility to apprise the physician of the severity, extent, duration, and systemic effect of the periodontal therapy.

MEDICAL CONSIDERATIONS

Due to hyperglycemia, ketoacidosis, and vascular wall disease, the uncontrolled diabetic patient has a reduced capacity to wound heal or to manage infection. Hyperglycemia may reduce granu-

locyte / phagocyte function and facilitate the growth of certain microorganisms. Ketoacidosis delays granulocyte migration to the wound and decreases phagocytic function. The narrowing of the vascular walls may lead to decreased blood flow to injuries, therefore reducing oxygen tension and decreasing granulocyte mobilization.[106,110,111]

The diabetic is known to have accelerated vascular wall changes leading to microangiopathy and macrovascular disease. Microangiopathy leads to diabetic retinopathy (leading cause of blindness in the United States) and renal failure (25% of dialysis patients are diabetic). Macrovascular disease (atherosclerosis) is of earlier onset, more widespread, and of greater severity in the diabetic patient. One must be aware that the diabetic patient will often be more susceptible to hypertension (cerebrovascular accidents), coronary atherosclerotic heart disease (myocardial infarction and angina pectoris), renal failure, and ulcerations (and gangrene) of the lower extremities (feet and toes).[112] Often the patient will be on medications for the aforementioned problems. Precautions should be taken even in the controlled diabetic for potential medical complications (Table 17-4).

Lastly, the diabetic patient suffers from a neuropathy that may manifest intraorally as paresthesia or burning tongue. Extraorally, dysphagia, muscle weakness, decreased gastric motility, impotence, and bladder weakness may also occur. These symptoms are noted in over 50% of diabetic patients (NIDDM or IDDM).[17]

PERIODONTAL MANAGEMENT OF THE DIAGNOSED DIABETIC PATIENT

Noninsulin-Dependent Diabetic (Controlled)

In periodontal treatment planning, the controlled NIDDM patient is treated as a healthy normal patient. Periodontal procedures may be performed if no active signs or symptoms of diabetes are apparent. Awareness of the medical complications associated with diabetes should be understood and monitored. Patients should take oral hypoglycemic medications as prescribed, and diet control is a continual must. Patient self-monitoring of glucose levels is generally encouraged. Confirm that the patient regularly visits his/her physician to assess blood glucose levels.

Periodontal surgical procedures in this population can safely be performed. Again, other medical complications of diabetes should be monitored. If surgical procedures may alter the patient's ability to maintain a well-balanced diet, dietary supplements (semisoft or liquid) should be recommended. Close monitoring of wound healing and blood glucose levels is advised.

TABLE 17-4 *Management of medical complications of diabetes mellitus*

Hypertension
- Do not perform routine periodontal therapy if patient is hypertensive (diastolic >105 mm Hg) or is not under adequate medical management
- Monitor blood pressure at each appointment
- Initiate stress and anxiety reduction protocol
- If diastolic >105 mm Hg, refer for medical evaluation
- If diastolic >115 mm Hg, emergency referral to physician
- Do not exceed 3 carpules of xylocaine epinephrine 1:100,000. Inject slowly and aspirate carefully. Do not use xylocaine with epinephrine if the procedure is <30 minutes in duration
- Know interactions of medications prescribed to the patient to control hypertension and the steps of control of the individual patient
- Elevated blood pressure will create increased bleeding at the operative site

Cerebrovascular accident (CVA)
- No treatment unless patient is 6 months post CVA
- Recommend a medical consultation if periodontal therapy is long term or extensive
- Monitor blood pressure closely
- Initiate stress and anxiety reduction protocol
- Schedule shorter morning appointments
- Minimize vasoconstrictors (do not exceed 3 carpules of xylocaine 1:100,000 epinephrine and do not use 1:50,000 epinephrine)
- Post-CVA patients are often on medications for hypertension and anticoagulation (ASA, Persantine, or Coumadin); check for drug interactions and need for alternative periodontal therapy. Coumadin patients should be at 1½ times control to treat periodontally
- Do not dismiss the patient until all hemorrhage is well controlled

Coronary atherosclerotic heart disease (CAHD) *(includes angina or myocardial infarction)*
- No treatment unless patient is 6 months post-MI (consult with physician)
- Schedule shorter, morning appointments
- Institute stress and anxiety reduction protocol (may need oral premedication, ie, valium 5 to 10 mg)
- Administer local anesthetics with no greater than 1:100,000 epinephrine and do not exceed 3 to 5 carpules
- Angina pectoris (stable) patients are safe to treat periodontally; do need to have fresh nitroglycerin available in case of emergencies
- Do not treat unstable angina patients unless in conjunction with medical advice (angina within the past month is considered unstable)
- Be aware of medication interactions and their effect on periodontal therapy (ie, anticoagulants, ASA, digitalis, etc)

Renal disease
- Recommend medical consultation prior to therapy
- Avoid medications metabolized exclusively by the kidney (ie, phenacetin, streptomycin, tetracycline); use ASA and acetaminophen with caution
- Monitor blood pressure closely
- Hospitalize for severe infections
- Design periodontal therapy for long-term maintenance; extraction of questionable teeth is recommended
- Use clean surgical technique to minimize tissue trauma and infection
- Encourage meticulous home care and frequent supportive periodontal therapy

Retinopathy
- If diagnosed for acute narrow-angle glaucoma, Valium is contraindicated

blood glucose levels are elevated, especially in cases of denture stomatitis.[33] Treatment of *Candida albicans* in the diabetic includes: *(1)* topical antifungal agents, or systemic antifungal agents (if under physician consultation) and *(2)* close evaluation of antibiotic therapy so as to not encourage fungal overgrowth.

"Burning mouth," glossodynia, or dental neuropathy has also been noted in the diabetic patient.[120,121] One must rule out pernicious anemia as the cause. Due to increased inflammation, soft tissues may be more sensitive and tender; therefore, adequate home care may not be performed. Recommendations are:

1. Rinse with topical analgesic
2. Rinse with equal parts elixir of diphenhydramine (Benadryl), kaolin (Kaopectate), and xylocaine viscous
3. Gentle, frequent supportive periodontal therapy
4. Meticulous home care with ultrasoft brushes

Lastly, there has been a recent report of high incidence of benign migratory glossitis (BMG) in the diabetic patient. If the diagnosis of BMG is made, further investigation into related diabetes should also be made.[122] Oral lichen planus incidence has had similar reporting.

TABLE 17-6 *Treatment of diabetic emergencies*

Hyperglycemia (diabetic acidosis) — gradual onset caused by inadequate insulin

Conscious patient
- Immediate medical consultation
- Hospitalization if warranted

Unconscious patient
- Basic life support (open airway, administer oxygen, check for circulation, monitor vital signs)
- Call for medical assistance
- Start an intravenous line (if available) to augment medical management
- Hospitalization and blood glucose monitoring

Hypoglycemia (insulin reaction-shock) — onset is sudden and is caused by excessive insulin and inadequate carbohydrate intake

Conscious patient
- Recognize signs/symptoms of glucose insufficiency (see Table 17-7)
- Give oral carbohydrates:
    sugar
    orange juice (better to add 2–4 tablespoons of sugar)
    candy bar
    cola (12 oz has 40 g of sugar)
    glucola 75–100 g of sugar — couple of oz every 5–10 min
- Recovery time: after oral carbohydrate load, wait 1 hour in the office to assess patient recovery
- If no change or if patient is not cooperative, administer parenteral carbohydates:
    — intramuscular glucagon (1 mg): patient should respond within 10–15 min
    — intravenous dextrose (50 mL in 50% concentration): patient should respond within 5 min
    — start oral carbohydrates when tolerated
- Call for medical assistance and probable hospitalization

Unconscious patient
- Basic life support
- Call for emergency medical assistance
- Administer carbohydrate in the most effective method available:
    — IV: dextrose 30–50 mL of a 50% concentration over 2–3 min. Response should be within 5–10 min
    — IM: glucagon 1 mg. Response should be within 0–15 min
    — IM (or subcutaneous): epinephrine 0.5 mg 1:1,000 **only** if no dextrose or glucagon available. Every 15 min until conscious
    — oral: only if previous methods are unavailable (eg, small amounts of cake icing under the tongue to avoid airway obstruction)

MANAGEMENT OF DIABETIC EMERGENCIES IN THE DENTAL PRACTICE

There are essentially two major types of diabetic emergencies that can occur in the dental office: chronic and acute. Chronic emergencies relate to the chronic medical complications to which the diabetic patient is subject: atherosclerosis, angina, myocardial infarction, hypertension, CVA, renal failure, and infection control[123] (see Table 17-4). The second major emergency is the acute form, which may manifest as hyperglycemia or hypoglycemia.

Hyperglycemia

Hyperglycemia is not likely to be encountered as an emergency state in the dental office. Clinical manifestations are more likely to be witnessed in the juvenile onset or "brittle" (ketosis-prone) diabetic. Clinical symptoms include: polydipsia, polyphagia, polyuria, excessive weight loss, fatigue, headache, blurred vision, abdominal pain, nausea and vomiting, constipation, dyspnea, mental stupor, and progression to loss of consciousness or diabetic coma. Signs of hyperglycemia are indicative of dehydration or are "dry" in character: hot, dry skin; deep, rapid (Kussmal) respirations; acetone breath; florid facies; tachycardia; and hypotension.[23] Because the onset of hyperglycemia is slow, the dental office should provide early recognition and referral. Management of the acute emergency is usually supportive. If the patient is still conscious, phy-

sician referral should be immediate. If the patient is unconscious, basic life support should be immediately provided (open airway, administer oxygen, check circulation, and summon medical aid). If possible, an intravenous infusion of normal saline should be started to provide a lifeline for the emergency team. Hospitalization and insulin with close blood glucose monitoring should follow (Table 17-6).

Hypoglycemia

Hypoglycemia is a more likely acute emergency in the dental office. It is the most common form of diabetic emergency and may occur suddenly. Although there are several forms of hypoglycemia (functional hyperinsulinism, enzyme deficiencies, exogenous, etc), this section will deal with hypoglycemia as seen in the diabetic (Table 17-7).

The initial stages of hypoglycemia are that of mental confusion, sudden mood changes, and decreased spontaneity in conversation (diminished cerebral function). Next, CNS signs and symptoms of hunger, nausea, and increased gastric motility occur. As the hypoglycemia progresses, signs are "wet" (increased epinephrine activity): sweating, tachycardia, piloerection, wet, cold skin, and bizarre behavior patterns (uncooperative, belligerent). If the hypoglycemic event is allowed to progress, the patient will become hypotensive, hypothermic, lose consciousness, and possibly go into seizures.[123]

TABLE 17-7 *Signs and symptoms of hypoglycemia*

Mild stage
Sudden mood change (ie, depression and lethargy)
Decreased mentation
Decreased ability to respond verbally
Hunger
Nausea
Paresthesia

Moderate stage
Wet, cold skin
Tachycardia
Bizarre behavior patterns (belligerence, poor judgment, uncooperativeness)
Anxiety and disorientation
Piloerection

Severe stage
Unconsciousness
Hypotension
Hyperthermia
Rapid, thready pulse
Seizures or tonic, clonic movements

Insulin shock occurrence is sudden in many cases and will have to be handled in the dental office. If recognized early, recovery is dramatic and rapid. Management should be as listed in Table 17-5.

Insulin shock is a serious life-threatening emergency if not recognized and treated by the dental team. It is imperative that all diabetic periodontal patients (especially insulin-dependent) be monitored for early insulin shock recognition. Periodontal disease is often a reflection of underlying systemic disorders; thus it becomes our professional obligation and duty to monitor not only the periodontal aspects but the etiologic contributor as well.

QUICK REVIEW

I. Diabetes mellitus
- Virtually every practicing dentist will encounter undiagnosed or known diabetic patients in his or her practice.
- Uncontrolled diabetes is associated with increased oral infections (candidiasis), recurrent or multiple periodontal abscesses, gingival hyperplasia, rapid alveolar bone loss, delayed wound healing, and an increased caries rate.
- Many controlled diabetics will respond favorably to periodontal therapy; a small group, however, may manifest a life-long susceptibility to periodontal destruction.
- The screening test of choice in periodontal patients may be the glycosylated hemoglobin test.
- Developing trends in medical treatment for diabetes may soon result in disease prevention and an overall reduction in complications presently associated with the disease.

II. Clinical periodontal therapy in the diabetic patient
- The initial recognition of diabetes mellitus may occur via recognition of oral manifestations.

- The diabetic patient has reduced capacity for wound healing and infection management due to hyperglycemia, ketoacidosis, and vascular wall disease.
- The dental clinician should be aware of the classification of the diabetic patient and know how to alter periodontal therapy accordingly.
- The diabetic patient who is uncontrolled should not receive routine periodontal therapy without medical intervention and advice. **Dentists should not diagnose diabetes**, but should screen and refer as indicated.
- Insulin-dependent diabetics may require alteration in insulin dosage prior to periodontal procedures that may alter carbohydrate ingestion.
- The dental team is responsible for recognition of oral tissue changes associated with diabetes mellitus.
- Hypoglycemia or insulin shock (reaction) is a life-threatening emergency for which initial recognition and treatment in the dental office is a necessity.

REFERENCES

1. Siperstein MD: The glucose tolerance test: A pitfall in the diagnosis of diabetes mellitus. *Adv Intern Med* 1975;20:297.
2. Cahill GF Jr, Arky RD, Perlman AJ: *Diabetes Mellitus.* New York: Scientific American, Inc, 1990.
3. Anonymous: Diabetes mellitus: Brief history. Diabetes mellitus: A collection of monographs. Kalamazoo, Mich: The Upjohn Company, 1968.
4. Smith U: Insulin action — Biochemical and clinical aspects. *Acta Med Scand* 1987;222:7.
5. Ramamurthy NS, Greenwald RA, Schneir M, Golub LM: The effect of alloxan diabetes on prolyl and lysyl hydroxylase activity in uninflamed and inflamed rat gingiva. *Arch Oral Biol* 1985;30:679.

6. Lichton IJ, Bullard LR, Sherrell BU: A conspectus of research on nutritional status in Hawaii and Western Samoa — 1960–1980 with references to diseases in which diet has been implicated. *World Rev Nutr Diet* 1983;41:40.
7. Sugarman JR: Prevalence of diagnosed hypertension among diabetic Navajo indians. *Arch Intern Med* 1990;150:359.
8. Murrah VA: Diabetes mellitus and associated oral manifestations: A review. *J Oral Pathol* 1985;14:271.
9. Harrison GA, Schultz TA, Schaberg SJ: Deep neck infection complicated by diabetes mellitus. Report of a case. *Oral Surg Oral Med Oral Pathol* 1983;55:133.
10. Rich LM, Caine MR, Findling JW,

Shaker JL: Hypoglycemic coma in anorexia nervosa. Case report and review of the literature. *Arch Intern Med* 1990;150:894.
11. Tarn AC, Smith CP, Spencer KM, Bottazzo GF, Gale EA: Type I (insulin dependent) diabetes: A disease of slow clinical onset? *Br Med J* 1987; 294:342.
12. Atkinson MD, Maclaren NK: What causes diabetes? *Sci Am* 1990; July:62.
13. Albrecht M, Banoczy J, Tamas G Jr: Dental and oral symptoms of diabetes mellitus. *Community Dent Oral Epidemiol* 1988;16:378.
14. Thorstensson H, Falk H, Hugoson A, Olsson J: Some salivary factors in insulin-dependent diabetics. *Acta Odontol Scand* 1989;47:175.

15. Murrah VA, Crosson JT, Sank JJ: Parotid gland basement membrane variation in diabetes mellitus. *J Oral Pathol* 1985;14:236.

16. Harrison R, Bowen WH: Periodontal health, dental caries, and metabolic control in insulin-dependent diabetic children and adolescents. *Pediatr Dent* 1987;9:283.

17. Goteiner D, Vogel R, Deasy M, Goteiner C: Periodontal and caries experience in children with insulin-dependent diabetes mellitus. *J Am Dent Assoc* 1986;113:277.

18. Albrecht M, Banoczy J, Baranyi E, Tamas G Jr, Szalay J, Egyed J, Simon G, Ember G: Studies of dental and oral changes of pregnant diabetic women. *Acta Diabetol Lat* 1987; 24:1.

19. Listgarten MA, Ricker FH Jr, Laster L, Shapiro J, Cohen DW: Vascular basement lamina thickness in the normal and inflamed gingiva of diabetics and non-diabetics. *J Periodontol* 1974;45:676.

20. Reyna J, Richardson JM, Mattox DE, Banowsky LH, Nicastro-Lutton JL: Head and neck infection after renal transplantation. *J Am Med Assoc* 1982;247:3337.

21. Lipsky BA, Pecoraro RE, Larson SA, Hanley ME, Ahroni JH: Outpatient management of uncomplicated lower-extremity infections in diabetic patients. *Arch Intern Med* 1990;150:790.

22. Archer CB, Scott GW, Rosenberg WMC, MacDonald DM: Progressive bacterial synergistic gangrene in patient with diabetes mellitus. *J R Soc Med* 1984;77(Suppl 4):1.

23. Baranda L: Facial erythema and edema in a diabetic man. *Arch Dermatol* 1986;122:329.

24. Rhodus NL: Detection and management of the diabetic patient. *Compend Contin Educ Dent* 1987;8:73.

25. Ureles SD: Case report: A patient with severe periodontitis in conjunction with adult-onset diabetes. *Compend Contin Educ Dent* 1983;4:522.

26. Bartolucci EG, Parkes RB: Accelerated periodontal breakdown in uncontrolled diabetes. Pathogenesis and treatment. *Oral Surg Oral Med Oral Pathol* 1981;52:387.

27. Akintewe TA, Kulasekara B, Adetuyibi A:Periodontitis diabetica. A case report from Nigeria. *Trop Geogr Med* 1984;36:85.

28. Harvey PM: Control of severe periodontitis with reduction of infection and some recovery of clinical attachment in a patient with initially undiagnosed diabetes. *J New Zealand Soc Periodont* 1986;61:12-17.

29. Van Dis ML, Allen CM, Neville BW: Erythematous gingival enlargement in diabetic patients: A report of four cases. *J Oral Maxillofac Surg* 1988;46:794.

30. Hurt WC, Rees TD: Adjunctive therapy. In: *Proceedings of the World Workshop in Clinical Periodontics.* Chicago: American Academy of Periodontology; 1989:X-18.

31. Sammalkorpi K: Glucose intolerance in acute infections. *J Intern Med* 1989;255:15.

32. Williams RC Jr, Mahan CJ: Periodontal disease and diabetes in young adults. *J Am Med Assoc* 1960; 172:776.

33. Phelan JA, Levin SM: A prevalence study of denture stomatitis in subjects with diabetes mellitus or elevated plasma glucose levels. *Oral Surg Oral Med Oral Pathol* 1986;62:303.

34. Larkin G, Frier BM, Ireland JT: Diabetes mellitus and infection. *Postgrad Med J* 1985;61:233.

35. Villeneuve ME, Treitel L, D'Eramo G: Dental care for the person with diabetes mellitus. *Diabetes Educ* 1985;11:44.

36. Correll RW, Jensen JL, Rhyne RR: Painless, irregularly shaped erythematous area on the middorsum of the tongue. *J Am Dent Assoc* 1985;111:793.

37. Fisher BM, Lamey PJ, Samaranayake LP, MacFarlane TW, Frier BM: Carriage of Candida species in the oral cavity in diabetic patients: Relationship to glycaemic control. *J Oral Pathol* 1987:16:282.

38. Manouchehr-Pour M, Bissada NF: Periodontal disease in juvenile and adult diabetic patients: A review of the literature. *J Am Dent Assoc* 1983;107:766.

39. Hugoson A, Thorstensson H, Falk H, Kuylenstierna J: Periodontal conditions in insulin-dependent diabetics. *J Clin Periodontol* 1989;16:215.

40. Rosenthal IM, Abrams H, Kopczyk A: The relationship of inflammatory periodontal disease to diabetic status in insulin-dependent diabetes mellitus patients. *J Clin Periodontol* 1988;15:425.

41. Tervonen T, Knuuttila M: Relation of diabetes control to periodontal pocketing and alveolar bone level. *Oral Surg Oral Med Oral Pathol* 1986;61:346.

42. Bernick SM, Cohen DW, Baker L, Laster L: Dental disease in children with diabetes mellitus. *J Periodontol* 1975;46:241.

43. Cianciola LJ, Park BH, Bruck E, Mosovich L, Genco RJ: Prevalence of periodontal disease in insulin-dependent diabetes mellitus (juvenile diabetes). *J Am Dent Assoc* 1982; 104:653.

44. Rylander H, Ramberg P, Blohme G, Lindhe J: Prevalence of periodontal disease in young diabetics. *J Clin Periodontol* 1987;14:38.

45. Kjellman O, Henriksson CO, Berghagen N, Andersson B: Oral conditions in 105 subjects with insulin-treated diabetes mellitus. *Swed Dent J* 1970;63:99.

46. Gislen G, Nilsson KO, Matsson L: Gingival inflammation in diabetic children related to degree of metabolic control. *Acta Odontol Scand* 1980; 38:241.

47. Gusberti FA, Syed SA, Bacon G, Grossman N, Loesche WJ: Puberty gingivitis in insulin-dependent diabetic children. I. Cross-sectional observations. *J Periodontol* 1983;54: 714.

48. Sarnat H, Eliaz R, Feinman G, Flexer Z, Karp A, Laron Z: Carbohydrate consumption and oral status of diabetic and nondiabetic young adolescents. *Clin Prev Dent* 1985;7:20.

49. Leeper SH, Kalkwarf KL, Strom EA: Oral status of "controlled" adolescent type I diabetics. *J Oral Med* 1985;40: 27.

50. Barnett ML, Baker RL, Yancey JM, MacMillan DR, Kotoyan M: Absence of periodontitis in a population of insulin-dependent diabetes mellitus (IDDM) patients. *J Periodontol* 1984;55:402.

51. Ervasti T, Knuuttila M, Pohjamo L, Haukipuro K: Relation between control of diabetes and gingival bleeding. *J Periodontol* 1985;56:154.

52. Cohen DW, Friedman LA, Shapiro J, Kyle GC, Franklin S: Diabetes mellitus and periodontal disease: Two-year longitudinal observations, Part I. *J Periodontol* 1970;41:709.

53. Galea H, Aganovic I, Aganovic M: The dental caries and periodontal disease experience of patients with early onset insulin dependent diabetes. *Int Dent J* 1986;36:219.

54. Belting CM, Hiniker JJ, Dummett CO: Influence of diabetes mellitus on the severity of periodontal disease. *J Periodontol* 1964;35:476.

55. Hove KA, Stallard RE: Diabetes and the periodontal patient. *J Periodontol* 1970;41:713.

56. Nichols C, Laster LL, Bodak-Gyovai LZ: Diabetes mellitus and periodontal disease. *J Periodontol* 1978;49: 85.

57. Bacic M, Plancak D, Granic M: CPITN assessment of periodontal disease in diabetic patients. *J Periodontol* 1988;59:8 6.

58. Glavind L, Lund B, Löe H: The relationship between periodontal state and diabetes duration, insulin dosage and retinal changes. *J Periodontol* 1968;39:341.

59. Piche JE, Swan RH, Hallmon WW: The glycosylated hemoglobin assay for diabetes: Its value to the periodontist. Two case reports. *J Periodontol* 1989;60:640.

60. Campbell MJA: Epidemiology of periodontal disease in the diabetic and nondiabetic. *Aust Dent J* 1972; 17:274.

61. Sheridan P: Diabetes and oral health. *J Am Dent Assoc* 1987;115:741.

62. Wilson TG Jr: Periodontal diseases and diabetes. *Diabetes Educ* 1989; 15:342.

63. Golub LM, Wolff M, Lee HM, McNamara TF, Ramamurthy NS, Zambon J, Ciancio J: Further evidence that tetracyclines inhibit collagenase activity in human crevicular fluid and from other mammalian sources. *J Periodont Res* 1985;20:12.

64. Golub LM, Lee HM, Lehrer G, Nemiroff A, McNamara TF, Kaplan R, Ramamurthy NS: Minocycline reduces gingival collagenolytic activity during diabetes. Preliminary observations and a proposed new mechanism of action. *J Periodont Res* 1983;18:516.

65. Kaplan R, Mulvihill J, Ramamurthy N, Golub L: Gingival collagen metabolism in human diabetics. *J Dent Res* 1982;61:275.

66. Johnson RB, Thliveris JA: Effect of low-protein diet on alveolar bone loss in streptozotocin-induced diabetic rats. *J Periodontol* 1989; 60:264.

67. Mathiassen B, Nielsen S, Ditzel J, Rodbro P: Long-term bone loss in insulin-dependent diabetes mellitus. *J Intern Med* 1990;227:325.

68. El Deeb M, Roszkowski M, Hakim I: Tissue response to hydroxylapatite in induced diabetic and nondiabetic rats. *J Oral Maxillofac Surg* 1990;48:476.

69. Mashimo PA, Yamamoto Y, Slots J, Park BH, Genco RJ: The periodontal microflora of juvenile diabetics. Culture, immunofluorescence, and serum antibody studies. *J Periodontol* 1983;54:420.

70. Sastrowijoto SH, Hillemans P, van Steenbergen TJM, Abraham-Inpijn L, de Graaf J: Periodontal condition and microbiology of healthy and diseased periodontal pockets in type I diabetes mellitus patients. *J Clin Periodontol* 1989;16:316.

71. Sandholm L, Swanljung O, Rytomaa I, Kaprio EA, Maenpaa J: Morphotypes of the subgingival microflora in diabetic adolescents in Finland. *J Periodontol* 1989;60:526.

72. Monefeldt K, Tollefsen T: Serum IgG antibodies reactive with lipoteichoic acid in adult patients with periodontitis. *J Clin Periodontol* 1989;16:519.

73. Morinushi T, Lopatin DE, Syed SA, Bacon G, Kowalski CJ, Loesche WJ: Humoral immune response to selected subgingival plaque microorganisms in insulin-dependent diabetic children. *J Periodontol* 1989;60:199-204.

74. Zambon JJ, Reynolds H, Fisher JG, Shlossman M, Dunford R, Genco RJ: Microbiological and immunological studies of adult periodontitis in patients with noninsulin-dependent diabetes mellitus. *J Periodontol* 1988;59:23-31.

75. Miller ME, Baker L: Leukocyte functions in juvenile diabetes mellitus: Humoral and cellular aspects. *J Pediatr* 1972;81:979.

76. McMullen JA, Van Dyke TE, Horoszewicz HU, Genco RJ: Neutrophil chemotaxis in individuals with advanced periodontal disease and a genetic predisposition to diabetes mellitus. *J Periodontol* 1981;52:167.

77. Manouchehr-Pour M, Spagnuolo PJ, Rodman HM, Bissada NF: Comparison of neutrophil chemotactic response in diabetic patients with mild and severe periodontal disease. *J Periodontol* 1981;52:410.

78. Bissada NF, Manouchehr-Pour M, Haddow M, Spagnuolo PJ: Neutrophil functional activity in juvenile and adult onset diabetic patients with mild and severe periodontitis. *J Periodont Res* 1982;17:500.

79. Golub LM, Nicoll GA, Iacono VJ, Ramamurthy NS: In vivo crevicular leukocyte response to a chemotactic challenge: Inhibition by experimental diabetes. *J Infect Immun* 1982;37:1013.

80. Iacono VJ, Singh S, Golub LM, Ramamurthy NS, Kaslick R: In vivo assay of crevicular leukocyte migration. Its development and potential applications. *J Periodontol* 1985;56:56.

81. Manouchehr-Pour M, Spagnuolo PJ, Rodman HM, Bissada NF: Impaired neutrophil chemotaxis in diabetic patients with severe periodontitis. *J Dent Res* 1981;60:729.

82. Reuterving CO, Hagg E, Gustafson GT: Root surface caries and periodontal disease in long-term alloxan diabetic rats. *J Dent Res* 1986; 65:689.

83. Falk H, Hugoson A, Thorstensson H: Number of teeth, prevalence of caries and periapical lesions in insulin-dependent diabetics. *Scand J Dent Res* 1989;97:198.

84. Tenovuo J, Alanen P, Larjava H, Viikari J, Lehtonen OP: Oral health of patients with insulin-dependent diabetes mellitus. *Scand J Dent Res* 1986;94:338.

85. Thorstensson H, Falk H, Hugoson A, Kuylenstierna J: Dental care habits and knowledge of oral health in insulin-dependent diabetics. *Scand J Dent Res* 1989;97:207.

86. Modelevsky S: Oral surgery management of patients with common endocrine diseases. *J Mo Dent Assoc* 1984;64:32.

87. Lundstrom IM: Incidence of diabetes mellitus in patients with oral lichen planus. *Int J Oral Surg* 1983; 12:147.

88. Lowe NJ, Cudworth AC, Clough SA, Bullen MF: Carbohydrate metabolism in lichen planus. *Br J Dermatol* 1976;95:9.

89. Lozaza-Nur F, Luangjarmekorn L, Silverman S Jr, Karam J: Assessment of plasma glucose in 99 patients with oral lichen planus. *J Oral Med* 1985;40:60.

90. Plemons J, Rankin K, Rees T, Cortes E, Glass M: Systemic abnormalities in patients with erosive lichen planus. *J Dent Res* 1990;69:150 (Abstr no. 331).

91. Firkin DJ, Ferguson JW: Diabetes mellitus and the dental patient. *N Z Dent J* 1985;81:7.

92. Hardy SL, Brennand CP, Wyse BW: Taste thresholds of individuals with diabetes mellitus and of control subjects. *J Am Dietetic Assoc* 1981; 79:286.

93. Singer DE, Coley CM, Samet JH, Nathan DM: Tests of glycemia in diabetes mellitus. Their use in establishing a diagnosis and in treatment. *Ann Intern Med* 1989;110:125.

94. DePaola LG, Kutcher MJ, Bowers GM: The dentist's role in the detection of the undiagnosed diabetic patient. *Compend Contin Educ Dent* 1989;187-195.

95. Tsutsui P, Rich SK, Schonfeld SE: Reliability of intraoral blood for diabetes screening. *J Oral Med* 1985;40:62.

96. Gram-Hansen P, Eriksen J, Mourits-Andersen T, Olesen L: Glycosylated haemoglobin (HbA$_{1c}$) in iron- and vitamin B$_{12}$ deficiency. *J Intern Med* 1990;227:133.

97. Newman WP, Laqua D, Engelbrecht D: Impact of glucose self-monitoring on glycohemoglobin values in a veteran population. *Arch Intern Med* 1990;150:107.

98. Heinemann L, Sonnenberg GE, Hohmann A, et al: Pulsatile insulin infusion and glucose-homeostasis in well-controlled type I (insulin-dependent) diabetic patients. *J Intern Med* 1989;226:325.

99. Rizza RA: New modes of insulin administration: Do they have a role in clinical diabetes? *Ann Intern Med* 1986;150:126.

100. Lomasky SJ, D'Eramo G, Shamoon H, Fleischer N: Relationship of insulin secretion and glycemic response to dietary intervention in non-insulin-dependent diabetes. *Arch Intern Med* 1990;150:169.

101. Watts NB, Spanheimer RG, DiGirolamo M, Gebhart SS, Musey VC, Siddiq YK, Phillips LS: Prediction of glucose response to weight loss in patients with non-insulin-dependent diabetes mellitus. *Arch Intern Med* 1990;150:803.

102. Quatraro A, Consoli G, Magno M, Caretta F, Nardozza A, Ceriello A, Giugliano D: Hydroxychloroquine in decompensated, treatment-refractory noninsulin-dependent diabetes mellitus. A new job for an old drug? *Ann Intern Med* 1990;112:678.

103. Bakris GL: Effects of diltiazem or lisinopril on massive proteinuria asso-

ciated with diabetes mellitus. *Ann Intern Med* 1990;112:707.

104. Wilkin T, Armitage M: Markers for insulin dependent diabetes: Towards early detection. *Br Med J* 1986; 293:1323.

105. National Diabetes Data Group: Classification and diagnosis of diabetes mellitus and other categories of glucose intolerance. *Diabetes* 1979;28:1039.

106. Carranza FA: Periodontal pathology. *Glickman's Periodontology.* Philadelphia: WB Saunders Co, 1990.

107. Olefsky JM: Diabetes mellitus. In: Wyngarrden JB, Smith LH, eds. *Cecil Textbook of Medicine.* Philadelphia: WB Saunders Co, 1985.

108. Little JW, Falace DA: Diabetes. In: *Dental Management of the Medically Compromised Patient.* St Louis: CV Mosby Co, 1984;197.

109. Otomo-Corgel J: Periodontal treatment for medically compromised patients. In: Carranza FA, ed. *Glickman's Periodontology.* Philadelphia: WB Saunders Co; 1990:573.

110. Blonde L, Re R: Endocrinologic diseases. In: Tullman MJ, Redding SW, eds. *Systemic Disease in Dental Treatment.* New York: Appleton-Century-Crofts; 1982:238-247.

111. Cogen RB: Diabetic patients in dentistry. In: Thornton JB, Wright JT, eds. *Special and Medically Compromised Patients in Dentistry.* Littletown, Mass: PSG Publ Co; 1989:113.

112. Saadoun AP: Diabetes and periodontal disease: A review and update. *Periodont Abstr* 1980;28:116.

113. Rothwell BR, Richard EL: Diabetes mellitus: Medical and dental considerations. *Spec Care Dent* 1984;4:58.

114. Ainamo J, et al: Rapid periodontal destruction in adult humans with poorly controlled diabetes. A report of 2 cases. *J Clin Periodontol* 1990;17:22.

115. Binder A, et al: Sjögren's syndrome: Association with type-I diabetes mellitus. *Br J Rheum* 1989;28:518.

116. Otomo-Corgel J: Periodontal management of the geriatric patient. In: Carranza FA, ed. *Glickman's Periodontology.* Philadelphia: WB Saunders Co; 1990:590.

117. Hill LV, et al: Association of oral candidiasis with diabetic control. *J Clin Pathol* 989;42:502.

118. Bartholomew GA, et al: Oral candidiasis in patients with diabetes mellitus. A thorough analysis. *Diabetes Care* 1987;10:607.

119. Van der Westhuijzen AJ, et al: A rapid y fatal palatal ulcer: Rhinocerebral mucormycosis. *Oral Surg Oral Med Oral Pathol* 1989;68:32.

120. Zegarelli DJ: Burning mouth: An alternative explanation for some patients with diabetes mellitus and pernicious anemia. *Ann Dent* 1987; 46:23.

121. Hatch CL: Glossodynia as an oral manifestation of diabetes mellitus. *ENT J* 1989;68:782.

122. Wysocki GP, Daley TD: Benign migratory glossitis in patients with juvenile diabetes. *Oral Surg Oral Med Oral Pathol* 1987;63:68.

123. Malamed SF: *Diabetes Mellitus: Hyperglycemia and Hypoglycemia.* St Louis: CV Mosby Co; 1982:187.

Intravenous Sedation

CURRENT CONCEPTS by Joseph A. Giovannitti, Jr

CLINICAL APPLICATION by Dan M. Loughlin

C U R R E N T   C O N C E P T S

PREOPERATIVE RISK FACTORS

When drugs are administered to patients to produce conscious sedation, the observed effects are the culmination of a series of altered physiologic functions. In a true sense, we produce pathophysiologic changes when we administer these agents, some of which are desirable and some of which are undesirable. Many factors determine how a drug or drug combination will affect the various functions of the human body. These factors include the preexisting medical condition of the patient, the nature and duration of the present illness, drug interactions, age, nutritional status, environmental factors, and genetically determined factors that may render patients more susceptible or resistant to the effects of a particular drug. In order to maximize the desirable effects produced by these agents and minimize the undesirable effects, a clinician must accurately assess the patient's preanesthetic condition, be thoroughly familiar with the pharmacodynamics of the drugs used, and be properly trained to continuously monitor the effects produced by these agents. In addition, the clinician should be trained to correct any significant pathophysiologic changes produced by the administration of these drugs. The office team should be experienced and well trained, and there should be sufficient backup resources in the event of an emergency. Without these basic precautions, inadvertent but significant changes in a patient's physiologic function may lead to injury or even death.

Care should be taken to avoid the anesthesia pitfalls that may lead to an adverse outcome. Without a doubt, the most common cause of anesthetic misadventures is an inadequate preoperative evaluation. This in turn may lead to technique failure due to improper technique selection, overdosage, or drug interaction. Exposing a medically compromised patient to the risks of deep sedation or general anesthesia when conscious sedation will do is just asking for trouble. On the other hand, using conscious sedation when general anesthesia is indicated may lead the practitioner to push the technique beyond the limits of good practice. This invariably leads to overdosage, airway obstruction, and cardiorespiratory depression. Inadequate or improper monitoring also contributes highly to anesthetic morbidity and mortality. The mere presence of an electronic monitor does not guarantee the patient's safety and may sometimes provide a false sense of security. Certain knowledge is required for proper interpretation, and during conscious sedation no monitor should be a substitute for verbally and visually ascertaining the patient's level of consciousness, comfort, and cooperation. Finally, anesthetic management may break down in the resuscitative phase. Inadequate treatment of an adverse event may further increase the risk and hinder the outcome.

RISK MANAGEMENT

When we as practitioners decide to provide anesthetic services to our patients, we become high risks in the eyes of our malpractice insurance carriers. Regardless of the arguments on either side of this issue, we must logically manage the inherent risks. Good risk management starts with good patient relations. The frequency of litigation is inversely proportional to the level of our relationship. Therefore, we should answer questions honestly, state facts objectively, avoid conclusions or guarantees, and constantly assure and reassure the patient. Patients have a right to know what they might reasonably expect from the proposed treatment. They should be provided with a written narrative detailing the treatment to be rendered, the inherent risks, possible complications and the

secondary costs they may incur, the goals of treatment, and the expected outcome or prognosis. The most common reasons for litigation are when professional practice goes beyond the limits of our expertise, and / or because we are directly responsible for the behavior of our employees. It goes without saying then, that the temptation to push an anesthetic technique beyond the limits of our training is to be avoided at all costs, and that it is our responsibility to see that our staff is properly trained as well. This is done by adhering to a certain standard of care through the demonstration of current practice standards, knowledge of the current literature, and by attending continuing education in the field.

Risk management for dental anesthesia consists of the prevention of anesthetic morbidity and mortality. This is done by first performing a comprehensive pretreatment evaluation to assess the patient's physical condition and identify potential risk factors. Next, thoroughly familiar drugs and techniques should be used on indicated patients only. Continuous physiologic and visual monitoring is essential throughout treatment. Office preparedness should be achieved by using sufficient, properly trained personnel and by maintaining appropriate emergency drugs, equipment, and facilities. Fully documented records must be maintained as well. A **written anesthetic record** must be kept that accurately reflects the results of physiologic monitoring over time, represents an accurate documentation of treatment, provides a justification of the appropriate technique, and draws no conclusions. It should also record injuries or subjective complaints and medication errors. In the event of an adverse outcome, the involved syringes, vials,

and malfunctioned equipment should be saved for later inspection. The written anesthesia record is a legal document that will provide the main defense in the event of litigation. It should therefore be as detailed as possible. It should not contain unexplained time gaps, conflicting entries, or any alterations or obliterations. Any information that comes to light after the fact should be written as an addendum to, and not as a part of, the original anesthesia record

MONITORING

The three organ systems most commonly affected by sedative drugs are the central nervous system, the respiratory system, and the cardiovascular system. Since sedative drugs can produce significant life-threatening changes in physiologic function, patients receiving these agents must be continuously monitored so that unwanted changes can be observed and corrected before injury occurs.

Central Nervous System

It is important that the clinician be aware of the extent to which sedative drugs depress the CNS since it is known that the risk of morbidity and mortality increases dramatically with excessive CNS depression and the onset of unconsciousness. This additional risk is related to the loss of protective reflexes and excessive cardiorespiratory depression, frequent companions of the unconscious state.

Consciousness has been operationally defined as the ability of a patient to respond rationally to command while maintaining his / her protective reflexes. An inportant component of this definition is that the elicited response be an appropriate one. A patient capable of gross body movement and vocalization on physical stimulation may or may not be conscious. Therefore, it is important to note that in order for a patient to meet the criteria for consciousness, the response to a command must be proper and must follow the command within a reasonable period of time. If the response does not occur in this fashion, the clinician must assume that the patient is unconscious and take appropriate action.

The extent to which the CNS is depressed following the administration of a sedative drug is affected by a number of factors that may change with time. For example, physical stimulation that occurs during an operative procedure is a natural antidote to the CNS depressant effects of some drugs. A patient judged to be conscious during a procedure may become sufficiently depressed in the absence of stimulation to become unconscious. This fact is often overlooked by those who would interrupt a procedure to answer a telephone call or examine another patient, only to return to find a previously sedated but conscious patient in an unconscious state. Thus, consciousness must continuously be reassessed throughout the perianesthetic period.

There are many electroencephalographic (EEG) techniques that are available today for monitoring electrical activity in the brain. These include conventional electroencephalography, computer-averaged evoked potentials, and power spectrum analysis. **Computer-averaged evoked potential recordings** have been used to study, among other things, the time course of recovery following brief exposures to nitrous oxide in a dental setting.[1] This recording technique proved to be a more sensitive indicator of the CNS depressant effects of nitrous oxide than previously used techniques and may become an important research tool in the study of drugs used to control pain and anxiety in dentistry. However, these monitoring devices are far too expensive and technically sophisticated to be used in a clinical setting for anything but research purposes.

Cerebral function monitors are commercially available that record and average EEG power spectrum. These devices are a first attempt to produce clinical instrumentation capable of assessing cortical function during anesthesia. However, there are no studies defining clinical correlates of averaged power spectrum, thus making interpretation of the information generated by these instruments difficult. For the purposes of IV conscious sedation, there currently is no substitute for the verbal and visual assessment of the patient's level of consciousness.

Respiratory System

Most emergencies associated with the anesthetic management of dental patients involve the respiratory system. As CNS depression occurs, minute ventilation decreases. With continued CNS depression and unconsciousness, other factors such as upper airway obstruction (usually by the tongue) worsen air exchange. The net result is hypoxemia and hypercarbia.

The Physiological Significance of Hypoxemia and Hypercarbia Oxygen is essential for the aerobic metabolism of glucose via the citric acid cycle and electron transport system. This pathway is much more efficient than anaerobic pathways in the production of the biological substrate, ATP. When aerobic metabolism is replaced by anaerobic metabolism, cells with high energy utilization (neurons, myocardial cells, and nephrons) cannot continue to function and may suffer structural damage. For example, in the absence of oxygen, the cerebral cortex soon stops functioning and irreversible brain damage occurs. As has often been stated, hypoxemia not only stops the machine, it wrecks the machinery!

Causes of Hypoxemia Hypoxemia refers to a reduction of the oxygen tension in arterial blood. There are three major physiologic causes of hypoxemia: decreased alveolar oxygen tension, increased shunting, and decreased mixed venous oxygen content.[2,3] **Decreased alveolar oxygen tension** is the result of inadequate ventilation. It is commonly caused by airway obstruction, hypoventilation, breathing less than 21% oxygen (room air), and an uneven distribution of alveolar ventilation with respect to pulmonary blood flow.

Untreated upper airway obstruction, either partial or complete, may ultimately lead to asphyxia. In the unconscious patient, the tongue will frequently obstruct the air flow. This obstruction can usually be corrected with a simple, but often life-saving, head tilt and/or jaw thrust maneuver. However, managing an obstructed airway in patients with short necks, limited cervical extension, retrognathia, and/or obesity may be extremely difficult. These conditions should be noted in the preanesthetic period.

Hypoxemia results from hypoventilation because the available hemoglobin is insufficiently oxygenated. Drugs may produce hypoventilation by a reduction in the tidal volume, respiratory rate, or by increasing the physiologic deadspace. In like manner, any factor that decreases the inspired oxygen tension to a level below that of ambient air (21%) will lead to hypoxemia. Conversely, increasing the inspired oxygen concentration will increase the alveolar oxygen tension and thus the arterial oxygen tension. However, increasing the inspired oxygen concentration does nothing to correct the ventilatory status of the patient. During sedation and anesthesia, drug-induced hypoventilation and its attendant risks may exist even when hypoxemia is absent.

The second major cause of arterial hypoxemia is the **shunting of blood** from the right side of the heart to the left side without becoming oxygenated. Slightly less than 2% of blood is normally shunted without it becoming oxygenated.[2] This is called the anatomical shunt and is made up of blood from the bronchial, coronary, and pulmonary circulations. Additional shunting may be associated with general anesthesia due to the production of atelectasis. The collapsed alveoli will not contribute to arterial oxygenation, and hypoxemia will ensue. Shunting can be differentiated from ventilation / perfusion inequalities in that PaO_2 will increase with 100% oxygen breathing in ventilation / perfusion problems but not with shunting.

The third major cause of hypoxemia is **decreased mixed venous oxygen content.** Anything that increases the amount of oxygen that is removed from hemoglobin by the tissues will lead to hypoxemia. Increased metabolic rate such as occurs with fever or hyperthyroidism will significantly increase oxygen consumption. This lowers the mixed venous oxy-

gen content, and hypoxemia will occur unless the body compensates by increasing the cardiac output.

Decreased mixed venous oxygen content is most commonly produced by decreased cardiac output. If cardiac output is diminished, more oxygen is extracted from the blood per unit time and the mixed venous oxygen content is lowered. Therefore, any drug-induced hypoperfusion state or syncopal episode places the patient at risk for hypoxemia. Objective therapy to correct hypoperfusion is directed at the restoration of tissue blood flow. In many instances, cerebral blood flow can be reestablished by simply placing the patient in a supine or head-down position. Supportive drug therapy may be indicated in cases unresponsive to positioning.

A final cause of decreased mixed venous oxygen content is anemia. The reduction in functional hemoglobin concentration causes the tissues to extract a greater proportion of oxygen from the blood. The ensuing hypoxemia can be corrected by increasing the hemoglobin concentration through transfusion. Anemia can usually be detected by laboratory testing, and appropriate preventative measures can be taken. Another form of anemia, methemoglobinemia, can be produced by certain drugs such as prilocaine, an intermediate-acting amide local anesthetic. A metabolite of prilocaine can produce significant methemoglobinemia when 500 mg (seven dental cartridges) or more of the drug are administered.[4]

Hypercarbia Carbon dioxide is an end-product of the aerobic metabolism of glucose. It is eliminated from the body primarily by the lung. The arterial carbon diox-

ide tension is a measure of the adequacy of pulmonary ventilation. There is an inverse relationship between minute ventilation and the arterial carbon dioxide tension such that a decrease in minute ventilation produces an increase in $PaCO_2$, and vice versa. Hypercarbia, or increased $PaCO_2$, is associated with increased sympathetic activity and direct myocardial depression, both of which may lead to serious cardiac dysrhythmias. Furthermore, increases in $PaCO_2$ result in decreases in alveolar oxygen tension. Every 1 mm Hg rise in alveolar carbon dioxide tension is associated with a concomitant reduction in alveolar oxygen tension. In fact, the $PaCO_2$ rarely will exceed 100 mm Hg in a patient who is breathing room air since the resultant alveolar oxygen dilution produces severe hypoxemia. Therefore, any drug-induced hypoventilatory state must be corrected with positive pressure ventilation in order to prevent hypercarbia and hypoxemia. Uncorrected hypoventilation will result in respiratory acidosis, hypoxemia, and potentially fatal cardiac dysrhythmias.

Monitoring Respiratory Function

Traditionally, respiratory function has been assessed by **counting the respiratory rate.** A normal adult respiratory frequency is 12 to 20 respirations per minute. For children, 20 to 26 respirations per minute is normal. Though monitoring respiratory frequency is useful for determining the impact of certain drugs (such as the opioids) on ventilation, it alone does not provide enough information about a patient's ventilatory status. **The tidal volume must** also be estimated to assess minute ventilation tidal volume × respiratory rate). In the dental setting, without the aid of a respirometer, the tidal volume may be difficult to estimate. This can be done, however, by watching and/or feeling the chest rise and fall with each breath, or by auscultation using a precordial stethoscope. **Estimating the adequacy of the patient's minute ventilation** can be accomplished by simulating the patient's breathing pattern for a period of time. Using his or her own breathing pattern as a control, the clinician can judge the adequacy of the patient's minute ventilation. If the minute ventilation is judged to be inadequate, intervention is indicated.

Some clinicians rely on a **patient's color as a sign of ventilatory status.** The lips, oral mucosa, nail beds, and blood are frequently examined for signs of cyanosis, which is indicative of hypoxemia. However, this is not always a reliable sign. Cyanosis occurs when 5 g of hemoglobin are deoxygenated.[2] A patient with a normal hemoglobin (12 to 15 g%) will exhibit cyanosis at higher arterial oxygen tensions than an anemic patient (hemoglobin < 10 g%), since a smaller percentage of a normal patient's hemoglobin will be reduced when cyanosis is clinically evident.

Pulse Oximetry The technological advances in recent years that have made it possible to noninvasively monitor the percentage of arterial hemoglobin saturated with oxygen has revolutionized anesthesia monitoring and improved patient safety. Pulse oximetry works by measuring the light absorbance at red and infrared light sources from oxygenated and reduced hemoglobin in a pulsatile capillary bed and compares the ratio of the absorbances with a built-in calibration function that converts it to percent hemoglobin

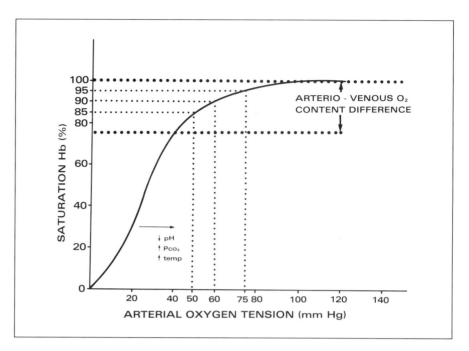

Fig 18-1 *Oxyhemoglobin dissociation curve. Arterial hypoxemia (PaO_2 = 75 mm Hg) occurs when the pulse oximeter reads 95% saturation.*

saturation.[3] The percentage of hemoglobin saturated with oxygen is correlated to the arterial oxygen tension by the oxyhemoglobin dissociation curve (Fig 18-1). Due to the unique shape of the curve, the arterial oxygen tension will fall sharply while the oximeter will show only minor saturation decreases. For example, the PaO_2 may fall from 100 mm Hg to 75 mm Hg (hypoxemia), but the oximeter reading will only change from 97% saturation to 95% saturation. The clinician should study the curve diligently to gain an understanding of the significance of the pulse oximeter readings.

Arterial hemoglobin oxygen saturation may be a more relevant indicator of tissue oxygenation than arterial oxygen tension. Factors such as temperature, arterial carbon dioxide tension, pH, and 2,3-diphosphoglycerate may cause the oxyhemoglobin dissociation curve to be shifted to the right or left, thereby decreasing or

increasing, respectively, the affinity of hemoglobin for oxygen. In the case of elevated body temperature, the curve would shift to the right, hemoglobin would be more prone to give up its oxygen to the tissues, and oxygen saturation would decrease while PaO_2 remained the same. This change could not be appreciated by measuring arterial oxygen tension alone.

Any event that significantly reduces vascular pulsation may limit the accuracy of the pulse oximeter.[3] Digital perfusion may be diminished or lost with hypothermia, hypotension, blood pressure cuff inflation, and infusion of vasoactive drugs. In addition, significant quantities of methemoglobin, bilirubin, carbon monoxide, skin pigmentation, and intravenous dyes such as methylene blue will cause the instrument to give false readings.[3] Another limitation of the pulse oximeter is that it does not function as a ventilation monitor. The oximeter does not reflect changes in the arterial oxygen tension in the hyperoxic state. In other words, when the patient is breathing supplemental oxygen, the PaO_2 may range up to 600 mm Hg. The pulse oximeter will read 100% saturation. The PaO_2 could fall all the way to 105 mm Hg and the oximeter would still read 100% saturation. Obviously, in this scenario, something serious is happening with ventilation, yet there is no indication of such from the pulse oximeter because the patient is breathing supplemental oxygen. Therefore, for the purposes of IV conscious sedation, supplemental oxygen is not routinely needed and should be used only when indicated.

Capnography The capnograph is the ultimate ventilation monitor. It measures end-expired carbon dioxide using infrared absorption spectroscopy.[3] The end-expired carbon dioxide correlates directly to the arterial carbon dioxide tension. Capnographs are now available that will measure end-expired carbon dioxide through a nasal cannula, thus eliminating the need for direct tracheal sampling. This technological advance makes capnography practical for assessing the ventilatory status of patients during conscious sedation. The capnograph will aid in the detection of apnea, airway obstruction, hyperventilation, hypoventilation, air embolism, pulmonary embolism, malignant hyperthermia, esophageal intubation, and bronchospasm.

Cardiovascular System

Changes in heart rate and rhythm, myocardial contractility, and peripheral vascular resistance are common during certain dental procedures.[5] In some situations, these changes can pro-

duce cardiovascular decompensation, leading to injury or death. Preexisting disease states, certain drugs and drug interactions, psychological and physical stress, hypoxemia, and hypercarbia contribute to these changes in cardiovascular function. The extent to which these changes will be tolerated depends on the cardiovascular reserve of the patient. Therefore, preoperative assessment of the patient's cardiovascular reserve is perhaps the most important measure a dentist can take to prevent cardiovascular emergencies associated with the anesthetic management of a dental patient.

Monitoring Cardiovascular Function Significant changes in cardiovascular function require immediate recognition and management. Tissue blood flow, and therefore oxygen delivery, is affected by a number of factors, including autoregulatory mechanisms, cardiac output, temperature, vascular disease states, body position, and vasoactive drugs. The cardiac output is the primary determinant of tissue blood flow and is monitored clinically by an assessment of the heart rate and rhythm and the systemic blood pressure. In addition, color of the skin, mucous membranes, and nail beds can indicate inadequate tissue blood flow. Pallor is indicative of reduced tissue blood flow, while cyanosis signals ventilatory deficiencies.

Assessment of Heart Rate and Rhythm The carotid or radial arteries can be manually palpated to assess the heart rate and rhythm. A qualitative assessment of the pulse can be made by noting the intensity of the pulse with each beat. A thready pulse that is barely perceptible is indicative of a limited stroke volume and/or

peripheral vasoconstriction that may be compensatory to a drop in cardiac output. Also, bradydysrhythmias, tachydysrhythmias, and ectopic beats can be detected. A trained clinician can obtain a significant amount of information about a patient's cardiovascular status by the simple palpation of a peripheral artery.

Digital pulse meters are available that provide a continuous display of the heart rate. However, patient movement introduces significant artifact, which may compromise the accuracy of the monitor. Also, pulse meters provide information about the rate only and do not assess rhythm or pulse quality. More sophisticated digital pulse monitors display a pulse wave in addition to the heart rate, which helps to qualitate the pulse. All pulse meters are subject to the effects of temperature, anxiety, and drugs on digital blood flow.

Cardiac dysrhythmias are often observed during certain dental procedures. A continuous **electrocardiographic (ECG) analysis** is useful for monitoring these changes. Small portable ECG monitors make ECG monitoring more feasible in a dental office. Although useful in detecting cardiac dysrhythmias, these monitors provide limited information about the cardiovascular status of the patient, especially in the hands of a poorly trained clinician. Therefore, an ECG monitor should be used as an adjunct to, and not as a substitute for, conventional monitoring techniques such as blood pressure and peripheral pulse.

A **precordial stethoscope** is an inexpensive monitoring device that can provide a relatively large amount of information about a patient's cardiorespiratory function. With this instrument, respiration and heart rate and rhythm may be continuously and simultaneously monitored. Furthermore, the operator's attention is not directed away from the patient to a remote monitor, as it frequently is when automated blood pressure monitors and ECG units are in use.

Assessment of Systemic Blood Pressure

Every dental patient should have a systemic blood pressure determination prior to the initiation of any dental treatment. This is essential to safe practice because of the extremely high incidence of hypertensive disease in the US population. Excessive anxiety, pain, and vasoactive drugs such as epinephrine and levonordephrin can precipitate life-threatening emergencies in patients with uncontrolled hypertension. The frequency with which this measure is repeated during the perianesthetic period depends on the physical status of the patient as well as the anesthetic technique used.

Preoperative blood pressure and pulse determinations during a nonstressful appointment is required to establish a baseline for emergency management. Intraoperative changes in these parameters can only be rationally managed relative to the norm. If the baseline is lacking, treatment becomes haphazard and the patient is exposed to further risk.

The clinician should not rely solely on automated blood pressure devices during anesthetic management. Although these monitors are extremely convenient and can be set to cycle at almost any interval, total dependence on them can lead to disaster. The dentist and other staff members should always be able to determine the blood pressure manually through the auscultation, palpation, and oscillation methods. This is prudent not only in cases of electrical failure, but also because automated cuffs sometimes have a tendency to delay reading or read error in low perfusion states. The ability to manually check the blood pressure as a backup can be life-saving.

DRUGS USED IN INTRAVENOUS CONSCIOUS SEDATION

The following section covers drugs used to bring about conscious sedation and their effects and precautions for use.

Benzodiazepines

Mechanism of Action
Benzodiazepines have specific anxiolytic, anticonvulsant, sedative, muscle relaxant, and amnestic properties. These effects are mediated through specific benzodiazepine receptors that have been identified in the brain and spinal cord.[6] The location of these receptors parallels that of the major inhibitory neurotransmitter in the brain, ie, gamma-aminobutyric acid (GABA). These sites are predominantly located in neuronal surface membranes and are distributed widely throughout the central nervous system.[7] Benzodiazepines combine in a selective, stereospecific manner with these receptor sites. They appear to intensify the physiological inhibitory effects of GABA via interference with GABA reuptake. The resultant accumulation of GABA produces neuronal membrane hyperpolarization.[8]

Midazolam (eg, Versed) has twice the affinity for the benzodiazepine receptor as diazepam (eg, Valium).[9] This accounts in part for the higher potency and greater amnestic and anticonvulsant effects of midazolam.[10]

Respiratory Effects
Although benzodiazepines exhibit a high margin of safety, their clinical effects are highly variable. Therefore, when used for intravenous conscious sedation, they must be carefully titrated to clinical effect rather than administered as a bolus injection. Both diazepam and midazolam produce respiratory depression in a dose-related fashion. The depressant effect is caused by direct action on the central nervous system by decreasing the ventilatory response to carbon dioxide. This respiratory depression is markedly worsened in patients with chronic obstructive lung disease when midazolam is used.[11,12] In contrast, when diazepam and midazolam are slowly titrated intravenously to a fixed clinical endpoint, no clinically significant ventilatory changes are evident.[13,14]

Cardiovascular Effects
Diazepam and midazolam have little effect on hemodynamic stability. Glisson et al[15] studied the effects of midazolam on plasma epinephrine and norepinephrine levels during induction of general anesthesia. They found that midazolam suppressed plasma elevations of epinephrine and norepinephrine. This indicates that midazolam, like diazepam,[5] may be of value in attenuating catecholamine surges during stress.

Pharmacokinetics
The pharmacokinetic profile of the benzodiazepines conforms to a classic two-compartment model, that is, distribution from a central compartment to a peripheral compartment along a concentration gradient, and then elimination. The rate of distribution depends upon the lipid solubility of the drug. The distribution phase is reversible and rapid for benzodiazepines. The elimination phase is irreversible and slow since it is governed by the rate of biotrans-

formation of the drug. Termination of activity for the benzodiazepines is caused by a combination of redistribution into the tissues and metabolic biotransformation.

The extreme lipid solubility of midazolam produces a very rapid onset. The distribution half-life ($t_{1/2dist}$) for midazolam is 6 to 15 minutes. Midazolam's short duration of action is attributed to its very high rate of metabolic clearance and rapid rate of elimination. The elimination half-life ($t_{1/2elim}$) for midazolam is 1 to 4 hours, which exceeds that of other benzodiazepines. In addition, the metabolites of midazolam are inactive.[16]

By contrast, diazepam has a slower rate of distribution than most benzodiazepines ($t_{1/2dist} = 30$ to 66 minutes) and therefore has a somewhat slower onset than midazolam. The elimination half-life for diazepam is 24 to 57 hours, which is at least 10 times slower than for midazolam. Diazepam also has two active metabolites: desmethyldiazepam ($t_{1/2elim} = 41$ to 139 hours) and oxazepam, which both produce sedative effects.[16] Termination of clinical activity for diazepam occurs primarily through redistribution. However, the combination of active metabolites and the long elimination half-life accounts for the residual "hangover" effects seen clinically after diazepam administration.

A number of factors influence the pharmacokinetic profile of the benzodiazepines. For example, the elimination half-life for diazepam and midazolam is prolonged in **elderly patients** because of their impaired total metabolic clearance rate.[17] The number of benzodiazepine receptors may also be decreased. Therefore, the dose requirement for diazepam and midazolam is lower in the elderly patient.

The extremely **obese patient** also presents a management problem because the elimination half-life of both diazepam and midazolam increases along with the volume of distribution. However, higher than usual dosages may be required to counteract the rapid redistribution of the drugs into fatty tissues. Thus, in the obese patient, higher drug doses may be necessary to produce the desired effect, and the recovery period may likewise be more prolonged.

There is often concern when drugs are administered to **patients with chronic renal failure** because the free fraction of drug that is normally eliminated in the urine may still be active. A decrease in plasma proteins, especially serum albumin, as is often seen in renal failure, results in an alteration in protein binding capacity. Since the benzodiazepines are highly protein bound, renal failure could increase the free fractions of midazolam and also of diazepam and its metabolites. This could result in more profound and prolonged effects. Therefore, the dose of diazepam and midazolam should be reduced in patients with chronic renal failure.[18]

Use in Intravenous Conscious Sedation Diazepam and midazolam have been used extensively as primary agents, and in combination with opioids, for intravenous conscious sedation in dentistry. The properties of diazepam and midazolam are compared in Table 18-1.

Diazepam Diazepam is water insoluble and is therefore compounded in 40% propylene glycol. This vehicle has been implicated in a significant incidence of pain during IV injection and venous irritation. The long elimination half-lives of its two active metabolites tends to prolong recovery by producing residual sedation and "hangover" effects. Despite these negatives, diazepam has been the mainstay for years as the principal drug for IV conscious sedation in dentistry. Its safety record has been remarkable, and it is decidedly less expensive than midazolam.

Midazolam Compared with diazepam, midazolam has some significant advantages. Because it is water soluble, there is little or no pain during intravenous injection, and the incidence of venous irritation is virtually nonexistent. Midazolam has a more rapid onset and produces more profound sedation and better amnesia than diazepam. Although patients who receive midazolam may be slightly more somnolent at the end of a procedure, and the return to "ambulatory fitness" may be slightly longer,[19] the short elimination half-life and the lack of active metabolites make overall recovery from midazolam sedation

TABLE 18-1 *Midazolam and diazepam comparison*

PROPERTY	MIDAZOLAM	DIAZEPAM
Water solubility	Yes	No
Pain on injection	No	Yes
Venous irritation	<1%	5%–30%
Distribution half-life	6–15 min	30–66 min
Elimination half-life	1–4 h	24–57 h
Metabolites	Inactive	Active

extremely rapid when compared with diazepam. With all else being equal, the water solubility and short elimination half-life of midazolam make it the superior drug for IV conscious sedation for outpatient procedures.

The recommended dose-range for IV conscious sedation with diazepam and midazolam is 0.15 to 0.3 mg/kg and 0.05 to 0.075 mg/kg, respectively. However, a more appropriate method of sedation with diazepam and midazolam is slow titration of the drug until a predetermined clinical endpoint is reached. Cardiorespiratory depression should be absent when this titration method is used. Should readministration become necessary, 25% of the initial dose of either drug will generally return the patient to the baseline level of sedation.

Precautions for Use The incidence of adverse reactions to benzodiazepines is infrequent. Nausea, vomiting, coughing, and "hiccoughs" have occasionally been noted. Respiratory depression with prolonged somnolence may also occur infrequently with midazolam. These effects have been rapidly and effectively reversed with physostigmine administration and with the specific benzodiazepine antagonist flumazenil.[20,21]

Caution should also be observed when managing elderly patients with benzodiazepines. In general, dosages should be reduced by at least 25%, and there is a less frequent need for drug readministration. Cardiac output is diminished in the elderly patient, thereby delaying the onset of sedation with these drugs after IV administration. Reduced plasma volume, protein binding, and CNS function act to increase the potency of the drugs. Reduced metabolic rate, hepatic and

renal clearance, and a higher percentage of body fat tend to slow metabolism and elimination and allow for drug accumulation. This increases the duration of action of the benzodiazepines and prolongs the interval between readministration.

Benzodiazepines must never be used for IV conscious sedation without individualization of dosage. Prior to IV administration in any dose, oxygen and resuscitative equipment for the maintenance of a patent airway and support of ventilation should be readily available. Patients should be continuously monitored for early signs of hypoventilation or apnea. Neither diazepam nor midazolam should be administered by rapid or single-bolus IV injection. This mode of administration has resulted in serious cardiorespiratory events, predominantly in older, chronically ill patients, and/or with concomitant use of other cardiorespiratory depressant agents. Midazolam especially has been associated with respiratory depression, apnea, respiratory and/or cardiac arrest in this age group, sometimes resulting in death. These events have almost always been a consequence of improper midazolam administration as well as violations of the tenets of diligent anesthesia care.

Adverse reactions such as agitation, involuntary movement, hyperactivity, and combativeness have been reported with the benzodiazepines. These reactions may be due to inadequate or excessive doses or improper administration. However, consideration should be given to the possibility of cerebral hypoxia or true paradoxical reaction.

In summary, the water solubility and rapid clearance of midazolam make it a clear choice over diazepam for IV conscious sedation.

Additionally, midazolam produces a more profound and prolonged amnestic effect than diazepam. This effect does not necessarily correlate with the clinical sedation level, thus, patients are more likely to experience amnesia without having to be heavily sedated.

Opioid Analgesics

Mechanism of Action Opioid analgesics exert their multitude of effects primarily through interaction with four major types of receptors found in the central nervous system and in the spinal cord (Table 18-2). The mu and kappa receptors are associated with analgesia; delta receptors are thought to be associated with alterations in affective behavior; and sigma receptors are involved in the dysphoria and psychotomimetic effects associated with some opioids.[22] The opioid analgesics are thus classified according to their relationship with the various receptors. The first group, opioid agonists, are drugs that bind to mu, kappa, and delta receptors. The second group, opioid agonist-antagonists, are agonists at some receptors and antagonists at others. The third group, opioid antagonists, have no agonist activity at any of the receptors.

Opioid Agonists Morphine is the prototype opioid analgesic against which all other drugs in this class are compared. Drugs in this class seem to have preferential affinity for mu receptors, but they are active to varying degrees at the other receptor sites as well. Opioid agonists exert their primary action on the CNS and the bowel.[23] In the CNS they produce the desirable effects of analgesia without drowsiness, alterations in mood, and the loss of consciousness. Morphine can relieve almost

TABLE 18-2 *Opioid analgesics and opioid receptors*

DRUG	RECEPTOR			
	MU	KAPPA	DELTA	SIGMA
Agonists				
Morphine	+ +	+		
Meperidine	+	+ +		
Fentanyl	+ +			
Agonist-antagonists				
Nalbuphine	-	+		+
Butorphanol		+		+
Antagonists				
Naloxone	−	-	-	-

```
* + +  =  strong agonism.
  +    =  agonism.
  −    =  strong antagonism.
  -    =  antagonism.
```

any type of pain, regardless of its origin or intensity. This is accomplished by raising both the patient's pain threshold and pain tolerance. During IV conscious sedation, the increased pain threshold, mood elevation, and indifference are valuable commodities to be exploited. As an aside, most opioid agonists produce constriction of the pupil through an excitatory action on the Edinger-Westphal nucleus of the oculomotor nerve. Miosis is pathognomonic of opioid agonists, and no tolerance develops to this effect.

Side Effects Opioid agonists produce some undesirable effects such as respiratory depression and nausea and vomiting. Morphine is a primary and continuous respiratory depressant that affects both respiratory rate and tidal volume. Morphine decreases the responsiveness of the medullary respiratory centers to increasing concentrations of carbon dioxide. The usual ventilatory response to increased carbon dioxide tension is to increase ventilation and return the carbon dioxide levels to normal. The stimulus to breathe is obtunded in a dose-related fashion with morphine as carbon dioxide levels rise. If the respiratory

depression is significant, patients may be forced to rely on their hypoxic ventilatory drive; that is, they breathe only in response to low arterial oxygen concentrations. It should be remembered then that in the treatment of opioid-induced respiratory depression, 100% oxygen administration could produce apnea. The ventilatory status must be monitored closely and positive pressure ventilation should be instituted if necessary.

Although all drugs in this class have the potential for emetic effects, morphine is most commonly implicated. The emetic effect occurs primarily through direct stimulation of the chemoreceptor trigger zone in the medulla. This dopaminergic effect can sometimes be countered by dopaminergic blocking drugs such as phenothiazines. There also appears to be a vestibular component to the nausea and vomiting seen with opioids in that rapid positional changes may induce emesis.

Opioid agonists are cardiovascularly stable drugs that produce no major effect on blood pressure, heart rate, or heart rhythm in the recumbent patient.[23] Peripheral vasodilation does occur, however, as a result of histamine release. Thus, when patients are returned

to an upright position, postural hypotension and syncope may occur. Morphine and meperidine promote the most histamine release and are the most likely candidates for postural hypotension. The cerebral circulation is affected indirectly in the presence of respiratory depression. If carbon dioxide levels rise, the cerebral blood vessels dilate and intracranial pressure increases.

Opioid agonists also have some interesting effects on the gastrointestinal tract and other smooth muscle. In the GI system, motility is decreased and smooth muscle tone is increased in the stomach and first part of the duodenum. This causes a major delay in gastric emptying, which is the basis for opioid-induced constipation. Similar increases in smooth muscle tone occur in the small and large intestines. Biliary tract pressure increases often with spasm at the sphincter of Oddi. Opioid agonists also increase smooth muscle tone in the ureter and bladder, which results in urinary retention. The volume of urine may also be affected since the secretion of antidiuretic hormone is stimulated.

Constipation, urinary retention, and biliary spasm are therefore side effects to be considered seriously when opioid agonists are used for sedation. In susceptible individuals, these side effects can override any potential benefit from the drug and should be avoided at all costs. The prudent course of action would be to eliminate them entirely or use a drug in the agonist-antagonist group that is not associated with these effects.

The histamine-releasing opioid agonists, morphine and meperidine, may exacerbate or induce an acute asthmatic attack. They also may produce pruritis, sweating, urticaria, and flushing of the face, neck, and upper thorax.

The above discussion of opioid agonists applies specifically to morphine and generally to meperidine (eg, Demerol) and fentanyl (eg, Sublimaze), two useful agonists for IV conscious sedation. Some minor differences exist that warrant further discussion.

Meperidine Meperidine was first studied as an atropine-like agent.[23] It was discovered to have analgesic activity similar to morphine. Meperidine is a weaker agent than morphine; 80 to 100 mg of meperidine is equivalent to 10 mg of morphine. It interacts more strongly with the kappa opioid receptor, and its duration of action is less than morphine. Properties unique to meperidine are its profound antisialogue effect, and tachycardia following IV administration. A metabolite of meperidine, normeperidine, is associated with toxic effects such as tremors, muscle twitching, and convulsions. High doses of meperidine may therefore cause an excitatory sequence of events. Meperidine is contraindicated in patients taking MAO inhibitors due to an alteration in the rate of metabolic transformation. Inhibition of MAO causes an accumulation of normeperidine, which can lead to delirium, hallucinations, seizures, hyperpyrexia, or respiratory depression.

Fentanyl Fentanyl is an extremely potent analgesic which is 80 to 100 times as potent as morphine.[23] It acts primarily at the mu receptor, and it produces the most profound respiratory depression of the drugs discussed in this class. However, its short duration of action makes it useful as a sedative agent for shorter dental procedures. *Fentanyl produces little if any euphoria or mood alteration; it becomes easy to overdose patients with fentanyl if this fact is not appreciated.* Inexperienced clinicians, expecting to see mood elevation with fentanyl, will readminister the drug until severe respiratory depression occurs. Fentanyl does not produce histamine release and may be used in asthmatic patients, providing that respiratory depression is avoided. Fentanyl has been associated with chest-wall rigidity, or stiff-chest syndrome.[24,25] This occurs through the enhancement of dopaminergic transmission. Although all opioid agonists can do this, fentanyl seems more prone to this effect. Chest-wall rigidity is usually associated with the rapid administration of high doses, but it has been reported with as little as 25 μg of fentanyl.[25] This effect can be antagonized by naloxone.

Opioid Agonist-Antagonists

Two drugs in this group are useful for IV conscious sedation: nalbuphine (eg, Nubain) and butorphanol (eg, Stadol).

Nalbuphine Nalbuphine is a competitive antagonist at the mu receptor, but it has partial agonistic properties at the kappa and sigma receptors (see Table 18-2). Nalbuphine is equipotent with morphine, but in contrast to the dose-dependent respiratory depression seen with morphine, there is a ceiling or plateau effect to the respiratory depression of nalbuphine. Nalbuphine produces no histamine release or minimal biliary constriction and is cardiovasculary stable.[26]

Butorphanol Butorphanol has no effect on the mu receptor, but it acts as a partial agonist at the kappa and sigma receptors (see Table 18-2). It is a potent drug in that 2 mg of butorphanol is equivalent to 10 mg of nalbuphine or morphine. While respiratory depression can occur, it also exhibits a ceiling effect. Butorphanol does not cause histamine release or biliary constriction, but unlike nalbuphine, it increases pulmonary arterial pressure and the cardiac index.[27] The increased work of the heart may preclude its use in patients with significant cardiac disease.

Any drug that stimulates the sigma receptors has the potential for psychotomimetic effects, which are described as uncontrollable or strange thoughts, anxiety, nightmares, and hallucinations. These are not common in therapeutic dose ranges, but their incidence may increase with increasing dosages. Both nalbuphine and butorphanol may produce these effects, but it is unlikely in the doses used for IV conscious sedation. Agonist-antagonist drugs are contraindicated in opioid-dependent patients due to the possibility of precipitating a withdrawal syndrome.

Opioid Antagonists Only one drug in this group has any clinical relevance. Naloxone (eg, Narcan) is a competitive antagonist at all of the opioid receptors. It is indicated in the reversal of any and all of the adverse effects seen with the opioids. However, its routine use to speed recovery following sedation is not recommended. Generally speaking, naloxone exerts no pharmacologic effects other than its action at the receptor sites. However, naloxone also antagonizes the effects of endogenous opioids on the neural systems that are involved in the regulation of blood pressure. There have been reports of severe hypertension and cardiac dysrhythmias following naloxone administration, possibly related to the recurrence of pain and subsequent sympathetic discharge.[28] Therefore, its use should be confined to those instances where the benefits outweigh the risks.

Precautions for Use Opioid analgesics are contraindicated in cases of closed-head injury where intracranial pressure may be elevated. The carbon dioxide retention that may occur with opioids could further increase intracranial pressure and produce disastrous results. These drugs should also be used with caution in patients with severe restrictive or obstructive pulmonary diseases. Further increasing carbon dioxide levels in patients with chronically elevated arterial carbon dioxide could effectively knock out the respiratory drive. Caution should be used with asthmatic patients as well. Opioids that release histamine, such as morphine and meperidine, could precipitate an acute asthmatic episode during treatment. Therefore, opioids are relatively contraindicated in the presence of respiratory disease.

Drug interactions between opioid analgesics and other drugs may be cause for concern. The CNS, cardiovascular, and respiratory system depression associated with opioids can be potentiated by benzodiazepines, phenothiazines, tricyclic antidepressants, and MAO inhibitors. Dosages should be appropriately reduced in these instances. The combination of meperidine with an MAO inhibitor is potentially life-threatening and is to be avoided.

Antiemetics

Antiemetics are really antipsychotic agents that happen to have antiemetic effects. They consist of two drug groups, the phenothiazines and the butyrophenones, both of which have similar pharmacologic properties.[29] Promethazine (eg, Phenergan) and prochlorperazine (eg, Compazine) are phenothiazine derivatives. Droperidol (eg, Inapsine) is a butyrophenone. Of the three agents, droperidol is probably the most effective antiemetic agent.

Pharmacologically speaking, these drugs are ganglionic and alpha-adrenergic blocking agents, anticholinergic, antidopaminergic, antihistaminic, antiemetic, and antipsychotic. They also potentiate the effects of other CNS depressants. Postural hypotension is common with rapidly changing position from supine to upright. Because of the variety of actions, drug interactions are also common with the antiemetics. In combination with epinephrine, the alpha-blocking properties of the phenothiazines could allow the beta effects of epinephrine to predominate, possibly resulting in a precipitous drop in blood pressure.

The anticholinergic effects of the antiemetics can lead to problems either alone or in combination with other anticholinergic drugs such as tricyclic antidepressants, antihistamines, and atropine. A central anticholinergic syndrome characterized by anxiety, agitation, disorientation, restlessness, delirium, or stupor may occur. While rarely life-threatening, this syndrome can be extremely disruptive and is to be avoided at all costs.

Other potentially disheartening side effects of the antiemetics are extrapyramidal reactions. These are mediated through the dopaminergic blocking effects of the drugs. It is ironic that the same mechanism that produces the desirable effect of emesis control also produces the undesirable effects of extrapyramidal reactions. These are characterized by Parkinsonian-like tremors at rest, akathisia (compelling need to be in constant motion), dystonia (facial grimacing and torticollis), and tardive dyskinesia (sucking and smacking of the lips, lateral jaw movements, darting of the tongue).

It should be obvious that due to the potential variety of adverse effects, antiemetic drugs are to be used only as an adjunct to IV conscious sedation. The routine prophylactic use of antiemetic agents is not necessary since the incidence of nausea and vomiting associated with conscious sedation is rare. The risks of routine administration far outweigh the perceived benefits, thus relegating these drugs to the role of adjuncts in susceptible individuals.

Antisialagogues

The role of antisialagogues in anesthetic practice probably evolved from the early days of ether anesthesia when excessive airway secretions caused significant management problems. **Atropine** and **scopolamine** were used to produce a dry field, reduce the incidence of laryngospasm, and improve visualization of the airway. These drugs are parasympatholytic or vagolytic agents. Among other things, they reduce salivary flow, increase the heart rate, and cross the blood/brain barrier to produce sedation. Scopolamine produces much more sedation than atropine and is still used as a sedative agent in some techniques. However, it produces the central anticholinergic syndrome quite frequently and therefore has no real value in dental sedation. Atropine may also produce the syndrome, but the incidence is less.

Glycopyrrolate (eg, Robinul) is a quaternary amine that is too large to cross the blood/brain barrier. Therefore, it does not produce sedation or the central anticholinergic syndrome. Additionally, it is a more prolonged drying agent than atropine and its cardiac acceleratory effects are less. Because of this, glycopyrrolate should be the antisialagogue of choice.

As with the antiemetics, the antisialagogues are only adjuncts to the sedative technique. Sedation with a benzodiazepine alone or in combination with an opioid will produce sufficient drying in the vast majority of cases. The routine administration of an antisialagogue is not warranted because of the potential for producing tachycardia or CNS side effects. If salivation is a problem even after sedation has been administered, glycopyrrolate is the drug of choice. Atropine should be relegated to the emergency drug kit for the treatment of bradycardia associated with hypotension.

A comparative summary of useful drugs for IV conscious sedation is provided in Table 18-3.

TABLE 18-3 *Comparative summary of useful intravenous drugs*

DRUG	DOSE	ONSET	DURATION
Benzodiazepines			
Diazepam	0.15–0.3 mg/kg	0.5–1 min	45 min
Midazolam	0.05–0.075 mg/kg	1–2 min	30–60 min
Opioid analgesics			
Morphine	0.05–0.1 mg/kg	5–10 min	2–4 h
Meperidine	0.3–0.6 mg/kg	2–4 min	30–45 min
Fentanyl	0.001–0.002 mg/kg	30 s	30–60 min
Nalbuphine	0.05–0.1 mg/kg	2–3 min	2–4 h
Butorphanol	0.007–0.014 mg/kg	2–3 min	2–4 h
Antiemetics			
Promethazine	12.5–25 mg		2–3 h
Prochlorperazine	5–10 mg		2–3 h
Droperidol	0.625–1.25 mg		3–6 h
Antisialagogues			
Atropine	0.2–0.4 mg	1 min	8–12 h
Glycopyrrolate	0.1–0.2 mg	1–2 min	2–3 h

CLINICAL APPLICATION

WHY INTRAVENOUS SEDATION?

The use of intravenous sedation is indicated for the reduction of stress with its undesirable sequela. However, intravenous sedation is not a cure-all for stress reduction but is one pharmacologic technique in a host of considerations for stress reduction in the dental office. Appropriately used it is a very effective tool.

Stress in the dental office is primarily the physical result of pain and the psychological result of fear and anxiety. In the risk/benefit ratio evaluation, the risks associated with the sequela of stress are far greater than the risks associated with the proper administration of IV conscious sedation. Stress can precipitate an acute medical emergency in the susceptible individual. Extensive dental procedures, because of their potential to produce stress, are cited as indications for sedation.

Specific principles of conscious sedation must be observed for patient safety. The patient must remain conscious. The conscious patient has been defined as one who has intact protective reflexes, including the ability to maintain an airway, and who is capable of rational response to questions or requests. The safety of the patient is dependent on his/her protective reflexes remaining intact, particularly the ability to clear and maintain an airway. Rational response to verbal requests is the single best monitor of the state of consciousness. Proper IV sedation technique can predictably place a patient in a conscious, cooperative, and nonapprehensive state.

STRESS REDUCTION PROTOCOL

It is important to note that stress reduction starts with the initial patient contact by the office staff and is carried on through treatment and into the posttreatment phase. The basic principles of a stress reduction protocol as suggested by Monheim,[30] Malamed,[31] and others should be followed:

1. Recognize anxiety and diagnose risk
2. Premedicate the evening before a dental appointment
3. Premedicate 1 hour before a dental appointment if necessary
4. Schedule short morning appointments
5. Be prompt, efficient, and organized
6. Inform the patient completely of the procedures to come
7. Maintain adequate pain control during the procedure
8. Follow through with postoperative pain and anxiety control

Recognize Anxiety and Diagnose Risk

The diagnosis of a potential medical risk patient should be determined from the medical history and physical evaluation. Consultation is required for those who are determined to be at risk. The dentist and entire office staff should be alert to note any signs or symptoms suggesting increased anxiety and fear. In addition to the obvious signs such as nervousness, sweating, increased blood pressure and pulse rate, or stated comments on the health history, the direct asking of the patient in a nonthreatening and supportive manner concerning his / her feelings about dental care will nearly always elicit the information being sought.

Premedicate the Evening Before a Dental Appointment

It is most important that the patient have a good night's sleep before the appointment. A well-rested patient is significantly better able to resist anxiety and tolerate stress. The oral benzodiazepines are ideal for this: diazepam, lorazepam, and triazolam are very effective. Triazolam perhaps is preferred for the exceptionally nervous patient who may have significant problems sleeping.

Premedicate 1 Hour Before a Dental Appointment if Necessary

For a few exceptionally nervous patients with some medical compromise it may be of additional benefit to administer an oral benzodiazepine an hour or so before the dental appointment. This is particularly helpful for those who acknowledge profound fear of the intravenous needle. It must be made absolutely clear that the patient is not to drive an automobile but must be escorted to and from the office by a responsible adult. Diazepam is perhaps an ideal medication for this purpose. Triazolam is not recommended unless the patient is in the dental office.

Schedule Short Morning Appointments

Early morning appointments permit the patient to undergo the procedure when he / she is most rested and stress tolerant. Also, the patient will have had minimal time to dwell on the upcoming procedure and work himself / herself into a state of anxiety and fatigue that would significantly decrease his / her stress tolerance.

Also, for the medically compromised patient, the length of the appointment should be kept minimal. As the length of the appointment increases, so does the stress level. Multiple short appointments with ample recovery time between are recommended.

Be Prompt, Efficient, and Organized

Do not keep the patient waiting. The anxiety of waiting an uncue length of time can be greater than that produced by the actual dental procedure. Some studies have shown that the greatest number of medical emergencies in the dental office occur in the waiting room and restroom. Be orderly and efficient in going about your tasks; this is not a time to show confusion on either the part of the dentist or office staff. The patient must be made to feel secure. He / she must believe that the therapist and staff are competent and his / her welfare is their foremost objective. Unpleasant sights such as the dental syringe, surgical instruments, bloody gauzes, or any object that might stimulate fear must be kept from view. Unfavorable sounds and odors produce all sorts of imagined threats.

Inform Patient Completely

Today's patient is generally well informed via fairly accurate lay and consumer publications, and his / her confidence must be gained through honest professional competence. Describing the proposed procedure thoroughly in general terms that can be understood will markedly decrease anxiety and fear. Fear of the unknown is a potentially great threat. Treat the patient the way you would like to be treated.

Adequate Pain Control During Therapy

Profound local anesthesia in the majority of cases is the one most important factor in anxiety control. Without it, all other aspects of anxiety management are of little value. Pain will stimulate the release of catecholamines with their undesirable effects, especially on the medically compromised patient. Painful stimuli of the oral cavity, although rare, can cause a reflex vagal efferent activity resulting in bradycardia, hypotension, and marked decreased cardiac output.[32]

Postoperative Pain and Anxiety Control

Once the procedure is completed, the welfare of the patient cannot be forgotten. Carefully review postoperative and postsedation instructions pretreatment with the patient and then posttreatment with the patient and accompanying adult. Describe what to expect as far as pain and side effects from the procedure so the patient will not become unduly alarmed if there is some pain, bleeding, swelling, some facial discoloration, lethargy, etc. Appropriate oral analgesics must be prescribed. If appropriate, administer one of the long-acting local anesthetics prior to office departure.

The patient will feel more secure if he/she has a means of readily contacting the therapist should questions or problems arise. It is important that the patient be telephoned 2 or 3 hours following the procedure to enquire as to his/her well-being and ask if there are any questions or problems.

RECOMMENDED DRUGS FOR PERIODONTAL SEDATION

Nearly all requirements for IV sedation induced in the periodontal office can be fulfilled with the following drugs:

1. Benzodiazepines:
   — diazepam
   — midazolam
2. Narcotics:
   — morphine
   — meperidine
   — nalbuphine
   — butorphanol
3. Antisialagogue:
   — glycopyrrolate

Used appropriately, these drugs are predictable in producing the desired effects with minimal undesirable side effects. By using a limited number of drugs, one can become very familiar with their pharmacologic action, indications, contraindications, and precautions.

DETERMINANTS OF RATE AND LENGTH OF SEDATIVE EFFECT

The serum concentration of a drug with IV administration depends primarily on the rate/quantity of injection. The drug is then distributed most rapidly to those tissues that are most vascular. Brain, heart, liver, and kidney are highly perfused and concentrate the drug rapidly. The rate and degree with which a sedative drug then exerts a clinical effect is primarily determined by two factors: the amount of administered drug that is free or unbound to plasma proteins, and its degree of lipid solubility. The rate of onset of sedation is directly related to the rate at which the unbound drug crosses the blood/brain barrier, which is determined by its degree of lipid solubility to affect a specific neuronal receptor. In time the drugs redistribute to less vascular tissues such as muscle, fat, skin, and bone, and the clinical effect of the drug decreases. Clinical recovery occurs during this redistribution phase. The rate of redistribution of the drug away from the specific neuronal receptors in the CNS largely determines the rate of clinical recovery and not the rate of metabolic breakdown or elimination of the drug from the body. For the drugs to be discussed, metabolism to inactive products plays only a minor role in their duration of effect. Some of the metabolic breakdown products actually have similar pharmacologic actions and a longer duration of action than the parent drug, particularly in the case of diazepam and to a lesser extent for meperidine. Repeat doses of medication will have a greater and a longer clinical effect relative to the dosage due to partial saturation of CNS receptor sites and inactive tissue sites such as muscle, fat, etc.

The sedatives and narcotics discussed can produce sedation, hypnosis, anesthesia, coma, and death, depending on the quantity and rate of administration and patient susceptibility.

SELECTION OF A DRUG OR COMBINATION OF DRUGS

The selection of a particular drug or combination of drugs will be determined by the degree of patient anxiety; the degree of stressfulness of the procedure; length of the procedure (longer procedures being more stressful); systemic status of the patient (the selection or nonselection of certain drugs can be affected by the patient's medical and physical status); and medications the patient is taking (various medications are incompatible or may produce an undesirable response with certain sedative medications — see contraindications and precautions and specific drug pharmacology).

To fulfill all the criteria of an ideal sedative, the agent would decrease fear and anxiety, have a very wide margin of safety between the therapeutic and toxic dose level, be predictable in its effects, elevate the pain threshold, produce euphoria, and promote an amnestic response. Additionally, it may be desired to have an antisialagogue effect. No single drug presently performs all of these functions, and in many cases all of these results may not be desirable for specific procedures and specific patients. For example, it is not always necessary to have a dry field or anterograde amnesia. With the drugs and techniques described, the clinician is able to tailor the sedation to a specific patient and specific response. Benzodiazepines will reduce apprehension and fear, narcotics will produce analgesia and euphoria and elevate the pain threshold, and antisialagogues will produce a dry field.

For relatively short procedures with moderate anxiety, effective sedation is adequately achieved with unidrug sedation using diazepam or midazolam. When appropriate, midazolam is the drug of choice. A combination of drugs or polydrug therapy is indicated when additional requirements for effective patient management and sedation are present. If a dry field is required, the appropriate antisialagogue may be added; the use of glycopyrrolate is a significant advantage, as it does not cross the blood/brain barrier. The addition of a narcotic is most de-

sirable for the excessively apprehensive patient and for long procedures or fairly traumatic procedures. Midazolam most likely will replace diazepam for dental IV sedation once more experience with its use is gained and it is accepted for the patient under 18 years old.

CONTRAINDICATIONS AND PRECAUTIONS
(Table 18-4)

Contraindications for IV sedation are not to be confused with situations in which precautions should be taken. There are no systemic contraindications to the intravenous route of drug administration. There are, however, two contraindications to local use: the inability to locate a suitable vein and a patient proven to be highly susceptible to phlebitis. Systemic contraindications are related to the drugs used and the patient's medical status and therefore would be the same for all routes of drug administration.

INTRAVENOUS VERSUS OTHER ROUTES OF ADMINISTRATION

Drugs may be administered by the oral, rectal, intramuscular, and intravenous routes to produce sedation, hypnosis, and general anesthesia. The clinical effects are due to dosage and rate of administration. Each route has its advantages and disadvantages. The primary disadvantage of the oral, rectal, and intramuscular routes is the use of arbitrary dosage.

The intravenous route, used properly, is the safest means of drug administration. A drug injected in the arm takes approximately 30 seconds to reach the

brain. It takes midazolam and diazepam approximately 30 to 40 seconds to cross the blood/brain barrier to initiate their pharmacologic effects. The clinical effects of midazolam and diazepam are noted in approximately 60 to 90 seconds from the time of injection. *Drugs that rapidly pass the blood/brain barrier to effect their pharmacologic action can be accurately titrated in incremental doses until the desired effect is obtained.*

Although the narcotic analgesics, meperidine, morphine, butorphanol, and nalbuphine are not titrateable, the patient's response to the sedatives permit a more accurate assessment of narcotic dosage since a relatively equal tolerance generally exists between these classes of drugs. *The significant advantage of the intravenous route of drug administration is that there is no dosage guessing as exists with the oral or intramuscular routes. The dangers of overdosage or inconvenience of underdosage are avoided.*

PRESEDATION PREPARATION

Medical history and physical evaluation. The pretreatment/presedation appointment or appointments are used to determine the patient's general medical status, ability to physically and psychologically tolerate the stress of the dental procedure, need for medical consultation, need for conscious sedation, the conscious sedation technique and drugs to be used, degree of sedation required, and time allotted for the procedure

The medical and dialogue history and physical evaluation for the conscious IV sedation patient

TABLE 18-4 *Contraindications and precautions to conscious IV sedation*

Contraindications
- Local
  - inability to locate a suitable vein
  - patient who has proved to be highly susceptible to phlebitis
- Systemic
  - specific drug allergy
  - hepatic porphyria (barbiturates)
  - monoamine oxidase inhibitors (meperidine)
  - alcohol
  - recreational drug usage and drug addicts
  - severe respiratory depression
  - pyloric stenosis (morphine, meperidine, fentanyl)
  - pregnancy and lactating mothers
  - glaucoma
  - uncontrolled diabetic
  - auricular flutter or supraventricular tachycardias (meperidine, scopolamine, atropine)

Precaution category patient
- Cardiovascular disease
  - hypertension
  - hypotension
  - angina
  - postmyocardial infarction
  - congestive heart failure
- Pulmonary disease
  - asthma
  - bronchitis
  - emphysema
- Endocrine disorders
  - diabetic
  - thyroid disease (hyperthyroidism, hypothyroidism)
  - adrenal cortical insufficiency
- Drugs the patient is taking
  - cardiac drugs (antihypertensives, antiarrhythmic)
  - CNS depressants (alcohol, barbiturates, tranquilizers, tricyclic antidepressants, narcotics, antihistamines, cold medications)
  - appetite depressors
  - steroids
  - oral contraceptives
  - sodium warfarin
- Drug abusers-addicts
- Drug metabolism and elimination
  - liver disease
  - renal disease
  - prostatic hypertrophy
- Age
  - children
  - elderly
  - debilitated
- Psychiatric patients
- Glaucoma
- Epilepsy
- Alcohol withdrawal psychosis
- Local aberrant arteries

Handling the precaution category patient:
- Requires additional care and consideration, but sedation is not contraindicated
  - medical consultation
  - administer drugs at reduced rate and total dosage
  - do not give certain drugs
  - substitute alternate drugs
  - discontinue present medications for specific period of time
  - carefully select intravenous vessel

are the same as for the general dental patient. If it is felt a special history is required for IV sedation other than for specific drug allergies, drug incompatibilities, history of susceptibility to phlebitis, and noting the presence of superficial veins, a proper history is not being taken. Stress and its sequela are the primary etiological factors for precipitating a medical emergency in the dental office. Evaluation and preparation of the patient for IV sedation begins with the initial patient visit. The dentist must determine if the patient represents an increased medical risk due to his/her medical, physical, or emotional status or the medications he/she may be taking. If the patient is found to be at increased risk, the dentist must determine what modifications can be instituted to decrease that risk to an acceptable level for dental office treatment. Medical consultation may be required as well as use of the stress reduction protocol as applicable. To be managed safely, some patients may require treatment in a hospital. Ultimately, the dentist is responsible for the safety and welfare of the patient.

The medical history is reviewed again on the day of the procedure because there can be a delay between the initial history and surgical treatment.

Instructions prior to sedation. Treatment and its contingencies and complications are reviewed before the sedation appointment. The patient is given written instructions that are thoroughly reviewed regarding presedation and postoperative and postsedation care. This decreases anxiety and apprehension.

Treatment room preparation. The treatment room should present a pleasant atmosphere that is conducive to sedation and has a minimum of distractions,

movement, and sounds. The intravenous equipment, monitoring equipment, and surgical instruments should be conveniently arranged, hidden from patient view and ready for use.

Patient preparation. Prior to the patient's entering the treatment room, verify that a responsible adult will escort him/her home and remain with him/her while he/she is under the influence of the medication. The patient is asked to void and to remove any false eyelashes, heavy eye makeup, contact lenses, fingernail polish, or false nails for the oximeter sensor. The patient is placed in the semireclined or dental contour chair position.

Measurement of vital signs. Blood pressure and pulse rate are taken in addition to the baseline vital signs originally recorded. The manual sphygmomanometer or automated blood pressure cuff is left in place. Variations in readings at this time relative to baseline values are most likely the result of the emotional tension of the anticipated procedure.

TECHNIQUE[33]

Selection of venipuncture site. Utmost caution must be observed in selecting a venipuncture site. Intra-arterial injection with barbiturates and tranquilizers can cause arterial spasm, with occlusion and subsequent gangrene of the distal extremities. Topazian[34] gives an excellent review of the precautions to observe in avoiding accidental intra-arterial injection. One should be familiar with the normal and abnormal vascular and nerve anatomy of the antecubital fossa, forearm, wrist, and hand. A site should be chosen where there is the least chance of accidentally penetrating an artery. Superficial vessels should be

selected, and blind probing with the needle should be avoided. The injection site is palpated prior to tourniquet placement to demonstrate the absence of arterial pulse. Occasionally, an injection site is not visible until the tourniquet is placed and the vessel is engorged. Although not as reliable, palpation for arterial pulse is accomplished at this time. The tourniquet should not be placed too tight and the arm should not be hyperextended to obliterate the arterial pulse.

The largest, straightest vein available should generally be selected for venipuncture. A thick-walled, large, straight vein will have greater resistance to drug and needle irritation, greater blood flow for increased drug dilution, will not require the immobilization of the wrist or antecubital fossa, and offers the decreased possibility of an accidental intra-arterial injection. The order of venipuncture site selection is:

1. Forearm
2. Back of the hand (no diazepam)
3. Dorsal and lateral wrist
4. Antecubital fossa

Following are the signs of an intra-arterial injection:

1. Unusual pain with vessel penetration
2. Pain distal to injection site
3. Color of blood
4. Blood backing up in the tubing
5. Pulsation of blood

Components of infusion. Drugs may be administered intravenously by direct and indirect methods. The direct method of injecting medications into a vein followed by needle removal is contraindicated. *The indirect method of injecting medications via a* *continuous infusion is the only method recommended.* It provides maintenance of a patent vein for drug reinforcement or emergency drug administration and decreases venous irritation due to drug dilution.

The components of an infusion setup consist of a bottle or plastic container of intravenous fluid, an administration unit with an adjustable flow rate control and injection site, and a butterfly needle. A 23-gauge needle may be used if minimally irritating drugs are being injected (no diazepam or barbiturates should be used with 23-gauge needles). A 21-gauge needle usually is selected to maintain an adequate flow rate. A 21-gauge needle will permit a flow rate of 13 mL versus 3 mL for a 23-gauge needle. A large needle relative to vessel diameter will cause increased irritation.

The intravenous fluid container is suspended, preferably by a ceiling attachment, at least 2 to 3 feet above the heart level, behind the patient away from his/her direct line of vision. This permits a more unobstructed treatment room. The components of the infusion setup must be carefully and aseptically connected together.

Tourniquet application. The tourniquet usually works best if applied proximal to the antecubital fossa, but occasionally it works best when placed a few inches proximal to the anticipated puncture site. The tourniquet is applied to prevent venous return but not so tightly as to obstruct arterial flow. Too-tight application obliterates the arterial pulse and prevents venous engorgement, which is required for easy venipuncture. The tourniquet is applied with the free ends pointing away from the venipuncture site to avoid its contamination and allow for proper removal. A 1-inch flat rubber strap, a 1-inch Penrose drain, or velcro tourniquet are the preferred tourniquets. A blood pressure cuff is a good tourniquet and may be used following blood pressure measurement by holding the pressure midway between the systolic and diastolic pressure.

Venous engorgement. The primary factor for venous engorgement is proper placement and tension of the tourniquet. Engorgement of the vein is aided if the patient hangs his/her arm down to one side while at the same time repeatedly closing and opening a fist. Venous spasm may prevent filling and distention, which can be countered by rubbing with an alcohol sponge or lightly slapping the puncture site. In difficult cases, a warm moist towel can be applied to the area. Occasionally a patient who had what appeared to be adequate veins at the presedation appointment will not at the sedation appointment. This is due to preoperative anxiety and increased circulating catecholamines.

Palpation for pulse. The anticipated venipuncture site should be palpated to verify a lack of pulse and to rule out an artery prior to tourniquet placement. Occasionally a suitable vein is not obvious prior to tourniquet placement. The selected vessel should then be palpated and demonstrated to be free of arterial pulse following tourniquet placement and prior to venipuncture. Correct tourniquet application and arm positioning are necessary.

Puncture site preparation. The site is scrubbed vigorously with a 70% isopropyl alcohol sponge for a minimum of 60 seconds. Mechanical cleansing is probably as important as the action of the alcohol. A circular motion is used from the center to the periphery. The alcohol is allowed to dry prior to needle penetration.

Vein penetration. With the patient maintaining a clenched fist, the arm is gripped with the left hand (or right hand if left-handed) and using the thumb the skin is stretched distally to immobilize the vein and facilitate penetration. The venipuncture is made by directing the needle at approximately 30 degrees to the surface of the skin. The skin and underlying tissues are firmly penetrated to reach but not to penetrate the vein. The needle is lowered until almost parallel with the skin surface and the vein is entered slowly. With experience the operator will be able to feel when the needle enters the venous lumen. Entry is verified by flushing blood back into the tubing or, if using a syringe, by aspirating back on the syringe. The needle, nearly parallel to the skin surface, is carefully advanced approximately two thirds its length for stability, avoiding venous wall penetration. The needle is advanced only with the tourniquet in place.

Release of tourniquet. The tourniquet is released by pulling on the correct free end away from the injection site. This prevents dislodgement of the needle and possible contamination of the injection site.

Start of infusion. The drip is opened or the fluid from the syringe is injected to clear the butterfly needle and tubing of blood and to verify a free flow. The infusion should never be started with the tourniquet in place. The air-free tubing of the administration unit is connected to the female end of the butterfly needle tubing if a syringe was used. The drip is left wide open for maximum drug dilution and to assure no infiltration at the injection site. The infusion is now ready for addition of the drug.

Immobilization. An armboard or commercial immobilizer is required for immobilization when the antecubital fossa or wrist areas are used. Commercial immobilizers are more comfortable than a rigid board. Specially designed arm slings on some dental chairs are also helpful to immobilize and stabilize the elbow and wrist.

Preparation of drugs. It is strongly recommended that each medication be drawn into a separate syringe. This allows for specific control over the administration of each individual drug. Commercial labels are available with printed names and individual colors for each drug. The total milligram content and milligram / milliliter is written on the label which is placed on the syringe. Preparation of drugs is as follows:

Diazepam: 10 mg (5 mg / mL) undiluted, 5 mg / mL
Midazolam: 5 mg diluted to 5 mL in a 5-mL syringe, 1 mg / mL
Meperidine: 25 mg diluted to 5 mL in a 5-mL syringe, 5 mg / mL
Morphine: 5 mg diluted to 5 mL in a 5-mL syringe, 1 mg / mL
Nalbuphine: 5 mg diluted to 5 mL in a 5-mL syringe, 1 mg / mL
Butorphanol: 2 mg diluted to 4 mL in a 5-mL syringe, 0.5 mg / mL
Glycopyrrolate: 0.2 mg, undiluted

Administration of drugs. The fundamental principles and guidelines recommended in administering the drugs were well established by Jorgensen and Hayden.[35] The sequence of drug administration is as follows:

1. Titrate the sedative (diazepam or midazolam) to establish baseline
2. Administer fixed dose of antisialagogue (glycopyrrolate, if indicated)
3. Slowly administer a fixed proportionate dose of the narcotic relative to the amount of sedative required to achieve the baseline

The arm-brain circulation time is approximately 30 seconds and the sedatives discussed rapidly cross the blood / brain barrier, exerting their clinical effect in 1 to 3 minutes from the time of administration. Only drugs that rapidly cross the blood / brain barrier to effect their pharmacologic action can be accurately and safely titrated. Because of the rapid pharmacologic effect of diazepam and midazolam, they can be slowly titrated in incremental doses until a desired level of sedation is achieved. This level was referred to as the *baseline* by Jorgensen.[35] He defined it as the first sign of cortical depression, a state of light or mild sedation. It can be recognized by the patient's exhibiting symptoms of drowsiness, dizziness, blurring of vision, and heavy eyelids. The patient may also blink his / her eyelids excessively and have difficulty in enunciating clearly. A small test dose of the medication is first administered. The sedative is then slowly titrated to achieve the desired clinical effect (the baseline). If a dry mouth is desired, a fixed dose of the antisialagogue is now slowly administered. If the additional effect of a narcotic is desired, it is added now. A predetermined proportionate dose of the narcotic is given slowly, relative to the amount of sedative required to achieve the baseline. The narcotics morphine, meperidine, butorphanol, and nalbuphine cannot be accurately titrated as they do not cross the blood / brain barrier rapidly and their full pharmacologic effects are not immediately evident. The full effect of the narcotics takes about 7 to 10 minutes. Immediate signs indicating dose limitations are not evident because of this slow effect. It is safe to give a fixed proportionate dose of the narcotic relative to sedative dosage because an equal tolerance gener-

ally exists to the sedatives and narcotics.

A test dosage (a few drops) of diazepam or midazolam is administered with the IV infusion wide open and rapidly running near its point of venous entry. With the drugs well diluted, less pain and phlebitis are experienced. This is particularly significant for diazepam with its irritating diluents. The patient is observed for 3 to 5 minutes for unusual local or systemic reactions. Pain at the venipuncture site may indicate seepage into the tissue spaces. Pain distal to the venipuncture site may indicate an intra-arterial injection. A continuous wide-open drip is required for maximum drug dilution to minimize venous wall irritation. Drug dilution will minimize the damage potential should seepage into the tissue spaces or an intra-arterial injection occur. It is paramount that the infusion setup not be removed when an intra-arterial injection is suspected it will be needed in local treatment. The test dosage and observation period provide an opportunity for an acute drug reaction to become apparent. This is a safety factor as little medication has been administered.

Drug administration, with the drip wide open, is continued at the maximum rate of 1 mg of diazepam and 0.25 mg of midazolam every 30 seconds until the baseline is achieved. During the titration, the patient and monitors are observed closely. Subjective inquiries of "What do you feel?" and "How do you feel?" are made. If an antisialagogue effect is desired, a fixed dose is now slowly administered. If a narcotic is used, a fixed proportionate dose relative to the sedative dosage required to achieve the baseline is now slowly administered. Following a test dose, meperidine is administered at the rate of 5 mg every 30 seconds and morphine and nalbuphine at the rate of 0.5 mg every 30 seconds until the fixed proportionate dose is reached. The vessel is flushed following administration of the drug. The drip rate is reduced to 5 or 6 drops / min, an adequate rate to maintain a patent infusion. There are no absolute maximum dosages for IV conscious sedation. However, dosages approaching 20 mg for diazepam and 10 mg for midazolam are usually more than sufficient for an initial titration. With experience and during 2½ to 3½ hour procedures, an accumulative of 30 mg of diazepam or 15 mg of midazolam may be carefully administered with periodic reinforcement. No more than 50 mg of meperidine or 5 mg of morphine is usually required with the initial administration, while 75 mg and 7.5 mg, respectively, may be given over a 2½ to 3½ hour procedure.

There are some situations in which the patient's response to sedative medications potentially may be exaggerated. This may occur in the presences of certain medications such as various antihypertensives, antiarrhythmics, CNS depressants, and various physical conditions such as hypothyroidism, debilitation, the elderly, the young, etc. In these patients the drugs are titrated more slowly to fully assess the maximum pharmacologic response. In some of these conditions the depth of sedation could be fairly deep even with a relatively small dose. In others the length of recovery may be prolonged or significant postural hypotension is potentiated. Additional care must be observed in uprighting and ambulating this patient. The responsible accompanying adult must also be cautioned. In the case of a marked drug response, intraoperative hypotension, or de-

layed recovery, one should suspect possible hypoglycemia, hypothyroidism, or adrenal insufficiency.

Monitoring. Monitoring is a process that provides us with a continuous, accurate, and immediate evaluation of the patient's basic physiological status, response to therapeutic procedures, effects of emotional and physical stress, and effects of administered sedative medications. It should provide us with information warning of an undesirable trend in physiologic status, the presence of an acute emergency and physiologic response to therapeutic intervention. It is determined by observation, touch, listening, conversation, and evaluation of the circulatory, respiratory, and central nervous systems.

With the recent availability of noninvasive sophisticated monitoring equipment at a reasonable cost, the minimal acceptable mechanical monitoring equipment for routine use are the pulse oximeter, a continuous pulse meter, an automatic mechanical blood pressure determining device, and a precordial stethoscope. However with the use of these devices, a significant note of caution is in order. There is a tendency and a great danger to become overly reliant on these wonderful monitoring devices. It has been estimated that 90% of all anesthesia-related problems are human related; the monitoring equipment by itself will not prevent an untoward event. With the combined use of the mechanical monitoring devices and the intelligent use of our senses, accurate monitoring of the conscious sedated patient is possible.

The sedated patient is *never* left unattended, and preferably both the dentist and the assistant trained in monitoring stay in attendance. Maximum drug effect

is determined by a number of factors. One factor that is seldom mentioned or realized is the role that the degree of stimulation the patient is undergoing plays. For example, a patient who is at a proper level of sedation while the dentist performs the procedures may be oversedated when not stimulated. Surgical stimulation of a patient under conscious sedation will increase respiratory rate and volume and antagonize the hypoventilation that may be present with the benzodiazepines and narcotics. The degree of stimulation the patient is undergoing will also affect the level of sedation, the maximum drug effect. The trained monitoring assistant should engage the patient in continuous conversation, observing him / her and the monitors closely and assuring proper head and neck position. With in-office sedation, it is imperative to have an attentive assistant trained to closely observe the patient's respiratory, circulatory, and central nervous systems.

Reinforcement. Reinforcement, or administration of additional medication, is frequently required for long procedures and occasionally when the patient is inadequately sedated, either intentionally or unintentionally. Approximately ⅕ to ¼ the initial dose of diazepam or midazolam will be adequate and is titrated at the same previous slow rate. In the multidrug technique with long, stressful procedures or very apprehensive patients, additional narcotic may be required in addition to the benzodiazepine. The same proportionate dosage of narcotic is used, staying on the low side, and is administered very slowly.

The precaution category patient who has systemic disease or who is taking various medications is intentionally undersedated initially when his/her response to sedatives and narcotics is in question. The therapist waits for maximum drug effect to occur and determines if additional medication is required.

Inadequate sedation may unintentionally occur when the level or degree of sedation is misjudged. Additional medication is then administered as described above.

Discontinuation of infusion. The infusion is discontinued when the procedure has been completed, the patient has been brought to an upright position, and the stability of the patient and his/her vital signs has been verified.

Dismissal of patient. The vital signs, particularly the blood pressure and pulse rate, must be checked prior to dismissing the patient and should be near baseline values prior to dismissal. Postural hypotension may be noted, which may be due to a prolonged semireclined position or possibly to the effects of narcotics on the peripheral vasculature. To avoid postural hypotension the patient is brought to the walking stage in phases.

Nausea may result from postural hypotension, narcotics, or swallowed blood. Administration of oxygen at a 3- to 6-L flow rate by means of a nasal canula or hood will enhance the rate of recovery from these side effects. No patient should be allowed to leave the office if he/she cannot walk unassisted. The stable patient is escorted from the office by an assistant and the accompanying adult. The postoperative and post-sedation instructions are thoroughly reviewed with the accompanying adult prior to office departure. A later telephone inquiry of patient well-being is wise and thoughtful and is an excellent aid in establishing patient rapport.

COMPLICATIONS

Local Complications

Local complications are of concern and range from a minor hematoma to intra-arterial injection. Good technique and careful selection of the venipuncture site prevent serious complications.

Hematoma. A hematoma is the leakage of blood from a vein into the interstitial space. It can be recognized by a localized swelling and/or bluish discoloration and is usually of little significance. The use of pressure is the initial treatment, followed by the application of hot, moist packs to aid in dissolution.

Localized infiltration. Infiltration of the medications into the perivascular or subcutaneous tissues can cause localized discomfort and even significant pain, especially if a large amount of sodium pentobarbital or diazepam is involved. It is prevented by selecting a large, straight vessel, needle well threaded in the vein, and properly stabilized elbow or wrist if one of those vessels used. Dilution of the sedatives with a fast drip and close observation of the injection site minimizes the possibility of extensive tissue injury should an infiltration occur.

Superficial red vessel. Superficial vessels may become red and itch soon after injection of the narcotic. This is due to histamine release stimulated by morphine and meperidine. This is not an allergic reaction and is of little consequence. It is treated by flushing the vessel with intravenous fluid.

Phlebitis. Phlebitis is inflammation of a vein and is caused by trauma of venipuncture, presence of an indwelling needle, irritating drugs, and possibly infection. The usual symptom is tenderness or pain along the route of the vein.

The overlying tissue may turn red, causing patient concern. The vein may contain a blood clot (thrombophlebitis) and feel ropelike. Phlebitis in the arm is usually a benign condition best treated by immobilization, elevation, application of moist heat, and use of analgesics, anti-inflammatory agents, and antibiotics if infection is suspected. Phlebitis that does not clear within 48 to 72 hours with conservative therapy should be referred to a physician.

Pain at or proximal to the injection site. A burning sensation may occur in the area of the venipuncture. This may be due to venospasm or drug irritation. The venospasm is probably secondary to the trauma of needle insertion and it soon fades. Some drugs, notably diazepam due to its diluent, can produce a marked burning sensation, especially when injected undiluted into a small vessel. The sensation soon dissipates if the vessel is well flushed with the intravenous fluid.

Intra-arterial injection. Intra-arterial injection, especially with sodium pentobarbital and diazepam, can cause arterial spasm or thrombosis leading to gangrene and loss of fingers, hand, or forearm. This is the most serious local complication that can arise from intravenous administration of drugs. It is best treated by prevention and good technique. Signs of an intra-arterial injection include severe pain extending distally from the injection site, slowing of the drip, blood rising in the tubing, pulsation of blood in the tubing and a brighter color of the blood. These signs are not always present and that is why good venpuncture technique is so important.

Systemic Complications

Atropine flush. This is a red blush

like appearance of the face, neck, and upper chest due to the atropine-induced vasodilation and the microcirculation of this area. It is not an allergic reaction and is totally innocuous and will soon subside without intervention.

Postural hypotension. This is primarily prevented by getting the patient upright and in the sitting position and then to the standing position slowly and purposefully. The patient taking antihypertensives and sedated with narcotics is significantly more susceptible. The accompanying adult must be cautioned about this possibility and instructed in its prevention.

Vasovagal syncope. Vasovagal syncope is associated with altered central homeostatic mechanisms, including decreased cardiac return with decreased arterial oxygen tension. They do not return to normal for 20 to 60 minutes even though the vital signs are normal. If sedatives or narcotic are administered during this altered hemostatic state, inadequate venous return leading to decreased cardiac output and cerebral and coronary perfusion can occur, leading to a potentially fatal outcome.

Central anticholinergic syndrome. This syndrome is manifested by restlessness, agitation, excitement, belligerent behavior, disorientation, delirium, tachycardia, or stupor and coma. It is due to the inhibition of acetylcholine at central sites. Classically it is produced by scopolamine but can also be produced by atropine, the major psychosedatives such as phenergan, and the benzodiazepines. Its chance of occurring is enhanced if the patient is taking tricyclic antidepressants or when major psychosedatives are combined with scopolamine or atropine. It is prevented by using glycopyrrolate only as an antisialagogue. Glycopyrrolate has not been shown to cause the reaction because it does not cross the blood/brain barrier. If scopolamine is to be used, use minimal dosage (0.25 mg maximum) but do not use in young, elderly, or debilitated patients or in conjunction with major psychosedatives and tricyclic antidepressants.

With mild to moderate symptoms it is treated by calming and reassuring the patient. Perhaps some physical restraint may be necessary to prevent injury. If the reaction is severe it is treated by physiostigmine titrated in 1-mg doses.

Extrapyramidal reaction. This is characterized by symptoms resembling Parkinson's disease: uncontrolled movement of voluntary muscle groups producing involuntary yawning and protrusion of the tongue, and twisting and turning movements of the head, neck, and extremities. Parkinson's disease is thought to be due to a deficiency of dopamine in the CNS (dopamine stimulates an inhibiting system responsible for central modulation of muscular activity). Psychosedatives, especially the major psychosedatives, are dopaminergic blocking agents. Extrapyramidal reaction is best prevented by not using major psychosedatives, and it has only rarely been implicated with minor psychosedatives.

Benzatropine in 1-mg doses administered intravenously or orally has been recommended by Bennett[36] to treat the condition. Intravenously it acts nearly immediately and orally in 20 to 30 minutes. Benzatropine is an anticholinergic that acts primarily in the CNS to block the unopposed facilitory system.

Deep sedation/excessive sedation/unconsciousness/light anesthesia/overdosage. Overdosage with IV drug administration is due to an inadequate history taking and/or physical evaluation, poor technique, poor judgment, and the extremely rare instance of hypersensitivity to the drugs. It is characterized by difficult arousability or inability to arouse, minimal responsiveness or unresponsiveness to verbal commands, shaking, and various physical stimuli.

One should be concerned with diminished protective reflexes, particularly the gag reflex, and partial or complete airway obstruction by allowing the head to slump forward, bending the neck with relaxation of the tongue and pharyngeal musculature, and vomiting with subsequent aspiration. All dental work should be stopped and complete and undivided attention given to the patient. Airway maintenance is controlled by placing one or two fingers under the chin to tip the head backward, extending the neck and thus providing a patent airway. This is perhaps the most important act in assuring the safety of the deeply sedated and unconscious patient. Respiratory depression may not be present. With deep sedation, give supplemental oxygen to prevent hypoxemia. Vomiting is managed/prevented first by instructing the patient to have nothing by mouth 4 hours prior to the procedure. Should vomiting occur, the patient is placed in a slightly head down position with the head and upper body turned to the right side. High volume suction and a pharyngeal aspirator need to be available for aspiration of vomitus.

Respiratory depression. Mild respiratory depression is treated by properly positioning the patient's head and neck to maintain an open airway, asking the patient to take deep regular breaths, giving oxygen via a nasal canula or mask, and continuously monitoring vital signs. With moderate respiratory depression, you may be able to partially assist breathing with some positive pressure. Deep respiratory depression is treated by proper positioning of the head and neck to maintain an open airway, oxygen, assisted ventilation, positive pressure breathing, drug therapy as indicated by the degree of depression and the drug at cause, and continuous monitoring of vital signs.

Circulatory depression. Circulatory depression is treated by elevating the patient's legs higher than the heart and by IV fluid administration. For cardiac arrest, evaluation, and treatment, refer to Standards for Cardiopulmonary Resuscitation (CPR) and Emergency Cardiac Care (ECC).

Air embolism. Small amounts of air introduced intravenously are usually not significant; however, they are significant in the patient with congenital heart defects, atrial septal defects, ventricular septal defects, and patent ductus arteriosus. A small air bubble that shifts from the venous to the arterial side, a possibility with these defects, can cause CNS damage.

REFERENCES

1. Herwig LD, Jones DL, Milam SB: Correlates of recovery from nitrous oxide exposure (abstr). IADR, Dallas, TX, 1984.
2. Shapiro BA, Harrison RA, Walton JR: *Clinical Application of Blood Gases.* Chicago: Year Book Medical Publ; 1977:88-91.
3. Chen L, Marshall BE: The diagnosis and management of perioperative hypoxemia. In: Barash PG, ed. *ASA Refresher Courses in Anesthesiology.* Philadelphia: JB Lippincott Co; 1988:43-44, 47-51.
4. Milam SB, Giovannitti JA: Local anesthetics in dental practice. Gage TW, *Dent Clin North Am* 1984;28(3):493-508.
5. Dionne RA, Goldstein DS, Wirdzek PR: Effects of diazepam premedication and epinephrine-containing local anesthetic on cardiovascular and plasma catecholamine responses to oral surgery. *Anesth Analg* 1984;63:640-646.
6. Richter JJ: Current theories about the mechanisms of benzodiazepines and neuroleptic drugs. *Anesthesiology* 1981;54:66-72.
7. Study RE, Barker JL: Cellular mechanisms of benzodiazepine action. *J Am Med Assoc* 1982;247:2147-2151.
8. Cheng SC, Brunner EA: Inhibition of GABA metabolism in rat brain synaptosome by midazolam (RO 21-3981). *Anesthesiology* 1981;55:41-45.
9. Gerecke M: Chemical structure and properties of midazolam compared with other benzodiazepines. *Br J Clin Pharmacol* 1983;16(Suppl I):11-16.
10. DeJong RH, Bonin JD: Benzodiazepines protect mice from local anesthetic convulsions and death. *Anesth Analg* 1981;60:385-389.
11. Forster A, Gardaz JP, Suter PM, Gemperle M: Respiratory depression by midazolam and diazepam. *Anesthesiology* 1980;53:494-497.
12. Gross JB, Zebrowski ME, Carel WD, Gardner S, Smith TC: Time course of ventilatory depression after thiopental and midazolam in normal subjects and in patients with chronic obstructive pulmonary disease. *Anesthesiology* 1983;58:540-544.
13. Southorn P, Rehder K, Didier EP: Midazolam sedation and respiratory mechanisms in man (abstr). *Anesthesiology* 1981;55:A367.
14. Power SJ, Morgan M, Chakrabarti MK: Carbon dioxide response curves following midazolam and diazepam. *Br J Anaesth* 1983;55:837-841.
15. Glisson SN, Belusko RJ, Kubak MA, Hieber MD: Midazolam on stimulatory responses to hypotension: Preinduction vs. during anesthesia (abstr). *Anesthesiology* 1982;57:A365.
16. Arendt RM, Greenblatt DJ, DeJong RH: In vitro correlates of benzodiazepine cerebrospinal fluid uptake, pharmacodynamic action and peripheral distribution. *J Pharm Exp Ther* 1983;227:98-106.
17. Smith MT: Pharmacokinetics of midazolam in the aged. *Eur J Clin Pharmacol* 1984;26:381.
18. Vinik HR: Pharmacokinetics of midazolam in renal failure patients (abstr). *Anesthesiology* 1982;57(3A):A366.
19. Ochs MW, Tucker MR, White RP, Anderson JA: Recovery following sedation with midazolam or diazepam alone or in combination with fentanyl for outpatient surgery. *Anesth Prog* 1986;33:230-234.
20. Caldwell CB, Gross JB: Physostigmine reversal of midazolam-induced sedation. *Anesthesiology* 1982;57:125-127.
21. Lauven PM: Application of a benzodiazepine antagonist (RO 15-1788) under steady-state conditions of midazolam (abstr). *Anesthesiology* 1982;57(suppl):A325.
22. Chang KJ, Cuatrecasas P: Heterogeneity and properties of opiate receptors. *Fed Proc* 1981;40:2729-2734.
23. Jaffe JH, Martin WR: Opioid analgesics and antagonists. In: Gilman AG, Goodman LS, Rall TW, Murad F, eds. *The Pharmacological Basis of Therapeutics.* New York: MacMillan Publishing Co 1985:496-504, 513-517.
24. Vaughn RL, Bennett CR: Fentanyl chest wall rigidity syndrome — A case report. *Anesth Prog* 1981;28:50-51.
25. Ackerman WE, Phero JC, Theodore GT: Ineffective ventilation during conscious sedation due to chest wall rigidity after intravenous midazolam and fentanyl. *Anesth Prog* 1990;37:46-48.
26. Romagnoli A, Keats AS: Comparative hemodynamic effects of nalbuphine and morphine in patients with coronary artery disease. *Cardiovasc Dis Bull Texas Heart Inst* 1978;5:19-24.
27. Popio KA, Jackson DH, Ross AM, et al: Hemodynamic and respiratory effects of morphine and butorphanol. *Clin Pharmacol Ther* 1978;23:281-287.
28. Mills CA, Flacke JW, et al: Narcotic reversal in hypercapnic dogs: Comparison of naloxone and nalbuphine. *Can J Anaesth* 1990;37:238-244.
29. Bennett CR: Jorgensen memorial lecture: Drug interactions. *Anesth Prog* 1983;30:106-112.
30. Monheim L: *General Anesthesia in Dental Practice.* St Louis: CV Mosby Co, 1964.
31. Malamed SF: *Sedation: A Guide to Patient Management.* 2nd ed. St Louis: CV Mosby Co, 1989.
32. Milam S, et al: Faint in supine position. Selective review of the literature and a case report. *J Periodontol* 1986;

57:44.

33. Loughlin D, Furman T, Scamman F, Tibbetts L: Intravenous sedation. In: *Clinical Dentistry.* New York: Harper and Row;1979:chap 27.

34. Topazian RG: Accidental intra-arterial injections: A hazard of intravenous medication. *J Am Dent Assoc* 1970; 81:410.

35. Jorgensen NB, Hayden J Jr: *Sedation, Local and General Anesthesia in Dentistry.* 3rd ed. Philadelphia: Lea & Febiger, 1980.

36. Bennett CR: Management of adverse drug reactions in conscious-sedation. *Dent Clin North Am* 1984;28:509.

PART IV

Implant Dentistry

Presurgical Treatment Planning and Surgical Guidelines for Dental Implants

by Oded Bahat / Mark Handelsman

Introduction	Space availability
Diagnosis	Occlusal evaluation
Soft tissue evaluation	
Hard tissue evaluation	QUICK REVIEW
Interridge relationship	
	REFERENCES

INTRODUCTION

One of the important goals of implant therapy is to accurately place implants in predetermined sites such that optimal esthetics and function can be established in the final reconstruction. But optimal results can only be achieved if the patient's expectations are accurately determined and if attention is paid to the interplay between anatomical structures and the restorative needs. What is required is a *team approach,* to be established in the early phases of treatment planning. Members of this team should be the surgeon (periodontist or oral surgeon) and the restorative dentist. In compromised clinical situations, the team should include the laboratory technician, ear, nose, and throat (ENT) specialist when sinus pathosis is present, and speech ther-

apist when it is anticipated that the patient's phonetics may be affected. Other dental specialists, such as orthodontists, may be needed to help improve a site dimension and its relationship to the natural teeth.

An excellent approach to obtaining optimal esthetics and function is to plan the treatment in reverse. That is, the reconstruction should be viewed completely, and all steps to reach this goal should be simulated in the reverse order. When such an approach is practiced, mishaps such as maligned or misplaced implants and early implant failure can be avoided.

DIAGNOSIS

Periodontal and restorative evaluation for long-term prognosis of

the existing dentition should precede any implant therapy. The easier phase of this evaluation is the elimination of any hopeless teeth. A greater challenge is presented by the teeth that can respond favorably to combined periodontal and restorative treatment. Clinicians should follow the same guidelines that are used in the restoration of the perio-prosthetic patient, keeping in mind that the presence of implants adds complication .

The clinician should certainly question the value of individual teeth in the overall plan. This does not mean that indiscriminate extraction should be practiced. On the contrary, procedures such as minor tooth movement and root resection are extremely valuable in circumventing some of the restrictions of current implant therapy that may adversely affect the placement, angulation, and ult-mate long-term success of implants.

The interim healing period after implant placement should be given detailed attention. Although it is simpler to extract all hopeless teeth and place a removable partial or complete denture in the interim period, this approach increases transmucosal loading during the healing phase, relegates the patient to keeping his / her removable denture out of the mouth for 2 to 3 weeks immediately postimplant placement, and often provides less than optimal esthetics. Therefore, in various clinical situations the following staged approach is suggested.

Stage 1:
• Extract all hopeless teeth affecting therapy (however, keep hopeless teeth that will assist in support of a provisional fixed restoration)
• Initiate therapy for all pathoses
• Complete all adjunct therapy (eg, periodontal, endodontic, occlusal, orthodontic)

Stage 2:
• Place provisional restorations
• Place implants in predetermined sites

Stage 3:
• Expose implants and connect abutments
• Extract remaining hopeless teeth and all other teeth that

do not enhance the final reconstruction

In order to achieve the optimal outcome for the patient, the treatment team should evaluate the hard and soft tissue. The interplay between these two tissues plays a most important role in the success and failure of dental implants. They should be reviewed together and separately, since both their interrelations and their individual character may affect the esthetic outcome.

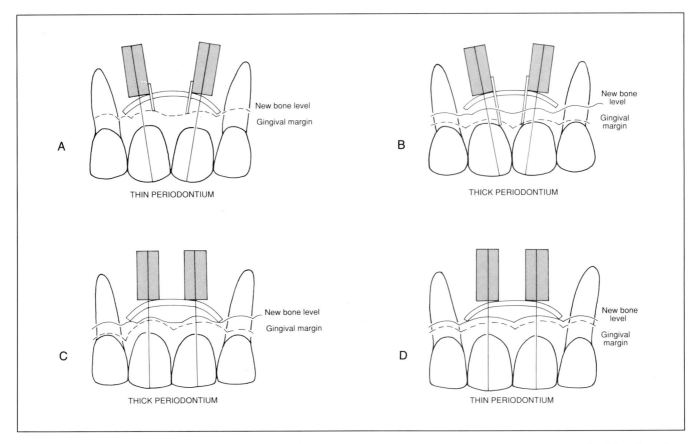

Fig 19-1 (A,B) *Converging the implants toward each other will vary the final position of the gingival level and will result in a more esthetic restoration. In the thin periodontium, a given interimplant distance will result in a gingival level apical to the gingival position in a thick periodontium. (C,D) Placement of implants parallel to each other will result in an apical gingival level as compared to its relative position when a convergence angle is established.*

SOFT TISSUE EVALUATION

The presence or absence of gingiva and its dimension (width and thickness) will have an influence on the final result, from flap elevation and transfer, to final healing, through the final reconstruction.

Gingiva-Mucosa Relationship

The thickness of the soft tissue dictates the length of the transepithelial abutment. The thickness of the gingiva affects the residual depth around the transepithelial abutment, thus influencing access for supportive periodontal treatment (maintenance).

Thin versus Thick Periodontal Tissues
(Fig 19-1)

In anterior areas, maintenance of the papilla is important for esthetic restorations. A thin periodontium is very unforgiving in this respect. Fixtures should be placed to scaffold the gingiva, which will optimize esthetics. Exact angulation of the fixture in the desired position is necessary to achieve this objective. Posterior areas are more forgiving because of reduced esthetic demands.

Width of Keratinized Tissue

Maintenance and long-term tissue health, along with patient comfort, might require that areas with no keratinized tissue be augmented with gingiva. This can be achieved either before or after implant placement.

HARD TISSUE EVALUATION

Bone

Lekholm and Zarb[1] classified bone according to the following:

Type 1: almost the entire jaw is composed of homogeneous compact bone.

Type 2: a thick layer of compact bone surrounds a core of dense trabecular bone.

Type 3: a thin layer of cortical bone surrounds a core of dense trabecular bone of favorable strength.

Type 4: a thin layer of cortical bone surrounds a core of low-density trabecular bone.

This classification was previously usable only *after* the surgical procedure to prepare sites for implants. Conventional radiographs do not allow accurate assessment of the bone quality within the jaw because the cortical plates tend to mask this information, and only since the introduction of the computed tomography scan has the operator been able to more accurately visualize *presurgically* the quality (degree of bone density) of the cancellous bone. Classifying bone type presurgically helps to plan the critical areas for placement.

In general, the implant surgical protocol suggested by Brånemark et al[2] is based on a sound biological and surgical foundation. However, in critical and compromised sites, any sequential enlargement of a site may invite overpreparation. Furthermore, in sites of poor bone quality, any inadvertent change in the direction of the implant may preclude the operator from initially stabilizing it. Therefore, the following modifications may be needed to ensure primary bone union[3] with the implant. The following guidelines are suggested.

1. Bicortical fixation. Anchoring the implant to both cortices will help achieve initial stabilization, especially in the posterior maxilla. Computed tomography scans can assist the surgeon in evaluating the exact length to the sinus floor.

2. Tight site. This prevents micromovement between the implant and bone. It is of great importance when bone quality is poor and when overpreparation negates initial implant stability. In these conditions, a reduction in sequential drilling is necessary. Only the largest-diameter twist drill should be advanced to the final length. Screw-tapping where appropriate should be avoided, or not carried the full length of the fixture preparation.

3. Countersinking. When the implant system requires countersinking, its depth should be evaluated compared to the dimension of the cortical plate. Traditional countersinking may result in destruction of the cortical plate and adversely affect initial stability and long-term loading. Other factors such as esthetic and mechanical requirements may affect the extent of countersinking, especially in sites adjacent to natural teeth. The CEJ of the adjacent tooth can usually be used as a guide to help determine this during the surgery. Countersinking below the CEJ will allow for adequate space for crown emergence, which is important for esthetics. The interocclusal distance should be evaluated to allow for adequate height for the restoration with optimal emergence profile for the restoration. Low-profile cover screws may be useful in avoiding transmucosal loading

4. Site selection. The most ideal site, preferably adjacent to an existing tooth, should have implants placed first, then one should proceed to the most compromised site. This approach reduces the possibility of damaging bone in more compromised areas adjacent to more desirable sites.

5. Implant angulation. Surgical stents are useful for determining optimal implant placement in compromised areas; they are essential in anterior areas but are also helpful in posterior areas. A radiopaque marker (catheter tubing or gutta percha) can be placed in a stent or the provisional acrylic resin restorations at the level of the edentulous ridge so

that during CT scanning additional information can be transferred onto the reformatted images. The marker will illustrate the desired position for implant placement. It will often be found that bone is not always directly apical to the predetermined site. The operator needs to interpret the images and think three-dimensionally in order to utilize the site optimally for implant placement. Therefore, the stent should not be relied on for initial drilling because the bone is not always directly apical to the occlusal table. By relying solely on a surgical stent for optimal placement, severe dehiscences and subsequent implant failure may result.

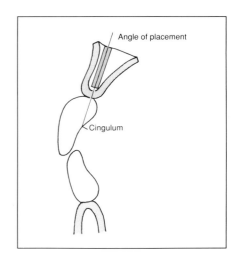

Fig 19-2 *Optimal ridge relationship will result in placement of the implant exiting towards the cingulum.*

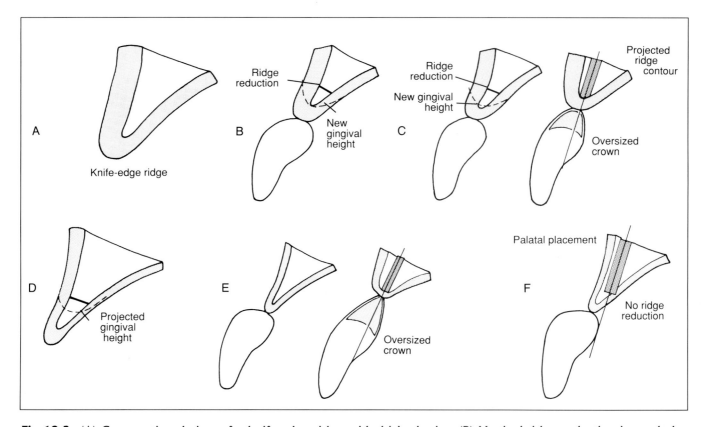

Fig 19-3 (A) *Cross-sectional view of a knife-edge ridge with thick gingiva.* (B) *Vertical ridge reduction is needed in order to accommodate implant placement. The gingiva will assume a more apical position and the restoration will be overcontoured apicocoronally.* (C) *The projected ridge contour will result in an oversized crown apicocoronally.* (D) *Cross-sectional view of knife-edge ridge and thin gingiva.* (E) *Ridge reduction in the presence of thin gingiva will result in a larger crown (apicocoronally) as compared to identical reduction in the presence of thick gingiva.* (F) *Lingual placement is an alternate approach to ridge reduction. It will result in overcontouring in a buccolingual direction.*

The ability to vary the angle of the implant is extremely important. Changes in angulation can be achieved by bodily moving the entry site and / or by tipping the direction of the implant. The first implant should be placed at its optimal angulation. Any deviation from the desired angle should be corrected prior to an attempt to parallel all the remaining implants. Continuous manipulation of the mandible into the centric relation position during placement will assist in evaluating whether optimal direction has been achieved.

Although the Lekholm / Zarb bone classification[1] is helpful, it should not be viewed as a single entity for decision making. Treat-ment decisions should also be re-lated to the adjacent teeth and the opposing jaw relationship, infor-mation which can be obtained by mounted casts on a semi-adjusta-ble or fully adjustable articulator, a well-constructed surgical stent, and three-dimensional CT radio-graphic reformations. These aids will not only assist in achieving a well-integrated implant but will also result in optimal function and esthetics. Therefore, the therapist should not hesitate to avoid or en-hance a site once the presurgical analysis deems it unfavorable. In order to illustrate this relationship of implant to hard and soft tissue, a visual approach for the interplay of ridge morphology and inter-ridge relationship is shown below.

INTERRIDGE RELATIONSHIP (Fig 19-2)

Ridge Morphology and Shape

Knife-Edge Ridge Reduction (Fig 19-3) In posterior areas, ridge reduction will allow for fix-ture placement totally covered with bone (no dehiscence), but the fixture length will be reduced. In the anterior maxilla, this is not always desired because reduction in ridge height will cause ridge deformity in an already compro-mised ridge.

Concavities Buccal and lingual concavities can cause dehiscence

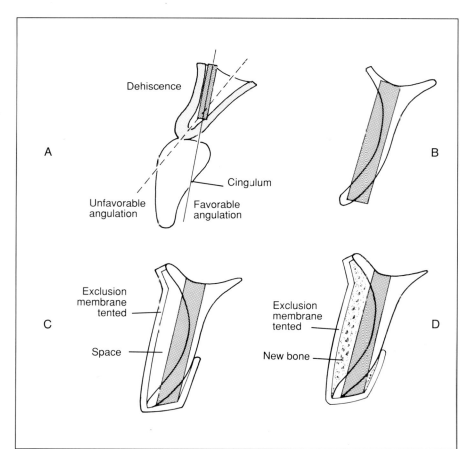

Fig 19-4 (A) The direction of the implant placement along the greater dimension of the ridge will result in unfavorable angulation. A labial dehiscence will occur when attempting to exit through the cin-gulum. (B) A labial dehiscence oc-curs as a result of optimal direction. (C) An exclusion membrane may be useful in order to augment bone on the labial aspect of a dehisced im-plant. Tenting the membrane will allow for space formation between the implant and the inner aspect of the flap. (D) New bone formation under the exclusion membrane.

and fenestration defects around implants and may result in failure of the implant. In the maxillary anterior area it may lead to excessive horizontal overlap, which further complicates the esthetic restorative and occlusal result.

Ridge Augmentation (Figs 19-4 and 19-5)

Ridge augmentation via advanced flaps with autogenous or alloplastic grafting material should be considered before or after placement of implants. The use of exclusion membranes for guided tissue regeneration over exposed implant fixture threads[4,5] should be considered when necessary. Ridge augmentation at the time of extraction with or without implant fixture placement should be evaluated before and upon extraction in order to avoid unfavorable ridge anatomy and dimension. (For further information, see chapter 2.)

Angle of Implant's Exit (Fig 19-6)

The skeletal and occlusal relationship, along with the degree of ridge resorption, will dictate the desired direction or angle of implant placement. This angle will not always accommodate the placement of the implant in the alveolar bone because of postextraction resorption patterns of the ridge. In the maxilla, resorption occurs in a posterior-superior direction, while the mandible resorbs in an inferior-posterior direction. In order to place the implant to exit through the desired central fossa and provide axial loading of the implant, periaxial cuts from the CT scan must be used to identify bony concavities and

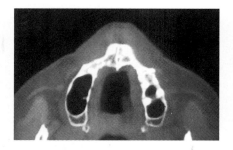

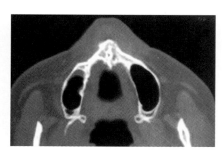

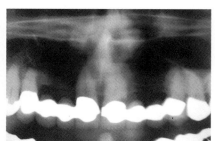

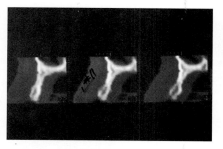

Figs 19-5a and b Two axial cuts show severe bone resorption and labial concavities in the maxillary anterior area.

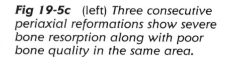

Fig 19-5c (left) Three consecutive periaxial reformations show severe bone resorption along with poor bone quality in the same area.

Fig 19-5d (right) Periapical radiographs of the maxillary anterior sextant.

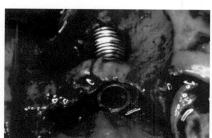

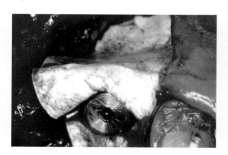

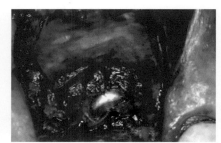

Fig 19-5e Optimal implant placement in the presence of severe concavity results in an 8-mm labial dehiscence. The implant must be stabilized by inferior and superior cortices.

Fig 19-5f An exclusion membrane is tented over the implant.

Fig 19-5g Four months after the initial surgery, the membrane is removed and the surgical site is exposed. The implant is covered entirely with bone and the concavity is obliterated.

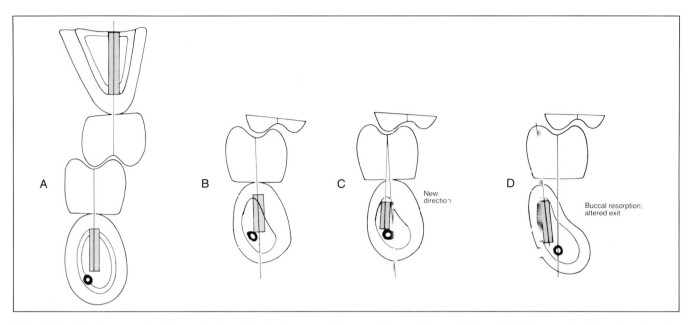

Fig 19-6 (A) *Favorable ridge relationship in the posterior maxilla and mandible will allow optimal occlusal and axial placement in both jaws. (B) A labial dehiscence will occur when optimal axial inclination in the presence of a knife-edge ridge in the mandible is attempted. (C) A new lingual angulation is suggested in order to avoid a labial dehiscence. The exit site remains favorable. (D) Exaggerated lingual inclination is required in the presence of severe labial resorption.*

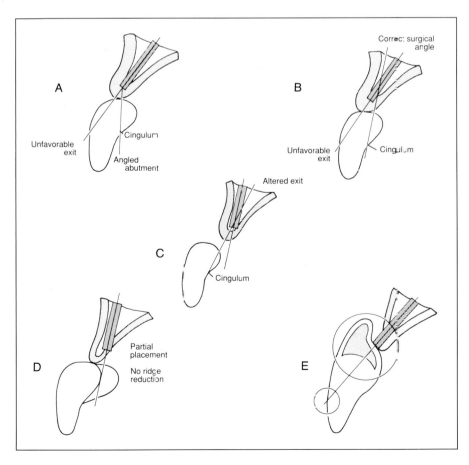

Fig 19-7 (A) *Angled abutment may correct for unfavorable exit in the presence of labial resorption and a thin maxillary anterior ridge. (B) An altered surgical inclination will avoid the need for an angled abutment and unfavorable exit. (C) Altering the angle of implant placement prevents the need for a lingually overcontoured restoration. (D) Lingual placement in the presence of a knife-edge ridge and labial resorption will result in an overcontoured restoration (buccolingually). (E) Unfavorable exit site and apicocoronal overcontouring is the result of implant placement along the narrow aspect of the ridge (compare to D).*

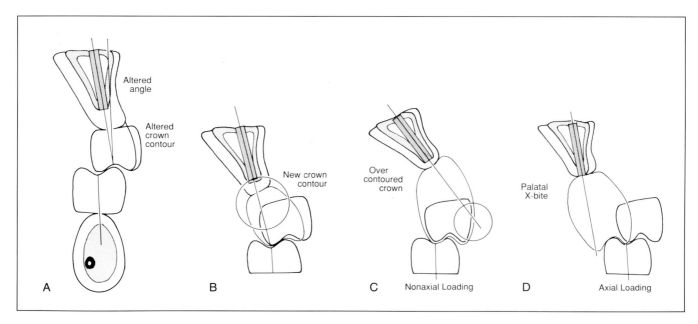

Fig 19-8 (A) *Altered angulation and crown contour is the result of labial resorption in the posterior maxilla.* (B) *Further labial resorption will necessitate additional crown contour modification with labial cantilevering.* (C) *Severe apical resorption may cause an angled residual maxillary ridge, nonaxial loading, and overcontouring in all dimensions, and an unfavorable exit will result.* (D) *Severe apical resorption may cause a vertical residual ridge. It will result in crossbite relationship, overcontoured crown, and favorable exit.*

correlate them to the desired occlusion.

To accommodate those anatomical changes, the starting point during the drilling sequence will not always begin in the center of the ridge. In the maxilla it will usually begin more palatally to accommodate buccal concavities and prevent dehiscences yet still provide the occlusal and esthetic demands.

The implant can thus be planned to be moved bodily, as compared to tipping, which will place the fixture within bone but will cause it to exit too buccally inclined. These changes will cause alteration in crown contour to compensate for the dimensional ridge loss (Figs 19-7 and 19-8).

Angle of Abutment (Figs 19-9a to e)

Angled abutments have become increasingly popular in order to correct undesirable placement of implants, but they present the problem of nonaxial loading forces. Nonaxial loading may contribute to mechanical failures of both suprastructure and implants. Recently, nonsegmented abutments[6] have been introduced in order to compensate for unesthetic crown contours. However, this type of abutment reduces access to the undersurface of the restoration (which increases bacterial accumulation) and introduces alloy subgingivally (which may not be as compatible as titanium). Furthermore, such abutments require a larger screw diameter that could cause unfavorable forces leading to implant overloading and subsequent fracture.

Interridge Distance

An accurate occlusal record is an essential aid for determining interridge distance at the centric relation or maximum intercuspation positions. This information will assist the team in evaluating the need for ridge reduction, ridge augmentation, or occlusal reduction via occlusal grinding. Clinically, the degree of jaw opening should be evaluated for surgical access.

Crestal Ridge—Mucobuccal Fold Relationship

The surgical execution and final placement becomes harder in clinical situations that present with alveolar ridge resorption apical to the level of the mucobuccal fold. Flap manipulation and implant angulation will be adversely affected.

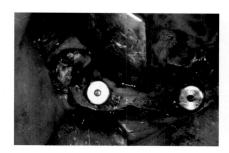

Fig 19-9a *A knife-edge ridge reduction will allow for implant placement.*

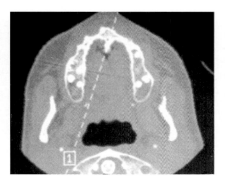

Fig 19-9b *Axial view shows a severe concavity in the maxillary anterior area.*

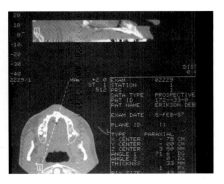

Fig 19-9c *Periaxial CT reformation illustrates similar clinical ridge deformity.*

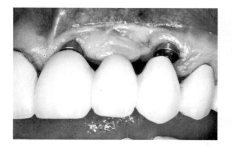

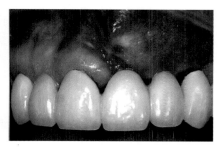

Fig 19-9d *(left) The placement of the implant along the severely resorbed ridge resulted in unfavorable angulation, ridge defect, and loss of interproximal papillae.*

Fig 19-9e *(right) Subsequent to surgical ridge reconstruction, an improved esthetic result is achieved. (Restorations by Dr. Lawrence Riskin.)*

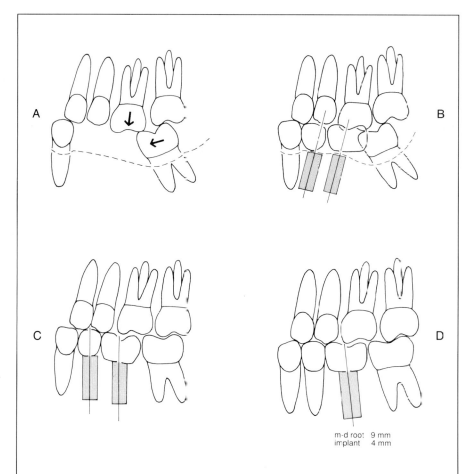

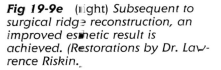

m-d root 9 mm
implant 4 mm

Fig 19-10 *(A) Loss of the mandibular first molar created a complex periodontal restorative and occlusal problem. (B) When implants are placed without prior orthodontic and occlusal correction, unfavorable implant angulation (to the distal) may result. (C) Prior to the implant placement, correction of the position of the second molar is indicated. Mesial inclination of the implant is suggested to accommodate the occlusal scheme. Repeated manipulation to centric relation position during placement will ensure an optimal occlusal relationship. (D) Placement of an implant in the molar area requires greater interimplant distance due to the greater mesiodistal dimension of the molar teeth. This also affects the contour of the final implant restoration because of the sharp emergence angle of the implant abutment.*

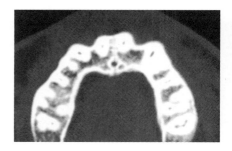

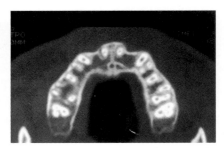

Fig 19-11a (left) *An axial view illustrating inadequate mesiodistal space for implant placement in the maxillary lateral positions.*

Fig 19-11b (right) *A similar view after orthodontic tooth movement.*

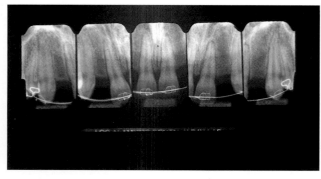

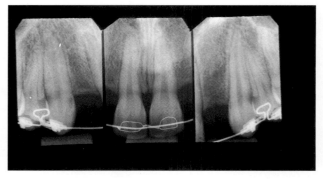

Figs 19-11c and d *Periapical radiographs before and after orthodontic tooth movement.*

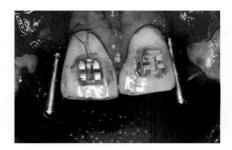

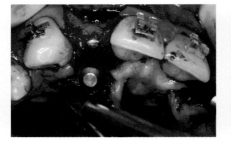

Fig 19-11e *The anticipated direction of the implants is evaluated intraoperatively.*

Figs 19-11f and g *Occlusal view of the implants illustrating the desired anticipated exit through the cingulum.*

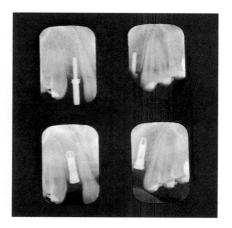

Fig 19-11h *Periapical radiographs illustrating the need for increased care not to damage adjacent teeth.*

Residual Ridge Relationship to Adjacent and Opposing Teeth
(Figs 19-10 and 19-11)

The relationship of the remaining dentition to the residual ridge should be evaluated intraorally, from mounted casts, and from CT scan analysis. When malalignment or extrusion occurs, it should be corrected during the diagnostic phase.

The implant should not be placed in a compromised site because of previous pathological processes that accompany partial edentulism. Thus, minor tooth movement, selective grinding, leveling the occlusal plane, and other similar procedures should always be done prior to implant placement.

When these presurgical treatment modalities are performed, careful evaluation of the future sites relative to the adjacent dentition is indicated. This is essential to prevent undue damage to the adjacent roots because of root angulation, convergence, etc.

Teeth (Fig 19-12)

Additional attention must be given to the remaining dentition before implant surgery because it influences the long-term prognosis for the final reconstruction.

Periapical pathosis should be eliminated in the initial phase of treatment, while periodontal bony defects on teeth adjacent to implant sites can be treated before or during implant placement.

When osseous resective surgery is indicated around the remaining dentition and is performed before implant placement, the surgeon should be cognizant of the degree of bone resection around the residual ridge so as not to jeopardize future implant sites. Overreduction of the ridge height and width will not permit an optimal implant site.

When there is inadequate clinical crown length adjacent to an edentulous ridge, careful evaluation prior to osseous resection is indicated. This is very important because of its adverse effect on the remaining height and width of the alveolar bone.

SPACE AVAILABILITY
(Figs 19-13 and 19-14)

Space analysis, especially for single-tooth replacement, is important. Converging roots, especially in the anterior maxilla region, can limit implant placement if no orthodontic movement was performed.

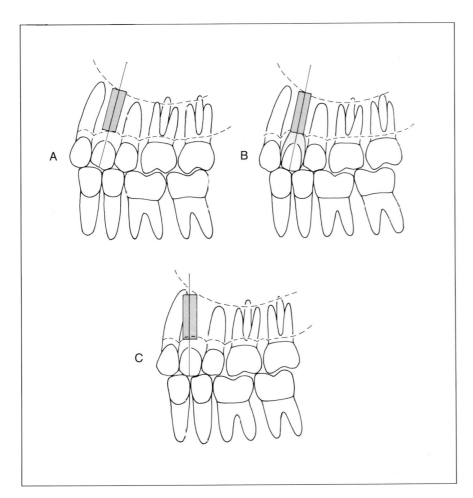

Fig 19-12 (A) Optimal placement of the implant at the maxillary first premolar region. (B) Due to vertical ridge resorption, an overcontoured crown is anticipated. (C) Incorrect angulation of the implant relative to the canine will result in root damage.

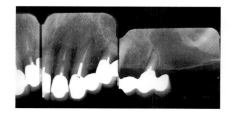

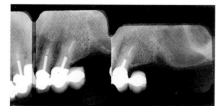

Figs 19-13a and b *Periapical radiographs before and after the loss of tooth 13. The distal aspect of tooth 13 borders on the anterior sinus wall.*

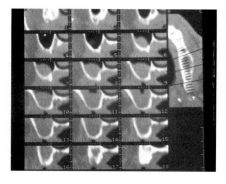

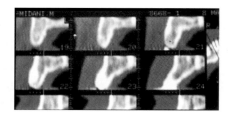

Figs 19-13c and d *Periaxial CT reformation of the maxillary left sextant. CT reformation of tooth 21 corresponds to the most mesial possible site. CT reformation of tooth 17 corresponds to the shallow residual socket and is unacceptable for implant placement. CT reformation of tooth 18 is therefore the most distal site, and only 6 mm of mesial distal space is present between the two anticipated sites.*

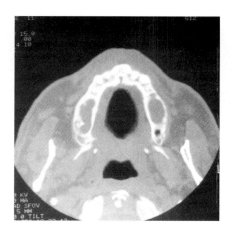

Fig 19-13e *An axial reformation illustrating a prominent sinus and severe ridge resorption distal to tooth 11.*

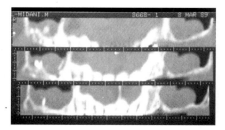

Fig 19-13f *Panoramic presentations of a resorbed maxilla, low sinus, and only 10 mm of mesiodistal space for implant placement distal to tooth 11. Therefore, interimplant and interimplant-tooth distance is reduced.*

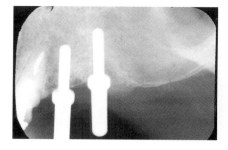

Fig 19-13g *Intraoperative radiographs illustrating two direction indicators at the anticipated angulation. The implant at tooth 12 position attempts to parallel the canine. The other implant parallels the anterior sinus wall. This forms a divergence exit that enables the accommodation of two implants in optimal occlusal relationship with adequate interimplant space.*

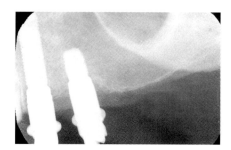

Fig 19-13h *(left) The second interoperative radiograph verifies the final implant location.*

Fig 19-13i *(right) A radiograph of the provisional cast restoration. A 1-mm clearance is established between the pontics and the residual ridge in order to avoid transmucosal loading in the healing phase.*

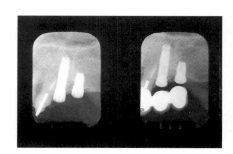

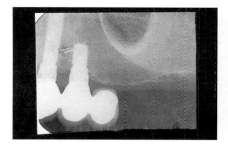

Fig 19-13j *A radiograph of the final reconstruction.*

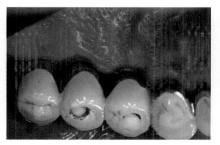

Figs 19-13k and l *Facial and lingual views of the final reconstruction. (Restorative dentistry courtesy of Dr L. Brucker.)*

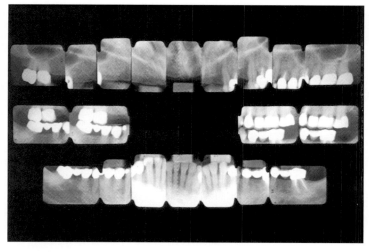

Fig 19-14a *Full-mouth radiographs illustrating an edentulous ridge from tooth tooth 2 to tooth 11.*

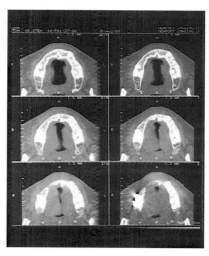

Fig 19-14b *Six axial CT reformations of the maxilla at different levels.*

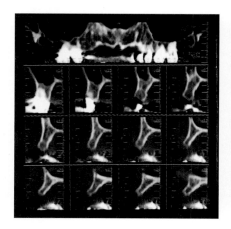

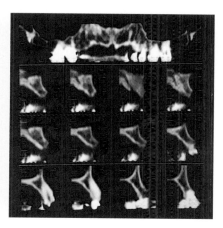

Figs 19-14c and d *Peri-axial reformations from tooth 2 to tooth 11 illustrating early moderate ridge resorption, adequate ridge height, and type 3 bone.*

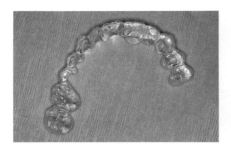

Fig 19-14e *A modified surgical stent to fit the crown preparations is useful during the surgery. (Courtesy of Dr Bruce Coye.)*

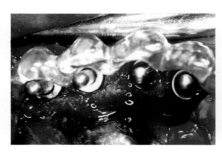

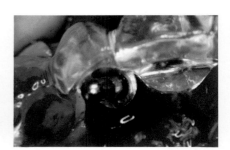

Figs 19-14f and g *Five implants are placed at sites corresponding to teeth 3, 4, 5, 6, and 10. The implants' directions are evaluated relative to the surgical stent.*

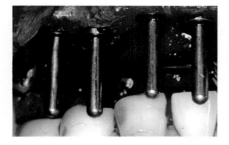

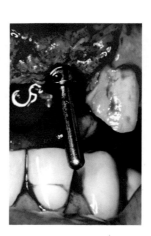

Figs 19-14h and i *The patient's jaw is manipulated to centric relation to further evaluate implant angulation and the degree of horizontal overlap.*

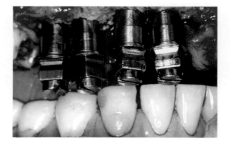

Fig 19-14j *Upon completion of implant placement, similar manipulation to centric relation is repeated. It is of great clinical significance if any deviation from the original desired angulation has occurred during the sequential site enlargement.*

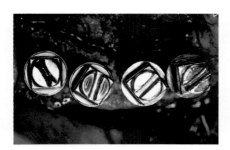

Fig 19-14k *Occlusal view shows final placement, optimal interimplant spacing, and the relationship between the implants and the alveolar ridge.*

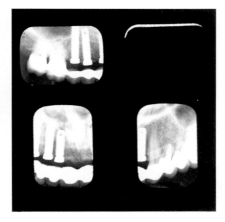

Fig 19-14l *Radiographs show the implant placement relative to the provisional fixed partial denture. Note the implant at the position of tooth 3 borders the anterior sinus wall.*

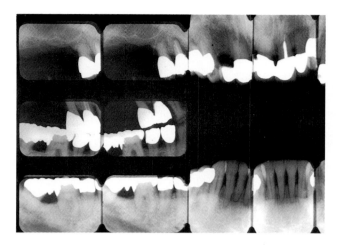
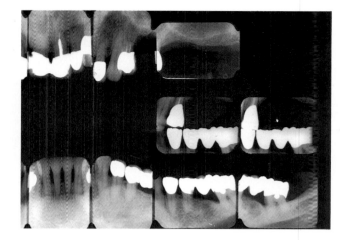

Figs 19-15a and b Radiographs show severe bone loss and low sinus distal to the second premolar.

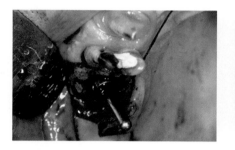
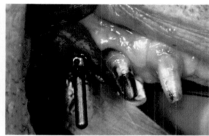
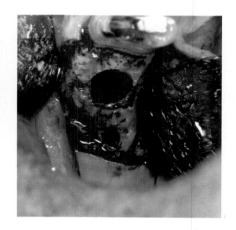

Figs 19-15c and d The implant's inclination at the second premolar position is evaluated preoperatively.

Fig 19-15e Completion of site preparation at tooth 4 position.

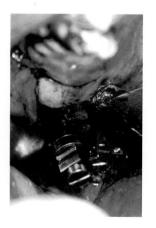
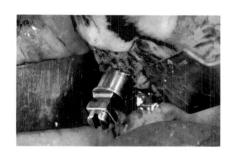

Figs 19-15f and g Right and left tuberosity implants are placed with a 20-degree inclination towards the mesial.

Figs 19-15h and i Lingual view of the provisional restorations spanning from the tuberosities to the second premolars.

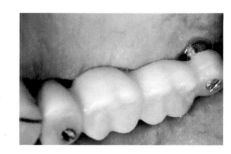
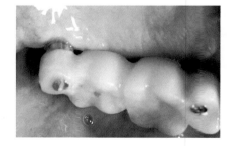

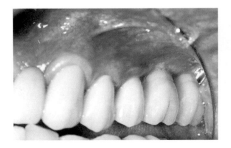 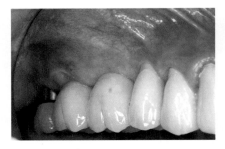 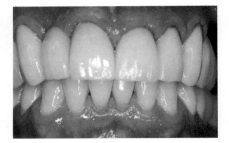

Figs 19-15j and k *Labial views of the final reconstruction 14 months after initial loading. (Restorative dentistry courtesy of Dr L. Brucker.)*

Fig 19-15l *Frontal view of the final reconstruction.*

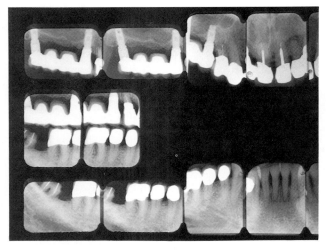 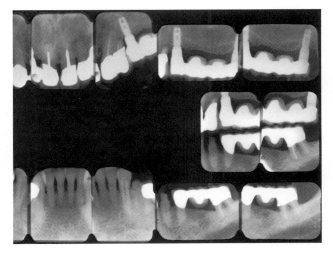

Figs 19-15m and n *Radiographs of the final reconstruction 18 months after completion.*

OCCLUSAL EVALUATION

The occlusal scheme for the reconstruction should be pre-planned because the occlusal load on the individual implants may adversely affect long-term prognosis. Thus, the interplay between the horizontal and vertical overlap, the strategic position of the implants and the remaining teeth, the nature of the reconstruction (fixed versus removable), and parafunctional activities, should all be determined before surgery.

The surgical site selection requires modifications when the original restorative protocol described by Brånemark et al[2] is modified. The team approach to build up ridges should be used when possible in placing implants in the posterior areas (Figs 19-15 and 19-16). This will reduce the cantilever effect on the reconstruction (in the area where the occlusal forces are greatest) and provide axial loading. It will also diminish the unesthetic results, often present when implant placement is relegated to resorbed anterior areas.

Giving due attention to the occlusal demands on the individual implants relative to their length, anatomical location, and quality and quantity of bone is crucial for success.

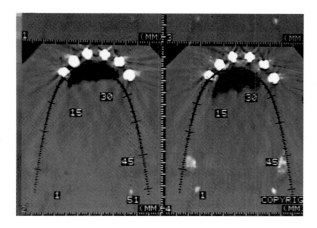

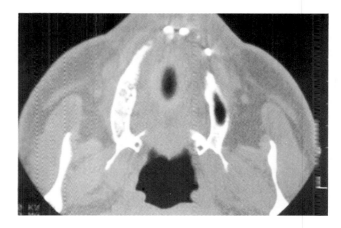

Fig 19-16a *Two axial cuts illustrating the initial plan for placement of six implants in the maxillary anterior area.*

Fig 19-16b *A more superior axial cut illustrating the lack of bone in this anterior area.*

Fig 19-16c *Four panoramic reformations show the absence of bone in the desired area. Only lingual to the midridge is a minimal ridge height present. A more acceptable ridge is present distal to teeth 6 and 12.*

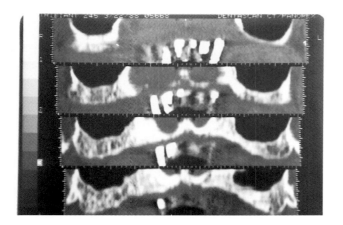

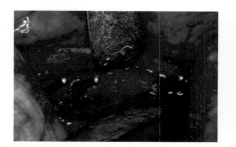

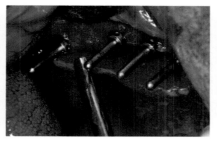

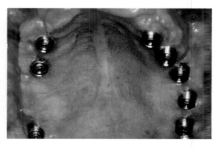

Figs 19-16d and e *The direction indicators show possible angulation at the position of teeth 12, 13, and 16, as well as teeth 1, 2, 3, 5, and 6.*

Fig 19-16f *The final distribution of the implants. It will allow a reconstruction supported by posteriorly placed implants without a posterior cantilever effect.*

QUICK REVIEW

- Planning for dental implants should include a member of the dental team who will participate in the patient's care.
- A restorative and, where appropriate, a periodontal examination should be performed.
- Both soft tissue and bone should be examined presurgically to assist in implant site selection.

- In some cases the soft or hard tissues may need to be augmented before, during, or after implant placement. In others, multidisciplinary care may be needed for optimal results.

REFERENCES

1. Lekholm U, Zarb GA: Patient selection and preparation. In: Brånemark PI, Albrektsson T, Zarb GA, eds. *Tissue-Integrated Prostheses: Osseointegration in Clinical Dentistry.* Chicago: Quintessence Publ Co; 1985:199-209.
2. Brånemark PI, Albrektsson T, Zarb GA, eds: *Tissue-Integrated Prostheses: Osseointegration in Clinical Dentistry.* Chicago: Quintessence Publ Co, 1985.
3. Hulth A: Current concepts of fracture healing. *Clin Orthop Related Res* 1989:249:265-284.
4. Becker W, et al: Bone formation at dehisced dental implant sites treated with implant augmentation material: A pilot study in dogs. *Int J Periodont Rest Dent* 1990:10:93-102.
5. Nyman S, et al: Bone regeneration adjacent to titanium dental implants using guided tissue regeneration: A report of two cases. *Int J Oral Maxillofac Implants* 1990:5:9-14.
6. Lewis SG, Beumer J, 3d, Perri GR, et al: Single tooth implant supported restorations. *Int J Oral Maxillofac Implants* 1988;3:25-30.

CHAPTER TWENTY

Special Radiographic Techniques for Implant Dentistry

by Vincent J. Iacono / Howard N. Livers

Recent successes in the development of new implant systems since the 1960s have contributed to the increasing popularity of dental implants within our profession.[1-3] It is now generally accepted that implants will become a reasonable alternative to removable prosthetic appliances for many patients. The advent of implants for partially edentulous patients has resulted in periodontists taking on an integral role in both the treatment planning and surgical phase for the insertion of implants in these patients. And with this increased use of implants by periodontists, several principles have been established in treatment planning for the prospective implant patient. First, because implant procedures are very technique-sensitive, they should be performed by teams of adequately trained individuals. Second, regardless of the implant system used, success is intrinsically dependent on the patient's health and cooperation, the design of

the prosthesis, and most importantly, the amount and quality of bone at the implant site.[4] This chapter addresses the latter principle with a discussion of the various techniques available to image the osseous structures in treatment planning for dental implants.

TYPES OF IMPLANTS

Many kinds of implants are available and they are generally classified by their shape and placement in the jaws. They include subperiosteal, transosteal, and endosseous implants.

Briefly, **subperiosteal implants** are in the form of a metal framework made from casts of the patient's jawbones. They are used in severely atrophic jaws where there is inadequate bone height to insert a root-form implant.

Transosteal implants are essentially a type of staple implant and are typically used in the man-

dibular anterior sextant as transmandibular implants.

Endosseous implants are the most common implants; they include many that osseointegrate (osseointegration being a histologic term coined by Brånemark[5] that has been defined as a direct structural and functional connection between ordered, living bone and the surface of a load-carrying implant, as observed at the light microscopic level). An osseointegrated fixture would be analogous to a nonresorbing ankylosed tooth. Endosseous implants include pins, blades, cylindric screws, and basket-shaped cylinders, with each manufacturer having its own modification of these designs. They are usually made out of titanium, or an alloy of titanium, aluminum (6%), and vanadium (4%), and may be sprayed with an apatite or titanium coating. The selection of a particular kind of implant is determined by a presurgical evaluation of the patient's needs and a thorough evaluation of the available bone at the edentulous site.

EXAMINATION OF THE OSSEOUS STRUCTURES

Evaluation of a prospective implant site requires adequate radiographs, which are necessary to determine the height, width, and quality of available bone and to determine the proximity of potential implant sites to the sinuses, foramina, mandibular canal, and adjacent teeth. The oral tissues and residual ridge should be visually and manually examined, including bone sounding, to assess the health of the oral tissues and the width of available bone, and to determine undercuts and exostoses.[4]

CONVENTIONAL RADIOGRAPHIC TECHNIQUES

Radiographic evaluation of an implant site may include panoramic, lateral, and occlusal views and periapical films. Periapical radiographs have been the most reliable indicator of alveolar support around the natural teeth. For the evaluation of bone for dental implants, however, they have proven to be of limited diagnostic usefulness. One area where periapical radiographs can be quite helpful in the presurgical evaluation is in the determination of the height of available bone in the posterior mandible when implants are planned for sites above the mandibular canal. When a precise paralleling technique is used as well as a radiopaque stent, periapical radiographs can be most accurate in assessing height of available bone at single implant sites.

According to Brånemark et al,[5] preoperative radiographic analysis should include a panoramic survey, a profile (lateral cephalometric) view, and intraoral views. In certain cases tomograms are indicated.

Panoramic Films

The panoramic film has become one of the most commonly used radiographs in treatment planning for the implant patient. It provides a general overview of the various anatomic structures. In the mandible, all borders are readily identifiable, and the locations of the mandibular canal and mental foramina can be approximated. In the maxilla, the nasal and maxillary sinuses and the canine septae are usually detectable. However, the panoramic film is not without its deficiencies and, in many instances, should not be used as the sole method for evaluating the osseous structures. For example, the image of the mandibular canal may vary with regard to sharpness and position from its true anatomic location. In addition, all images within the panoramic film may be magnified by as much as 10% to 25%.[6] Differences in magnification are attributed to the film moving in the same direction as the x-ray beam, but at a slower speed, which results in a foreshortening of the image in the direction of movement. Measurement of horizontal or anterior-posterior dimensions are therefore unreliable with a panoramic film. This problem may be partially rectified by using intraoral stents containing radiopaque markers of known dimension and then calculating the percentage of magnification.

Posterior to the mental foramen, the panoramic film also causes problems in determining the precise location of the mandibular canal. Since the x-ray beam is frequently aimed in an inferior-to-superior position through the mandible, localization of the mandibular canal in a buccal-lingual dimension may be difficult, if not impossible, due to the vagaries of the buccal object or Clark's rule.[6]

Lateral Cephalometric Films

Lateral or profile cephalometric films may be helpful in determining the height and width of the anterior mandible, anterior palate, and maxillary sinuses and are generally used when implants are being considered for sites in the anterior sextant of the mandible.[5]

Conventional Tomography

Conventional tomography is also used by many implant specialists. It is able to produce cross-sectional images perpendicular to the edentulous ridge by blurring all planes outside the field of focus. The images produced are by nature fairly blurry or indistinct due to the projection of three-dimensional images onto a two-dimensional surface, resulting in shadows from overlying structures.[7,8] At this time, however, new techniques are being developed for conventional tomography that reduce the blurring effect and result in accurate cross-sectional oblique images without the need for computer reformatting (personal communication, G. Barrack). Drawbacks in conventional tomography include the lack of built-in markers to identify each sectional image and the inability to cross reference between the tomograph and standard plane films. In addition, the conventional tomographic process is quite time-consuming.

COMPUTED TOMOGRAPHY AND MAGNETIC RESONANCE IMAGING

Three-dimensional computed tomography (CT) scans are used when accurate information regarding the topography of osseous structures is needed. For example, irregular, thin, or spiny osseous contours may be discernible from CT scans. In addition, soft tissue contour and dimension, continuity and density of the cortical plates, vertical height of the residual alveolar ridges, and density of the medullary space and basilar bone can be determined from CT images.[8-15]

Computed tomography is a radiographic technique that can display an image based on a gray scale using a television monitor. It is capable of producing a cross-sectional image of a slice of tissue that has been reformatted from a series of axial images or slices. The first clinically useful CT scanner was manufactured in the early 1970s and was aided in its development by G.V. Hounsfield.[7] The CT scanner can be broken down into four components: (1) the computerized patient bed; (2) a gantry containing an x-ray tube and a large array of x-ray-sensitive detectors; (3) microprocessors for data analysis; and (4) a television monitor and filming device for hard copies. The development of new x-ray-sensitive detectors has revolutionized the CT process. The latest scanners use a ring of detectors that surround the patient and remain stationary as the x-ray tube rotates, significantly reducing scan times.

Generally, each CT image or slice is 1.0 to 1.5 mm thick. The thinner the slice, the more noise or distortion. Each picture is usually created as a 512 × 512 dot matrix of data points, similar to a newspaper photograph. The density of each point is analogous to the amount of x-rays absorbed; it is stored as a CT number, assigned a level of gray, and displayed. The operator can vary the level of gray in accordance with the density of the structures being studied. This "window" can be expanded or condensed, so that individual structures can be assigned a level of gray from black to white to demonstrate small or large differences in density within a given field. The use of CT numbers enables the radiologist to measure the linear attenuation coefficient for air and water for a specific scanner. A constant value in calculating these numbers is $K = 1,000$. By convention, water is assigned a value of 0, soft tissue and muscle generally range from $+25$ to $+70$, and dense cortical bone is greater than $+1,000$. This numerical scale is referred to as the *Hounsfield scale.*

The CT scanner generally makes axial slices of a given area approximately 1.0 mm apart. These slices are usually made as close to parallel to the edentulous site or occlusal plane as possible. They are referred to as axial slices because they are made perpendicular to the long axis of the body. The microprocessor can then create a series of panoramic views, coronal views, or cross-sectional (oblique) views. The oblique views are most useful to the implant team. They illustrate the given structure in a cross section and are easily cross referenced to a master or scout film, giving specific sites numerical locators.

Computed tomography has recently been used to generate three-dimensional models of the osseous structures under examination. This may be most advantageous in the design of subperiosteal implants. When subperiosteal implants were first introduced, their design was based on an analysis of individual radiographs taken to determine osseous contours.[16] A metal framework was then fabricated from a cast, which was altered to compensate for soft tissue thickness. Because of the inaccuracies inherent to this approach, many of the early attempts using this technique failed due to discrepancies of bone-to-implant proximity.[17,18] Short of a two-surgery approach for the design (first surgery) and insertion (second surgery) of subperiosteal implants, the use of CT scans has become increasingly popular with the development of computer aided design–computer aided manufacture (CAD-CAM) of subperiosteal implants on CT-generated casts.

Another diagnostic technique that has been suggested as a possible aid for the evaluation of the osseous structures is magnetic resonance imaging (MRI). MRI, however, is more suited for the evaluation of soft tissues than for osseous structures (see chapter 3) and is currently considered to have little potential in implantology.

SUMMARY

Adequate radiographs and visual and manual examination of the prospective implant site are necessary to determine the amount and quality of available bone for selection of the appropriate implant. For the fully edentulous patient in whom several implants are planned for the anterior sextant of the mandible, panoramic, lateral, and occlusal films are generally sufficient for presurgical evaluation. When implants are planned for areas posterior to the mental foramina, CT scans are necessary

(1) to determine the distance between the superior cortex to mandibular canal; (2) to identify the mandibular canal in its buccal-lingual position using the reformatted cross-sectional oblique images; and (3) to determine the relative thickness of the crestal cortical plate and density of the body of cancellous bone.

When maxillary sites are being evaluated for implants, CT scans should be obtained because they provide the implant team with the most accurate assessment of the location of the sinuses and relative amount and quality of available bone. It may also be possible to use individual Hounsfield numbers to locate maxillary sites with the greatest bone density, which might allow for the prediction of a greater degree of osseointegration following insertion of the appropriate implant (personal communication, C. L. Berman).

Regardless of the radiographs used in the presurgical evaluation of the prospective implant site, unforeseen problems may occur at the time of surgery. This is due to the various shortcomings inherent to the imaging techniques currently available. The provider should be aware of the possibility of having to select implants of a different size and shape than planned, and/or to insert the fixtures at different locations.[4] At the time of surgery, it may be determined that the buccal-lingual width of the alveolar ridge may be too narrow for the axial placement of a root-form implant. The implant would have to be inserted at an angle to the ridge, or an implant of different design or dimension would need to be used.

Another fairly common problem is the lack of adequate cortical bone to engage clinical threaded fixtures. The selection of different implants and the preparation of antiaxial receptor sites affect the prosthetic phase of treatment. The patient should therefore not be given a guarantee as to the design and type of the final prosthesis before the surgical phase.

The need for accurate presurgical assessment of the quality and quantity of bone at a prospective implant site has resulted in a significant amount of research in various imaging techniques. These include the development of new formatting programs,[19] novel subtraction radiography, and absorptiometry techniques,[20] and methods to assess the status of bone metabolism.[20] The near future may see the inclusion of these potentially practical and significant techniques in implant dentistry.

QUICK REVIEW

IMPLANT RADIOGRAPHIC TECHNIQUES

Implant treatment planning — Imaging the osseous structures

- Regardless of the implant system used, success is intrinsically dependent on the patient's health and cooperation, the design of the prosthesis, and, most importantly, the amount and quality of bone at the implant site.
- Adequate radiographs are necessary to evaluate the implant site for its osseous status and proximity to vital structures.
- Manual examination of the residual ridge, including bone sounding, is of value to assess the width of available bone and presence of undercuts and exostoses.

- Radiographic assessment may include panoramic, lateral, and occlusal views and CT scans.
- The CT scan is rapidly becoming the most commonly used radiograph in imaging implant sites in the maxilla and in the posterior sextants of the mandible.
- All imaging techniques currently available have various shortcomings. The provider should therefore be aware of the possibility of unforeseen problems at the time of surgery and be prepared to use alternative implant treatment plans.
- The patient should not be given a guarantee as to the design and type of the final prosthesis before the surgical phase.

REFERENCES

1. Brånemark P-I, Hansson BO, Adell R, Breine U, Lindstrom J, Hallen O, Ohman A: Osseointegrated implants in the treatment of the edentulous jaw. Experience from a 10-year period. *Scand J Plast Reconstr Surg* 1977;11(Suppl 16):1. Also as a monograph from Almquist & Wiksell International, Stockholm.
2. Albrektsson T, Dahl E, Ehnbom L, et al: Osseointegrated oral implants. A Swedish multicenter study of 8139 consecutively inserted Nobelpharma implants. *J Periodontol* 1988;59:287-296.
3. Tetsch P, et al: Proceedings of a consensus conference on implantology, October 18, 1989, Mainz, West Germany. *Int J Oral Maxillofac Implants* 1990;5:182-187.
4. Iacono VJ: Dental implants. In: Genco RJ, Goldman HM, Cohen DW, eds: *Contemporary Periodontics.* St Louis: CV Mosby Co; 1990: 653-667.
5. Brånemark PI, Zarb G, Albrektsson T: *Tissue Integrated Prosthesis: Osseointegration in Clinical Dentistry.* Chicago: Quintessence Publ Co, 1985.
6. Serman NJ: Pitfalls of panoramic radiology in implant surgery. *Ann Dent* 1987;48:13-16.
7. Moss AA, Gamsu G, Genant HK: *Computed Tomography of the Body.* Philadelphia: WB Saunders Co; 1986:6-10.
8. Schwarz MS, Rothman SL, Chafetz N, Rhodes M: Computed tomography in dental implantation surgery. *Dent Clin North Am* 1987;33:555-597.
9. McGivney GP, Haughton V, Strandt JA, Eicholz JE, Lubar M: A comparison of computer-assisted tomography and data-gathering modalities in prosthodontics. *Int J Oral Maxillofac Implants* 1986;1:55-68.
10. Schwarz MS, Rothman S, Rhodes ML, Chafetz N: Computed tomography: Part I. Preoperative assessment of the mandible for endosseous implant surgery. *Int J Oral Maxillofac Implants* 1987;2:137-141.
11. Schwarz MS, Rothman S, Rhodes ML, Chafetz N: Computed tomography: Part II. Preoperative assessment of the maxilla for endosseous implant surgery. *Int J Oral Maxillofac Implants* 1987;2:143-148.
12. Wishan MS, Bahat O, Krane M: Computed tomography as an adjunct in dental implant surgery. *Int J Periodont Rest Dent* 1988;8(1):30-47.
13. Casselman JW, Quirynen M, Lemahieu SF, Baert AL, Bonte J: Computed tomography in the determination of anatomical landmarks in the perspective of endosseous oral implant installation. *J Head Neck Pathol* 1988;7:255-264.
14. Andersson JE, Svartz K: CT-scanning in the preoperative planning of osseointegrated implants in the maxilla. *Int J Oral Maxillofac Surg* 1988;17:33-45.
15. Berman CL: Osseointegration, complications, prevention, recognition, treatment. *Dent Clin North Am* 1989;33:635-663.
16. Gershkoff A, Goldberg NI: *Implant Dentures; Indications and Procedures.* Philadelphia: JB Lippincott Co, 1957.
17. Truitt HP, James RA, Lindley PE, Boyne P: Morphologic replication of the mandible using computerized tomography for the fabrication of a subperiosteal implant. *Oral Surg Oral Med Oral Pathol* 1988;65:499-504.
18. Truitt HP, James RA, Altman A, Boyne P: Use of computer tomography in subperiosteal implant therapy. *J Prosthet Dent* 1988;59:474-477.
19. Shimura M, Babbush CA, Majima H, Yanagisawa S, Sairenji E: Presurgical evaluation for dental implants using a reformatting program of computed tomography: Maxilla/mandible shape pattern analysis (MSPA). *Int J Oral Maxillofac Implants* 1990;5:175-181.
20. Hausmann E: A contemporary perspective on techniques for the clinical assessment of alveolar bone. *J Periodontol* 1990;61:149-156.

Choice of Implant System and Clinical Management

C U R R E N T   C O N C E P T S by Niklaus P. Lang

C L I N I C A L   A P P L I C A T I O N by Thomas G. Wilson, Jr

C U R R E N T   C O N C E P T S

For many years, it was the desire to replace missing teeth in partially or fully edentulous patients by inserting artificial prosthetic abutments that could be firmly anchored in the jawbone. Initially, implant dentistry based its clinical performance on clinical observations and the experience of a few pioneers in the field. Subsequently, however, carefully conducted longitudinal studies as well as basic laboratory studies on wound healing, tissue integration of biomaterials, and microbiological aspects have provided the scientific basis for a predictable and successful incorporation of oral implants.

In essence, four implant systems that differ substantially in their nature of tissue integration have been developed:

1. Subperiosteal implants. These implants may be considered *first generation implants.* Their development goes back into the 1930s and 1940s.[1,2] The system was simple and involved the subperiosteal placement of a cast chrome-cobalt frame. These implants served as a basis for complete denture retention with reported degrees of success from only 6% after 7 years[3] to 93% after 5 years.[4] Because of this high risk of failures, they have been replaced by the later generations of dental implant systems.

2. Transmandibular implants. These implants are placed subperiosteally with transmandibular fixation and were developed especially for the fully edentulous, sometimes resorbed and atrophic mandible. Although this system is a later development,[5] its basis for a successful tissue incorporation is questionable. A gold alloy (70% Au, 5% Pt, 12.8% Ag, 12.2% Cu) with a homogeneous crystal structure is used. Although this metal does not seem to corrode, the incorporation into the living bone does not lead to a tight adaptation of the surrounding bone, which results in a questionable long-term prognosis.

3. Endosseous implants (fibro-osseous integration). These implants may be designated as *second generation implants.* Various forms and materials have been advocated for numerous implant systems. It was thought that the masticatory forces should be distributed over a bone mass with adequate surface for retention. Furthermore, it was claimed that implants should be designed to fit the great variety of anatomical relations in the maxilla and the mandible. In addition, it was realized that the metal alloys that had been used for many years should be replaced by new materials with better biocompatibility and improved physical features. Linkow[6] developed a blade implant system. These implants were encapsulated into connective tissue, which was termed *fibro-osseous integration.* Some authors claimed that this represented an acceptable healing pattern,[7] while others considered the presence of soft tissue between the bone and the implant an undesirable relation similar to a pseudoarthrosis.[8] Other systems that did not use titanium or other metals for the implant but used bioglasses, such as Al_2O_3, appeared to heal likewise. The "shock absorbing" effect of this "pseudo-periodontal ligament" was generally considered a functionally acceptable implant/bone interface.[9]

4. Endosseous implants (osseointegration). Osseointegration is the latest development in implant dentistry, although its scientific basis goes back to the 1960s.[9,10] An intimate bone-to-implant contact was preferred over the fibro-osseous integration to provide a permanent, firm anchorage of the implant body in the jawbone in order to equally deflect masticatory forces and transfer them to a broad base in the jawbone. Generally, titanium implants are used to achieve such an anchorage, which was first reported by Brånemark et al.[11] Subsequently, this intimate bone-to-implant contact was documented in undecalcified histologic ground sections by Schroeder et al.[12] While these authors referred to the intimate contact anchorage as "functional ankylosis," Brånemark et al later created the term *osseointegration,* defined as "a direct structural and functional connection between bone and the surface of a load carrying implant."[13] Osseointegrated implants may be considered *third generation implants.* In recent years, they have clearly become the preferred system in clinical practice over the previous generations. The main emphasis in basic and clinical research in this field has been placed on understanding the biological properties and improving clinical success of osseointegrated dental implants. This is the reason why these implants will be emphasized in this review.

PREREQUISITES FOR SUCCESSFUL OSSEOINTEGRATION

There is agreement in the literature that functional ankylosis or osseointegration depends on a few essential principles, which include *(1)* the selection of implant materials, *(2)* the surface properties of implants, *(3)* the surgical preparation of the implant recipient site, and *(4)* the control of loading forces during healing.[8,12-15]

Selection of Implant Materials

To promote optimal tissue integration of an implant, its design and the material chosen for the machining are of essential significance. Biocompatibility, resistance to corrosion, and adequate physical properties must be optimized. Although many materials, including stainless steel, chrome-cobalt alloys, precious metal alloys, aluminum oxides, and bioglasses, have been tested predominantly in vitro, pure titanium has emerged as the metal of choice for the construction of dental implants.[16,17] Titanium is a highly reactive metal initiating the spontaneous formation of an oxide layer upon contact with air, water, or electrolytes.[16] This titanium oxide layer is most resistant to corrosion. Hence, this surface layer of titanium oxide will effectively protect the titanium against chemical attacks even in biological liquids. In vivo studies[16] have clearly indicated that the corrosion for titanium was 250 times lower than for gold and 35 times lower than for chrome-cobalt alloys. Since a complete absence of corrosion does not exist in nature, minimal corrosion, or rather "chemical compatibility," may also implicate biocompatibility.[17] Indeed, further physicochemical properties of elements, such as their intrinsic toxicity and their capability to bind macromolecules, are additional factors to consider when evaluating the biocompatibility of materials. It is unlikely that for elements such as titanium, zirconium, and niobium, binding reactions between metal hydroxides and/or metal ions will occur with proteins and result in potentially toxic products. Titanium with its protective surface layer of TiO_2 therefore represents an ideal material for implantation, at least from a corrosion as well as biocompatibility standpoint.

Functional loading of implants will result in the transfer of masticatory forces to the jawbone;

hence, the stiffness of an implant body should be similar to that of the alveolar bone proper. When an endosteal implant body is placed into the bone structure, it is essential that the bone defect created by the placement be as small as possible and that the functional deformation of the mandible not be compromised. Compared to stainless steel, aluminum oxides, or bioglasses,[14] titanium yields a stiffness that is closer to that of cortical bone. Moreover, titanium may easily be machined as hollow bodies with or without additional perforations, resulting in a stiffness which is even more adapted to that of cortical bone.[14]

Surface Properties of Implants

The physical nature of the implant surface appears to have a major impact on the ankylotic anchorage of the implant in bone. Numerous retentive shapes have been developed for different implant systems to provide adequate *macroretentions* for achieving primary stability during the healing phase. Most commonly, screw threads of various shapes and inclinations have been advocated.[8] Furthermore, perforations and/or fenestrations are prepared in several implants systems.[14] For some systems, macroretentions provide the only stability in addition to friction, while other systems also include microretentions to improve the bonding strength of the interface region. Such *microretentions* include surface coatings resulting in a rough surface. For example, titanium plasma coatings applied to implants increase the surface area at the implant/bone interface at least by a factor of six, thereby increasing the surface available for ankylotic anchorage.[12] Following healing, removal torques for pol-

ished titanium implant surfaces appear to be much lower than for rough surfaces.[18] Hence, implants with rough surfaces will also be more resistant to shearing forces than smoothly polished implants. Resistance to shearing forces may be an essential indicator for successful osseointegration. Commercially pure titanium incorporated for at least 100 days developed a resistance against pulling and shearing forces which resembled that of trabecular bone and indicated some kind of a chemical bonding between bone and titanium.[19] It was suggested that the observed bone-titanium adhesion was based on a possible chemisorption onto the titanium oxide layer, inducing a growth stimulation of bone.

In order to improve the tight bone-to-implant interface, hydroxyapatite coatings were promoted. It has been demonstrated,[20] however, that 32 weeks following the incorporation of implants coated with hydroxyapatite the bond between the implant body and the hydroxyapatite appeared ruptured, indicating that the bonding strength between hydroxyapatite and bone is greater than the bonding strength between the former and titanium. In addition, recent in vivo experiments have also shown that hydroxyapatite coatings may be locally resorbed and replaced by connective tissue, resulting in a surface locally covered by fibrous tissue rather than by ankylotic adhesion of bone.[20] It is not known, however, to what extent the local resorption of hydroxyapatite coatings will influence the prognosis and clinical outcome of implants. Even though the biological properties of hydroxyapatites and their so-called bioactive capacities may render these materials interesting for further studies, there is no scientific evidence pro-

viding documentation for additional benefits of hydroxyapatite coatings over rough titanium surfaces.[21]

Surgical Preparation of the Recipient Site

The chemical and physical properties of implant materials and their design can markedly affect the integration into host tissues. In addition, the surgical technique required for preparation of the implant recipient site is crucial for the healing of the tissues, thereby affecting implant integration in its early stages as well. Unfortunately, the techniques for the placement of endosseous implants have been dominated by dogmatic prerequisites based on deductive thinking rather than on scientific evidence. One of these was the claim that implant fixtures must be submerged under the mucosal tissues at the time of installation in order to predictably achieve osseointegration.[11] Consequently, after a tissue integration period of 3 to 6 months, a second surgical intervention was necessary to gain access to the fixtures for the installation of prosthetic abutments. Recently, it has been demonstrated in a controlled experiment[22] that nonsubmerged or one-stage titanium implants osseointegrate with equal predictability as do submerged or so-called two-stage titanium implants. Furthermore, epidemiologic surveys[23,24] as well as prospective clinical trials[25] document a high success rate of up to 98% for the tissue integration of nonsubmerged implants. In comparison with results of surveys of submerged implants, these success rates are quite similar.[26]

There is general agreement that the most critical aspect of the surgical intervention is the preparation of the implant bed. Because of its physical nature, drilling of bone generates considerable amounts of heat, which may result in bone necrosis. Low drilling speeds (under 800 rpm)[24] and abundant irrigation with chilled sterile saline may minimize bone tissue injury.[8,24] Furthermore, the use of drilling instruments of progressively increasing diameter will also help to minimize thermal trauma.

In order to achieve *primary stability* of the implant and to minimize the gap between the bone and the implant, it is essential to prepare the recipient site in congruence with the implant. Primary stability will assure optimal conditions for the promotion of the remodeling process of the intervening thin bony layer damaged during the drilling process. Thus, new bone will grow and replace the damaged bone, resulting in an intimate bone-to-implant contact with a gap of only approximately 20 μm or less between the bone cells and the titanium oxide layer.[18,27] If an implant lacks primary stability, healing will occur by fibrous replacement of the damaged bone, resulting in a fibrous encapsulation of the implant rather than osseointegration.

Control of Loading Forces

Other very important factors influencing osseointegration of implants are the timeframe following installation and the magnitude of loading forces applied to an implant.[28,29] The presence of a fibrous or a mineralized interface between bone and implant seems to depend on the timing of the postoperative loading of implants. Osseointegration appears to require 3 to 6 months of quiescence.[28]

Research in the field of implant loading remains sparse, and no

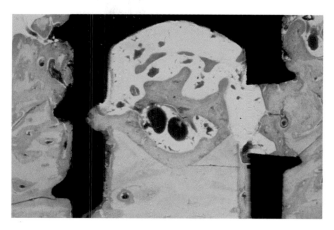

Fig 21-1 *Overview of osseointegrated one-stage implant. The outline of the surgical preparation is visible. Close distance from the walls of the implant bed to the implant surface results in primary stability. (Slide courtesy of ITI, Waldenburg, Switzerland.)*

scientific data are available to postulate clear-cut requirements. Even following successful osseointegration, the bone / implant interface may still change as a result of excessive loading or the application of high shearing forces. This may lead to micromotions of the implant in relation to the surrounding bone, provoking bone resorption in the immediate vicinity and subsequent repair by ingrowth of fibrous tissue. It may be anticipated that physical properties of implant materials or designs (solid versus hollow) may modify the potentially deleterious effects of excessive masticatory forces.

TISSUE INTEGRATION

Endosteal dental implants are artificial, inorganic tooth substitutes exogenously introduced into an endosseous receptor site with the expectation that the surrounding tissues will adapt to them physiologically, allowing function during mastication (Fig 21-1).

Dental implants are not de-signed to interface with the tissues at the recipient site in the same way that natural teeth relate to periodontal tissues. Placing implants in an osseous environment in which cementum progenitor cells are missing precludes a functional periodontal ligament from developing. Thus, all current evidence suggests that the presence of these progenitor cells is a prerequisite for the formation of a periodontal ligament.[30-33] It has recently been shown that a periodontal ligament may also form around the surface of titanium implants, provided that progenitor cells originating from a periodontal ligament of a residual root tip left in close contact with the implant surface are allowed to migrate along the implant surface.[34,35] The possibility of implant incorporation mediated by a cementum layer on the implants via a functionally oriented ligament to the surrounding bone is, therefore, a reality, although thus far no such attachment apparatus has been demonstrated, to form around titanium implants installed under routine clinical conditions.

Whether or not such tissue integration will lead to a new generation of dental implants remains to be explored in future research projects.

Bone/Implant Interface

The intimate contact of bone at the implant interface shows all the features of a *functional ankylosis*,[12] which has also been designated as osseointegration.[13] Since the implant bed should be prepared carefully in congruence with the implant fixture to be installed, a minimal distance between surrounding bone and implant surface is created, thereby excluding other tissues from proliferating in an apical direction between the implant bed and its surface. As a result of postsurgical immobilization, only bone cells may fill this gap and proliferate toward the implant surface. At the same time, they may be expected to replace bone cells that have undergone necrosis as a result of surgical trauma.[21] As pointed out before, the physical and chemical surface properties may have a major effect on the bone apposition to the implant surface. Rough titanium plasma coated surfaces appear to show preferable bone/implant interfaces,[24] requiring greater removal torques than smooth surfaces[18] (Fig 21-2). Hence, even an osseoinductive effect of such surfaces has been postulated.[24] Furthermore, the nature of the bone/implant interface depends on the structure and nature of the bone of the recipient site. Obviously, a much higher degree of intimate contact with lamellar or mineralized bone may be expected when the implant is placed into compact bone as compared to cancellous bone.

In light microscopic studies analyzing quantitatively undecalcified ground sections in which the

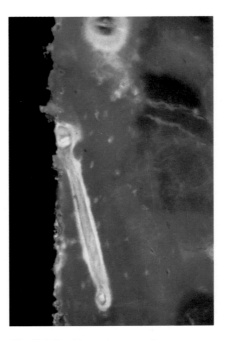

Fig 21-2 *Osseointegration on a rough titanium surface. Direct contact of bone to the titanium plasma surface. Capillary in direct contact with implant surface (original magnification x 65). (Slide courtesy of ITI, Waldenburg, Switzerland.)*

cut implant remained in place during the histological processing, a surface coverage around titanium implants of up to 90% mineralized lamellar bone was demonstrated for cortical bone.[21] Such a contact may only be seen for approximately 50% of the implant surface in cancellous bone, the remaining surface being in direct contact with nonmineralized bone marrow.[22] These contact relationships are similar irrespective of whether an implant fixture had been allowed to heal in a submerged environment or in open contact with the oral cavity.[22]

In light microscopic sections, a fine white interface layer may occasionally be observed.[20] This layer, which is 1 to 10 μm in width, does not yield stain, nor does it contain tissues. It is commonly

considered a sign of a direct bony anchorage, while larger gaps exceeding the dimension of 10 μm are generally representative of the formation of a fibrous tissue layer between the mineralized bone and the implant surface. The small-dimension separation gaps are generally interpreted as artifacts. However, recent ultrastructural studies using a newly developed technique for the processing of intact bone/titanium interfaces revealed that these gaps contain collagen with a very low mineral content.[21] Because of the technical difficulties in obtaining adequate undecalcified sections of massive titanium implants, information on the ultrastructure of the interface with the surrounding tissues is sparse. Nevertheless, the titanium oxide layer appears to be covered with a very thin layer of approximately 100 Å, containing proteoglycans and glycosaminoglycans.[36] Collagen filaments originating from the surrounding bone were observed at a distance of 20 to 40 μm from the interface.[36] In contrast to the findings by Albrektsson et al,[36] Listgarten et al[37] were able to document, in nondemineralized sections, an intimate contact between the hydroxyapatite crystalites from the bone matrix and the titanium surface without any evidence of a nondemineralized zone between the titanium and the bone. They were also able to confirm this bone-to-titanium relationship in demineralized sections. Collagen fibrils extended close to and, in some regions, were in direct contact with the titanium surface.[37] Scanning electron microscopic images confirmed the results from light microscopic studies and further documented the intimate apposition of mineralized bone to rough titanium surfaces.[24]

Most of the studies on tissue integration were performed on unloaded dental implants. However, the ankylotic contact between bone and titanium appears to be even more intimate and the bone denser following occlusal loading.[24] Following the placement of a hollow cylinder titanium implant into a monkey jaw, a non-lamellar, mineralized substance closely resembling osteocementum with cementocyte-like cells (as opposed to a lamellar bone structure) was observed around the apical termination of the implant after 16 months of functional loading. This was interpreted as functional adaptation of the recipient bone.[24] Conclusively, the term osseointegration does represent a multidirectional force-transmitting attachment of the implant in the bony housing.

Supracrestal Connective Tissue

All dental implants, regardless of their relationship to the alveolar bone (that is, regardless of whether the healing pattern is by fibro-osseous incorporation or by osseointegration) will penetrate through the supracrestal region in which a close contact of the gingival connective tissue or the alveolar mucosa with the implant surface has to be expected. As opposed to natural teeth, no layer of extrinsic fibrous cementum can be expected on the implant surface due to a lack of the appropriate progenitor cells. The tight seal of the soft tissue collar around the implant abutment penetrating into the oral cavity appears to be mediated by a distinct region of supracrestal fibers running more or less parallel with the long axis of the implant abutment in an apicocoronal direction[38-40] (Fig 21-3).

Several reports have indicated that the surface topography of dental implants will significantly affect the orientation of the su-

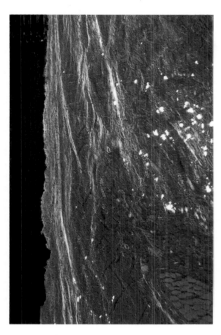

Fig 21-3 *Fibers running parallel with the long axis of the implant, thereby providing an effective seal around the implant post (original magnification x 65). (Slide from Buser et al.[40])*

pracrestal fibers. While smooth implant surfaces are almost always associated with a fiber orientation parallel to the long axis of the implant,[39-41] rough surfaces such as titanium plasma coatings appear to result in a perpendicular fiber arrangement almost mimicking the insertion of functionally oriented dentogingival fibers.[40,41] Furthermore, in in vitro studies,[42] the different orientation of fibroblasts toward a smooth or a rough and porous surface, respectively, was demonstrated. Fibroblasts became oriented at acute angles to smooth surfaces, whereas they assumed almost perpendicular orientations toward the surface of porous implants.

It has also been postulated that the orientation of the supracrestal fibers may be affected by the tissue characteristics and hence also

by the mobility of the mucosa surrounding the implant.[40] Where implants had been placed into an area with keratinized oral mucosa (gingiva), which is firmly connected with the periosteum, the orientation of the supracrestal fibers tended to be perpendicular to a rough plasma-coated implant surface.[40] By contrast, the supracrestal fibers ran parallel to the implant surface when the implant was surrounded by (nonkeratinized) alveolar mucosa. The clinical significance of the presence or absence of keratinized mucosa for the longevity of a dental implant is not yet fully elucidated. Results from longitudinal studies, however, raise some doubt as to the necessity of the presence of keratinized mucosa (gingiva) for maintaining healthy peri-implant structures.[43]

The dense network of supracrestal connective tissue in which fibers running parallel with the implant surface in an apicocoronal direction appear to splice with circumferentially oriented fibers, seems both to provide an effective seal around the implant abutment and to mediate the formation of an epithelial attachment. Some inflammatory cell infiltrates may be seen in the area adjacent to the junctional epithelium, while apical to the junctional epithelium the supracrestal region appears free from an inflammatory infiltrate[37] (Fig 21-4).

Epithelial Attachment

The epithelial contact around an implant corresponds to the structural relationship encountered between it and the natural teeth. Like that tissue adjacent to teeth, the oral epithelium is continuous with the oral sulcular epithelium covering the lateral surface of the gingival sulcus just below the free gingival margin. The apical part

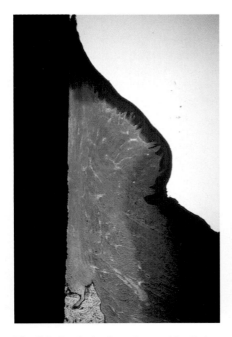

Fig 21-4 *Apical to the epithelial attachment the connective tissue is free from inflammation. Epithelial lining does not reach the alveolar crest (original magnification x 8). (Slide from Buser et al.[40])*

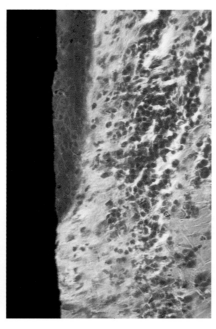

Fig 21-5 *Junctional epithelium. Apical termination of junctional epithelium cells adjacent to supracrestal fiber region (original magnification x 200). (Slide courtesy of ITI, Waldenburg, Switzerland.)*

this functional adaptation of the junctional epithelium around implants manifests itself also in the presence of plasminogen activator, an enzyme normally restricted to junctional epithelium around natural teeth.[49]

It is evident that the subepithelial connective tissue fiber network is essential for mediating a tight implant-epithelial junction and thus providing an optimal functional seal and a protective mechanism against peri-implant infection. An adequate keratinized mucosa is, therefore, thought by many clinicians to be essential for maintaining healthy peri-implant tissues.[40,41]

PERI-IMPLANT INFECTIONS

It has become universally accepted that bacterial plaque and its products are not only the cause of gingivitis and periodontitis but also the major etiologic factor for dental caries, provided that adequate substrates such as sucrose are available.[50] It is evident that bacterial plaque also plays a key role in determining healthy or diseased conditions around implant abutments. Since the oral diseases mentioned represent opportunistic infections,[51] the colonization of implant surfaces as well as the characterization of the subgingival microbiota associated with well-maintained or failing implants is of great interest.

Early Colonization of Endosseous Implants

Few longitudinal studies have investigated the sequence of colonization of newly placed implant surfaces with health-associated or periodontopathic microorganisms. Moreover, it is not known

of the sulcus, however, is lined by a few layers of nonkeratinizing squamous epithelium known as junctional epithelium around natural teeth (Fig 21-5). As around teeth, the junctional epithelium is attached to the implant surface by means of a basal lamina and hemidesmosomes. On the basis of freeze-fractured gingival preparations, the ultrastructure of the interface of the junctional epithelium to vitallium implants was demonstrated.[44] Moreover, by using epoxy resin implant replicas, Listgarten and Lai[38] documented the implant/epithelium interface with a basal lamina and hemidesmosomes between the junctional epithelium and the adjacent implant surface.

In vitro, the attachment of epithelial cells to titanium surfaces via hemidesmosomes and a basal lamina-like structure was shown.[45] Similar findings were reported for aluminum oxide ceramic implants inserted in dogs[46] and for polymethacrylate dental implants.[47] All these studies confirm that junctional epithelium is capable of attaching itself to a variety of hard surfaces, even including clean calculus,[48] by means of hemidesmosomes and a basal lamina. These structures appear virtually identical to those observed at the dentoepithelial junction around natural teeth. Although junctional epithelium around teeth is derived from reduced enamel epithelium, it originates from oral epithelium around dental implants. Recently, it has been shown that whether the initial colonization of implants is influenced by the presence or absence of remaining teeth and / or the presence or absence of periodontal infections.

The development of the microbial complex associated with hollow cylinder implants was studied in edentulous patients from the day of implantation up to 180 days.[52] A total of 114 samples of 9 sites in 5 patients were evaluated by darkfield microscopy and cultured anaerobically. On the average, 86% of the microorganisms were identified as coccoid cells and more than 80% of the cultivated bacteria were gram-positive facultative cocci in preoperative swab samples obtained from the mucosal surfaces at the area of implantation. Following implantation, no significant changes in the proportions of bacteria were detected, except in one site. After 21 days, this particular site showed a steady decrease in the percentages of coccoid cells associated with a simultaneous increase in the proportion of rods. At day 120, small spirochetes were found for the first time concomitantly with the formation of pus and other clinical signs of a developing peri-implant lesion such as bleeding on probing and a probing depth of 6 mm. None of the other sites showed any signs of inflammation throughout the duration of the study. Spirochetes were never seen in the clinically healthy sites. Black-pigmenting gram-negative rods (Bacteroides) were detected only infrequently and in small proportions; no trend of increase was apparent at any site over 180 days. This clearly indicates that the bacterial colonization of newly placed implants follows a pattern similar to that known for the colonization of natural teeth.[52] Lastly, the microbiota found as early as 1 week after placement of implants appears

similar to that found on mucosal surfaces.

Further longitudinal studies over 5 years on the microflora associated with osseointegrated implants in 18 edentulous patients, 53 implants have revealed a health-associated microbiota, with 53% of the organisms cultured being facultatively anaerobic cocci and 17% being facultatively anaerobic rods. Gram-negative anaerobic rods were found in only 7%. Fusobacterium species and Prevotella intermedia (Bacteroides intermedius) were both enumerated in 9% of the samples, while Porphyromonas (Bacteroides) gingivalis and spirochetes were never observed in these clinically successful sites. Repeated microbiological and clinical data after 3, 4, and 5 years following implantation showed a stable microbiota associated with healthy peri-implant tissues.[53] Since the presence of natural teeth may influence the composition of the subgingival microbiota around implants,[54] it is conceivable that the early colonization with presumptive periodontopathogens could be more frequently encountered in patients with untreated or poorly controlled periodontal disease. Further studies should elucidate the possible role of periodontal pockets serving as a reservoir for pathogenic bacteria colonizing implant surfaces.

Microbiota Associated With Failing Implants

In recent years, several cross-sectional studies have successfully associated tissue-integrated dental implants with a predominantly gram-positive facultatively anaerobic microbiota.[54-59] Yet limited data are available on the microbiota associated with failing implants.[58,60] In a recent study,[58] samples from five patients with suc-

cessfully incorporated implants serving as abutments for overdentures for more than 1 year were compared to samples from seven patients with clinically failing implants (Fig 21-6). These unsuccessful sites were characterized by probing depths exceeding 5 mm, suppuration, and visible loss of alveolar bone in the crestal area around the implant as visualized on radiographs. These sites harbored a complex microbiota with a large proportion of gram-negative anaerobic rods. Black-pigmenting gram-negative anaerobic rods (Bacteroides) and Fusobacterium were regularly found, and spirochetes, fusiform bacteria, as well as motile and curved rods were a common observation in the darkfield microscopic specimens of the failing sites. Control samples from healthy sites in the same patients harbored small amounts of bacteria, predominantly coccoid morphotypes. Spirochetes were absent. Fusiform bacteria and motile and curved rods were found occasionally, but only in small proportions. Both these control sites in unsuccessful patients and the sites in successful patients yielded a similar microbiota. The striking difference between successful and failing implant sites was not only a 20-fold lower total bacterial count (CFU/mL) in the successful sites, but also a microbiota with remarkable qualitative differences. Since the microbiota associated with peri-implant infections closely resembled that of a chronic adult periodontitis,[58-60] peri-implant infections should be considered as site-specific opportunistic infections.[60]

Experimental Peri-implantitis

A decade ago, animal models were introduced to study the microbiota associated with deve-

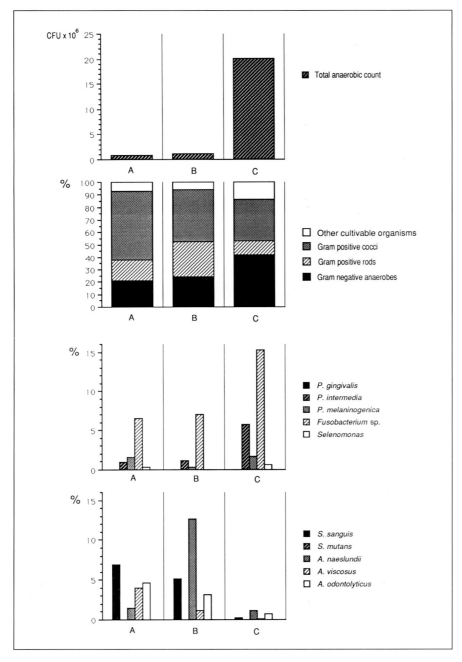

Fig 21-6 *Microbiota associated with healthy peri-implant tissues in successful patients (A) and in unsuccessful patients (B) with failing implant sites (C). Total number of colony forming units (CFU x 10μm) and percentages of bacterial groups and species are given. The microbiota associated with failing implants is predominantly gram-negative and anaerobic (Prevotella intermedia and Fusobacterium species), while healthy implant sites are characterized by a predominantly gram-positive facultatively anaerobic microbiota.*

oping periodontitis. In cynomolgus monkeys, plaque retaining ligatures were tied around experimental teeth and the composition of the subgingival microbiota was sequentially analyzed using continuous anaerobic culturing techniques.[61] The increase in proportions of surface translocating bacteria, such as *Capnocytophaga* species, preceded the proportional increase of *P. gingivalis* and *P. intermedia.* High proportions of these organisms could be associated with signs of clinical attachment and radiographic bone loss, that is, with the transition of gingivitis to periodontitis, *Capnocytophaga* appeared more prominent in the early phases of the study (ie, the development of gingivitis).

Recently, another clinical, microbiological, and radiological study was performed in the cynomolgus monkey.[62] The purpose of this ligature-induced periodontitis model was to compare the etiologic factors and the pathogenic sequence of events of peri-implant infections with those observed in periodontitis (Figs 21-7 and 21-8). Plaque accumulation and concomitant development of gingival inflammation progressed in a fashion similar for both ligated teeth and ligated implants. Consequently, increased probing depths were observed in both models with equal severity. Subtraction radiographic images[63] also revealed a similar loss of crestal bone density adjacent to the ligated teeth or the ligated implants, respectively. Lesions of equal size and shape were identified in histologic specimens at the termination of the study. The bacterial plaque development occurred at almost identical rates in both ligated teeth and ligated implants. Approximately 40% of the subgingival microbiota consisted of spirochetes and motile rods as

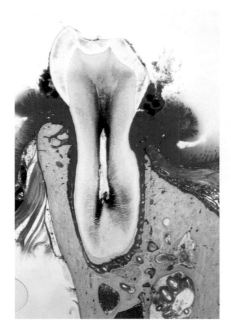

Fig 21-7 *Ligature-induced periodontitis in a cynomolgus monkey. Note loss of connective tissue fiber attachment and bone loss as a result of the plaque accumulation for 8 months (original magnification ×2.5).*

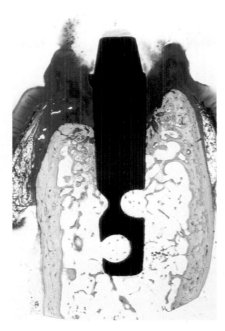

Fig 21-8 *Ligature-induced peri-implantitis in a cynomolgus monkey. Note loss of alveolar bone in an angular pattern as a result of the plaque accumulation for 8 months (original magnification ×2.5).*

early as 2 months in both models. The data from the cultural studies also yielded similar percentages of black-pigmenting gram-negative anaerobic rods *(Bacteroides)* around ligated teeth and ligated implants.[62] These studies indicated that implant failures after osseointegration has taken place (ie, after 4 to 6 months) are most likely the result of a bacterial infection rather than an effect of occlusal overload.

Therapy of Peri-implant Infections

Stable implants have a subgingival microbiota very similar to that of healthy gingival tissues. Also, peri-implant infections seem to harbor the same pathogenic microorganisms associated with

chronic adult periodontitis.[58] Therefore, antimicrobial therapy to eliminate the pathogenic microbiota appears to be the obvious modality for peri-implant infections. Presently, only few well-controlled double blind studies are available on the treatment outcomes of various antimicrobial regimens. Thus, recommendations can only be made on the basis of case reports and anecdotal evidence. Systemic antibiotics, such as metronidazole or omidazole, in combination with or without simultaneous administration of amoxicillin, have been successful in the treatment of recurrent periodontitis, refractory lesions, and rapidly progressive periodontitis. Such regimens may also be effective in arresting peri-implant infections.[64] Systemic tetracycline

has also been shown to effectively eradicate black-pigmenting Gram-negative anaerobic rods *(Bacteroides)* from subgingival implant sites.[65]

In addition to systemic antibiotic administration, regular applications of antiseptic agents such as chlorhexidine are valuable adjunctive treatment options.[66]

Periodontal flap surgery to gain access to the defect may be advocated in more advanced cases of peri-implant infections (Fig 21-9). Although implant surfaces cannot be instrumented like natural teeth, strong and abundant irrigations with either sterile saline or chlorhexidine should be sufficient to clean implant surfaces from bacterial deposits and hence to initiate healing in the presence of optimal supragingival plaque control. Also, alveolar bone may be regenerated adjacent to cleaned titanium implants using the principle of guided tissue regeneration.[67,68] It is evident that meticulous plaque control must accompany these efforts for regenerating new bone into peri-implant defects (Fig 21-10).

Prevention of Implant Failures

There is convincing evidence that bacterial plaque not only leads to gingivitis and periodontitis[50] but may also induce the development of peri-implant infections, resulting in loss of bone around osseointegrated dental implants.[62] As the infection encompasses a greater and greater radius, more and more bony support is lost, eventually leading to the loss of the implant if the infection is left untreated. Hence, regular maintenance visits are a prerequisite for long-term clinical success. Early diagnosis and interference with a developing peri-implant lesion may prevent further deteriora-

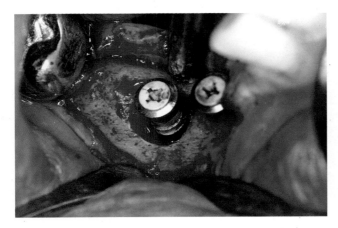

Fig 21-9 *Peri-implant infection in a patient 4 months after the installation of an endosseous implant. Craterlike defect around the implant prior to the placement of a barrier membrane for bone regeneration according to the principle of guided tissue regeneration. (From Lekmann et al.[68])*

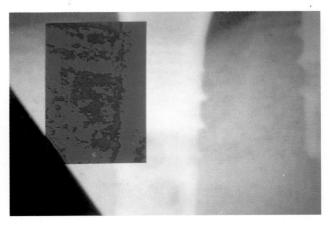

Fig 21-10 *Regeneration documented on a set of subtraction radiographs obtained at the time of membrane placement and 6 months thereafter. Blue pseudocolor indicates increase in bone density. Adjacent to the implant the defect of Fig 21-9 appears completely filled. (From Lekmann et al.[68])*

tion. Since implant surfaces are usually rough and since screw threads or other macroretentions may provide optimal retention for plaque accumulation, regular plaque control practices are of utmost importance. Personal oral hygiene practices must be modified and adjunctive aids for oral hygiene must be adapted to the altered morphology of dental implants compared to natural teeth. Specially designed interproximal brushes have been shown to penetrate up to 3 mm into a gingival sulcus or pocket[69] and hence may also efficiently clean the peri-implant sulcus. In addition to mechanical plaque control, daily rinses using 0.1% chlorhexidine digluconate[66] provide a welcome adjunct, thereby supporting the concept of a plaque-free peri-implant region. Calculus deposits are difficult to remove from the implant surfaces, hence their formation should be prevented by effective plaque control. Residual calculus deposits may be carefully chipped off with curets. During

maintenance visits, implant surfaces should be polished using rubber cup and polishing paste. A recent report[53] on stable osseointegrated implants indicated that regular maintenance visits and supporting therapy maintained a predominantly coccoid microbiota (83%) with no spirochetes present in darkfield microscopy over a period of 3 to 5 years. The analysis of the cultural data yielded a predominantly gram-positive facultatively anaerobic microbiota (< 70%) associated with stable implants. During the entire observation period of up to 5 years, periodontopathic microorganisms were seen in low frequencies (< 10% of the samples), and when present, in very low proportions (< 3%). *P. gingivalis* was absent in all samples. This study, therefore, confirms the necessity of maintaining a nonpathogenic ecosystem around dental implants in order to prevent implant failures from occurring following successful osseointegration.

REGENERATION OF ALVEOLAR BONE

Guided Tissue Regeneration

In periodontal therapy, surgery aimed at regenerating periodontal tissues lost as a result of periodontal disease has been developed and termed *guided tissue regeneration* (GTR) (for a review see Nyman et al[70]). This new principle is based on the hypothesis that different types of cells that surround the surgical wound region proliferate into the wound area, determining the outcome of the healing process. By the placement of barrier membranes, preference can be given to those cells to repopulate the wound that have the potential to regenerate the desired type of tissue. At the same time, cells that may negatively interfere with the regenerative process can be excluded from proliferating into the wound. A further prerequisite for successful GTR is the creation of an adequately dimensioned space allowing the formation of desired type of tissue.

The principle of GTR was first developed to regenerate periodontal tissues, but it may also be applied outside the periodontium.[71] Bone tissue was successfully regenerated to cover denuded parts of dental implants in experimental animals[72,73] and in humans.[67,74] Also, alveolar ridge augmentation was successfully completed in animals[75] as well as in humans.[67,76] Hence, a new concept is practicable to regenerate bone in areas with inadequate volume or height prior to, concomitant with, or following the installation of a dental implant.

Alveolar Ridge Enlargement

Histological samples obtained from implant bed preparations documented the normal structure and morphology of newly regenerated bone tissue[76] according to the principle of guided tissue regeneration. In the same report,[76] 12 cases of insufficient alveolar bone prior to implant placement were presented. Depending on the space provided by the placement of the membrane, between 1.5 and 5.5 mm of alveolar crestal width could be gained 6 to 10 months following the regenerative surgery. However, in 25% of the cases, the membranes had to be removed prematurely because of the development of an abscess. From this study[76] it appears that

the biological principle of GTR is highly predictable for alveolar ridge enlargement prior to placement of implants. Technical factors such as flap design, placement of membranes providing sufficient space for bone regeneration, flap closure, and postsurgical infection control may influence the outcome of the healing process. Nevertheless, it should be realized that bone regeneration for the enlargement or augmentation of the alveolar ridge created by the GTR procedure results in the formation of new bone originating from the host's own local tissue. This must certainly be preferred over various other tissue augmentation techniques involving the placement of various types of autografts and allografts.

C L I N I C A L   A P P L I C A T I O N

OVERVIEW

The introduction of osseointegration has made dental implants a popular topic for both dental professionals and the general public. This popularity has led to placement of more and more fixtures. While many implant systems are available, conflicting information from both the dental literature and manufacturers has complicated the clinician's choice. It appears that changes in implant design or material can have a significant impact on the degree of success. Systems that initially looked promising have later been found to fail routinely, this often despite well-documented animal histology and good intent by those proposing the implant. In addition, prosthetic options and

vendor service must be considered before choosing an implant system.

Part of this problem resulted because there was little attempt to systematically document successes and failures of the implants until the 1978 National Institutes of Health Conference.[77] Once this process of gathering information was completed, it became apparent that fibro-osseous systems (non-osseointegrated blades and subperiosteal implants for the most part) had a failure of up to 50% at 10 years.[73] At about the same time, Brånemark et al[13] introduced the concept of a tight interface of bone to a titanium surface, which they termed osseointegration. This Swedish group's high percentage of long-term success (in the anterior edentulous mandible) spawned a number of systems with

similar features. Some of these systems are screw form such as the Brånemark System, some are cylindrical, and others are combinations. Initially these systems were made from titanium; later many of the designs were made available covered with some form of hydroxyapatite.

As a result of the knowledge gained from the Brånemark System, it is now clear that successful osseointegration requires the following: (1) the implant must be composed of a biocompatible material and (2) the placement must be atraumatic to the bone. Initial loading of the implant decreases the success rate. Several systems presently available allow these criteria to be met and each offers advantages and disadvantages in terms of surgical procedure and/or prosthetic reconstruction.

The choice of system for the individual practitioner and patient is difficult. At present the systems of choice are ITI (Straumann Institute, Waldenberg, Switzerland) and Brånemark (Nobelpharma AB, Nobel Industries, Sweden). The ITI system is suggested because of the simplicity of placement, its hollow design, and plasma sprayed surface (which increases the area available for osseointegration), the superb dealer support, and the fact that it is placed with a single-stage surgery. The Brånemark System offers a long-term record of success in the anterior mandible and can be used in immediate extraction sites and where protection of the implant to avoid early loading would be a problem.

Examination and treatment planning for dental implants are covered in chapter 19, while basic surgical procedures are dealt with very adequately in other books.[8,24,79] Therefore, this chapter covers specific strategies for improving implant placement, guided tissue regeneration around dental implants, and augmenting deficit bony edentulous ridges to enhance later implant placement. Sections on supportive periodontal treatment (SPT) for dental implants and on complications associated with implants and possible solutions are also included.

IMPROVING IMPLANT PLACEMENT

Anterior Mandible (Totally Edentulous Patients)

Incisions For the ITI System, incisions that bisect the remaining keratinized gingiva mesiodistally with vertical releasing incisions,

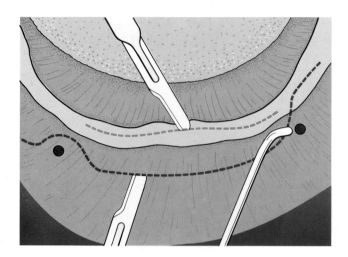

Fig 21-11 *Midcrestal (for ITI) or vestibular (for Brånemark) incisions are preferred in the anterior mandible. Before distal extensions of the flap are made, the mental foramen should be located.*

when needed, are preferred. For the Brånemark System, incisions should be made well into the buccal vestibule. For Brånemark placement, start with a partial thickness dissection, then direct the blade toward the ridge to form a full-thickness mucoperiosteal flap. The incision line should be semilunar and care should be taken to avoid severing the mental nerve. This nerve can be best preserved by carefully exploring with a curet until the mental foramen is found (Fig 21-11). Exploration is performed after the anterior part of the incision has been made and carried back to the area previously occupied by the canines. The clinician should be aware that while the mental foramen usually indicates the most anterior position, occasionally the nerve will run forward a few millimeters then trace back posteriorly before exiting the mandible. Once the foramen is located, the incision can be carried to the ridge crest mesial of the foramen. If further flap retraction is required, the incision on the crest of the ridge (assuming the inferior alveolar nerve is not immediately subad-

jacent) can be extended distally and the flap further elevated.

Stents If tooth placement is to be altered, the patient's denture (Fig 21-12) or a duplication of their existing denture or of a new denture waxup (Fig 21-13) provides an acceptable guide for implant placement. This stent can be hollowed out from the lingual or facial or have holes to guide the appropriate drill to proper alignment. For best results, the patient should wear his / her maxillary denture (if he / she has one) during this stage of the surgery. The center of the top of the handpiece can then be placed just lingual to the incisal edges of the maxillary teeth to provide another alignment guide. For duplicated stents, the ridge lap portion of the stent is trimmed from canine to canine until only the most coronal portion touching the ridge remains. This provides a fairly stable posterior base and when the flap is sutured to itself on the lingual surface allows for visualization of the operative field. The stent should have at least one anterior tooth left to align with the maxillary denture. The

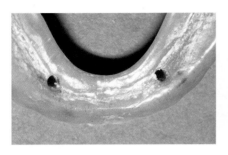

Fig 21-12 *Guide holes have been drilled in the patient's existing denture.*

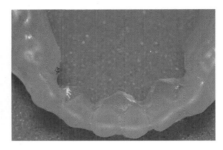

Fig 21-13 *Because teeth on the new denture were to be moved anteriorly in relation to the patient's existing denture, a waxup was made of the proposed prosthesis. This waxup was used to fabricate a stent with lingual cutouts used to guide drills during implant surgery.*

space should be left between two of the anterior implants to place a clip.

Posterior Mandible (Partially or Totally Edentulous Patients)

Implant success in this sextant is less predictable than in the mandibular anterior region because there is usually less available bone and the cortical plate is often thin. For this sextant implants with a large surface area for bony contact such as the ITI System should be considered first if adequate bone is available.

surgeon can then hold the posterior flanges of the guide during use. Correct alignment should place the implant(s) within the bony housing, within the confines of the proposed restoration, parallel to each other and lingual to the maxillary teeth.

Number of Implants Two implants provide the minimum support needed for a prosthesis in these cases. Often, when the patient's chief complaint is soft tissue impingement by their existing denture, two implants will not provide adequate stability to prevent some continued tissue trauma in posterior areas. In these cases, or when bone heights are minimal or there is opposing natural dentition, three to five implants should be considered. O-rings have proven to successfully retain the denture over two implants when the patient wants only minimal additional support. Fixed removable or bar and clip prostheses work well when additional support is needed. When this last approach is used, at least three implants should be consid-

ered to provide additional stability of the denture.

Alignment The following information assumes implant sites are not available in the posterior mandible. However, both the anterior and posterior sextants should be used when increased stability and function are needed if adequate bone is available.

Fixed removable. The most distal implants in this sextant are placed approximately 3 to 5 mm anterior to the mental foramen. Any additional implants can be spaced evenly between these two most distal fixtures and if possible should be aligned with individual teeth in the stent. Enough space should be left between individual implants to provide access for oral hygiene and prosthetic devices; 8 mm between implant centers is suggested.

Bar and clip. When only two implants will be used to support a bar, the implants must be far enough to the anterior so that the bar will not interfere with the tongue or the floor of the mouth.

When a bar and clip is used with three or more implants, adequate

Incisions For those cases using two-stage implants, buccal vestibular incisions are suggested (Fig 21-14). If possible, 1 to 2 mm of interproximal soft tissue should be retained around adjacent teeth. Vertical incisions crossing the ridge to the lingual and straight line incisions away from the implant site can be used if greater visibility is desired. These straight-line incisions should be made within the lingual gingiva but away from the gingival sulcus when possible. If the ITI System is employed, midcrestal incisions with vertical or straight line releasing incisions should be used. Suturing the lingual flap to the anterior teeth or soft tissue will keep the flap out of the surgical field and therefore simplify implant placement.

Guided tissue regeneration is often required in this sextant. Flaps should be larger than normally used and any vertical incisions should be distant from the material used for guided tissue regeneration.

The mental foramen should be located with a curet whenever feasible to increase the chances of avoiding both the mental and inferior alveolar nerves and to give a more accurate assessment of the height of bone coronal to this structure.

Stents In edentulous cases, stents constructed in a fashion similar to that used in mandibular anterior regions are employed. In this sextant, guide holes are ideally placed in the central fossa of the teeth on the stent. If enough teeth remain to stabilize the stent in a partially edentulous patient, a hemimandibular guide is preferred because it allows placement of a bite block on the opposite side of the dental arch while the stent is in use.

In cases where implants will be placed under provisional or existing permanent fixed restorations, a stent can be made to fit the prepared teeth. However, it is often simpler to drill holes in the existing restoration than to construct a new stent (Fig 21-15). Direction of the implant can be accurately predicted by use of metal pins glued to the stent and then used as radiographic markers (Fig 21-16) (Higginbottom F: Personal communication, 1989).

Number of Implants The longer the implants or the greater their combined surface area, the fewer needed. No significant difference in implant-to-implant or implant-to-tooth connections have been found in the short term, but the implant-to-implant prosthetic connections may have a better long-term outlook. When implants and teeth are connected, it is suggested that the teeth have permanently cemented metal copings and that the implant prosthesis serve as a superstructure. When using a screw-retained prosthesis, only one screw is usually needed; this permits simple retrieval of the superstructure.

Alignment There are two prob-

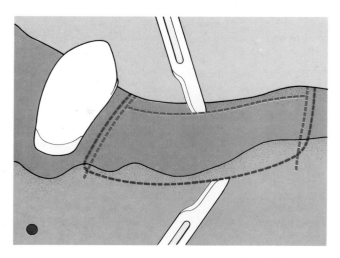

Fig 21-14 *Midcrestal incisions are preferred for ITI and a buccal vestibular approach for Brånemark. A collar of the soft tissue should be left around adjacent teeth if possible. Care should be taken to avoid the mental nerve.*

lems unique to the posterior mandible: the position of the inferior alveolar nerve and the unavailability of an apical (inferior) cortical plate. The latter of these two situations makes Brånemark implants less predictable in this sextant when compared to the anterior mandible. In a few cases the nerve can be moved, and occasionally the facial or (usually) lingual cortical plate can be engaged, but these options are not often available.

To minimize the chance of damaging the nerve, combinations of computerized tomograms, panographic radiographs, and preoperative and intraoperative periapical radiographs can be used to aid in positioning implants (see chapter 19).

Computerized tomograms help to determine the shape of the mandible in cross section and to locate the approximate position of the inferior alveolar canal and mental foramen. Panographic radiographs provide a useful two-dimensional image familiar to the dentist. Unless the precise magnification of the image seen on the panograph is known, one should assume a 25% magnification error. Preoperative periapical radiographs with metal markers on the stent aid implant alignment, while intraoperative films with metal guide markers reveal the coronoapical relation of the implant site relative to the inferior alveolar canal and other adjacent structures.

Placement 5 mm mesial or distal from adjacent teeth to the center of the implant is preferred, with at least 8 mm between the centers of adjacent implants. In cases where the mandibular second premolar is the most anterior missing tooth, placing the first implant 5 mm distal to the first premolar and the molar implant 10 mm distal to that implant will usually place the implant in the center of the prosthetic teeth.

When using a Brånemark implant, if a cortical plate of bone is not engaged, there are several steps that can be taken to increase the probability of success: minimal countersinking, tapping only about one third of the implant depth (when the cancellous bone is thin), stopping the implant

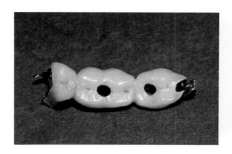

Fig 21-15 *Guide holes have been made in the patient's existing prosthesis to help align implant drills.*

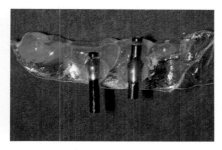

Fig 21-16 *Metal pins have been attached to a plastic stent. Radiographs will show alignment of the pins to the adjacent teeth and permit more accurate fabrication of guide holes in the stent. (Stent courtesy of Dr Donald E. Dobbs.)*

just as the last screw thread is covered by bone, and in very delicate bone using 4-mm-diameter implants. These procedures work well with conventional Brånemark implants. Even though 7-mm Brånemark implants will frequently succeed in this sextant, they should be avoided when possible, and an 8-mm ITI implant used instead.

Maxillary Arch (Partially or Totally Edentulous Patients)

In the maxilla, the prognosis for Brånemark implants is more guarded than that for similar fixtures.[80] Therefore, ITI implants are suggested where their placement is practical. The denser the bony housing, the better the prognosis. As a result of failures in this area,

7-mm Brånemark implants are rarely suggested in the maxillary arch. Inadequate bony housing is frequently found in this arch, and guided tissue regeneration is often appropriate.

Incisions For patients receiving Brånemark implants in whom the incision line will not create an esthetic deformity and guided tissue regeneration is not anticipated, a buccal incision similar to that described in the anterior mandible can be used. When an ITI implant is used, a midcrestal approach is preferred (Fig 21-17). Increased access on the facial surface can be achieved with straight line, or where necessary, intrasulcular incisions around the adjacent teeth. For patients who may require guided tissue regeneration, a split-thickness flap with a palatal approach is often helpful (Fig 21-18).

Stents Stents used for the maxillary arch are similar to those described for the mandibular arch, with a few exceptions. These exceptions include a cutout on the

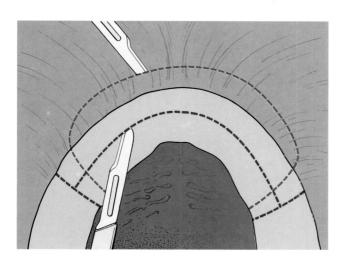

Fig 21-17 *When the patient has a low lip line and two-stage implants are to be placed, a buccal vestibular incision is used. With ITI implants a midcrestal incision is used.*

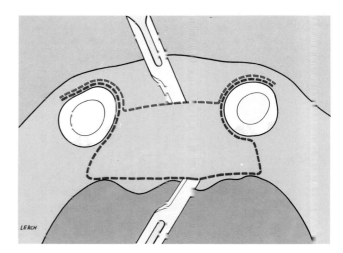

Fig 21-18 *When esthetics is a concern, either a midcrestal or palatal approach with a split-thickness dissection to the bone crest can be used.*

palatal aspect for flap retention and placement of guide holes for anterior teeth being made without the cutaways used in the mandibular arch.

Placement Because of increased esthetic concerns and diminished quality and quantity of bone, placement in the maxilla is often more problematic than in the mandible.

In the anterior region the use of coated stents in conjunction with computerized tomography is helpful in preplacement treatment planning. These stents can be barium coated by the radiologist then used with the computerized tomogram. Later, the barium is removed and the same device is used as a surgical stent.

Number of Implants The number of implants is governed by the need for esthetics, function, and the bone available for optimal placement. Because of the higher failure rate in the maxilla seen with the Brånemark System compared to the mandible, it is often prudent to place more of these implants than the minimal number

needed for proper function. Some placement problems in the maxillary arch may be reduced by recent advances in grafting techniques.

Alignment Resorption patterns in the maxilla often dictate that implants be placed lingual to their natural counterparts or that guided tissue regeneration be used to improve placement. Bone enhancement can be performed before, during, or after implant placement.

Single-Tooth Replacement

Incisions For implants placed in areas of esthetic concern, a midcrestal (for ITI) or palatal (for Brånemark) incision should be used. When additional retraction is necessary on the facial aspect, an intrasulcular releasing incision around the adjacent teeth can be used (see Fig 21-18).

Stents Stents often speed single-tooth replacement where very wide or very narrow edentulous sites are found (Fig 21-19). These stents are best fabricated and used

with radiographic direction markers before the guide hole is drilled. This approach will minimize the chances of hitting adjacent teeth during implant site preparation.

Alignment When esthetics is of concern, proper implant alignment is vital. The following guidelines are designed to enhance the esthetics of the final prosthesis by optimizing implant placement.

Buccolingual position. The position of the implant in a buccolingual direction depends on available bone and the type of prosthetic abutment to be used for the final restoration. For a conventional Brånemark abutment, the center of the fixture should project through the lingual cingulum of anterior teeth and in the central fossa of posterior teeth. If a tapered cylinder Brånemark abutment or ITI implant is to be used, then the center of the implant should exit at the lingual incisal edge of anterior teeth and in the central fossa of the posterior dentition.

Mesiodistal position. In cases where the distance between ad-

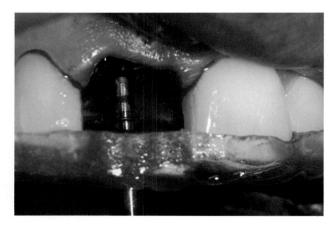

Fig 21-19 *A stent which has a guide hole rests on adjacent teeth and aides in drill alignment. (Slide courtesy of Dr Frank L. Higginbottom.)*

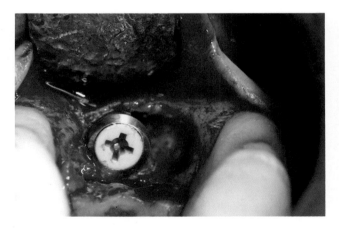

Fig 21-20 *This ITI implant, which replaced a left maxillary lateral incisor, was positioned closer to the central incisor than to the canine. This placement matched the location of the right incisor. Guided tissue regeneration was used to regenerate the lost bone seen in the photograph.*

jacent teeth will allow fabrication of a restoration the same size and shape of the missing tooth, the implant should be placed in the center of the edentulous space. In spaces of 6 mm or less, placement becomes difficult both because of lack of access for implant instruments and the root / implant proximity often created. In edentulous spaces wider than the extracted tooth, careful presurgical planning, often including a waxup, is often needed to achieve the desired esthetic result (Fig 21-20).

Occlusoapical position. The implant should be placed far enough apically to achieve the proper emergence profile on the implant prosthesis. To obtain this goal with Brånemark implants, the coronal end of the implant should be located a minimum of 3 mm apical to a line connecting the free gingival margins on the adjacent teeth. The wider the space between adjacent teeth, the more apically the coronal portion of the implant must be carried to enhance esthetics (Goldberg P: Personal communication, 1990). For ITI implants, 1 mm of facial bone must be available to prevent gin-

gival recession. Additionally, ITI implants should be placed 1 mm more apical than normal in areas of esthetic concern.

Number of Implants One implant for each missing tooth is indicated in most single-tooth replacements. For single-tooth replacement in the maxillary anterior sextant, an ITI Hollow Cylinder with a 15-degree angled head can be used. The angle of the implant head often allows better use of available bone, and the 5-mm bevel helps to create an esthetic restoration with a favorable emergence profile.

GUIDED TISSUE REGENERATION AROUND DENTAL IMPLANTS

The concept of excluding the epithelium and connective tissues of the gingiva from healing surgical wounds around natural teeth was introduced to dentistry in 1979.[81]

The goal of this therapy is to regenerate lost periodontal attachment apparatus (alveolar bone, periodontal ligament, and cementum). Details of this concept, which is now termed *guided tissue regeneration,*[82] can be found in chapter 11.

Guided tissue regeneration (GTR) was later applied to osseointegrated dental implants, the goal of treatment in these cases being generation of bone. The original work on this subject was published by Dahlin and co-workers in 1989.[72] In this study a polytetrafluorethylene (PTFE) membrane was placed to cover Brånemark dental implants in an animal model. Several screw threads of each implant were left uncovered by the bony housing. In the experimental site, the membrane was draped over the implant and then covered with a soft tissue flap that included the periosteum; the control site received no membrane. When the stage-two surgery was performed, the experimental areas had bone growth that covered the previously exposed threads in almost every case. The differences in bone growth between the experimental and control sites were statistically significant.

Before the introduction of GTR it was suggested that one wait several months following tooth extraction before placing implants.[83] Others suggested that placing dental implants into fresh or recent extraction sites was possible only under certain limited conditions.[84-86] These conditions usually required a large amount of preexisting bone in the potential implant site. These concepts were changed when the idea of using a PTFE membrane in immediate extraction sites was introduced by Lazzara.[74]

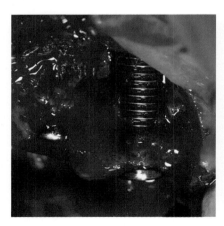

Fig 21-21 *This implant was placed with a large dehiscence. At uncovering, the implant was mobile and was removed.*

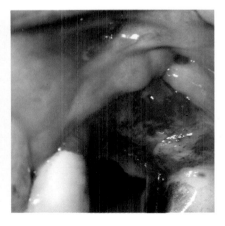

Fig 21-22 *A large soft tissue defect was left under a piece of e-PTFE periodontal material that had migrated through the soft tissue.*

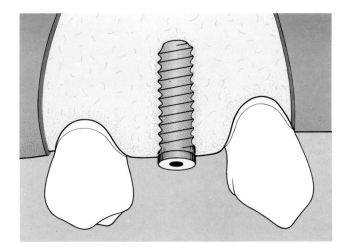

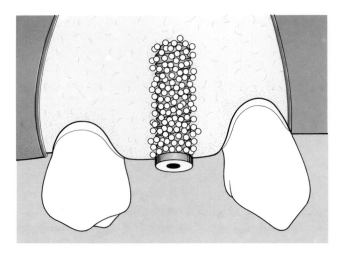

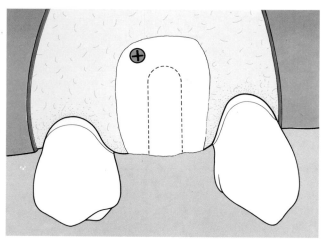

Fig 21-23a (above left) *A full-thickness mucoperiosteal flap is raised and the extraction site is debrided.*

Fig 21-23b (above right) *The implant is placed and a graft of freeze-dried bone is placed over exposed portions of the implant body.*

Fig 21-23c (left) *e-PTFE augmentation material is trimmed to fit over the implant, under the flap, and away from adjacent teeth. It is then held in place with sutures or screws.*

Immediate and Recent Extraction Sites and Dehiscences

This section deals with the clinical application of PTFE membranes in dehiscences and in immediate or recent extraction sites. In addition, a technique to use this membrane for preserving and regenerating bone in immediate extraction sites or in deficient ridges will be discussed.

Rarely does bone grow to cover an implant dehiscence around a titanium implant between first- and second-stage surgery. These exposed areas have typically created problems for the patient, ranging from difficulty in cleaning the area, to discomfort, to loss of the implant (Fig 21-21).

Initially, Gore-Tex Periodontal Material (e-PTFE periodontal material) (W. L. Gore & Associates) was used in fresh extraction sites as a tent placed over the implant and bone but subadjacent to the soft tissues (including the periosteum). While bone usually regenerated quite well using this approach, the shape memory in the material often resulted in migration of the membrane through the soft tissues during healing and occasionally left an unwanted soft tissue defect. This was especially true when the material was left in place until the stage-two surgery (Fig 21-22).

Presently, a new material called Gore-Tex Augmentation Material (e-PTFE augmentation material) (W. L. Gore & Associates) is suggested for these areas. This material has less shape memory and was designed especially for use with dental implants. This new material works well and often results in significant bony regeneration when primary flap closure is achieved at surgery and the material stays covered (Figs 21-23 to 21-25). GTR is also possible around ITI implants (Figs 21-26a to c). The material occasionally becomes uncovered, and in approximately 10% of these cases, infection is seen. These infections can destroy bone around the implants and

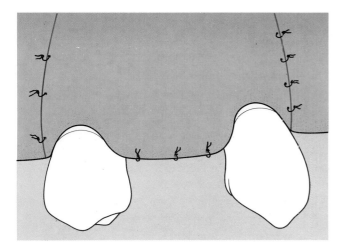

Fig 21-23d *Primary flap closure is achieved.*

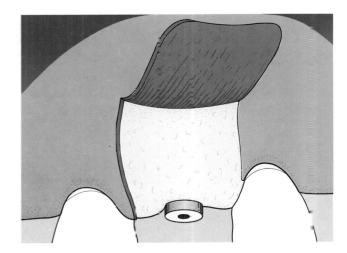

Fig 21-23e *Upon reopening, bone generation has occurred.*

may contribute to implant loss (Figs 21-27a and b).

Initial suggestions to hold the e-PTFE augmentation material in place with the implant cover screw created retrieval problems. Presently, it is suggested that a tent of e-PTFE augmentation material be placed over the implant and the site where bone generation is desired. Primary soft tissue closure seems important and often necessitates releasing incisions or scoring the periosteal surface with a scalpel blade to achieve sufficient flap mobility. If the material becomes exposed within the first 30 to 45 days after placement, the patient is continued on twice daily chlorhexidine rinses and the material is removed 30 to 45 days after placement. If the material becomes uncovered after 30 days, it is removed as soon after discovery of the problem as possible.

One of the keys to successfully generating bone under these membranes is to allow space for hard tissue to fill. In some extraction sites the remaining bony anatomy holds the membrane away from the implant, providing adequate space. Additional space, where needed, can be provided by the use of freeze-dried bone or specially designed screws designed to hold space.

Early experiences with GTR led to the guidelines seen in Table 21-1.

TABLE 21-1 *Preliminary guidelines for guided tissue regeneration around root form osseointegrated dental implants*

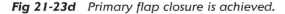

1. Use guided tissue regeneration with two-stage titanium implants in immediate extraction sites. One-stage or two-stage titanium implants may be indicated for use in areas of deficient ridge.
2. Site selection:
   • There should be enough bone to initially stabilize the implant.
   • Thick soft tissues over the implant site are optimal because less exposure of the material occurs.
   • Primary closure of soft tissues over the material is suggested.
3. e-PTFE augmentation material is suggested for two-stage placement, while e-PTFE periodontal material is used around one-stage implants.
4. The use of the material to form a tent over the implant is preferred to securing the material with the fixture's cover screw.
5. Care during the healing phase:
   • When using a method that involves initial primary closure, any material that comes uncovered should be suspect and carefully observed.
   • Material that becomes uncovered before 30 to 45 days (after placement) should be removed 30 to 45 days after placement.
   • Material that becomes uncovered after 30 to 45 days should be removed as soon as the exposure is discovered.
   • Twice daily use of chlorhexidine rinses is suggested as a routine for 4 weeks after surgery and should be reinstituted if membrane exposure occurs at a later date.
   • Antibiotics are suggested beginning before surgery and for 3 weeks postoperatively.

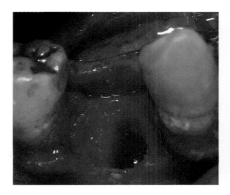

Fig 21-24a *A clinical case seen after extraction and debridement.*

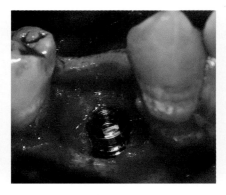

Fig 21-24b *The implant in place.*

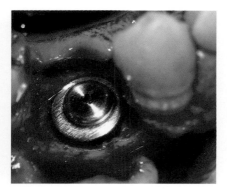

Fig 21-24c *The bone graft is placed and a titanium washer placed to act as a space holder. (Washer courtesy of Dr William E. Becker.)*

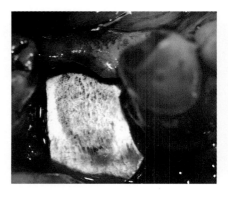

Fig 21-24d *The trimmed e-PTFE augmentation material in place.*

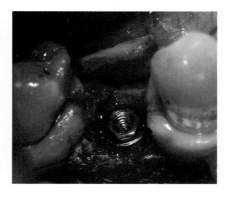

Fig 21-24e *At stage-two surgery, bone regeneration was found completely encasing the body of the implant.*

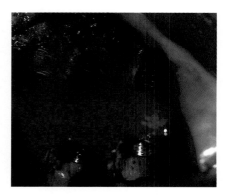

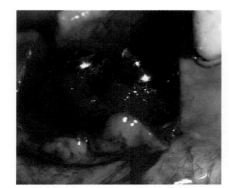

Fig 21-25a (above left) *Implants were placed in sockets of extracted maxillary premolars. Bone grafts and e-PTFE augmentation material were placed.*

Fig 21-25b (below left) *Original radiograph.*

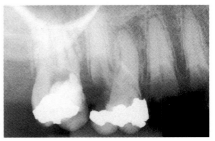

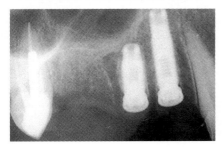

Fig 21-25c (above right) *The area seen originally in Fig 21-25a, uncovered 6 months later. Hard tissue that clinically and radiographically appeared to be bone had generated around the implants.*

Fig 21-25d (below right) *Radiograph 6 months after implant placement.*

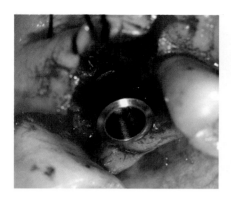

Fig 21-26a *An ITI implant placed into an edentulous ridge deficient on the lingual surface.*

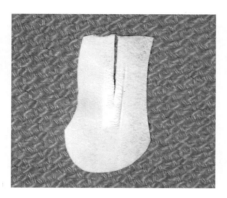

Fig 21-26b *A piece of e-PTFE periodontal material, designed for freestanding premolars, shaped and split to fit around the ITI implant.*

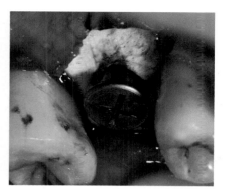

Fig 21-26c *The material placed and sutured to the facial surface.*

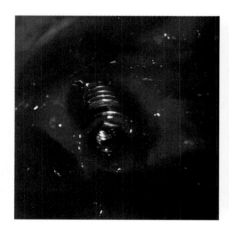

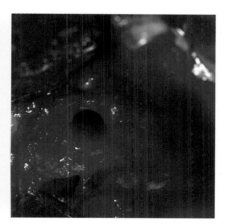

Fig 21-27a *(left) An implant at placement before bone graft and e-PTFE augmentation material were placed.*

Fig 21-27b *(right) The tissue around the e-PTFE augmentation material placed over the implant became infected. It went unreported by the patient. The implant was lost.*

BONY RIDGE ENHANCEMENT

An adequate amount of residual bone is often not available to initially stabilize an implant, thereby allowing the use of GTR. In these cases, adequate bone can often be gained by using GTR before implant placement. In these cases, the residual socket (or ridge) should be completely debrided of soft tissue after flap retraction; then marrow penetrations are made. Space for regeneration is created by the use of e-PTFE periodontal material or e-PTFE augmentation material. The newly created space is held by various means including specially designed screws and can be filled with freeze-dried bone or other materials. The surgical area is allowed to heal for 6 to 9 months and then an implant can be placed (Figs 21-28a to d). The e-PTFE material should be treated like that used around implants. This usually results in a dense bony housing suitable for implant stabilization.

SUPPORTIVE PERIODONTAL TREATMENT FOR OSSEOINTEGRATED IMPLANTS

Osseointegrated implants have an intimate association with the bone when viewed under a light microscope. These implants have a greater longevity than do their fibro-osseous counterparts.[78] This longevity may be related both to the bony interface with the implant and, in those made from titanium, to the hemidesmosomal attachment seen between implant and soft tissue.[87] This is an epithe-

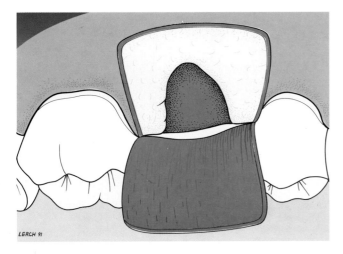

Fig 21-28a *This cracked molar's roots extended into the maxillary sinus. The tooth was extracted.*

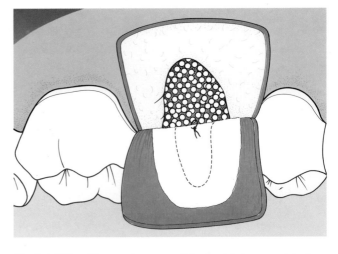

Fig 21-28b *The socket was filled with freeze-dried bone and covered.*

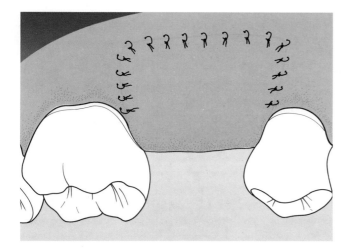

Fig 21-28c *The area 30 days after placement and just prior to removal.*

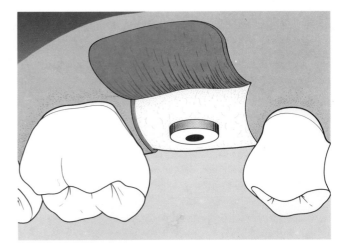

Fig 21-28d *The area 6 months later at stage-one implant surgery. The bone was very dense and was found at the level of the original extraction site.*

lial attachment similar to that seen around teeth.

The few studies done on the microbiology of the ecosystem around osseointegrated implants[55,58,88] suggest that periodontal-like breakdown is possible around these teeth. This breakdown can be termed peri-implantitis.

Diagnosis of Peri-implantitis Around Root Form Osseointegrated Implants

1. Radiographs. Periapical radiographs are helpful in diagnosing problems around these implants. If the clinician needs a right-angle view of the entire implant, it may be necessary to remove the overlying prosthesis or to make a specially designed holder. However, in most cases a combination of periapical and vertical bite-wing radiographs will provide adequate information on the bone / implant interface. Right-angle radiographs are needed because the thin line that is often seen around failing implants can be easily obscured by small changes in angulation (see chapter 5). One study showed that Brånemark implants can be expected to lose about 0.5 to 1 mm of bone the first postoperative year and then 0.06 to 0.08 mm per year afterwards. Changes greater than these should be viewed with alarm.[89]

2. Sound. An osseointegrated titanium implant produces a ringing sound when struck with a metal instrument. This can be used as one of the diagnostic criteria for health. To accomplish this, the overlying prosthesis must be removed, which may not be possible or practical to perform at each SPT visit. It should be noted that this parameter may be positive even after significant bony support has been lost around the implant.

3. Probe. There is a question about whether implants should be probed, because little evidence exists of a direct connective tissue interface. Probing may then strip away the epithelial attachment. Despite this warning, probing seems a reasonable approach to ascertain gingival health and to take pocket probing depths. The information provided would be improved if a known probing force could be used so the clinician could be consistent. A plastic probe is suggested to avoid scratching the implants (Fig 21-29), but unfortunately no such probe with a constant force is currently available.

4. Gingival bleeding, color, and tone. No bleeding should be seen upon probing. This parameter is particularly important because patients with poor oral hygiene tend to have more rapid breakdown around implants than patients who clean well.[89] Gingival color should be the same as around a healthy tooth. The tissue tone should be tight even though some osseointegrated implants do well despite a lack of gingiva. At present, however, the literature and clinical experience suggest that a band of keratinized tissue is desirable.[90]

5. Plaque and calculus. The

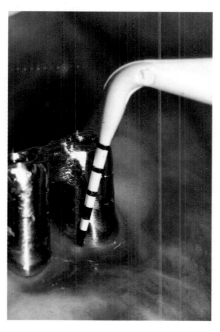

Fig 21-29 *A plastic probe used to check pocket probing depths (Prodentec).*

presence or absence of plaque and calculus on these implants should be noted, and these deposits should be removed at each SPT visit.

6. Occlusal factors. Osseointegrated implants can successfully support greater loading than fibro-osseous implants of similar size. However, one should still avoid excessive occlusal loads because these forces (especially in the form of bruxing) may accelerate breakdown.[89] This seems to hold true despite the fact that some would argue that the quantity and quality of bone actually increases around the implant in the patient who has parafunctional habits.

7. Prosthesis check. The implant prosthesis should be checked to ensure that there is no movement and that the screws or cement seals remain tight; otherwise, fracture may occur. Small changes in the prosthetic device can be translated into very detrimental effects on the implants themselves.

8. Microbiologic monitoring. A recent study by Mombelli and co-workers[58] studied healthy and failing titanium implants in the same mouth. They found microbes similar to those seen in healthy crevices around teeth in the sulci surrounding successful implants. Around failing implants they saw bacteria much like those found around teeth with periodontitis. This type of monitoring may be useful in the recalcitrant case but is not suggested as a routine.

Prevention of Peri-implantitis

Supragingival and subgingival deposits should be removed at each SPT visit. Plaque can be removed using Super Floss (Oral-B) or gauze or with a fine pumice in a rubber cup (Fig 21-30).[91] Calculus on these surfaces is not as tenacious as on natural teeth and usually can be readily removed. Use of specially designed rigid plastic or titanium instruments can be used for this purpose (Fig 21-31). Care should be used with the titanium curet to break away the calcium but not to scratch the implant surface. Avoid ultrasonic scalers and interdental brushes with exposed metal because these tend to scar the implant surface.[92] A chlorhexidine mouthrinse can help to clean prostheses that have large surfaces approximating the soft tissues as well as the implants themselves. This mouthrinse, along with metronidazole, may help to reduce gingival hyperplasia seen around these implants[91]; however, a gingival graft is occasionally neces-

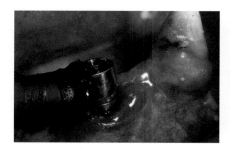

Fig 21-30 *Fine pumice in a rubber cup can be used to remove bacterial plaque from implants.*

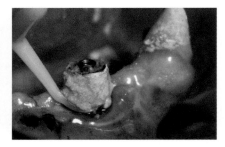

Fig 21-31 *Several plastic instruments are available for calculus removal but none work well.*

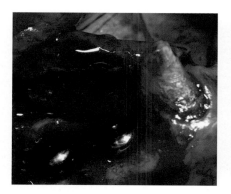

Fig 21-32a *Implants at the time of placement in a patient previously diagnosed as having refractory periodontitis.*

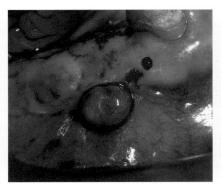

Fig 21-32b *A few days later, the patient presented with localized swelling and tenderness around the most mesial implant. Various antibiotics were used but the problem continued.*

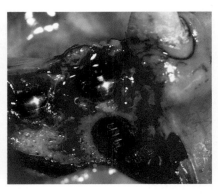

Fig 21-32c *Thirty days after placement the area was opened and the mesial implant, which was mobile, was removed. Cultures taken during this period identified an antibiotic appropriate for use during stage-two surgery.*

Fig 21-33a *A peri-implant infection had destroyed the bone circumferentially around this implant. The area was opened and debrided with titanium curets, and the implant was cleaned with chlorhexidine.*

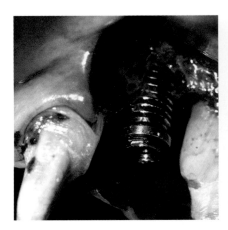

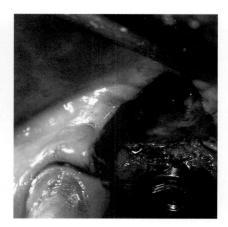

Fig 21-33b *The implant 3 months after guided tissue regeneration. The tissue around the implant is hard but may not be bone.*

sary to eliminate this condition. Little information on correct SPT intervals for totally edentulous patients is available, but for now these patients should be placed on SPT 3 months after stage-two surgery and seen every 3 months for the first year. If the peri-implant tissues are stable, then previously edentulous patients can be seen every 6 months. Patients with remaining teeth should be seen on an average of every 3 months.

At home patients should be encouraged to use manual methods for personal oral hygiene. These include toothbrushes (regular or single tuft rotating) and gauze or specially designed dental floss. Chlorhexidine can be used where manual methods are found wanting.

Failure of Osseointegrated Systems

Long-term information is available only on the Brånemark Sys-

tem at present. These implants fail in one of two ways: very rapidly or very slowly. The rapid failures (most within the first year) are the most common and are usually because of failure to osseointegrate or prematurely placing strong mechanical forces on the fixtures. Other failures due to material breakdown have been reported. The rapidly failing implant is often doomed; however, removal of excess loads, if discovered early, along with guided tissue regeneration where indicated, may allow retention of the implant (see the following section). Slowly progressing bone loss can be treated by more conventional methods to control the inflammatory process. These include reinforcement of oral hygiene, soft tissue curettage, and flap operations with guided tissue regeneration when appropriate. This slow bone loss appears radiographically like that seen around a tooth.

COMPLICATIONS

Despite efforts to provide a sterile field and routine prescription of postoperative antibiotics, postinsertion infections do occur. Some lead to implant loss. The infection may occur around the implant or an e-PTFE membrane used for guided tissue regeneration.

There is some evidence that aggressive periodontitis around remaining teeth serves as a nidus for infection.[93] In such cases, prescribing appropriate antibiotics before and after surgery would seem prudent (Figs 21-32a to c).

When the infection is found, it should first be treated by a change in antibiotics, which often rectifies the situation. When no positive response is seen, the area should be opened surgically and debrided. Often GTR can accompany this operation (Figs 21-33a and b). If the implant is mobile or becomes mobile at a later date, it is removed.

QUICK REVIEW

CHOICE OF IMPLANT SYSTEM AND CLINICAL MANAGEMENT

I. Prerequisites for successful osseointegration
- Titanium is the biomaterial of choice. The formation of an oxide layer protects against corrosion.
- Macroretentions and microretentions appear necessary for adequate anchorage. Rough surfaces are superior to smooth surfaces.
- Primary stability must be obtained to minimize the gap between the bone and the implant. Careful preparation at low speed (< 800 rpm) of the implant bed and abundant irrigation for cooling are necessary.
- Postoperative loading of the implants must be avoided for at least 3 months.

II. Peri-implant infection
- Bacterial colonization occurs rapidly after implant installation (or abutment placement). Bacteria are recruited from ecological niches of the oral cavity. Pathogens are sparse.
- A microbiota consisting predominantly of gram-negative anaerobic bacteria resembling that seen associated with advanced periodontitis is encountered at failing implant sites.
- Antibacterial therapy, including chemical plaque control with chlorhexidine and systemic antibiotics such as metronidazole, may control a developing infection. Flap surgery in combination with or without GTR may be advocated.

Quick Review continues on page 372.

QUICK REVIEW
(continued)

- Regular supportive therapy is a prerequisite for success. Chemical plaque control may also be advocated as an adjunctive preventive measure.

III. Regeneration of alveolar bone
- The GTR principle may be applied to regenerate alveolar bone.
- Depending on the placement of a barrier membrane, substantial amounts of the host's own local bone may be regenerated.

IV. Clinical overview
- Titanium osseointegrated root form implants should be the clinician's first choice.
- Because of its single-stage placement, increased attachment, surface, and titanium construction, the clinician should consider the ITI System. The preferred forms are the Hollow Screw and the Hollow Cylinder.
- In immediate extraction sites, or where early implant loading may be a problem, the Brånemark System is suggested.

V. Improving implant placement

Anterior mandible (totally edentulous patient)
- Incisions — midcrestal: ITI, facial vestibule, Brånemark
- Stents — duplication of the new or existing denture or guide holes in the existing denture
- Number of implants
  - two: used for patients having problems with denture displacement
  - three to four: can be used with bar and clips to provide more stability
  - four to six: used with a fixed / removable prosthesis
- Alignment
  - fixed removable: place most posterior fixtures 3 to 5 mm anterior to mental foramen (assumes no posterior implants), implants at least 8 mm center to center
  - bar and clip: place most distal implants in a similar manner to fixed removable placement then leave space for a wide clip between more anterior implants (assumes three or more implants)

Posterior mandible (partially or totally edentulous patient)
- Incisions — midcrestal for ITI; for Brånemark in the buccal vestibule if bony anatomy not well known (for possible guided tissue regeneration)
- Stents
  - for edentulous cases make similar to that described for the anterior mandible, but guide holes in central fossa
  - for fixed removable cases use an existing provisional or permanent bridge where possible
- Number of implants — the more the implant-to-bone surface, the fewer implants needed
- Alignment
  - care should be taken to avoid the inferior alveolar nerve and when using solid screw implants to engage the lingual or labial cortical plates where possible
  - implants should be placed approximately 5 mm from adjacent teeth with 8 mm between premolar implants (10 mm for molars)

Maxillary arch (partially or totally edentulous patient)
- Incisions — Brånemark: buccal when no esthetic problem, palatal with esthetic problems or expected guided tissue regeneration; ITI: midcrestal except where two-stage guided tissue. regeneration is expected, then palatal
- Stents — similar to those for mandibular arch except that palate is removed to hold the flap and guide holes are used instead of grooves.
- Number of implants — the poorer quality of bone in the maxilla may require placement of more Brånemark implants than in the mandible for the same degree of success.

QUICK REVIEW
(continued)

CHOICE OF IMPLANT SYSTEM AND
CLINICAL MANAGEMENT

- Alignment — maxillary ridges resorb to the lingual complicating implant placement, often necessitating guided tissue regeneration.

Single-tooth replacement

- Incisions — midcrestal or palatal where esthetics are of concern or GTR is anticipated
- Stents — usually needed when teeth are very close together or widely spaced
- Alignment
  (1) buccolingual
    - for Brånemark, using the original abutment cylinder, the center of the implant should exit the lingual cingulum of anterior tooth and the central fossa of posteriors
    - for single-tooth Brånemark abutment or ITI implants, the center should exit just lingual to or just even with the incisal edge
  (2) mesiodistal: alignment should allow construction of a natural looking prosthesis
  (3) occlusoapical: where esthetics is a concern, the coronal end of the implant should be located a minimum of 3 mm apical to a line connecting the free gingival margins of adjacent teeth. The wider the interdental space, the more apically the coronal portion of the implant should be placed
  (4) number of implants: usually one implant per missing tooth
VI. Guided tissue regeneration (GTR) around dental implants and bony ridge enhancement
- Bone can be generated (or regenerated) around dental implants using the guidelines similar to those used for GTR around natural teeth.

- Gore-Tex Augmentation Material e-PTFE augmentation material (a modified polytetrafluoroethylene membrane) can be used to allow bone to form around implants in fenestrations, dehiscences, or in immediate or recent extractions sites.
- Gore-Tex Periodontal Material (e-PTFE periodontal material) can be used to enhance localized bony deficiency to improve chances for implant success.
VII. Supportive periodontal treatment for osseointegrated implants
- Diagnosis of peri-implantitis
  - radiographs: right-angle periapical or bitewings preferred
  - sound: a ringing noise is made when osseointegrated implants are struck by a metal instrument
  - probe: implants should be probed at each SPT visit
  - gingival bleeding, color, and tone should be noted
  - plaque and calculus should be recorded
  - occlusal factors: premature contacts and high stress loads should be removed
  - prosthesis check: the overlying prosthesis should be checked at each SPT visit
  - microbiologic monitoring: this may be needed around failing implants
- Prevention of peri-implantitis SPT for osseointegrated implants
  (1) supragingival and subgingival deposits should be removed at each visit
    - remove soft deposits with fine pumice and a rubber cup
    - remove calculus with a plastic scaler
  (2) reinforce oral hygiene
VIII. Failure / complications
- Osseointegrated implants may fail rapidly or slowly.
- GTR can help lengthen the service of some failing implants

REFERENCES

1. Wahl G: Neuere Möglichkeiten zur Kontrolle enossaler Einheilungsvorgänge in der zahnärztlichen Implantologie mit Hilfe der Szintigraphie. Med. Thesis, Bonn, 1985.

2. Dahl GSA: Om möjligheten för implantation i käken av metall-skelett som bas eller retention för fasta eller avtagbara proteser. *Odontol Tidskr* 1943;51:400-449.

3. Köle H: Erfahrungen mit Gerüstimplantaten unter die Schleimhaut und Haut zur Befestigung von Prothesen und Epithesen. *Fortschr Kiefer Gesichtschir* 1965;10:76-89.

4. Bodine RI, Yanase RT: Thirty year report on 28 implant dentures inserted between 1952 and 1959. Proc Int Symp on Preprosth Surg, Palm Springs, California, 1985.

5. Bosker H: *The Transmandibular Implant.* Thesis, University of Utrecht, The Netherlands, 1986.

6. Linkow LI: The multipurpose blade: A three-year progress report. *J Oral Implantol* 1981;9(4):509-529.

7. Weiss CM: Tissue integration of dental endosseous implants: Description and comparative analysis of the fibro-osseous integration and osseous integration systems. *J Oral Implantol* 1986;12:169-214.

8. Brånemark PI, Zarb GA, Albrektsson T: *Tissue-Integrated Prostheses: Osseointegration in Clinical Dentistry.* Chicago: Quintessence Publ Co, 1985.

9. Schulte W: Das enossale Tübinger Implantat aus Al$_2$O$_3$ (Frialit). Der Entwicklungsstand nach 6 Jahren. I. and II. *Zahnärztl Mitt* 1981;71:1114, 1181.

10. Albrektsson T, Brånemark P-I, Hansson HA, Lindström J: Osseointegrated titanium implants. *Acta Orthop Scand* 1981;52:155-170.

11. Brånemark P-I, Breine U, Adell R, Hansson BO, Lindström J, Olsson A: Intraosseous anchorage of dental prostheses. I. Experimental studies. *Scand J Plast Reconstr Surg* 1969;3:81-100.

12. Schroeder A, Pohler O, Sutter F: Gewebsreaktion auf ein Titan-Hohlzylinderimplantat mit Titan-Spritzschichtoberfläche. *Schweiz Mschr Zahnheilk* 1976;86:713-727.

13. Brånemark P-I, Breine U, Adell R, Hansson BO, Lindström J, Olsson A: Osseointegrated implants in the treatment of the edentulous jaw. Experience from a 10-year period. *Scand J Plast Reconstr Surg* 1977;11(Suppl 16):1-132.

14. Sutter F, Schroeder A, Buser D: The new concept of ITI hollow-cylinder and hollow-screw implants: Part 1. Engineering and design. *Int J Oral Maxillofac Implants* 1988;3:161-172.

15. Buser D, Schroeder A, Sutter F, Lang NP: The new concept of ITI hollow-cylinder and hollow-screw implants: Part 2: Clinical aspects, indications and early clinical results. *Int J Oral Maxillofac Implants* 1988;3:173-181.

16. Steinemann SG: Corrosion of titanium and Ti-alloys for surgical implants. Proc 5th Inernat Conf Deutsche Ges Metallkunde. Titanium, Science and Technology, Oberursel, 1985:1373-1379.

17. Steinemann SG, Perren SM: Titanlegierungen für Implantate-physikochemische Prinzipien. Deutscher Verb für Materialprüfung. 5th Lecture Series DVM Workgroup for Implants, Berlin, 1985:63-73.

18. Carlsson L, Röstlund T, Albrektsson B, Albrektsson T: Removal torques for polished and rough titanium implants. *Int J Oral Maxillofac Implants* 1988;3:21-24.

19. Steinemann SG, Eulenberger J, Mäusli PA, Schroeder A: Adhesion of bone to titanium. *Adv Biomat* 1986;6:409-414.

20. Buser D, Schenk RK, Steinemann S, Fiorellini JP, Fox C, Stich H: Influence of surface characteristics on bone integration of titanium implants. A histomorphometric study in miniature pigs. *J Biomed Mater Res* 1991 (In press).

21. Albrektsson T, Sennerby L: Direct bone anchorage of oral implants: Clinical and experimental considerations of the concept of osseointegration. *Int J Prosthodont* 1990;3:30-41.

22. Gotfredsen K, Rostrup E, Hjörting-Hansen E, Budtz-Jørgensen E: Histological and histomorphometrical evaluation of tissue reactions adjacent to endosteal implants in monkeys. *Clin Oral Impl Res* 1991;2:30-37.

23. Babbush CA, Kent JN, Misiek DJ: Titanium plasma-sprayed (TPS) screw implants for the reconstruction of the edentulous mandible. *J Oral Maxillofac Surg* 1986;44:274-282.

24. Schroeder A, Sutter F, Krekeler G: *Orale Implantologie. Allgemeine Grundlagen und ITI-Hohlzylindersystem.* Stuttgart, New York: Georg Thieme, 1988.

25. Buser D, Weber HP, Lang NP: Tissue integration of non-submerged implants. 1-year results of a prospective study with 100 ITI hollow-cylinder and hollow-screw implants. *Clin Oral Impl Res* 1990;1:33-40.

26. Albrektsson T, Zarb G, Worthington P, Eriksson AR: The long-term efficacy of currently used dental implants: A review and proposed criteria of success. *Int J Oral Maxillofac Implants* 1986;1:11-25.

27. Schenk R, Willenegger H: Zur Histologie der primären Knochenheilung. Modifikationen und grenzen der Spaltheilung in Abhängigkeit von der Defektgrösse. *Unfallheilk* 1977;80:155-160.

28. Brunski JB: The influence of force, motion and related quantities on the response of bone to implants. In: Fitzgerald R Jr, ed. *Non-Cemented Total Lip Arthroplasty.* New York: Raven Press; 1988:7-21.

29. Brunski JB: Biomechanics of oral implants: Future research directions. *J Dent Educ* 1988;52:775-787.

30. Nyman S, Gottlow J, Karring T, Lindhe J: The regenerative potential of the periodontal ligament. An experimental study in the monkey. *J Clin Periodontol* 1982;9:257-265.

31. Gottlow J, Nyman S, Karring T, Lindhe J: New attachment formation as the result of controlled tissue regeneration. *J Clin Periodontol* 1984;11:494-503.

32. Aukhill I, Simpson DM, Suggs C, Pettersson E: In vivo differentiation of progenitor cells of the periodontal ligament. An experimental study using physical barriers. *J Clin Periodontol* 1986;13:863-868.

33. Aukhill I, Iglhaut J: Periodontal ligament cell kinetics following experimental regenerative procedures. *J Clin Periodontol* 1988;15:374-382.

34. Buser D, Warrer K, Karring T, Stich H: Titanium implants with a true periodontal ligament: An alternative to osseointegrated implants? *Int J Oral Maxillofac Implants* 1990;5:113-116.

35. Buser D, Warrer K, Karring T: Formation of a periodontal ligament around titanium implants. *J Periodontol* 1990;61:597-601.

36. Albrektsson T, Brånemark P-I, Hansson HA, Ivarsson B, Jönsson U: Ultrastructural analysis of the interface zone of titanium and gold implants. *Adv Biomat* 1982;4:167-177.

37. Listgarten MA, Buser D, Steinemann S, Donath K, Weber HP, Lang NP: Light and transmission electron microscopy of the intact interface between bone, gingiva and non-submerged titanium-coated epoxy resin implants. *J Dent Res* 1991(accepted for publication).

38. Listgarten MA, Lai CH: Ultrastructure of the intact interface between an endosseous epoxy resin dental implant and the host tissues. *J Biol Buccale* 1975;3:13-28.

39. van Drie HJY, Beertsen W, Grevers A: Healing of the gingiva following installment of Biotes® implants in Beagle dogs. *Adv Biomat* 1988;8:485.

40. Buser D, Stich H, Krekeler G, Schroeder A: Faserstrukturen der periimplantären Mukosa bei Titanimplantaten. Eine tierexperimentelle Studie am

Beagle-Hund. *Z Zahnärztl Implantol* 1989;5:15-23.

41. Schroeder A, van der Zypen E, Stich H, Sutter F: The reactions of bone, connective tissue, and epithelium to endosteal implants with titanium-sprayed surfaces. *J Maxillofac Surg* 1981;9:15-25.

42. Inoue T, Cox JE, Pilliar RM, Melcher AH: Effect of the surface geometry of smooth and porous-coated titanium alloy on the orientation of fibroblasts in vitro. *J Biomed Mater Res* 1987; 21:107-126.

43. Adell R, Lekholm U, Röckler B, Brånemark P-I: A 15-year study of osseointegrated implants in the treatment of the edentulous jaw. *Int J Oral Surg* 1981;10:387-416.

44. James RA, Schultz RL: Hemidesmosomes and the adhesion of junctional epithelial cells to metal implants—A preliminary report. *Oral Implantol* 1974;4:294-302.

45. Gould TRL, Brunette DM, Westbury L: The attachment mechanism of epithelial cells to titanium in vitro. *J Periodont Res* 1981;16:611-616.

46. McKinney RV Jr, Steflik DE, Koth DL: Evidence for junctional epithelial attachment to ceramic dental implants. A transmission electron microscopic study. *J Periodontol* 1985;56:579-591.

47. Peterson LJ, Pennel BM, McKinney RV Jr, Klawitter JJ, Weinstein AM: Clinical, radiographical, and histological evaluation of porous rooted polymethylmethacrylate dental implants. *J Dent Res* 1979;58:489-496.

48. Listgarten MA, Ellegaard B: Electron microscopic evidence of a cellular attachment between junctional epithelium and dental calculus. *J Periodont Res* 1973;8:143-150.

49. Schmid B, Spycher I, Schmid J, Lang NP: Plasminogen activator in human gingival tissues adjacent to titanium dental implants. *Clin Oral Implant Res* 1991 (In press).

50. Socransky SS, Tanner ACR, Haffajee AD, Hillman JD, Goodson JM: Present status of studies on the microbial etiology of periodontal disease. In: Genco RJ, Mergenhagen SE, eds. *Host Parasite Interactions in Periodontal Diseases.* Washington, DC: American Society of Microbiology; 1982 1-12.

51. Listgarten MA: The role of dental plaque in gingivitis and periodontitis. *J Clin Periodontol* 1988;15:485-487.

52. Mombelli A, Buser D, Lang NP: Colonization of osseointegrated titanium implants in edentulous patients. Early results. *Oral Microbiol Immunol* 1988;3:113-120.

53. Mombelli A, Mericske-Stern R: Microbiological features of stable osseointegrated implants used as abutments for overdentures. *Clin Oral Implant Res* 1990;1:1-7.

54. Quirynen M, Listgarten MA: The distribution of bacterial morphotypes around natural teeth and titanium implants ad modem Brånemark. *Clin Oral Implant Res* 1990:1:8-12.

55. Lekholm U, Ericsson I, Adell R, Slots J: The condition of the soft tissues at tooth and fixture abutments supporting fixed bridges. A microbiological and histological study. *J Clin Periodontol* 1986;13:558-562.

56. Apse P, Ellen RP, Overal CM, Zarb GA: Microbiota and crevicular fluid collagen as activity in the osseointegrated dental implant sulcus: A comparison of sites in edentulous and partially edentulous patients. *J Periodont Res* 1989;24:96-105.

57. Bower RC, Radny NR, Wall CS, Henry PJ: Clinical and microscopic findings in edentulous patients 3 years after incorporation of osseointegrated implant-supported bridgework. *J Clin Periodontol* 1989;16:530-587.

58. Mombelli A, Van Oosten MA, Schürch E Jr, Lang NP: The microbiota associated with successful or failing osseointegrated titanium implants. *Oral Microbiol Immunol* 1987;2:145-151.

59. Rams TE, Roberts TW, Tatum H, Keyes PH: Subgingival bacteriology of periodontally healthy and diseased human dental implants. *J Dent Res* 1984;63:200 (abstr no. 267).

60. Krekeler G, Petz K, Nelissen R: Mikrobielle Besiedlung der Zahnfleischtaschen am künstlichen Titanpfeiler. *Dtsch Zahnärztl Z* 1986;41:569-572.

61. Kornman KS, Holt SC, Robertson PB: The microbiology of ligature-induced periodontitis in the cynomolgus monkey. *J Periodont Res* 1981;16:363-371.

62. Brandes R, Beamer B, Holt SC, Kornman K, Lang NP: Clinical-microscopic observation of ligature-induced "periimplantitis" around osseointegrated implants. *J Dent Res* 1988;67: 287(abstr no. 1397).

63. Brägger U, Bürgin W, Lang NP, Buser D: Digital subtraction radiography for the assessment of changes in periimplant bone density. *Int J Oral Maxillofac Implants* 1991;6:160-167.

64. Van Winkelhoff AJ, Rodenburg JP, Goené RJ, Abbas F, Winkel EG, de Graaff J: Metronidazole plus amoxicillin in the treatment of *Actinobacillus actinomycetemcomitans* associated periodontitis. *J Clin Periodontol* 1989;16:128-131.

65. Duckworth J, Brose M, Avers R, French C, Savitt E: Therapeutic implications of the bacterial pathogens associated with dental implants. *J Dent Res* 1987;66:114(abstr no. 57).

66. Lang NP, Brecx MC: Chlorhexidine digluconate—An agent for chemical plaque control and prevention of gingival inflammation. *J Periodont Res* 1986;21(Suppl 16):74-89.

67. Nyman S, Lang NP, Buser D, Brägger U: Bone regeneration adjacent to titanium dental implants using guided tissue regeneration: A report of two cases. *Int J Oral Maxillofac Implants* 1990;5:9 14.

68. Lekmann B, Brägger U, Fourmousis I, Hämmerle C, Lang NP: Guided tissue regeneration for the treatment of a periimplant infection. A case report. *Clin Oral Implant Res* 1991(In press).

69. Waerhaug J: The interdental brush and its place in operative and crown and bridge dentistry. *J Oral Rehabil* 1976;3:117-113.

70. Nyman S, Lindhe J, Karring T: Reattachment new attachment. In: Lindhe J, ed. *Textbook of Clinical Periodontology.* Copenhagen: Munksgaard; 1989:450-476.

71. Dahlin C, Linde A, Gottlow J, Nyman S: Healing of bone defects by guided tissue regeneration. *Plast Reconstr Surg* 1988;81:672-676.

72. Dahlin C, Sennerby L, Lekholm U, Linde A, Nyman S: Generation of new bone around titanium implants using a membrane technique: An experimental study in rabbits. *Int J Oral Maxillofac Implants* 1989;4:19-25.

73. Becker W, Becker B, Handelsman M, Celletti R, Ochsenbein C, Hardwick R, Langer B: Bone formation at dehisced dental implant sites treated with implant augmentation material: A pilot study in dogs. *Int J Periodont Rest Dent* 1990;10:93-101.

74. Lazzara R: Immediate implant placement into extraction sites: Surgical and restorative advantages. *Int J Periodont Rest Dent* 1989;9(5):332-313.

75. Seibert J, Nyman S: Localized ridge augmentation in dogs: A pilot study using membranes and hydroxyapatite. *J Periodontol* 1990;61:157-165.

76. Buser D, Brägger U, Lang NP, Nyman S: Regeneration and enlargement of jaw bone using guided tissue regeneration. *Clin Oral Implant Res* 1990;1:22-32.

77. National Institutes of Health: Dental Implants. NIH Consensus Development Conference, 1988.

78. Smithloff M, Fritz ME: The use of blade implants in a selected population of partially edentulous adults. A 15-year report. *J Periodontol* 1987;58:589.

79. Hobo S, Ichida E, Garcia LT: *Osseointegration and Occlusal Rehabilitation.* Chicago: Quintessence Pub Co, 1989.

80. Albrektsson T, Dahl E, Ehnbom L, et al: Osseointegrated oral implants. A Swedish multicenter study of 8 139 consecutively inserted Nobelpharma implants. *J Periodontol* 1988;59:287.

81. Kahnberg KE: Restoration of mandibular jaw defects in the rabbit by subperiosteally implanted Teflon mantle leaf. *Int J Oral Surg* 1979;8:449.

82. Nyman S, Gottlow J, Lindhe J, Karring T, Wennsrom J: New attachment formation by guided tissue regeneration. *J Periodont Res* 1987;22:252.

83. Lekholm U, Zarb GA: Patient selection and preparation. In: Brånemark P-I, Zarb GA, Albrektsson T, eds. *Tissue-Integrated Prostheses: Osseointegration in Clinical Dentistry.* Chicago: Quintessence Publ Co; 1985:199.

84. Barzilay I, Graser GN, Caton J, Shenkle G: Immediate implantation of pure titanium threaded implants into extraction sockets. *J Dent Res* 1988;67: 234.

85. Golec TS: Extraction of teeth with simultaneous implant placement. *Pract Periodontal Aesthetic Dent* 1989; 1:14.

86. Langer B, Sullivan DY: Osseointegration: Its impact on the interrelationship of periodontics and restorative dentistry: Part I. *Int J Periodont Rest Dent* 1989;9:84.

87. Gould TR, Westbury L, Brunette DM: Ultrastructural study of the attachment of human gingiva to titanium in vivo. *J Prosthet Dent* 1984;52:418.

88. Becker W, Becker BE, Newman MG, Nyman S: Clinical and microbiologic findings that may contribute to dental implant failure. *Int J Oral Maxillofac Implants* 1990;5:31.

89. Lindquist LW, Rockler B, Carlsson GE: Bone resorption around fixtures in edentulous patients treated with mandibular fixed tissue-integrated prostheses. *J Prosthet Dent* 1988; 59:59.

90. Albrektsson T: A multicenter report on osseointegrated oral implants. *J Prosthet Dent* 1988;60:75.

91. Newman MG, Flemmig TF: Periodontal considerations of implants and implant-associated microbiota. National Institutes of Health. NIH Consensus Development Conference: Dental Implants, 1988:57.

92. Thomson-Neal D: *A pilot study to evaluate the effects of various prophylactic treatments on titanium, sapphire and hydroxylapatite coated implants via SEM.* Masters Thesis, Louisiana State University, 1988.

93. Malmstrom HS, Fritz ME, Timmis DP, Van Dyke TE: Osseo-integrated implant treatment of a patient with rapidly progressive periodontitis. A case report. *J Periodontol* 1990;61:300.